CARDIOVASCULAR DISEASE IN THE ELDERLY

DEVELOPMENTS IN CARDIOVASCULAR MEDICINE

Reiber, J.H.C., Serruys, P.W., Siager, C.J.: Quantitative coronary and left ventricular cineangiography. ISBN 0-89838-760-4.
Fagard, R.H., Bekaert, I.E., eds.: Sports cardiology. ISBN 0-89838-782-5. DICM 52.
Reiber, J.H.C., Serruys, P.W., eds.: State of the art in quantitative coronary arteriography. ISBN 0-89838-804-X. DICM 53.
Roelandt, J., ed.: Color doppler flow imaging. ISBN 0-89838-806-6. DICM 54.
van de Wall, E.E., ed.: Noninvasive imaging of cardiac metabolism. ISBN 0-89838-812-0. DICM 55.
Leibman, J., Pionsey, R., Rudy, Y., eds.: Pediatric and fundamental electrocardiography. ISBN 0-89838-815-5. DICM 56.
Higter, H., Hombach, V., eds.: Invasive cardiovascular therapy. ISBN 0-89838-818-X. DICM 57.
Serruys, P.W., Meester, G.T., eds.: Coronary angioplasty: a controlled model for ischemia. ISBN 0-89838-819-8. DICM 58.
Tooke, J.E., Smaje, L.H., eds.: Clinical investigation of the microcirculation. ISBN 0-89838-833-3. DICM 59.
van Dam, Th., van Oosterom, A., eds.: Electrocardiographic body surface mapping. ISBN 0-89838-834-1. DICM 60.
Spencer, M.P., ed.: Ultrasonic diagnosis of cerebrovascular disease. ISBN 0-89838-836-8. DICM 61.
Legato, M.J., ed.: The stressed heart. ISBN 0-89838-849-X. DICM 62.
Safar, M.E., ed.: Arterial and venous systems in essential hypertension. ISBN 0-89838-857-0. DICM 63.
Roeland, J., ed.: Digital techniques in echocardiography. ISBN 0-89838-861-9. DICM 64.
Dhalla, N.S., Singal, P.K., Beamish, R.E., eds.: Pathophysiology of heart disease. ISBN 0-89838-864-3. DICM 65.
Dhalla, N.S., Pierce, G.N., Beamish, R.E., eds.: Heart function and metabolism. ISBN 0-89838-865-1. DICM 66.
Dhalla, N.S., Innes, I.R., Beamish, R.E., eds.: Myocardial ischemia. ISBN 0-89838-866-X. DICM 67.
Beamish, R.E., Panagia, V., Dhalla, N.S., eds.: Pharmacological aspects of heart disease. ISBN 0-89838-867-8. DICM 68.
Ter Keurs, H.E.D.J., Tyberg, J.V., eds.: Mechanics of the circulation. ISBN 0-89838-870-8. DICM 69.
Sideman, S., Beyar, R., eds.: Activation metabolism and perfusion of the heart. ISBN 0-89838-871-6. DICM 70.
Aliot, E., Lazzara, R., eds.: Ventricular tachycardias. ISBN 0-89838-881-3. DICM 71.
Schneeweiss, A., Schettler, G.: Cardiovascular drug therapy in the elderly. ISBN 0-89838-883-X. DICM 72.
Chapman, J.V., Sgalambro, A., eds.: Basic concepts in doppler echocardiography. ISBN 0-89838-888-0. DICM 73.
Chien, S., Dormandy, J., Ernst, E., Matrai, A., eds.: Clinical hemorheology. ISBN 0-89838-807-4. DICM 74.
Morganroth, J., Moore, E. Neil, ed.: Congestive heart failure. ISBN 0-89838-955-0. DICM 75.
Heintzen, P.H., Bursch, J.H., eds.: Progress in digital angiocardiography. ISBN 0-89838-965-8.
Scheinman, M., ed.: Catheter ablation of cardiac arrhythmias. ISBN 0-89838-967-4. DICM 78.
Spaan, J.A.E., Bruschke, A.V.G., Gittenberger, A.C., eds.: Coronary circulation. ISBN 0-89838-978-X. DICM 79.
Bayes de Luna, A., ed.: Therapeutics in cardiology. ISBN 0-89838-981-X. DICM 81.
Visser, C., Kan, G., Meltzer, R., eds.: Echocardiography in coronary artery disease. ISBN 0-89838-979-8. DICM 80.
Singal, P.K., ed.: Oxygen radicals in the pathophysiology of heart disease. ISBN 0-89838-375-7. DICM 86.
Iwata, H., Lombardini, J.B., Segawa, T., eds.: Taurine and the heart. ISBN 0-89838-396-X. DICM 93.
Mirvis, D.M., ed.: Body surface electrocardiographic mapping. ISBN 0-89838-983-6. DICM 82.
Morganroth, J., Moore, E.N., eds.: Silent myocardial ischemia. ISBN 0-89838-380-3. DICM 88.
R. Vos: Drugs Looking for Diseases. Innovative Drug Research and the Development of the Beta Blockers and the Calcium Antagonists. 1991 ISBN 0-7923-0968-5.
S. Sideman, R. Beyar and A.G. Kleber (eds.): Cardiac Electrophysiology, Circulation, and Transport. Proceedings of the 7th Henry Goldberg Workshop (Berne, Switzerland, 1990). 1991 ISBN 0-7923-1145-0.
D.M. Bers: Excitation-Contraction Coupling and Cardiac Contractile Force. 1991 ISBN 0-7923-1186-8.
A.-M. Salmasi and A.N. Nicolaides (eds.): Occult Atherosclerotic Disease. Diagnosis, Assessment and Management. 1991 ISBN 0-7923-1188-4.
J.A.E. Spaan: Coronary Blood Flow. Mechanics, Distribution, and Control, 1991 ISBN 0-7923-1210-4.
R.W. Stout (ed.): Diabetes and Atherosclerosis. 1991 ISBN 0-7923-1310-0.
A.G. Herman (ed.): Antithrombotics. Pathophysiological Rationale for Pharmacological Interventions. 1991 ISBN 0-7923-1413-1.
N.H.J. Pijls: Maximal Myocardial Perfusion as a Measure of the Functional Significance of Coronary Arteriogram. From a Pathoanatomic to a Pathophysiologic Interpretation of the Coronary Arteriogram. 1991 ISBN 0-7923-1430-1.
J.H.C. Reiber and E.E. v.d. Wall (eds.): Cardiovascular Nuclear Medicine and MRI. Quantitation and Clinical Applications. 1992 ISBN 0-7923-1467-0.
E. Andries, P. Brugada and R. Stroobrandt (eds.): How to Face 'the Faces' of Cardiac Pacing. 1992 ISBN 0-7923-1528-6.
M. Nagano, S. Mochizuki and N.S. Dhalla (eds.): Cardiovascular Disease in Diabetes. 1992 ISBN 0-7923-1554-5.
P.W. Serruys, B.H. Strauss and S.B. King III (eds.): Restenosis after Intervention with New Mechanical Devices. 1992 ISBN 0-7923-1555-3.
P.J. Walter (ed.): Quality of Life after Open Heart Surgery. 1992 ISBN 0-7923-1580-4.
E.E. van der Wall, H. Sochor, A. Righetti and M.G. Niemeyer (eds.): What is new in Cardiac Imaging? SPECT, PET and MRI. 1992 ISBN 0-7923-1615-0.
P. Hanrath, R. Uebis and W. Krebs (eds.): Cardiovascular Imaging by Ultrasound. 1992 ISBN 0-7923-1755-6.
F.H. Messerli (ed.): Cardiovascular Disease in the Elderly. 3rd ed. 1992 ISBN 0-7923-1859-5.
J. Hess and G.R. Sutherland (eds.): Congenital Heart Disease in Adolescents and Adults. 1992 ISBN 0-7923-1862-5.
J.H.C. Reiber and P.W. Serruys (eds.): Advances in Quantitative Coronary Arteriography. 1992 ISBN 0-7923-1863-3.

CARDIOVASCULAR DISEASE IN THE ELDERLY

THIRD EDITION

EDITED BY

FRANZ H. MESSERLI
Ochsner Clinic and Alton Ochsner Medical Foundation
New Orleans, Louisiana

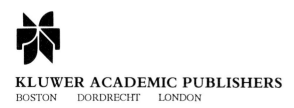

KLUWER ACADEMIC PUBLISHERS
BOSTON   DORDRECHT   LONDON

Distributors

for North America:
Kluwer Academic Publishers
101 Philip Drive
Assinippi Park
Norwell, Massachusetts 02061 USA

Distributors

for all other countries:
Kluwer Academic Publishers Group
Distribution Centre
Post Office Box 322
3300 AH Dordrecht, THE NETHERLANDS

Library of Congress Cataloging-in-Publication Data
Cardiovascular disease in the elderly / Franz H. Messerli, editor.—
  3rd ed.
      p.   cm.—(Developments in cardiovascular medicine; 129)
  Includes bibliographical references and index.
  ISBN 0-7923-1859-5
  1. Geriatric cardiology. I. Messerli, Franz H. II. Series:
Developments in cardiovascular medicine; v. 129.
  [DNLM: 1. Cardiovascular Diseases—in old age. W1 DE997VME
v.129]
  RC669.C278   1993
  618.9'7612—dc20
  DNLM/DLC
  for Library of Congress   92-23628
                                                  CIP

Copyright 1993 by Kluwer Academic Publishers

PRINTED IN THE UNITED STATES OF AMERICA.

CONTENTS

CONTRIBUTING AUTHORS

Richard R. Barager, M.D.
Tri-City Medical Center
3923 Waring Road
Suite D
Oceanside, CA 92056

Joyce P. Barnett, M.S., R.D./L.D.
Instructor
Department of Clinical Nutrition
Allied Health Sciences School
The University of Texas
Southwestern Medical Center
5323 Harry Hines Boulevard
Dallas, TX 75235-8877

David C. Booth, M.D.
Associate Professor of Medicine
University of Kentucky College of Medicine
and
Director, Cardiac Catheterization Laboratories
A.B. Chandler Medical Center
University of Kentucky
and
Chief, Cardiology Section
Lexington Veterans Affairs Medical Center

Mailing Address: Division of Cardiology
                   Rm MN670
                   University of Kentucky Medical Center
                   800 Rose Street
                   Lexington, KY 40536-0084

Donald J. Breslin, M.D.
Section of Vascular Medicine and Hypertension
Lahey Clinic Medical Center
Burlington, MA
and
Assistant Clinical Professor
Harvard Medical School
Boston, MA
Mailing Address: Section of Vascular Medicine and Hypertension
                   Lahey Clinic Medical Center
                   41 Mall Road
                   Burlington, MA 01805

Christopher J. Bulpitt, M.D.
Head
Division of Geriatric Medicine
Royal Postgraduate Medical School
Du Cane Road
London W12 ONN
England

K. Danner Clouser, Ph.D.
University Professor of Humanities
The Pennsylvania State University
Hershey, PA 17033

Jules Constant, M.D.
57 Tillinghast Place
Buffalo, NY 14216

Dwight Davis, M.D.
The Milton S. Hershey Medical Center
The Pennsylvania State University
Division of Cardiology
P.O. Box 850
Hershey, PA 17033

Anthony N. DeMaria, M.D.
Professor of Medicine
Chief, Cardiovascular Section
A.B. Chandler Medical Center
University of Kentucky
Lexington, KY 40536–0084

James R. Douglas, Jr., M.D.
Department of Anesthesiology
Ochsner Clinic and Alton Ochsner Medical Foundation
1514 Jefferson Highway
New Orleans, LA 70121

Leonard S. Dreifus, M.D.
Professor of Medicine
and
Director, Heart Station
Hahnemann University
M.S. 470
Broad and Vine
Philadelphia, PA 19102–1192

Jerome L. Fleg, M.D.
Staff Cardiologist
National Institutes of Health
National Institute on Aging
Gerontology Research Center
4940 Eastern Avenue
Baltimore, MD 21224

Astrid E. Fletcher, M.D.
Epidemiology Research Unit
Division of Geriatric Medicine
Royal Postgraduate Medical School
Du Cane Road
London W12 ONN
England

Noble O. Fowler M.D.
Department of Internal Medicine
Division of Cardiology
University of Cincinnati
Medical Center
Mail Location 542
231 Bethesda Avenue (Rm 3354)
Cincinnati, OH 45267-0542

Gary Gerstenblith, M.D.
Laboratory of Cardiovascular Science
Gerontology Research Center
National Institute on Aging
National Institutes of Health
and
Assistant Professor of Medicine (Cardiology)
Johns Hopkins Medical Institutions
Baltimore, MD

Mailing Address: Johns Hopkins Hospital
565 Carnegie Building
660 N. Wolfe Street
Baltimore, MD 21205

Tomasz Grodzicki, M.D.
Department of Internal Medicine
Section on Hypertensive Diseases
Ochsner Clinic and Alton Ochsner Medical Foundation
1514 Jefferson Highway
New Orleans, LA 70121

Peter R. Kowey, M.D.
Chief
Division of Cardiovascular Diseases
The Lankenau Hospital and Medical Research Center
and
Professor of Medicine
Thomas Jefferson University School of Medicine
Mailing Address: Lankenau Medical Office Building East
Suite 556
100 Lancaster Avenue west of City Line
Wynnewood, PA 19096

Edward G. Lakatta, M.D.
Chief, Cardiovascular Section
Gerontology Research Center
National Institute on Aging
National Institutes of Health
and
Associate Professor of Medicine (Cardiology)
Johns Hopkins Medical Institutions
and
Adjunct Associate Professor of Physiology
University of Maryland School of Medicine
Baltimore, MD
Mailing Address: Johns Hopkins Hospital
565 Carnegie Building
600 N. Wolfe Street
Baltimore, MD 21205

John H. Laragh, M.D.
Hilda Altschul Master Professor of Medicine
and
Director
Cardiovascular Center and Hypertension Center
and
Chief
Cardiology Division
Department of Medicine
The New York Hospital–Cornell Medical Center

Mailing Address: The New York Hospital–Cornell Medical Center
525 East 68th Street
New York, NY 10021

Carl J. Lavie, M.D.
Department of Internal Medicine
Section on Cardiology
Ochsner Clinic and Alton Ochsner Medical Foundation
1514 Jefferson Highway
New Orleans, LA 70121

Andrew B. Littman, M.D.
Department of Psychiatry
Behavioral Medicine Unit
Cardiovascular Health Center
Massachusetts General Hospital
Boston, MA 02114

T.A. Mabin, M.D.
Cardiac Clinic
Groote Schuur Hospital and University of Cape Town
Cape Town, South Africa
Mailing Address: MRC/UCT Ischaemic
Heart Disease Research Unit
Department of Medicine
University of Cape Town
Medical School
Department of Medicine
Observatory 7925
Cape Town, South Africa

Roger A. Marinchak, M.D.
Director, Electrophysiology Laboratory
The Lankenau Hospital and Medical Research Center
and
Associate Professor of Medicine
Thomas Jefferson University School of Medicine
Mailing Address: Lankenau Medical Office Building East
Suite 556
100 Lancaster Avenue west of City Line
Wynnewood, PA 19096

Barry M. Massie, M.D.
Professor of Medicine
University of California, San Francisco
Mailing Address: Department of Medicine
Cardiology Section, 111C
Veterans Administration
Medical Center
4150 Clement Street
San Francisco, CA 94121

P. de V. Meiring, M.D.
MRC/UCT Ischaemic
Heart Disease Research Unit
Department of Medicine
University of Cape Town Medical School
Observatory 7925
Cape Town South Africa

Franz H. Messerli, M.D.
Professor of Medicine
Tulane University School of Medicine
and
Department of Internal Medicine
Section on Hypertensive Diseases
Ochsner Clinic and Alton Ochsner Medical Foundation
1514 Jefferson Highway
New Orleans, LA 70121

Eric L. Michelson, M.D.
Professor of Medicine
and
Director
Division of Cardiology
Likoff Cardiovascular Institute
Hahnemann University
M.S. 470
Broad and Vine
Philadelphia, PA 19102-1192

Richard V. Milani, M.D.
Department of Internal Medicine
Section on Cardiology
Ochsner Clinic and Alton Ochsner Medical Foundation
1514 Jefferson Highway
New Orleans, LA 70121

Celia M. Oakley, M.D.
Professor of Clinical Cardiology
Royal Postgraduate Medical School
Hammersmith Hospital
Du Cane Road
London W12 ONN
England

John L. Ochsner, M.D.
Department of Surgery
Ochsner Clinic and Alton Ochsner Medical Foundation
1514 Jefferson Highway
New Orleans, LA 70121

Lionel H. Opie, M.D., Ph.D.
MRC/UCT Ischaemic
Heart Disease Research Unit
Department of Medicine
University of Cape Town Medical School
Observatory 7925
Cape Town South Africa

Mark Pecker, M.D.
Assistant Professor of Medicine
and
Assistant Attending Physician
Cardiovascular Center and Hypertension Center
The New York Hospital–Cornell Medical Center
Mailing Address: NYH–CUMC, Cardiovascular Center
                Starr 4
                525 East 68th Street
                New York, NY 10021

Carl J. Pepine, M.D.
Department of Medicine
Division of Cardiovascular Medicine
University of Florida
Box J–277, JHM Health Center
Gainesville, FL 32610–6103

Herman L. Price, M.D.
Department of Internal Medicine
Section on Cardiology
Ochsner Clinic and Alton Ochsner Medical Foundation
1514 Jefferson Highway
New Orleans, LA 70121

Stephen R. Ramee, M.D.
Director
Interventional Cardiology
Department of Internal Medicine
Section on Cardiology
Ochsner Clinic and Alton Ochsner Medical Foundation
1514 Jefferson Highway
New Orleans, LA 70121

Andrew P. Rees, M.D.
Department of Internal Medicine
Section on Cardiology
Ochsner Clinic and Alton Ochsner Medical Foundation
1514 Jefferson Highway
New Orleans, LA 70121

Seth J. Rials, M.D., Ph.D.
Cardiovascular Division
The Lankenau Hospital and Medical Research Center
Lankenau Medical Office Building East
Suite 556
100 Lancaster Avenue west of City Line
Wynnewood, PA 19096

James A. Schoenberger, M.D.
Roberts Professor and Chairman
Department of Preventive Medicine
Rush-Presbyterian-St. Luke's Medical Center
10th Floor Schweppe Sprague
1725 W. Harrison Street
Chicago, IL 60612

Frank W. Smart, M.D.
Department of Internal Medicine
Section on Cardiology
Ochsner Clinic and Alton Ochsner Medical Foundation
1514 Jefferson Highway
New Orleans, LA 70121

David W. Snyder, M.D.
Cardiology Consultants of Louisiana
East Jefferson General Hospital
4200 Houma Boulevard
Metairie, LA 70011

Kelly Anne Spratt, D.O.
Department of Medicine
Hahnemann University
M.S. 470
Broad and Vine
Philadelphia, PA 19102-1192

Dwight D. Stapleton, M.D.
Department of Internal Medicine
Section on Cardiology
Ochsner Clinic and Alton Ochsner Medical Foundation
1514 Jefferson Highway
New Orleans, LA 70121

John D. Swales, M.D.
Department of Medicine
Clinical Sciences Building
Leicester Royal Infirmary
P.O. Box 65
Leicester LE2 2PF
England

Nicholas P. Tsapatsaris, M.D.
Section of Vascular Medicine and Hypertension
Lahey Clinic Medical Center
Burlington, MA
Mailing Address: Department of Cardiology
Lahey Clinic Medicial Center
41 Mall Road
Burlington, MA 01805

Clifford H. Van Meter, M.D.
Department of Surgery
Ochsner Clinic and Alton Ochsner Medical Foundation
1514 Jefferson Highway
New Orleans, LA 70121

Hector O. Ventura, M.D.
Department of Internal Medicine
Section on Cardiology
Ochsner Clinic and Alton Ochsner Medical Foundation
1514 Jefferson Highway
New Orleans, LA 70121

Nanette K. Wenger, M.D.
Professor of Medicine
Department of Medicine
Division of Cardiology
Emory University School of Medicine
and
Director—Cardiac Clinics
Grady Memorial Hospital
Mailing Address: Emory University School of Medicine
Thomas K. Glenn Memorial Building
69 Bulter Street, S.E.
Atlanta, GA 30303

Christopher J. White, M.D.
Director
Cardiac Catheterization Laboratory
Department of Internal Medicine
Section on Cardiology
Ochsner Clinic and Alton Ochsner Medical Foundation
1514 Jefferson Highway
New Orleans, LA 70121

Christopher L. Wolfe, M.D.
Cardiology Division
Veterans Administration Medical Center
and
Department of Medicine and Cardiovascular
Research Institute
University of California, San Francisco
San Francisco, California

Mailing Address: University of California, San Francisco
858 40th Avenue
San Francisco, CA 94121

Robert Zelis, M.D.
Professor of Medicine and Physiology
The Milton S. Hershey Medical Center
The Pennsylvania State University
Hershey, PA 17033

Michael G. Ziegler, M.D.
Division of Nephrology
University of California, San Diego School of Medicine
Mailing Address: University of California Medical Center
225 Dickinson Street
H-781-B
San Diego, CA 92103–8341

FOREWORD TO THE FIRST EDITION

After a certain age, one is elderly, aged, venerable, and patriarchal. Or just plain old. When I became old, I did not know it. I do know it now because of a syndrome of which I had previously been unaware. It is quite simple—when it hurts, it works; when it doesn't hurt, it doesn't work!

Writing about the old is a preoccupation of the young, and that is as it should be because it is the young who must carry the burden of the old. I don't know the average age of the contributors to Franz Messerli's book, but I would guess it to be less than 50, which to me is positively pubescent!

For many years I thought geriatric medicine was nonsense, and today I still think some of it is. What changes with age is principally the attitude and purposes of the individual and how much energy he or she has to carry out those purposes. It isn't so much that the goals, ambitions, and desire to alter or improve the world disappear; they just diminish along with what it takes to accomplish them. Which brings me to one particular aspect of aging, that is, the cardiovascular system.

The first evidence of the cardiovascular system's aging is the failure of the heart to respond to the demands placed on it. The cardioinhibitory reflexes do not quite do their job, and the Starling responses are not quite as effective as they used to be. Blood pressure exceeds the most effective limits more often than it should. All these and other signs and symptoms imperceptibly lead to human twilight, a period that should be the richest in the journey through life.

The end stage is, of course, cardiac failure, myocardial infarction, stroke, or all three. I have had the latter two and am thoroughly enjoying life and the pseudo-arrogance, puffery, and pulling of rank that is vouchsafed to us all, if we could but accept it.

Still another aspect (not "parameter") of old age warrants attention: the difference between wearing out and disease. Teeth, eyes, and joints wear out, whereas coronary and cerebral vessels usually become diseased. We need medicine and surgery for the latter and the hygiene of good living for the former.

From the economic point of view, the next decade will see the number of old people exceeding the growth rate of all other sections of society. This abundance of healthy-old, sick-old, poor-old, and wealthy-old may create a new job market for the presently unemployed younger generation. Perhaps those unable to find work in the high-tech domain or the smokestack industry can be put to work making the elderly useful people, an accomplishment that in itself will add a special flavor to life that only the old can give.

As has come to be expected, the World Health Organization in 1982 concluded that aging was a problem. Having arrived at this conclusion, it responded by holding a 2000-delegate meeting in Vienna in the Hofburg Palace. I was astonished at the great number of delegates who turned out to be "national authorities on aging." One cannot help but marvel at the magnitude of animal tropism leading unerringly to potential power centers, which in the end often prove only to be centers of Brownian movement.

It is the physician's duty to guide the needs of both the healthy- and sick-old, just as the pediatrician cares for the healthy and sick child. I hope and believe that all physicians, not just geriatricians, will profit from this book. Some of the authors I know and greatly respect; the rest I take on faith and the good judgment of Franz Messerli, for I know that he himself is first rate.

IRVINE H. PAGE, M.D.
Hyannis Port, Massachusetts
Emeritus Director, Cleveland Clinic

By the time a man gets well into his seventies, his
continued existence is a mere miracle.
                              —Robert Louis Stevenson

It seems hardly possible that a third edition is needed after the second has
been in print for only three years. However, when I look at the evolution of
geriatric cardiology during these few years, the reasons become obvious.

More and more cardiologists have begun to realize that geriatric cardiology
has become a science and a clinical discipline of its own. Although at a first
glance such a "sub-subspecialization" may seem unfortunate, it has become
clear that most cardiac disorders present with different symptoms and signs,
require a different diagnostic and therapeutic approach, and also have a
different prognosis in the elderly when compared to younger and middle-
aged patients. Currently, Americans older than age 60 number more than 30
million and thereby constitute over 12% of the population. Cardiovascular
disorders now account for more than 50% of all deaths in the geriatric
population. This means that specific age-related disorders are more frequently encountered by the practicing physician, be it the general practitioner,
family practitioner, internist, or cardiologist. *Cardiovascular Disease in the
Elderly* provides a comprehensive, up-to-date guide to help the physician deal
with these problems. It is hoped that this text will lead the way in this
increasingly complex area.

Also, I have been heartened by the warm reception of the previous editions and by the excellent reviews that they received in the most prestigious medical journals. Clearly, however, a critical need emerged to add to, update, and improve the previous editions. Accordingly, most of the chapters have been completely rewritten, some by different authors. Four new chapters, one dealing with cardiac transplantation in the elderly, another discussing invasive cardiovascular procedures, a third on dietary considerations, and a fourth on ethical considerations, have been added. I realize that topics such as invasive cardiac procedures and cardiac transplantation are highly controversial and have therefore attempted to provide a counterbalance by asking Dr. Davis and associates to outline the ethical dilemmas involved. An attempt was made to thoroughly reference all chapters; inevitably, therefore, the third edition has a few more pages than previous editions.

In this third edition, the authors would like to honor the outstanding contribution to cardiovascular medicine of Dr. Irvine Page, who unexpectedly passed away before he could revise his foreword. We decided to let it stand unchanged from the previous edition.

Within the past several years, a variety of other monographs on geriatric cardiology have appeared in the medical literature. This has clearly attested to the timeliness of our endeavor and has also prompted us to make an effort to stay abreast of the competition. The third edition of *Cardiovascular Disease in the Elderly*, like its predecessors, will provide the practicing physician with a thorough yet concise guide to diagnosis and treatment of heart disease in the geriatric patient.

FRANZ H. MESSERLI, M.D., EDITOR
Ochsner Clinic
New Orleans, Louisiana

ACKNOWLEDGMENTS

I appreciate the skill and dedication of Susan Barker, Associate Editor of Special Projects, Marion Stafford, Medical Editor, and the medical editing staff at the Alton Ochsner Medical Foundation, without whom this book would not have been possible. I also thank Tammy Slack of Ochsner Clinic for her assistance in preparing the manuscript. I am grateful for the advice and guidance of Mr. Jeffrey K. Smith, Vice President and Publisher of Kluwer Academic Publishers.

CARDIOVASCULAR DISEASE IN THE ELDERLY

1. INTRODUCTION: OLDER PEOPLE AND CARDIOVASCULAR ILLNESS

MARK PECKER

JOHN H. LARAGH

You must help me, Doctor. I have so much to live for.
>   —Eva Babbit, age 89

"The very rich are different from you and me.
Yes, they have more money."
>   —Ernest Hemingway

The accumulation of years brings with it a variety of changes. Some changes are qualitative, such as the special love that only grandparents can provide for children. Other changes are quantitative, like the accrual of wisdom. But in the realm of medicine, aging tends to take on a shadowy connotation. Here, the alterations that occur are limiting, and the best that can be done is to hold one's own.

In medical terms, *aging* generally refers to a series of progressive and incremental losses of organic function. These losses may occur in discrete steps or gradually over time, owing to pathologic or vaguely defined physiologic mechanisms. There is great variability in patterns of aging, however, not only among individual people but among different organ systems within one individual. Thus, the loss of function that we consider to reflect "aging"

Franz H. Messerli (ed.), CARDIOVASCULAR DISEASE IN THE ELDERLY (Third Edition). Copyright © 1993 Kluwer Academic Publishers. ISBN 0-7923-1859-5. All rights reserved.

cannot be accurately predicted either by chronologic age or by any single physiologic "index of aging."

Although we cannot yet clearly define aging or predict how or when it will manifest itself in a particular person, we do know that some of the physiologic changes that occur as people age lead to serious health problems—problems that are rapidly becoming more widely recognized in our society and more expensive. A brief excursion into epidemiology will illustrate this observation.

STATISTICAL REALITIES

In the twentieth century, life expectancy in the industrialized world has increased dramatically. As a result, more than 15% of U.S. citizens are now older than 60, and more than 10% are over 65. In fact, half of all people over 65 who have ever lived in the United States are alive today [1]! Although this increase in longevity is due largely to decreases in infantile and juvenile mortality rates—maximal life span has not increased—older people's mortality rates have also lessened during the past 25 years. Thus, the U.S. death rate for those 85 or older decreased between 1966 and 1977 by 26%, a greater decline than was observed among younger people [2]. The reasons for this decline are not fully understood, but they probably include the fact that today's older population has access to better medical treatment. Advances in medical science as well as the greatly improved access to treatment brought about by the Medicare system have made excellent health care generally available to older people.

That the decrease in mortality is not a cosmetic statistic but rather a companion to improved health is suggested by the National Health Interview Survey (1972). This study found that over 80% of those 65 years of age and older reported no limitations of mobility, and that only about 5% were confined to their homes [3]. Thus, with improved health care, most older people continue to live and function independently. Stead and Stead's [4] distinction between the *independent* and *dependent* elderly is an attractive stratification scheme, particularly in view of the lack of age-specific criteria for any of the phenomena of aging. At the same time, the scheme does not distinguish among individuals in any discrete way. And it must be admitted that younger people as well as older people vary in terms of the degree of independence with which they function.

Still, it is clear that the proportion of those who are in some degree disabled increases markedly with age [5]. Less than a quarter of people over 65 and less than a fifth of those over 75 find themselves free of continuing chronic ailments [6].

The health problems of the elderly thus take on two major aspects. The first of these is scientific and social in nature, relating to the specific medical problems that are predominant or unique among the elderly. The second important factor revolves around the economic challenge that the rapidly growing numbers of older persons pose for our society.

AGING: INTRINSIC, OR THE RESULT OF PATHOLOGIC INSULT?

In their seminal work on normal human aging, Shock and his colleagues at the National Institute on Aging identified six general types or patterns of change with age [7]. One of the patterns identified by the Baltimore Longitudinal Study of Aging (BLSA) involves changes that have little or nothing to do with age or health or disease but reflect changes in society at large. The investigators cite, for example, the general reduction in dietary cholesterol intake that has occurred since the study began.

Shock and his associates termed a second pattern *stability*, or the absence of meaningful change in specific aspects of the person, such as resting heart rate or various personality characteristics. In a third pattern it was found that some declines in function reflect not aging per se but illnesses associated with age; declining testosterone levels found in earlier studies, for example, disappeared when subjects were screened for specific diseases.

Changes in physical or mental functioning that occur abruptly form a fourth pattern. Such sudden alterations are usually the result of overt pathology, although they may also reflect gradual, underlying changes in bodily structures or function. In contrast, a fifth pattern sees the aging exhibiting a slow, steady decline in function, as when people find their daily walks gradually becoming shorter, or find it necessary to keep increasing the strength of eyeglasses prescriptions.

Finally, Shock and colleagues described a sixth pattern in which people as they grow older are seen to engage in compensatory actions and behaviors designed to help them maintain function despite accumulating losses. Inasmuch as the abrupt changes seen in the aging usually reflect clearly defined pathology, it is the last two of these six patterns that are of particular interest to those concerned with exploring the causes of aging.

A major question in the pathophysiology of aging is whether a "biological clock" is intrinsic to living organisms and, if it is, to what extent a physiologic aging process could account for the loss of function we see in aging. The notion that we age physiologically finds some support in the fact that for each species there is a nearly fixed, maximal life span. This finite existence of the creature world has its correlate in the more controlled environment of tissue culture, where nontransformed cells survive only a finite number of passages. Also compatible with the concept of a biological clock is recent evidence that at least some forms of Alzheimer's disease have a genetic basis [8,9]

It is quite difficult to ascribe common clinical phenomena that involve integrated organ functions to physiologic, or intrinsic, aging. Consider blood pressure, for example. It has been established that among the populations of industrialized nations, blood pressure routinely rises with age. We might consider this elevation a fundamental part of growing old were it not for the fact that in some nonindustrial, tribal societies blood pressure uniformly does *not* rise with age [10]. Evidently, then, blood pressure elevation is not inherent in human aging.

In similar fashion, clinical research has documented a decline in renal function among the elderly, as measured by creatinine clearance. In the Baltimore study, creatinine clearance was seen to fall steadily with age despite the absence of disease; these results were obtained in both cross-sectional and longitudinal examinations [11]. The investigators concluded initially that deterioration in kidney function was intrinsic to aging. When they subjected the data to further analysis, however, they found that in some individuals, creatinine clearance did not fall at all over periods longer than 20 years [12]. The fact that animal research has linked age-related falls in renal function to a high rate of consumption of dietary protein suggests the influence of one or more intervening variables. In any event, it may be that people are no more predestined to show a decline in renal function as they grow older than they are to exhibit elevated blood pressure.

Clearly, it is not easy to distinguish between physiologic aging and the accretion of pathologic insults. It is particularly difficult to understand the deterioration that occurs over long periods in fairly uniform societies, where such "insults" may be as seemingly innocuous as moderate salt intake, daily stress, or the steady consumption of protein. In addition, intrinsic properties may themselves be pathologic: consider the possible effects of a genetic mutation responsible for sickle cell anemia or of a genetic combination pre-disposing to Alzheimer's disease. In fact, if we are going to consider aging itself to be a disease, any biological clock can be viewed as pathologic. In such a context, the distinction becomes academic and useful, perhaps, only in directing research efforts. What matters to clinicians is whether or not we can intervene in the aging process, if we want to.

HOMEOSTENOSIS

Whether the reasons for aging are inherent in the life cycle or related to specific environmental factors, aging organ systems are characterized by a reduced ability to perform or to compensate in response to stress. Weksler [13] has termed this relative loss of resilience *homeostenosis*, suggesting that it narrows the scope of derangements that can be tolerated in the individual's effort to maintain homeostasis. The impairments may be due both to a diminution of maximum function and to defective operation of regulatory mechanisms.

A chronic ailment such as degenerative joint disease may be one cause of homeostenosis, but evidence of lessened ability to perform may appear in the face of apparently normal function in the unstressed state. Good examples are the professional ballplayer in his early 30s who "loses a step," or the competitive swimmer whose performance peaks in her teenage years. A wide range of subclinical losses of function occur, some quite subtle. For example, when placed on a low-salt diet, older people come into sodium balance just as younger people do. However, they take longer to do so and lose more sodium in the process [14]. Similarly, muscle mass, bone density, brain reserve, maximum cardiac output, and hepatic clearance all tend to diminish with age, and often at ages that would be considered old only by the standards of the 1960s.

Homeostenosis is most prominent when stresses occur that require integrated responses of multiple organ systems. Because the circulatory system is central to homeostasis of all organ systems, understanding the alterations in function of the aging cardiovascular system is critical not just in the treatment of cardiac illness but in the general medical care of the elderly.

MULTIPLE ILLNESSES, MULTIPLE THERAPIES

Because older people are more likely than younger people to have chronic diseases, diagnosis in the elderly patient is often a double-edged sword. On the one hand, it is frequently difficult to establish a diagnosis because a multitude of medical problems preclude straightforward interpretation of the history or of physical or laboratory evaluations. Chest pain in the setting of cervical arthritis or shortness of breath in the setting of chronic pulmonary disease are two troubling examples in which cardiac disease can be over- or underdiagnosed. It has been our observation that digitalis is very often prescribed for elderly patients in whom heart failure has not been well documented.

On the other hand, a great number of medical problems present atypically in the elderly. These problems range from apathetic hyperthyroidism to infections that are unaccompanied by fever. The physician who treats older patients, therefore, must maintain a high index of suspicion for a wide variety of illnesses and must also take care to document thoroughly both the initial diagnosis and prescription and the ongoing therapeutic interventions.

Hand in hand with multiple illnesses go multiple therapies. The need for multilayered treatment, however, poses problems with respect to both pharmacologic and nonpharmacologic therapies. A good example can be seen in the elderly patient who has both arthritis and heart disease. For this person, diagnostic procedures, such as stress testing, and therapeutic regimens that involve strenuous exercise may have to be very carefully adjusted.

Cautionary statements about therapy in the elderly have tended to emphasize drug therapies, however, and with good reason. Although judicious pharmacologic therapy is often well tolerated, adverse drug reactions occur at least four times as often among the elderly as among younger people. Indeed, such reactions are seen in perhaps a quarter of hospitalized octogenarians.

There are several reasons for the heightened vulnerability of the elderly to the risks of drug therapy. First, they take more medicines. A recent survey of hypertensive outpatients at Parkland Memorial Hospital found that patients 65 years and older had on average four distinct diagnoses and were regularly taking 3 to 4 prescription drugs [15]. These numbers, as large as they are, are nevertheless among the lowest reported in similar studies of older patients.

The fact that older people simply take more medicines increases not only the risk of side effects from individual medications but also the risk of adverse drug interactions. A particularly common drug interaction in elderly patients with both arthritis and hypertension is the loss of hypertensive control caused by administration of nonsteroidal anti-inflammatory agents.

Several other factors are involved in the adverse reactions to drugs seen in the aging. Drug metabolism is often slower in older people as a result of the decreased renal function mentioned earlier. However, because reductions in muscle mass as well as lower protein intake are also common, routine measurements of creatinine and blood urea nitrogen (BUN) may not accurately reflect the lessened renal function. Thus it may be difficult both to prescribe and to monitor drug therapies in the appropriate dosages and frequencies. Hepatic reserve may also be diminished, although this does not usually have as marked an effect on drug metabolism as does diminished renal function.

The elderly are also likely to compensate less well for side effects such as the impaired mentation often brought on by sedatives or centrally acting antihypertensive agents, or the impaired renal function that accompanies the use of nonsteroidal anti-inflammatory agents. And finally, failure of short-term memory, not uncommon in the elderly, may result from overdosing as well as undermedication, further compromising a therapeutic regimen.

For all these reasons, the safe and effective use of medical therapy in the elderly patient requires careful titration of as few drugs as possible. The best motto for the clinician working with older patients is "Go slow, stay low."

THE SOCIAL CHALLENGE

Decreased ability to compensate for altered physiologic mechanisms and functioning comes at a time when the older person is likely to be challenged in the social arena as he or she has never been before. The aging confront major changes in life-style, including retirement, the death of family members and friends, and, for those who are institutionalized, the loss of independence and of familiar surroundings. In mobile societies like the United States, it is more the rule than the exception that the older person's children live a considerable distance away; as a result, family networks are often weakened. To cope with all these stresses, the aging person must find new resources—not an easy task for someone whose own mobility is reduced and who lives in a society that gives its greatest rewards to the young.

Although the younger adult may face any one of these challenges at any time in his or her life, it is rare for young or even middle-aged people—

who, on average, have reasonably good physical health and strength—to be besieged by so many problems at once. The onslaught that a younger person might be able to handle may overwhelm the older person whose physical capacities are less and whose options are often few. These psychosocial challenges may well affect not only the older person's reaction to physical illness but also his or her response to treatment.

Herein may lie some of the most meaningful differences between the old and the young. Younger people may not realize just how much support they have in their work, family, friends, leisure activities, and so forth, all of which stand them in good stead when they are ill. Older people, without the badge of "contributing member of society" awarded by the work role, as well as the financial security a job confers—and often without the social support of a spouse—are very alone. Friends die, so unless the aging are able to make new, young friends, their support systems are seriously damaged. Any way one looks at it, in our present social scene the older person is at a disadvantage.

Thus, when working with the elderly, interventions of a social nature may be just as therapeutic as physical treatment measures. As already noted, we do not yet know whether the observable physiologic differences between young and old reflect inherent or environmentally induced deterioration. But we do know the sources of many psychosocial insults to the aging human being, and dealing with them thus becomes as legitimately therapeutic as treatment by drugs, surgery, or other physical means.

OVERVIEW

The chapters of this book are organized in such a way as to enable the reader to review what is known about cardiac epidemiology and pathophysiology (chapters 2 and 3) and to consider physical findings in the older cardiovascular patient (chapter 3) before going on to explore, in the first major group of chapters (chapters 4–15), the symptomatology, diagnosis, and treatment of the most common cardiovascular disorders. Some noncardiac illnesses, such as diseases of the lungs or endocrine system, that may lead to cardiovascular difficulties in the elderly are also discussed (chapter 16).

A second group of chapters (chapters 17–24) examines issues of prevention, psychological adaptation to cardiovascular illness, ethical considerations, diet, exercise, and other interventions, including pharmacologic, surgical, and physical rehabilitative measures. A final chapter (chapter 25) familiarizes the reader with the controversies of cardiac transplantation in the geriatric population.

The authors of this book, whose chapters reflect clinical, academic, and research expertise, in general subscribe to the caveat that age is often not the primary determining factor in the way patients manifest the signs and symptoms of cardiovascular illness or respond to therapy. It is true that the aging present special problems of diagnosis and treatment, but in part because we do not yet know whether to attribute these problems to some inherent program for age-related change or to cumulative pathologic insult, it may be most useful to regard the older person as having the same basic difficulties as the younger adult, only more so. By combining our knowledge about people of all ages, gained through clinical practice and research, with psychosocial acumen attuned to the elderly person's life space, we may offer our patients the very best care possible.

REFERENCES

1. Dans PE and Ken MR. 1979. Gerontology and geriatrics in medical education. N Engl J Med 300:228–232.
2. Rosenwaike MA, Yaffe N, and Sagi PC. 1980. The recent decline in mortality of the extreme aged: An analysis of statistical data. Am J Public Health 70:1074–1080.
3. National Health Interview Survey 1972.
4. Stead EA Jr and Stead NW. 1980. Problems and challenges in the treatment of the aging patient. Dis-Mon 26(11):1–41.
5. Bourliere F and Vallery-Masson J. 1985. Epidemiology and ecology of aging. In JC Brocklehurst (ed), Textbook of Geriatric Medicine and Gerontology, 3rd ed. London: Churchill Livingston, pp 3–28.
6. Jeffreys M. 1985. The elderly in society. In JC Brocklehurst (ed), Textbook of Geriatric Medicine and Gerontology, 3rd ed. London: Churchill Livingston, pp 961–981.
7. Shock NW, Greulich RC, Andres R, et al. 1984. Normal Human Aging: The Baltimore Longitudinal Study of Aging. Washington, DC: U.S. Department of Health and Human Services, NIH Publication No. 84–2450.
8. St George-Hyslop PH, Tanzi RE, Polsky RJ, et al. 1987. The genetic defect causing familial Alzheimer's disease maps on chromosome 21. Science 235:846–847.
9. Tanzi RE, Gusella JF, Watkins PC, et al. 1987. Amyloid protein gene: cDNA, mRNA distribution, and genetic linkages near the Alzheimer locus. Science 235:880–884.
10. Freis ED. 1976. Salt, volume, and the prevention of hypertension. Circulation 53:589–595.
11. Rowe JW, Andres R, Tobin JD, et al. 1976. The effect of age on creatinine clearance in men: A cross-sectional and longitudinal study. J Gerontol 31:155–163.
12. Lindeman RS, Tobin JD, and Shock N. 1985. Rates of decline in renal function with age. J Am Geriatr Soc 33:278–285.
13. Weksler M. 1986. Biologic basis of and clinical significance of immune senescence. In I Rossman (ed), Clinical Geriatrics. Philadelphia: Lippincott, pp 57–67.
14. Epstein M and Hollenberg NK. 1976. Aging as a determinant of renal sodium conservation in normal man. J Lab Clin Med 87:411–417.
15. Anderson RJ. 1985. The control of hypertension in the elderly: Understanding the challenge, responsibility and opportunities for preventive interventions in the elderly. Parkland Memorial Hospital, University of Texas Health Sciences Center. Parkland Medical Grand Rounds, July 18. Unpublished.

2. EPIDEMIOLOGY

JOHN D. SWALES
ASTRID E. FLETCHER
CHRISTOPHER J. BULPITT

With advancing age, heart disease and stroke assume increasing importance as a cause of death in industrialized countries. Thus, while death from malignant disease is almost as important a cause of death in younger subjects, circulatory disease is responsible for more than half the deaths in people over 65 years old in the United States and Europe (table 2-1) [1–4].

TRENDS IN MORTALITY

Substantial declines in cardiovascular mortality have occurred in some countries since the late 1960s, both in middle-aged subjects and in the elderly [4–6]. Figure 2-1 shows the rates for circulatory disease mortality over the last 30 years in the United Kingdom (Scotland, Northern Ireland, England, and Wales) in men aged 65 to 74 years. Also shown is the decline for the U.S., Australia, and Finland. Within the U.K., the highest rate was in Scotland. This fell by 14% in comparison with a fall of 17% in England and Wales, and of only 7% in Northern Ireland. The most dramatic declines have occurred in the U.S. and Australia, both of which started with a very high rate and achieved reductions of over 30%. In 1950, Finland had the highest mortality from circulatory disease in the world, but it has reduced the rate by 16%. In women, for reasons that are not understood, quite large falls in circulatory-disease mortality have occurred for at least the last 40 years in

Franz H. Messerli (ed.), CARDIOVASCULAR DISEASE IN THE ELDERLY (Third Edition). Copyright © 1993 Kluwer Academic Publishers. ISBN 0-7923-1859-5. All rights reserved.

Table 2-1. Percentage of deaths ascribed to various
cardiovascular causes in four countries during 1979[a]

Cardiovascular cause	Age at death (years)			
	45–54	55–64	65–74	75+
All circulatory disease (ICD 390–459)				
United States	37	44	51	65
England and Wales	43	47	51	55
Australia	40	49	55	64
Japan	30	35	45	54
Acute myocardial infarction and ischemic heart disease (ICD 410–414)				
United States	23	28	32	35
England and Wales	30	32	31	24
Australia	27	34	36	30
Japan	5	7	8	7
Cerebrovascular disease (ICD 430–438)				
United States	4	5	8	13
England and Wales	6	7	11	16
Australia	7	8	8	9
Japan	16	19	25	29
Malignant neoplasms (ICD 140–208)				
United States	31	32	27	15
England and Wales	35	34	27	14
Australia	30	30	26	15
Japan	34	38	29	14

[a] Based on data published by the World Health Organization. ICD = International Classification of Diseases.
Source: Adapted from Whelton PK. 1984. J Hypertens 2:4 [3].

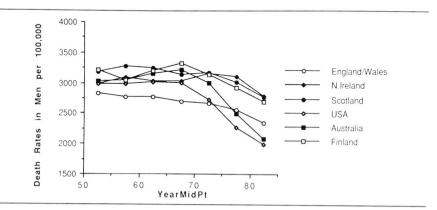

Figure 2-1. Rates for circulatory disease mortality in men aged 65–74 years over the last 30 years in the U.K. (Scotland, Northern Ireland, England and Wales), U.S., Australia, and Finland. YearMidPt = midpoint of year.

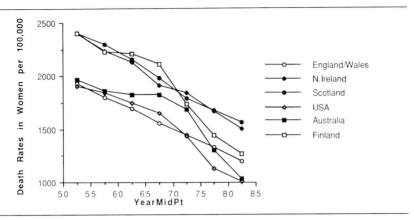

Figure 2-2. Rates for circulatory disease mortality in women aged 65–74 years over the last 30 years in the U.K. (Scotland, Northern Ireland, England and Wales), U.S., Australia, and Finland. YearMidPt = midpoint of year.

most European countries, including the U.K. Figure 2-2 shows that in the U.K. the fall was nearly 40%, comparable to that seen in the U.S.

Although it is generally accepted that modification of risk factors (cholesterol, blood pressure, and smoking), either through medical care or life-style changes, has contributed to the observed decline in circulatory disease, the magnitude of the contribution remains relatively small. It is clear that these factors alone are insufficient to account for the observed temporal changes. For example, stroke mortality has been declining since at least the 1950s in many countries, including the U.S. and England. The decline predated widespread use of antihypertensive therapy in the community. However, the fact that in women the incidence of circulatory disease has been documented to decrease consistently across countries with very different patterns of male circulatory-disease mortality suggests the influence of other etiologic factors. Patrick et al. [7] examined mortality from coronary heart disease (CHD) between 1945 and 1975 for white men and women in the U.S. CHD declined at the same rate in all female cohorts born between 1886 and 1910, while in men CHD mortality increased in all cohorts up until 1965, and then declined.

Goldman and Cook [8] concluded that 60% of the decline in ischemic heart disease mortality was attributable to life-style modifications directed at reducing serum cholesterol and abstaining from cigarette smoking. This does not explain the fall observed in women who showed little, if any, change in smoking habits over the same period. Goldman and Cook also believed that about 40% of the decline could be attributed to direct medical interventions for the management of ischemic heart disease and hypertension. Conversely, Bonita and Beaglehole [9] have argued that although a 40% reduction in stroke mortality was observed in the U.S. between 1970 and 1980, this was not fully accounted for by changes in population blood-pressure levels or in the proportions of threated and controlled hypertensives. They estimated that, at most, control of hypertension accounted for 25% of the observed decline.

In summary, risk-factor modification has probably made a contribution to the decline in cardiovascular disease observed in many countries, which may be as high as 50%. The decline in cardiovascular disease has occurred in older age groups (65+) as well as in the younger groups, suggesting that the effects of risk-factor modification persist well into later life. However, most preventative advice is targeted at middle-aged subjects, especially men. This is partly due to the relative paucity of risk-factor data in the elderly compared to the young. There are at present insufficient prospective studies to establish risk factors in the elderly, and no large intervention trials to examine the effects of changing risk factors.

We will review the evidence that the established risk factors for cardio-vascular disease in middle-aged subjects persist into old age. Special factors that may modify the natural history of cardiovascular disease should be considered in the elderly.

SPECIAL FACTORS IN THE ELDERLY

The incidence and expression of disease may be substantially different in older age groups. Several reasons accout for this:

1. *Changed pathophysiology of the elderly.* Pathophysiologic changes in the heart, arteries, kidneys, and central nervous system may all contribute to the incidence and nature of disease in elderly patients. It cannot be assumed, however, that all differences in disease between elderly and young people are attributable solely to this cause.
2. *Selective mortality.* Removal of persons at high risk (by premature death) may modify the role of risk factors in the surviving elderly.
3. *Multiple pathology.* The frequent presence of such conditons as arthritis and dementia in the elderly may, through modification of activity and diet, change the pattern of cardiovascular disease. Other conditions such as anemia or malnutrition may have a more direct impact.
4. *Altered life-style.* Malnutrition and self-neglect are more common in the elderly and may have an important impact upon disease.

CARDIOVASCULAR RISK FACTORS

A variety of epidemiologic studies have established cholesterol, blood pressure, smoking, overweight, and glucose intolerance as major risk factors for CHD in middle-aged subjects. Other risk factors include fibrinogen, social class (semiskilled and unskilled workers), ethnic origin, family history of premature CHD, a rapid pulse rate, high hematocrit, low physical activity, and type A personality. The major risk factors for cardiovascular disease have been established as a result of longitudinal population studies such as those conducted at Framingham [10], the Pooling Project [11], and the Whitehall Civil Servants' Project [12]. Information has also been provided for certain risk factors (such as blood pressure) by insurance data [13]. Conclusive data on the elderly are more sparse and have taken a long time to accrue.

Blood pressure

Natural history

Systolic blood pressure rises throughout life. Blood pressure levels are slightly lower in women than in men up to about age 50, when for both systolic and diastolic blood pressures elderly women have slightly higher blood pressure levels than men. Diastolic blood pressure declines from about age 50 to 60 onward [14]. While selective mortality of persons with a higher diastolic blood pressure level may contribute to an apparent decline in cross-sectional studies, this phenomenon can also be observed in longitudinal studies and represents a genuine population fall in diastolic blood pressure with increasing age. The mean rise in systolic blood pressure is 1 mmHg per year in elderly subjects. Thus, the net result of these divergent trends in blood pressure is increasing pulse pressure. The major contributory cause of this is probably reduced aortic compliance (see chapter 15). Thus, the high systolic and relatively low diastolic blood pressure observed in the elderly may indicate pathologic vasular changes that have already taken place rather than simply serving as risk factors for future cardiovascular events (see below).

Prevalence of high blood pressure

Blood pressure distribution curves in the elderly, as in younger subjects, are smooth and unimodal with no evidence of discontinuity. Likewise, in the elderly (younger than age 80) there is no discontinuity in the curve relating blood pressure and risk, so hypertension cannot be defined as a level of blood pressure at which increased risk occurs. The best definition of hypertension is the level of pressure above which treatment does more good than harm. One frequently used criterion for hypertension in the elderly is a blood pressure greater than or equal to 160 mmHg and a diastolic blood pressure (phase V, disappearance of sounds) greater than or equal to 90 mmHg, measured after a period of rest [15]. This definition was derived from the successful outcome of antihypertensive treatment in the European Working Party on High Blood Pressure in the Elderly (EWPHE) trial [16]. Patients with blood pressure below this level still show a gradient of risk and may or may not benefit from treatment. While few clinicians would treat blood pressures below this level pharmacologically, there is a case to be made for nonpharmacologic reduction of blood pressures that are even lower than these criteria. Although the increased risk in such subjects is small, their number far exceeds that of patients with higher blood pressure levels, so the overall population advantage of small reductions in blood pressure is substantial although individual risk may be only slightly improved.

Estimates of the prevalence of blood pressure are widely divergent for two reasons. The first difficulty is that casual blood pressures measured on a single occasion are usually higher than repeated blood pressure measurements. This phenomenon is due to regression toward the mean and habituation to the blood-pressure-measuring procedure; that is, the pressor response to measurement decreases when the subject is familiarized with the procedure. Thus, prevalence rates based upon measurements on a single occasion over-estimate the true figure. Hawthorne and coworkers [17] observed that the prevalence of diastolic hypertension (defined as a blood pressure greater than 99 mmHg) in men and women aged 45 to 64 fell from 15.6% to 5.5% on reexamination. Other studies [18,19] have also suggested that the apparent prevalence rate falls to about one third with repeated examination. The second difficulty is created by the increased proportion of the population now receiving antihypertensive medication. Thus, in the National Health and Nutrition Examination Survey (NHANES 1), 15% of white men aged 65 to 74 years were receiving antihypertensive medication [20]. Ten years later, this figure had risen to 30% in the National Health Epidemiologic Follow-Up Study (NHEFS). Among black women aged 65 to 74 in the latter study, antihypertensive medication had been prescribed for almost 60% [20]. The prevalence of hypertension in such a situation is difficult to estimate, since it critically depends upon doctors' beliefs about treatment rather than on more objective criteria. Using a criterion for hypertension of an average of three blood pressure measurements equal to or more than 140/90 mmHg on a single occasion or the taking of antihypertensive medication yields a prevalence in excess of 60% for subjects over age 65 [20].

Isolated systolic hypertension

The upward trend in systolic pressure and the fall in diastolic pressure give rise to increasing numbers of people whose systolic pressure meets the criterion for hypertension but whose diastolic pressure lies within the arbitrarily defined normal range. Isolated systolic hypertension is usually defined as systolic pressure equal to or greater than 160 mmHg and a diastolic pressure less than 90 mmHg. In the N-HANES Study [20], prevalence rates of 6.7%, 7.1%, 6.1%, and 11.6% were observed, respectively, in white men, white women, black men, and black women age 65 or older. Other large studies have yielded variable results for prevalence. The Evans County Study [21] reported a prevalence rate of 6% in men (average age 65) that rose to 21% in men over 80: the rate for women was 15% at 65 rising to 27% at 75 and 19% over 80. In the Hypertension, Detection and Follow-Up Program [19], the overall prevalence rate for men and women was 7%. Garland and coworkers [22] reported a rate of 3% in men and women aged 60 to 64 that rose to 11% in those 75 years of age or older.

The effect of repeated blood pressure measures on these prevalence figures is difficult to assess. Colandrea and coworkers [18] measured blood pressures repeatedly in 3245 subjects (average age: 69). The apparent prevalence of isolated systolic hypertension fell from 14% to 3% on repeated examinations. This fall, however, was due not only to systolic pressure falling below the criterion of 160 mmHg (which occurred in half of these subjects) but also to an increase in diastolic blood pressure in other subjects (14%) and concomitantly a fall in systolic and a rise in diastolic pressure in 6% of subjects. However, in this study, subjects with initial combined systolic and diastolic hypertension were not rescreened. Some of these subjects would show isolated systolic hypertension on second measurement; it seems likely that the apparent fall in prevalence of isolated systolic hypertension was overestimated. In a study of blood pressure in relation to dietary electrolytes intake in Belgium [23], 2211 subjects were examined on two occasions. Systolic and diastolic pressures were measured five times on each occasion. The prevalence of isolated systolic hypertension over 160 mmHg (diastolic pressure less than 95 mmHg) in subjects aged 60 or older decreased from 14.1% to 9.5% when readings on the two occasions were compared. In a study of nearly 6000 subjects in a younger age group (20 to 49 years) [24], the prevalence of isolated systolic hypertension (diastolic pressure less than 90 mmHg) fell from 1.7% to 0.4% between the first and last reading in six measurements over 25 minutes.

Selection of different cutoff points for diastolic and systolic pressure predictably has a major impact on the observed prevalence. Thus, reducing the cutoff point for diastolic pressure from less than 95 mmHg to less than 90 mmHg decreased the observed prevalence of isolated systolic hypertension from 3.2% to 2.3% in the Belgian studies [23], and from 13.4% to 8.4% in the Hypertension Detection and Follow-Up Program [19]. The claim that there has been a decrease in the prevalence of isolated systolic hypertension from the 1960s to the 1980s has not been confirmed on retrospective analysis of population data [23].

Risks of hypertension, age 65–74

Early, relatively small studies [25,26] suggested that hypertension in the elderly bore a fairly good prognosis. More recent and rigorously conducted longitudinal studies [18,20,22,27] have not confirmed this finding, and it is now clear that established hypertension is a risk factor for cardiovascular disease in the geriatric population as well.

The strongest evidence relating to both the prognosis of hypertension in the elderly and its treatment is provided by clinical trials. Two major randomized controlled trials have shown benefits from antihypertensive treatment in the elderly in the age range of 60 to 79 years: the EWPHE trial [16] and the Hypertension in Elderly Patients in Primary Care (HEP) [28]. The EWPHE trial included subjects over 60 years of age with a sitting blood pressure on placebo between 160 and 239 mmHg systolic *and* between 90 and 119 mmHg diastolic, while the HEP trial included patients aged 60 to 79 years with a sustained systolic pressure of either 170 mmHg or more *or* a diastolic (phase V) pressure of 105 mmHg or more. Stroke events (fatal and nonfatal) were significantly reduced by about 40% in both trials. Nonfatal cardiac events were not reduced in either trial, and cardiac mortality was only reduced in the EWPHE trial. The 40% reduction in stokes and a smaller benefit for cardiac events mirror the results from trials in younger subjects.

In most cases, hypertension in the elderly probably reflects elevated blood pressure over a period of years. Buck et al. [29] explored the effect on cardiovascular complications of age at onset of hypertension. The criterion for diagnosis of hypertension was a diastolic blood pressure of 90 mmHg or greater on two consecutive office visits. The excess risk among subjects with recently diagnosed hypertension compared with normotensive controls declined with age. The odds ratio for cardiovascular complications declined from 6.39 in male subjects aged 40 to 49 to 0.96 in subjects whose hypertension was first diagnosed in the age range of 60 to 65. The authors suggest that late-onset hypertension, as opposed to hypertension in the elderly, enjoys a better prognosis than hypertension first manifesting itself in younger subjects. It is important to emphasize, however, that hypertension in this study was diagnosed using as a criterion diastolic blood pressure only.

In young and middle-aged patients, there is a close relationship between systolic and diastolic pressure and cardiovascular risk. Each predicts cardiovascular events and death independently. However, in the elderly, systolic pressure predominates. Thus, when diastolic blood pressure is held constant, risk increases with systolic blood pressure, while when systolic blood pressure is held constant, diastolic blood pressure is a much weaker predictor of risk in the elderly [30].

Results from the 30-year follow-up of the Framingham Study have provided more detailed information on these relationships. The overall risk in both sexes of either cardiovascular events or death is 2 to 3 times higher in subjects with definite hypertension (blood pressure more than 160/95 mmHg) than in normotensive subjects (blood pressure less than 140/90 mmHg). Specific morbidity from coronary heart disease, stroke, transient ischemic attacks, congestive failure, and peripheral arterial disease [30] showed very similar patterns of increased risk (see table 2-2).

Isolated systolic hypertension is also a potent predictor of cardiovascular risk. Studies suggest that a high pulse pressure per se is not a risk factor. Dawber et al. [31] used the position of the dicrotic notch on the arterial pulse wave to assess arterial rigidity. Systolic blood pressure remained an independent risk factor in the Framingham cohort even when the influence of arterial rigidity measured in this way was adjusted for. Darne et al. [32] used the statistical technique of principal components analysis to generate two components. One reflected mean arterial pressure and the other pulsatility. More than 27,000 subjects aged 40 to 69 years were followed up for a mean

Table 2-2. Risk of coronary and cerebrovascular disease by hypertensive status according to age and sex, 30-year follow-up, Framingham study—average annual age-adjusted rate per 1000

	Coronary heart disease				Stroke and transient ischemic attacks			
	35–64[a] years		65–94[a] years		35–64[a] years		65–94[a] years	
Hypertensive status	Men	Women	Men	Women	Men	Women	Men	Women
Normal (<140/90 mmHg)	8	3	14	11	2	1	5	5
Mild (140–160/90–95 mmHg)	15	7	28	16	4	1	8	7
Definite (>160/95 mmHg)	21	10	41	22	9	3	16	15

[a] All trends significant at $p < 0.001$.
Source: Reproduced from Vokonas PS, Kannel WB, Cupples LA. 1988. J Hypertens 6:S7 [30].

period of 9.5 years. The steady component of blood pressure, as reflected by mean arterial pressure, was a strong risk factor for cardiovascular death in both sexes. In contrast, the pulsatile component was only a risk factor for cardiovascular disease independent of steady pressure, in women over 55 years of age.

In summary, both cross-sectional and longitudinal studies in the elderly have confirmed the importance of hypertension as a risk factor for cardio-vascular disease up to the age of 75 to 80. However, the relationship is modified in comparison with younger subjects, with a greatly predominant role for systolic blood pressure at least up to age 85. On the limited evidence available, it is possible that systolic hypertension in this context is acting as a predisposing factor for cardiovascular disease rather than as a marker for an increased pulse pressure or vascular damage. There are two large trials examining the effects of the treatment of isolated systolic hypertension in the elderly, the SHEP trial in the U.S. and the SYST-EUR trial in Europe. The SHEP trial has recently reported its results [33]. Active treatment significantly reduced the incidence of stroke by 36%, of nonfatal myocardial infarction plus coronary death by 27%, and of all cardiovascular events by 32%. The SYST-EUR trial is still underway [34].

In contrast, in the very elderly, studies on the prognostic significance of an elevated blood pressure provide conflicting evidence. An adverse effect of raised blood pressure has been shown in subjects with an average age of 82 years [35]. However, in other studies [36,37] a low blood pressure has also been related to a high mortality, although this may be a secondary effect of low pressure associated with cardiac disease, weight loss, or other conditions closely related to a poor survival.

Left ventricular hypertrophy
Electrocardiographically demonstrable left ventricular hypertrophy emerged as a strong predictor both of cardiac events and of mortality in the Framingham Study and in other longitudinal studies [10,38,39]. The development of

echocardiography afforded more precise and detailed documentation of hypertrophy. Studies using this investigation have demonstrated an even stronger association with morbidity and mortality and, moreover, have shown that this relationship is independent of blood pressure, age, or other cardiovascular risk factors. In one five-year follow-up study [40], echocardiographically demonstrable left ventricular mass was associated with a fourfold increase in morbid events in a mixed population of normotensive and hypertensive men.

The role of left ventricular mass as a risk factor in elderly subjects has been investigated in the Framingham cohort [41]. A group of subjects aged 59 to 90 were followed up for a four-year period. After adjustment for age, systolic blood pressure, smoking, total stroke, and high-density lipoprotein (HDL)cholesterol, the ratio of left ventricular mass to height remained significantly associated with CHD in both sexes. It is calculated that for each 50-g increase in left ventricular mass, the risk of a coronary event increased by 50%. A particular problem was presented by the higher number of technically suboptimal studies in elderly subjects. In the 30-year follow-up cohort of the Framingham Study [42], electrocardiographically assessed left ventricular hypertrophy was more closely correlated with CHD events and cerebrovascular disease events among the elderly population than it was in those younger than age 65.

Plasma lipids

Prevalence

Serum cholesterol levels rise with age up to age 60. Thus, while 15% of men and 12% of women in the 25- to 34-year-old age group have cholesterol levels above 240 mg/100 ml, this figure rises to 32% and 52%, respectively, in men and women aged between 65 and 74 [43]. The proportions fall thereafter.

Risks of hyperlipidemia

In middle-aged men, experimental evidence from trials shows that a 10% fall in serum cholesterol is associated with a reduction of 15% to 20% in CHD over a two-year period, while the prospective epidemiologic data give an estimate of a 30% reduction in CHD for a 10% fall in cholesterol accuring over several decades [44]. Early reports from the Framingham study, which suggested that this relationship was lost in the elderly, have not been confirmed by more recent analysis of the 30-year follow-up [45]. Risk factors for subjects aged 60 to 70 were analyzed. For men, the relative risk of high cholesterol was somewhat less in older than in younger subjects, although for women the relative risk was the same in both age groups. The absolute risk of an increase in cholesterol was greater in elderly subjects of both sexes, since the risk of coronary events is so much greater.

In contrast, in the Honolulu Heart Study, [46], the relative risk for men over age 65 followed up for an average of 12 years showed an increasing risk of CHD from the lowest to the highest quartile. The risk of the highest compared to the lowest quartile was 1.64 (95% confidence interval: 1.14 to 2.36). This was the same level of risk as in middle-aged men, and further analyses adjusting for the effect of other variables revealed no significant differences in the effects of cholesterol in middle-aged and elderly men.

The CHD risk conferred by total cholesterol persists in the very elderly. In a study [35] of subjects in long-term health care (average age: 82 years), total cholesterol was a significant independent predictor of new coronary events in both men and women, regardless of a history of previous coronary artery disease. Considering CHD mortality rather than incidence, total cholesterol was a significant predictor of CHD mortality among men and women aged 65 to 70, and it was also a significant predictor in women up to age 79 [47]. In the Glostrup Study [48], a cohort of 70-year-old men and women were followed for 10 years. Mortality from cardiovascular disease was significantly higher in the upper quartile than in the lower quartile of the cholesterol distribution, with a similar trend in women. Cancer mortality was significantly higher in the lower quartile of cholesterol than in the upper quartile, an association that has been well documented in many studies and is probably secondary rather than causal, although this remains disputed [49–51].

Other studies have reported either J or inverse relationships for cholesterol with total mortality [48,52,53] that are not explained solely by the association between a low cholesterol level and cancer risk. The average length of follow-up in these studies was less than five years, and in two of the studies [52,53] the average age of the subjects was over 80 years. In the study of women by Forette et al. [52], it was notable that women in the lowest quartile of cholesterol experienced a threefold increase in mortality within the first year of follow-up, suggesting that a low cholesterol is secondary to some other factor influencing death, perhaps malnutrition. However, these authors reported no correlation between cholesterol and body weight or plasma proteins. In a small study of very elderly men [54], significant correlations were reported for total cholesterol with body mass index, a better measure of nutrition than body weight. In the EWPHE trial [55], a significant inverse relationship was found between cholesterol (measured at entry to the trial) and total cardiovascular and noncardiovascular mortality (principally cancer). Subjects in the lowest fifth of the cholesterol distribution had the lowest body mass index and hemoglobin values.

The possibility that the relationship between cholesterol and CHD, though present, is diluted in the elderly is supported by data demonstrating age-related declines in the relationship in other longitudinal studies of younger subjects. However, the largest analysis has been carried out on the 356,222 asymptomatic male screenees for the Multiple Risk Factor Intervention Trial (MRFIT) [56]. The age range was only 35 to 57 years, but the large size of this population permitted comparison of different age groups. In an analysis of these data, Gordon and Rifkind [57] showed that mortality rates from CHD increased linearly with plasma cholesterol within a series of age strata. However, the relationship was steepest in the youngest age group and least steep in the oldest (55 to 57 years). The key question is how far these data can be extrapolated to the elderly. Unfortunately, the conclusion from such an extrapolation is critically dependent upon whether the relationship between cholesterol and CHD with age is linear or exponential. If the relationship is linear, the association between CHD events and cholesterol disappears at age 70 and even becomes negative at greater ages. If the relationship is exponential, a weakened association exists into ole age. Data from Framingham and other sources [35,45–48] suggest that the latter hypothesis is more likely to be correct, although the evidence is limited.

Even the demonstration of a weakened relationship between cholesterol and CHD would have important preventive implications. If risk is reversed by lowering cholesterol, the degree of risk reduction resulting from reduced blood cholesterol would be greatest in young subjects. However, since the incidence of CHD is so much greater in the elderly, the absolute benefits of reducing cholesterol would be much greater, even in the face of a weaker association with CHD. Thus, Gordon and Rifkind [57] calculate that a reduction in serum cholesterol from 285 mg per 100 ml to 200 mg per 100 ml in men aged 35 to 44, although it would reduce the risk of CHD by 77%, would only reduce coronary deaths by 1.8 per year per 1000 men treated. The 23% reduction in risk in elderly men aged 75 to 84, based on the assumption that the CHD–age relationship declines exponentially, would reduce coronary deaths by 12.7 per year per 1000 men treated. Interesting as Gordon and Rifkind's speculations are, it must be realized that they were extrapolated from a population aged 35 to 57; 80-year-old men do not have an average serum total cholesterol of 285 mg/dl but instead a level of only 190 to 207 mg/dl (4.9–5.3 mmol/l).

In men, total cholesterol plateaus before age 60 and declines thereafter. This implies not only that cholesterol-lowering strategies should start at a lower level of relative risk but also that the risk factor is falling anyway. Nevertheless, it is important to determine the benefits in the elderly, if any, of cholesterol-lowering strategies. We must remember that many men who are going to die from heart disease die before age 80. This is known as "exhaustion of the susceptibles," and the survivours may or may not require treatment. Elderly women may have more to gain from intervention than elderly men because at age 80 their average serum cholesterol is 230 to 236 mg/dl [58–61], and fewer women than men have died of heart disease at younger ages.

The weakness of the evidence on which extrapolations are based, the assumption of complete reversibility of risk, and the absence of adequate intervention trials in the elderly make Gordon and Rifkind's calculations a theoretical but perhaps useful illustrative example of possible gains in life expectancy that could be achieved by cholesterol-lowering strategies.

There are fewer data on the relevance of cholesterol subfractions to CHD in the elderly. Nevertheless, it appears that the positive relationships between low-density lipoprotein (LDL) cholesterol and CHD and between triglycerides and CHD are preserved in patients over age 50. In middle-aged subjects, the risk associated with a high level of triglycerides usually disappears when HDL cholesterol is taken into account; for subjects over age 50 in the Framingham Study, a weak independent relationship between triglycerides and CHD incidence remained in women but not in men after an adjustment for HDL cholesterol was made. Conversely, the concentration of HDL cholesterol is negatively related to the risk of CHD in patients over age 50. It is possible that these data conceal subgroups of patients at particularly high risk. This was suggested by the relatively high risk exhibited by men with high triglyceride and low HDL levels. These subjects are often overweight, have a high blood sugar, and are at high risk of developing diabetes mellitus. Risks of cholesterol subfractions are additive, so when HDL cholesterol is combined with other cholesterol measurements, prediction of CHD is enhanced.

In other studies, HDL cholesterol was a significant inverse predictor of risk in very elderly subjects (average 85 years) [53], and LDL was a positive predictor of risk [54]. High triglyceride values were associated with increased cardiovascular mortality in 70-year-old men in the Glostrup Study [48].

Body weight

In subjects aged 35 to 64 in the Framingham Study, relative weight—that is, ratio of weight to desirable weight as determined for gender and height groups studied by the Metropolitan Life Insurance Company in 1959—was related to the risk of CHD but not to the risk of cerebrovascular disease or intermittent claudication. In older subjects, this relationship with CHD was less strong [45]; although it reached statistical significance on univariate analysis and on bivariate analysis (adjusted only for age), it ceased to be significant on multivariate analysis in which adjustment was made for other risk factors, such as blood pressure and lipids. Univariate analysis revealed a stronger association between weight and CHD in men aged 65 to 94 than in women. It thus seems that the short-term risk of obesity is attributable to its association with blood pressure and lipids. Its role as an independent risk factor in the elderly still has to be established. The dilution of the association between obesity and CHD, which is seen particularly in elderly women but which also occurs in elderly men, may be attributable to an increased importance of other risk factors. However, it also should be borne in mind that there are important changes in body composition in the elderly that may lend a different significance to body weight. Thus, there is a decline in the proportionate contribution of skeletal muscle to body mass. Two reports

[62,63] have suggested that in younger hypertensive subjects the relationship between body mass and mortality is reversed. Whether this is also true of elderly subjects is unknown.

Cigarette smoking

Within populations with high CHD rates, smoking is an important risk factor for CHD. Several studies have also shown that elderly men who smoke are at increased risk either of developing CHD or of death. The relative risk for smoking and CHD incidence in the Honolulu Heart study for men over age 65 was 1.55 (95% confidence interval: 1.01 to 2.40). In the Glostrup study [48], 70-year-old men who smoked more than 15 g of tobacco daily had a poorer survival, while in a study of the very elderly both men and women who smoked had almost twice the risk of coronary events of non-smokers. In the Framingham Study [64], the effect of being a smoker at age 65 years was of borderline significance in both men and women; the relative risk for both sexes combined of smoking 20 cigarettes or more a day was 1.2 (95% confidence interval: 0.9 to 1.6).

A few experimental studies [65] have evaluated the effects of antismoking advice, mainly in middle-aged subjects, with no clear-cut benefit on CHD incidence. The benefits of giving up smoking are usually inferred from mortality rates in former smokers. Jajich and colleagues [66] examined the effects of smoking and smoking cessation in a community sample of elderly persons (65 to 74 years old) followed for five years. Smokers had a 50% excess mortality from CHD. Former smokers had mortality rates similar to nonsmokers, including those who had given up smoking in the previous 1 to 5 years. Smoking cessation has benefits other than reduction of CHD risk. Vetter and Ford [67] found that in a randomized controlled trial of subjects over 60 years of age who received antismoking advice, the intervention group had fewer episodes of breathlessness.

Other factors

The significance of blood sugar as a risk factor for CHD increases in the elderly [42]. In both men and women, glucose concentrations are related to CHD after correction for such factors as lipids, blood pressure, body weight, and smoking. There is also a weak relationship between cerebrovascular disease and blood glucose and a strong relationship with intermittent claudication in elderly subjects.

The additive nature of risk factors such as blood pressure, plasma lipids, glucose intolerance, and left ventricular hypertrophy has been demonstrated in younger subjects as well as in subjects over 65 years of age.

CONCLUSION

The evidence so far shows that the well-established risk factors of middle-aged populations persist in old age. In summary, the epidemiologic data suggest that, with regard to predicting risk from the age of 65 years, total cholesterol is a risk factor for CHD in men and women even though the relationship may be weaker than at younger ages. The relationship between cholesterol and total mortality in the very elderly follows a U- or J-shaped curve, probably as a result of other confounding factors. HDL cholesterol may be a better predictor of mortality than total cholesterol. Despite these considerations, there is little information from experimental data on cholesterol-lowering strategies in the elderly. Secondary prevention may be more relevant than primary prevention, since a high proportion of elderly subjects already suffer from the manifestations of CHD. The potential effects of intervention are based on extrapolation from epidemiologic investigations in younger subjects.

Blood pressure is a major risk factor for stroke and CHD in the elderly. The benefits of treating high systolic and diastolic pressure have been shown by randomized controlled trials in subjects up to age 80, although the benefits of reducing CHD are less than the predictions of epidemiologic studies. A high blood pressure in the very old probably remains a risk factor, although, as with cholesterol, prospective studies tend to be confounded by other factors. Trials are underway to examine the effects of treating systolic rather than diastolic blood pressure. Thus, when these results are reported, our understanding of the significance of isolated systolic hypertension should be greatly enhanced.

It is probable that smoking cessation should be encouraged in subjects in their 60s and 70s, although benefit has to be demonstrated in these and in older persons. Left ventricular hypertrophy and blood glucose are, if anything, more important as risk factors in the geriatric population.

The higher incidence of cardiovascular morbidity and mortality in the elderly than in other age groups suggests that the absolute number of patients who stand to gain is great, despite the fact that risk factors often are weaker and proportionate benefits from preventive intervention lower than in middle-aged patients. It is to be hoped that, in addition to longer-term follow-up studies in the elderly, intervention studies will throw light upon the role of these risk factors and demonstrate possible reductions of risk.

REFERENCES

1. Health Statistics in Older Persons. United States, 1986. Analytical and Epidemiological Studies. Series 3, no. 25. 1988. Hyattsvile, MD: U.S. Department of Health and Human Services, table 3, p 8.
2. Mortality Statistics: Cause. Review of Registrar General on Deaths by Cause, Sex and Age in England and Wales. 1988. London: HM Stationery Office, figure A, p 9.
3. Whelton PK. 1984. Essential hypertension—therapeutic implications of epidemiological risk estimation. J Hypertens 2 (Suppl 2):3–8.
4. World Health Statistics. 1988. Geneva: World Health Organization.
5. Simons LA. 1989. Epidemiologic considerations in cardiovascular diseases in the elderly: international comparisons and trends. Am J Cardiol 63:5H–8H.
6. Changes in Mortality Amongst the Elderly 1940–1978. Analytical Studies. Series 3, No. 22.

1982. Department of Health and Human Services Publication No. (PHS) 82–1406. Hyattsville, MD: U.S. Department of Health and Human Service, pp 6–13.

7. Patrick CH, Palesch YY, Feinleib M, et al. 1982. Sex differences in declining cohort death rates from heart disease. Am J Public Health 72:161–166.

8. Goldman L and Cook EF. 1984. Decline in ischemic heart disease mortality rates: an analysis of the comparative effects of the medical interventions and changes in life style. Ann Intern Med 101:825–836.

9. Bonita R and Beaglehole R. 1989. Increased treatment of hypertension does not explain the decline in stroke mortality in the United States, 1970–1980. Hypertension 13:I69–I73.

10. Kannel WB. 1989. Risk factors in hypertension. J Cardiovasc Pharmacol 13:S4–S10.

11. Pooling Project Research Group. 1978. Relationship of blood pressure, serum cholesterol, smoking habits, relative weight and ECG abnormality to incidence of major coronary events. The Final Report of the Pooling Project. J Chron Dis 31:201–306.

12. Rose G and Shipley M. 1986. Plasma cholesterol concentration and death from coronary heart disease: 10 year results of the Whitehall Study. Br Med J 293:306–307.

13. The Society of Actuaries and the Association of Life Insurance Medical Directors of America: Blood Pressure Study 1979. 1980. Boston: Society of Actuaries.

14. Acheson RM. 1973. Blood pressure in a national sample of US adults: Percentile distribution by age, sex and race. Int J Epidemiol 2:293–301.

15. Bulpitt CJ. 1989. Epidemiology. In FH Messerli and JD Swales (eds), Hypertension and the Elderly. London: Science Press, pp 1–7.

16. Amery A, Birkenhäger W, Brixko R, et al. 1985. Mortality and morbidity results from the European Working Party on High Blood Pressure in the Elderly trial. Lancet 1:1349–1354.

17. Hawthorne VM, Greaves DA and Beevers DG. 1974. Blood pressure in a Scottish town. Br Med J 3:600–603.

18. Colandrea MA, Friedman GD, Nichaman MZ, et al. 1970. Systolic hypertension in the elderly: an epidemiologic assessment. Circulation 41:239–245.

19. Curb JD, Borhani NO and Entwisle G. 1985. Isolated systolic hypertension in 14 communities. Am J Epidemiol 121:362–370.

20 Cornoni-Huntley J, La Croix AZ and Havlik RJ. 1989. Race and sex differentials in the impact of hypertension in the United States. The National Health and Nutrition Examination Survey 1. Epidemiologic Follow-Up Study. Arch Intern Med 149:780–788.

21. Wing S, Aubert RE, Hansen JP, et al. 1982. Isolated systolic hypertension in Evans County. Prevalence and screening consideration. J Chron Dis 35:735–742.

22. Garland C, Barret-Connor E, Suarez L, et al. 1983. Isolated systolic hypertension and mortality after 60 years. A prospective population based study. Am J Epidemiol 118:265–276.

23. Staessen J, Amery A and Fagard R. 1990. Isolated systolic hypertension in the elderly. J Hypertens 8:393–405.

24. Van Loo JM, Peer PG and Thien TA. 1986. Twenty-five minutes between blood pressure readings: the influence on prevalence rates of isolated systolic hypertension. J Hypertens 4:631–635.

25. Fry J. 1974. Natural history of hypertension. A case for selective non-treatment. Lancet 2:431–433.

26. Holme I and Waaler H. 1976. Five year mortality in the city of Bergen, Norway, according to age, sex and blood pressure. Acta Medica Scand 200:229–239.

27. Stokes J, Kannel WB, Wolf BA, et al. 1989. Blood pressure as a risk factor for cardiovascular disease. The Framingham Study 30 years of follow-up. Hypertension 13 (Suppl I):I-13–I-18.

28. Coope J and Warrender TS. 1986. Randomised trial of treatment of hypertension in elderly patients in primary care. Br Med J 293:1145–1151.

29. Buck C, Baker P, Bass M, et al. 1987. The prognosis of hypertension according to age and onset. Hypertension 9:204–208.

30. Vokonas PS, Kannel WB and Cupples LA. 1988. Epidemiology and risk of hypertension in the elderly: the Framingham Study. J Hypertens 6:S3–S9.

31. Dawber TR, Thomas HE and McNamara PM. 1973. Characteristics of the dichotic notch of the arterial pulse wave in coronary heart disease. Angiology 24:244–255.

32. Darne B, Girerd X, Safar M, et al. 1989. Pulsatile versus steady component of blood pressure: A cross-sectional analysis and a prospective analysis of cardiovascular mortality. Hypertension 13:392–400.

33. Co-operative Research Group. 1991. Prevention of stroke by antihypertensive drug treatment in older persons with isolated systolic hypertension. JAMA 265:3255–3264.
34. Amery A, Birkenhäger W, Bulpitt CJ, et al. 1991. Syst-Eur, 1991. A multicentre trial on the treatment of isolated systolic hypertension: objectives, protocol and organization. J Hum Hypertens 3:287–302.
35. Aronow WS, Herzig AH, Fritzner E, et al. 1989. 40 month follow up of risk factors correlated with new coronary events in 708 elderly patients. J Am Geriatr Soc 37:501–506.
36. Mattila K, Haavisto M, Rajala S, et al. 1988. Blood pressure and five year survival in the very old. Br Med J 296:887–889.
37. Coope J, Warrender TS and McPherson K. 1988. The prognostic significance of blood pressure in the elderly. J Hum Hypertens 2:79–88.
38. Weber JR. 1988. Left ventricular hypertrophy: its prime importance as a controllable risk factor. Am Heart J 116:272–279.
39. Devereux RB. 1990. Hypertensive cardiac hypertrophy. Pathophysiologic and clinical characteristics. In JH Laragh and BM Brenner (eds), Hypertension: Pathophysiology, Diagnosis and Management. New York: Raven Press, pp 359–377,
40. Casale PN, Devereux RB and Milner M. 1986. Value of echocardio-graphic measurement of left ventricular mass in predicting cardiovascular morbid events in hypertensive men. Ann Intern Med 105:173–178.
41. Levy D, Garrison RJ, Savage DD, et al. 1980. Left ventricular mass and incidence of coronary heart disease in an elderly cohort. The Framingham Heart Study. Ann Intern Med 110:101–107.
42. Stokes J, Kannel WB, Wolf PA, et al. 1987. The relative importance of selective risk factors for various manifestations of cardiovascular disease among men and women from 35 to 64 years old: 30 years of follow-up in the Framingham Study. Circulation 75 (Suppl V):V65–V73.
43. Expert Panel. 1988. Report of the National Cholesterol Education Program Expert Panel on Detection, Evaluation and Treatment of High Blood Cholesterol in Adults. Arch Intern Med 148:36–39.
44. Peto R, Yusuf S and Collins R. 1985. Cholesterol lowering trial results in their epidemiologic context (abstract). Circulation 72:III-451.
45. Castelli WP, Wilson PWF, Levy D, et al. 1989. Cardiovascular risk factors in the elderly. Am J Cardiol 63:12H–19H.
46. Benfante R and Reed D. 1990. Is elevated serum cholesterol level a risk factor for coronary heart disease in the elderly? JAMA 263:393–396.
47. Barret-Connor E, Suarez L, Khaw KT, et al. 1984. Ischaemic heart disease risk factors after age 50. J Chron Dis 37:903–908.
48. Agner E and Hansen PF. 1983. Fasting serum cholesterol and triglycerides in a ten year prospective study in old age. Acta Med Scand 214:33–41.
49. Isles CG, Hole DJ, Gillis CR, et al. 1989. Plasma cholesterol, coronary heart disease and cancer in the Renfrew and Paisley survey. Br Med J 298:920–924.
50. International Collaborative Group. 1982. Circulating cholesterol level and risk of death from cancer in men aged 40 to 69 years. Experience of an international collaborative group. JAMA 248:2853–2859.
51. Yaari S, Goldbourt U, Even-Sohar S, et al. 1981. Association of serum high density lipoprotein and total cholesterol with total, cardiovascular and cancer mortality in a 7 year prospective study of 10,000 men. Lancet 1:1011–1015.
52. Forette B, Tortrat D and Wolmark Y. 1989. Cholesterol as risk factor for mortality in elderly women. Lancet 1:868–870.
53. Nikkila M and Heikkinen J. 1990. Serum cholesterol, high density lipoprotein cholesterol and five year survival in elderly people. Age Ageing 19:403–408.
54. Deutscher S, Bates MW, Caines MJ, et al. 1986. Determinants of lipid and lipoprotein level in elderly men. Atherosclerosis 60:221–229.
55. Staessen J, Amery A, Birkenhäger W, et al. 1990. Is a high serum cholesterol level associated with longer survival in elderly hypertensives? J Hypertens 8:755–761.
56. Stamler J, Wentworth D and Neaton JD. 1986. Is relationship between serum cholesterol and risk of premature death from coronary heart disease continuous and graded? Findings in 356,222 primary screenees of the Multiple Risk Factor Intervention Trial (MRFIT). JAMA 256:2823–2828.

57. Gordon DJ and Rifkind BM. 1989. Treating high blood cholesterol in the older patient. Am J Cardiol 63:48H–52H.
58. Kesteloot H, Heyrman J, Geboers J, et al. 1988. Cardiovascular risk factor distribution above the age of 75 years in a Belgian community. Int J Epidemiol 17:520–524.
59. The Lipid Research Clinic Program Epidemiology Committee. 1979. Plasma lipid distributions in selected North American populations. Circulation 60:427–439.
60. Curb DJ, Reed DM, Yano K, et al. 1986. Plasma lipids and lipoproteins in elderly Japanese-American men. J Am Geriatr Soc 34: 773–780.
61. Foster TA, Hale WE, Srinivasan SR, et al. 1987. Levels of selected cardiovascular risk factors in a sample of geriatric participants—The Dunedin Program. J Gerontol 42:241–245.
62. Barrett-Connor E and Khaw KT. 1985. Is hypertension more benign when associated with obesity? Circulation 72:53–60.
63. Elliott P, Shipley MJ and Rose G. 1987. Are thin hypertensives at greater risk than obese hypertensives? J Hypertens 5:S517–S519.
64. Harris T, Cook E, Kannel WB, et al. 1988. Proportional hazards analysis of risk factors for coronary heart disease in individuals aged 65 or older. J Am Geriatr Soc 36:1023–1028.
65. World Health Organization European Collaborative Group. 1983. Multifactorial trial in the prevention of coronary heart disease: 3. Incidence and mortality results. Eur Heart J 4:141–147.
66. Jajich CL, Ostfeld AM and Freeman DH. 1984. Smoking and coronary heart disease mortality in the elderly. JAMA 252:2831–2834.
67. Vetter NJ and Ford D. 1990. Smoking prevention among people aged 60 and over: a randomised controlled trial. Age Ageing 19:164–168.

3. PATHOPHYSIOLOGY OF THE AGING HEART AND CIRCULATION

JEROME L. FLEG
GARY GERSTENBLITH
EDWARD G. LAKATTA

The structure and function of any organ system in an older person are the end products of the aging process, disease-related alterations, and life-style variables. In the heart and vasculature, the cumulative effects of these latter two variables often obscure the effects of aging per se. It is neverthe-less important to delineate true aging changes in cardiovascular structure and function because they serve as the backdrop upon which the specific cardiovascular diseases to be discussed in subsequent chapters are super-imposed. Such age-associated changes, although usually causing no overt manifestations themselves, may significantly alter the symptoms, signs, and clinical course of cardiovascular pathology in elderly patients. This chapter will attempt to delineate those changes in the heart and peripheral vasculature, at rest and during exercise, that are thought to represent "normal" aging.

EXCLUSION OF CORONARY ARTERY DISEASE
In this chapter, *normal* will denote individuals thought to be free from cardiovascular pathology by the best available criteria. The extent to which these individuals can be considered truly normal is determined by the level of certainty that they are free of recognizable disease. The major disease that must be excluded is coronary artery disease, which in a typical Western

Franz H. Messerli (ed.), CARDIOVASCULAR DISEASE IN THE ELDERLY (Third Edition). Copyright © 1993 Kluwer Academic Publishers. ISBN 0-7923-1859-5. All rights reserved.

nation accounts for 80% to 90% of all cardiac deaths. Fifty percent of deaths from all causes in Western countries can be attributed to either a coronary or cerebrovascular event.

Prevalence of coronary arteriosclerosis

Two extreme estimates of the prevalence of significant coronary atherosclerosis derive from postmortem and epidemiologic studies. Postmortem studies of people dying from random causes have revealed significant coronary narrowing in a major coronary vessel in up to 60% of hearts (figure 3-1A) [1]. This percentage seems to level off at 50 to 59 years in men and almost two decades later in women [2,3]. One interpretation of this figure is that men who are alive in their seventh, eighth, and ninth decades have no greater probability of having severe stenosis than their counterparts aged 50 to 60 years.

Epidemiologic studies in subjects aged 32 to 90 years, based on history and resting electrocardiograms, have found the prevalence of coronary artery disease to range from 2% to 30%, depending on the bracketing of the data for analysis. These studies use relatively insensitive criteria for the diagnosis of coronary disease in a given patient, and probably in a study population as well. The highest prevalence of coronary disease in the 75-plus-years bracket for a community-dwelling population is about 30% [4]. This figure is still somewhat below the 50% to 60% level expected from necropsy studies. Thus, the results of epidemiologic studies must be interpreted as indicating only the prevalence of *symptomatic* coronary artery disease.

The true prevalence of coronary artery disease includes individuals with occult disease in addition to those who are symptomatic. Stress thallium scans have been shown to be a useful tool in identifying individuals with occult coronary artery disease. In this technique, 1 mCi to 2 m Ci of thallium[201], an analogue of potassium, is injected into a peripheral vein at the peak of treadmill exercise. Immediately following exercise, the heart is imaged in several views with a gamma camera. Since the myocardium extracts thallium in proportion to its blood flow, a significant coronary arterial stenosis will decrease the amount of thallium reaching the myocardium it supplies.

One study has demonstrated that in 407 asymptomatic volunteers ages 40 to 96 years, the prevalence of coronary artery disease as assessed by a concordant abnormal electrocardiogram (ECG) and thallium response to maximal treadmill exercise increased from 2% in the fifth and sixth decades to 15% over age 80 (figure 3-1B) [5]. Conversely, concordant negative results declined from 85% in the fifth and sixth decades to 58% in the ninth.

Adding the 42% prevalence of silent abnormalities on exercise ECG/thallium testing to the 20% to 25% prevalence of clinically manifest coronary artery disease in the ninth decade gives an estimated disease prevalence of 62% to 67%, similar to that found in autopsy studies (figure 3-1A). The implication of this finding is that at least one half of all elderly people will have either

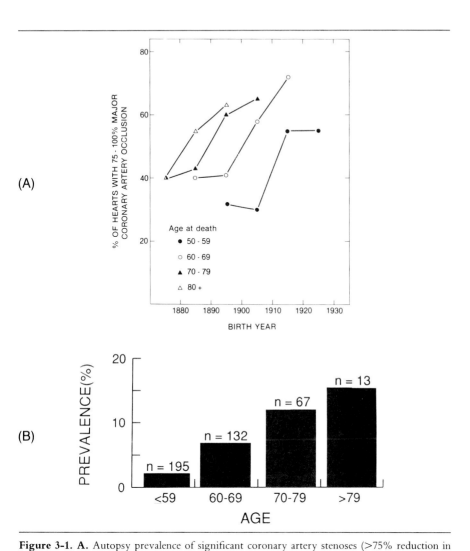

Figure 3-1. A. Autopsy prevalence of significant coronary artery stenoses (>75% reduction in luminal area) by decade of birth and age at death. Note that in all age groups, the prevalence of coronary artery disease at necropsy approaches 60% in the most recent cohorts. (Adapted from Elveback and Lie [1] by permission of the American Heart Association, Inc.)
B. Stepwise increase with age in the prevalence of exercise-induced silent myocardial ischemia, as defined by a concordant abnormal S-T segment and thallium[201] scintigraphic response to maximal treadmill exercise, in 407 apparently healthy volunteers. (From Fleg JL et al. [5] by permission of the American Heart Association, Inc.)

latent or overt disease and would have to be excluded from studies designed to examine the physiology of normal aging changes in humans. Within the bounds of normality, it should be recognized that additional factors such as the blood pressure level used to define hypertension at a given age, physical

Table 3-1. Structural alterations in the cardiovascular system that occur with age

Thickening and stiffening of large and medium-sized arteries
Concentric left ventricular hypertrophy
Modest left atrial enlargement
Modest aortic root dilation
Variable degree of fibrosis of left cardiac skeleton

fitness, nutritional status, and patterns of social behavior may also modify the results of investigation into the aging process of the "normal" cardiovascular system.

A main focus of this chapter will be those physiologic changes associated with aging per se that alter cardiovascular performance at rest and during stress.

CARDIAC ANATOMY AND ELECTROPHYSIOLOGY

Anatomy

Although the concept that the heart undergoes atrophy with advancing age has been espoused for four decades, recent evidence suggests that, if anything, the opposite may be true (table 3-1). From autopsy data of 7112 human hearts spanning 91 years, it was found that between the ages of 30 and 90 years, the heart weight increases an average of 1 to 1.5 g per year [6]. This study, however, included hearts from individuals with cardiovascular disease, raising the possibility that the increase in heart weight with age was related, at least in part, to the development of cardiovascular pathology. A recent autopsy study or 765 normal hearts from people ages 20 to 99 who were free from both hypertension and coronary atherosclerosis showed no relationship, in men, between age and heart weight, indexed to body surface area [7]. For women, however, indexed heart weight increased significantly with age, primarily between the fourth and seventh decades.

Echocardiography has made it possible to measure left ventricular wall thickness and chamber size very accurately, thus allowing accurate non-invasive assessment of left ventricular mass in normal subjects. In studies of normal men and women, an age-related increase in the left ventricular posterior wall thickness of approximately 25% has been found between the second and the seventh decades [8,9]. Figure 3-2A [9] shows the increase in left ventricular posterior wall thickness with age in 56 healthy active men age 25 to 80 years from the Baltimore Longitudinal Study, all of whom had been carefully screened to exclude cardiovascular disease and had resting blood pressures less than 140/90 mm Hg. Similar age differences in left ventricular posterior wall thickness are seen even when these variables are not corrected for body surface area (BSA).

Since ventricular hypertrophy usually occurs in response to an increased cardiac volume or pressure workload, it is reasonable to ask what the stimulus

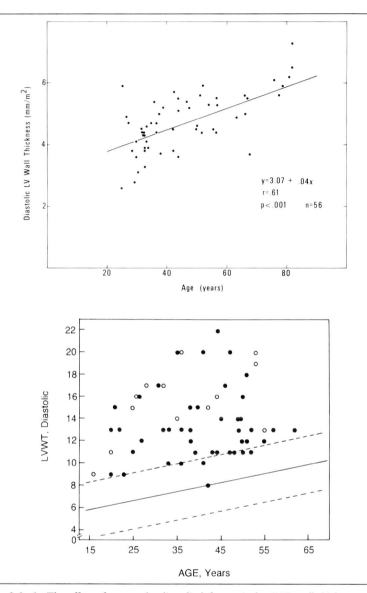

Figure 3-2. A. The effect of age on the diastolic left ventricular (LV) wall thickness measured echocardiographically in 56 healthy normotensive men. The wall thickness has been normalized for body surface area to correct for differences in body size. Adapted from Gerstenblith et al. [9] by permission of the American Heart Association, Inc.)
B. Comparison of the increase in LV diastolic wall thickness (LVWT diastole) with aging versus that induced by aortic valvular disease. The solid line represents the age regression in normal subjects, and the dotted lines indicate the 95% tolerance limits in this population. The closed circles denote patients with aortic stenosis, and the open circles patients with aortic regurgitation. It can be seen that the wall thickness in the majority of the patient group lies well above the age-adjusted normal limit. (From Sjogren [8], Ann Clin Res, 1972.)

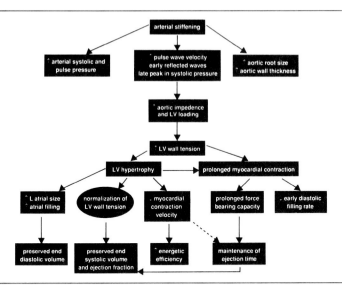

Figure 3-3. Proposed mechanism of age-associated changes on echocardiography. Structural changes in the arterial wall give rise to increases in systolic blood pressure and its harmonic component, aortic input impedance. These changes, in turn, lead to adaptive LV hypertrophy and aortic root dilatation. As a result of the thickened, less compliant state of the LV, early diastolic filling rate decreases, and a compensatory increase occurs in left atrial size and contribution to LV filling, allowing end-diastolic volume to be preserved.

for hypertrophy is in the hearts of apparently normal, older individuals. There is no evidence to suggest an increase in resting stroke volume or cardiac output with age. However, it has long been recognized that both systolic and mean blood pressures increase with age at rest and during exercise, at least in industrialized populations. Age-associated changes in the amount and composition of elastin and collagen within the walls of the large central arteries result in changes in pulse wave velocity and aortic impedance that also increase the load against which the aging left ventricle must eject its blood. The increased volume of blood in the ascending aorta due to age-related aortic dilatation [9] may be an additional stimulus for hypertrophy, since this larger volume of blood must be accelerated by the heart for ejection to occur. It should be kept in mind, however, that the degree of left ventricular hypertrophy seen with advancing age is mild compared to that seen in pathologic conditions (figure 3-2B). Nevertheless, the age-related decrease in mitral valve closing rate (E-F slope) [9,10] and the increase in left atrial size [10], both seen on echocardiography, are analogous to findings in hypertensive populations. A proposed framework for the age-related echocardiographic changes described above is found in figure 3-3.

In addition to the modest structural echocardiographic changes just discussed, additional common pathologic changes have been described in the senescent heart. Lipofucsin, a brownish lipid-containing substance, accumulates at the poles of the nuclei of myocardial cells. Basophilic degeneration, probably a by-product of glycogen metabolism, is found within the sarcoplasmic reticulum. The deposition of amyloid in the myocardium, usually in the atria, occurs in up to one third of elderly patients, and adipose deposition between muscle cells is also common. The endocardium and its specialized extensions, the cardiac valves, have generally been observed to thicken with advancing age. Calcium deposition is frequently noted in the aortic valve and the mitral annulus; in its extreme form, such calcification may result in clinically significant aortic stenosis and mitral regurgitation, respectively. It is important to note, however, that because these histologic changes are derived from autopsy series that undoubtedly included many individuals with coronary artery disease, their specificity as "aging" changes in cardiac structure is open to question, and their functional significance is uncertain.

Conduction system

With advancing age, there is an increase in elastic and collagenous tissue in all parts of the conduction system. Fat accumulates around the sinoatrial (S-A) node, sometimes producing a partial or complete separation of the node from the atrial musculature, which in extreme cases may be related to the development of sick sinus syndrome. Beginning by age 60 there is a pronounced "falling out" or decrease in the number of pacemaker cells in the S-A node, and by age 75 less than 10% of the cell number found in the young adult remain. A variable degree of calcification of the left side of the cardiac skeleton, which includes the aortic and mitral anuli, the central fibrous body, and the summit of the interventricular septum, occurs. Because of their proximity to these structures, the atrioventricular (A-V) node, A-V bundle, bifurcation, and proximal left and right bundle branches may be damaged or destroyed by this process, resulting in so-called primary or idiopathic block. However, in many instances, such conduction disturbances in the aged are associated with hypertensive, arteriosclerotic, or amyloid disease.

Electrocardiography

Based on the structural changes with age already described, it is not surprising that several features of the electrocardiogram are altered by "normal" aging. Although resting heart rate is not age related, the P-R and Q-T intervals of healthy men show small but significant increases with age [11]. The age-related increase in the P-R interval has recently been shown to be due to conduction delay occurring proximal to the bundle of His (figure 3-4A) [12]. Conduction time from the His bundle to the ventricle is not affected (figure 3-4B) [12]. A leftward shift of the QRS axis occurs with advancing age, perhaps reflecting a variable degree of fibrosis in the anterior

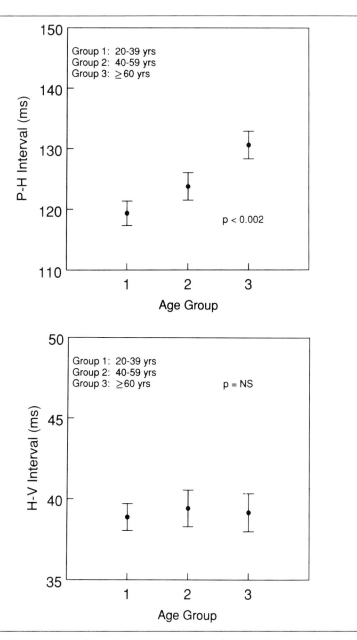

Figure 3-4. A. Age-associated increase in conduction time from the P-wave to the His bundle deflection, determined from the signal-averaged high-resolution surface ECG in normal subjects. **B.** In this same population, the conduction time from the His bundle to the ventricles is not related to age. (From Fleg JL, et al. [12]. Copyright © The Gerontological Society of America.)

fascicle of the left bundle branch as well as mild left ventricular hypertrophy. Despite the echocardiographic evidence of increased left ventricular mass in elderly subjects, QRS voltage actually declines with age. This apparent paradox is largely explicable by extracardiac factors such as changes in the heart's position in the thorax, senile emphysema, and chest wall deformities; partial replacement of cardiac muscle by fat or amyloid may also be contributory. Perhaps the most readily observed electrocardiographic changes related to age involve the repolarization process; the S-T segment becomes flattened, and the amplitude of the T-wave diminishes [11].

Cardiac arrhythmias

Even in apparently healthy populations, the prevalence of cardiac arrhythmias at rest, during routine daily activity, and with exercise has generally been found to increase with age. For example, in the Baltimore Longitudinal Study the prevalence of isolated ventricular ectopic beats on resting ECG increased from 2.5% in the third decade to 17% in the ninth. Because the resting electrocardiogram generally represents less than one minute's electrical activity out of a 24-hour day, far more accurate quantification of arrhythmias can be obtained by 24-hour ambulatory electrocardiography, i.e., Holter monitoring.

Studies of clinically normal subjects investigated by this technique have shown that the prevalence of supraventricular and ventricular ectopic beats increases with age. Isolated supraventricular and ventricular ectopic beats, usually less than one per hour, were found, respectively, in 88% and 78% of a population of 98 healthy men and women age 60 to 85 years, who were free of heart disease as determined by extensive noninvasive testing [13]. Supraventricular tachyarrhythmias were found in one third of the subjects; 26% displayed more than 100 supraventricular ectopic beats, and 17% displayed more than 100 ventricular ectopic beats over the 24-hour monitoring period. Ventricular couplets or short runs of ventricular tachycardia were detected in 15%. The prevalence of each of these arrhythmias was markedly higher than in healthy young subjects studied by other investigators. In contrast, sinus bradycardia of less than 40 per minute, long sinus pauses, and high-degree A-V block as well as atrial flutter to fibrillation were extremely uncommon or nonexistent in these carefully screened elderly subjects. Similar findings were noted in a recent study of clinically healthy subjects older than 80 years [14].

Exercise-related arrhythmias also increase dramatically with advancing age. In the Baltimore Longitudinal Study population, isolated supraventricular ectopic beats increased from 8% in the 20s to 76% in the 80s; corresponding figures for ventricular ectopic beats were 11% and 57%, respectively. Furthermore, short runs of nonsustained ventricular tachycardia were found in 3.8% of clinically normal volunteers older than age 65, a rate 25-fold that seen in younger subjects (figure 3-5) [15]. A recent analysis of 1160

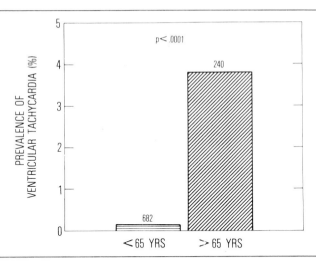

Figure 3-5. Prevalence of exercise-induced nonsustained ventricular tachycardia in asymptomatic volunteers from the Baltimore Longitudinal Study of Aging. Note the 25-fold higher prevalence in subjects older than 65 years versus younger than 65 years. (From Fleg JL and Lakatta EG [15].)

people confirmed a striking age-associated increase in frequent or repetitive ventricular ectopic beats in men but not in women [16]. No differences in the subsequent incidence of coronary events or syncope were noted over a mean 5.6-year follow-up between the 80 subjects with such complex exercise-induced ventricular arrhythmias and an age-matched control group free of these arrhythmias.

Chest roentgenology

Chest x-rays in the elderly may be difficult to interpret due to chest deformities caused by kyphoscoliosis and emphysema, which may alter the normal relationship between the heart and the chest cavity. Although the cardiothoracic ratio (CTR) on chest x-ray increases slightly with age in both cross-sectional and longitudinal studies, a CTR exceeding 50% in elderly subjects is rare in the absence of clinical heart disease and thus confirms the specificity of this finding even in senescence [15]. The small (2% to 5%) age-related increase in CTR has been found in some studies to be due primarily to a decrease in the transverse thoracic diameter, although a small increase in heart size has been observed in some longitudinal investigations [17]. An age-related dilatation of the aortic knob has also been found both cross-sectionally and longitudinally. The knob increased from 3.4 to 3.8 cm in men followed for 17 years from an initial average age of 48 years [17]. Aortic tortuosity and aortic knob calcification are also common findings on chest x-ray that do not by themselves imply cardiovascular disease. Recent data from Framingham suggest that aortic knob calcification has no prognostic significance in older subjects but confers a twofold increased risk for cardiac events in those younger than 65 years [18]. Intracardiac calcifications, on the other hand, may be due to a calcified aortic valve, mitral anulus, or ventricular aneurysm, constrictive pericarditis, or coronary artery calcification. Intracardiac calcifications, therefore, should not be attributed to normative aging.

Peripheral vasculature

Because the peripheral vasculature provides the delivery system by which blood pumped by the heart reaches the various body tissues, age-related changes in the blood vessels may limit the maximal perfusion of these tissues and affect cardiac performance as well. It is therefore essential that any discussion of the aging heart also consider the aging peripheral vasculature.

It has been suggested that peripheral vascular resistance (PVR), defined as mean arterial pressure divided by cardiac output, increases with age [19]. The mechanism of this generalized increase in PVR is not currently defined. By Ohm's law applied to the steady-state circulation, a primary decrease in cardiac output would lead to an increase in PVR. However, a wide spectrum of basal cardiac output exists among all people, including the elderly. Resting cardiac output in apparently healthy individuals has thus been found to decrease, to remain unchanged, or even to increase slightly [20] with advancing age. These variable results may account for the heterogeneity in PVR in older people. In one study, although cardiac output at rest decreased with age, the calculated increase in PVR in elderly people appeared greater than that which could be attributed to a reduction in cardiac output, suggesting a primary increase in PVR in the aged individuals studied [21]. Thus, when all people (i.e., both hypertensives and normotensives) are considered together, a picture emerges showing that mean arterial pressure and PVR increase and cardiac output decreases with advancing age. However, if patients with specific cardiovascular diseases, including hypertension, are excluded, the remaining elderly individuals have a resting cardiac output equal to that of younger subjects and have no marked increase in PVR [22]. Though normotensive by clinical criteria, most healthy populations still exhibit an age-associated increase in brachial systolic arterial pressure within the "clinically normal" range, while diastolic pressure remains relatively constant.

A full century ago, it was suggested that arterial walls stiffen with age in both animals and humans. Since that observation, numerous investigators have shown major aging changes in the composition of vessel walls, including increases in calcium and collagen content and degeneration of the internal elastic membrane. Macroscopically, both wall thickness and lumen diameter of the aorta increase. Peripheral arteries also increase in thickness, although the arterial wall thickness–radius ratio varies from site to site. It should be emphasized that the age-associated increase in arterial stiffness is secondary to a diffuse process occurring in the vessel wall and cannot be attributed to

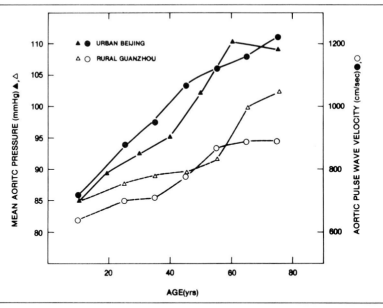

Figure 3-6. Change in mean aortic pressure (▲,△) and aortic pulse wave velocity (●,○) with age in normal subjects from urban Beijing, an area of high salt intake, and rural Guangzhou, an area of low salt intake. At any age, aortic pressure and pulse wave velocity are lower in the Guangzhou population. (Redrawn from Avolio et al. [23] by permission of the American Heart Association, Inc.)

atherosclerosis. Such vascular changes have already been documented in Asian populations, in whom clinical manifestations of atherosclerosis are uncommon (figure 3-6) [23]. Nonetheless, the histologic, morphologic, and stiffness changes found in the aging aorta are similar to those seen with essential hypertension.

The structural changes in the aorta and other large arteries are reflected clinically in a rise of the systolic pressure and widening of pulse pressure with advancing age. Pulse wave velocity also has consistently been found to increase with age in humans, indicating decreased arterial compliance. The carotid pulse contour is altered with age, demonstrating an increase in the second systolic maximum relative to the first. This is due to the presence of early reflected pulse waves.

Left ventricular pulsatile arterial load is characterized by the aortic input impedance and is a function of the peripheral vascular resistance, central aortic stiffness, and wave reflections; thus, the age-related changes in arterial properties may have an important effect on arterial impedance and thence myocardial afterload. Each of these components of arterial load changes with aging in man. Thus, the senescent human heart, due to increased arterial loading, requires greater left ventricular stroke work, increased wall tension, and myocardial oxygen consumption during systole. This may explain, at least in part, the age-associated increase in left ventricular mass found in echocardiographic and postmortem studies.

CARDIOVASCULAR PERFORMANCE AT REST

Systolic time intervals and ballistocardiography

In the 1950s and 1960s, noninvasive assessment of ventricular function was limited largely to ballistocardiography and systolic time intervals (STIs). These studies suggested increased ejection and relaxation times in hearts of older individuals.

Cardiac output (Fick, dye dilution)

Several studies over the past 25 years have shown that resting cardiac output and stroke volume determined by Fick or dye dilution techniques decline with age. In a group of 67 institutionalized men between ages 19 and 86 years, cardiac output fell an average of 1% per year, from a mean of 6.5 l/min in the third decade to 3.9 l/min in the ninth decade [21]. Stroke volume fell from 85 to 60 ml over the same time period. These decrements remained highly significant when corrected for age differences in BSA.

Such investigations of cardiac output are difficult to interpret for several reasons. First, as already noted, the invasive methodology employed in these studies cannot be considered to measure cardiac performance under true resting conditions. Age differences elicited under these conditions may represent differences in response to stress. Second, the individuals studied were not screened for the presence of occult coronary disease. Physical conditioning status also probably differed widely among the individuals. Furthermore, it is not valid to use cardiac output or stroke volume to measure intrinsic cardiac performance, since difference in preload or afterload may modify these measurements.

Echocardiography and radionuclide angiography

In the last 15 years, more direct techniques for the noninvasive assessment of ventricular function have allowed further insights into the effects of aging on cardiac performance. M-mode echocardiography allows accurate beat-by-beat measurement of left ventricular dimensions and septal and posterior wall thickness throughout the cardiac cycle. Gated radionuclide angiography is probably the most accurate technique for measuring global left ventricular function, both at rest and during exercise. Studies utilizing these techniques have been performed on carefully screened community-dwelling volunteers from the Baltimore Longitudinal Study [9,24]. Subjects who had a history of cardiac disease or who exhibited signs of cardiac disease by physical examination, chest x-ray, and resting electrocardiography were excluded from analysis. In addition, those subjects who exhibited ischemic electro-

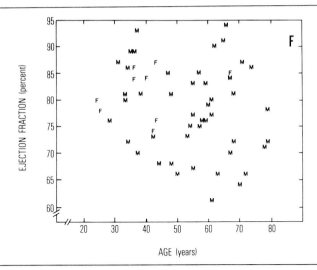

Figure 3-7. The effect of age on the resting LV ejection fraction determined by radionuclide angiography in 61 healthy men (M) and women (F) from the Baltimore Longitudinal Study. No age effect is seen. (From Rodeheffer et al. [24] by permission of the American Heart Association, Inc.)

cardiographic or thallium scintigraphic changes during maximal treadmill exercise, which suggests latent coronary artery disease, were also excluded, as were subjects who had systolic blood pressures greater than 140 mmHg or diastolic pressures greater than 90 mmHg. However, it is important to note than even in this select group, both systolic and mean blood pressure significantly increased from 20 to 80 years.

Ejection fraction

The most widely used index of overall cardiac pump performance is ejection fraction. This is determined by end-diastolic volume (preload), the resistance to emptying (afterload), and intrinsic muscle performance (contractility). As is evident in figure 3-7, resting ejection fraction does not decline between ages 25 and 80 years [18]. There is also no significant age change in end-diastolic volume determined by radionuclide angiography (figure 3-8A). This confirms prior M-mode and two-dimensional echocardiographic studies in the Baltimore Longitudinal Study population, which showed no change in resting end-diastolic dimension [9] or area [25] with age, respectively. Similarly, scintigraphic end-systolic volume is unrelated to age (figure 3-8B).

From a given end-diastolic volume, an age-related decrease in resistance to emptying is another factor that might mask a decrease in cardiac muscle function. This resistance to left ventricular emptying, or vascular impedance, is a complex function of central aortic compliance or stiffness, systemic

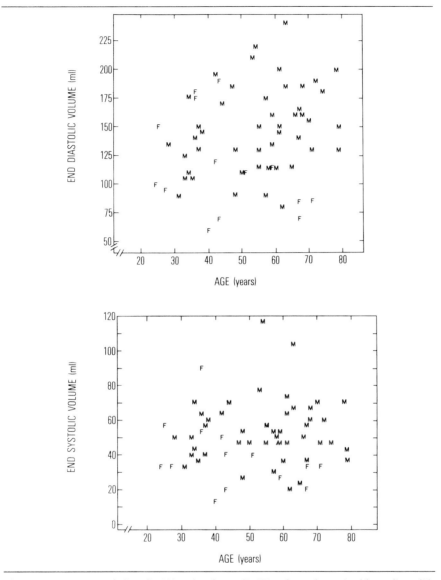

Figure 3-8. Resting end-diastolic (**A**) and end-systolic (**B**) volume determined by radionuclide angiography in the population from figure 3-7. Again, no age relationship is present. (From Rodeheffer et al. [24] by permission of the American Heart Association, Inc.)

vascular resistance, reflected pressure waves, and the inertial properties of blood. However, no evidence for a decrease in vascular impedance as a mechanism for the maintenance of normal cardiac pump function has been documented in the elderly.

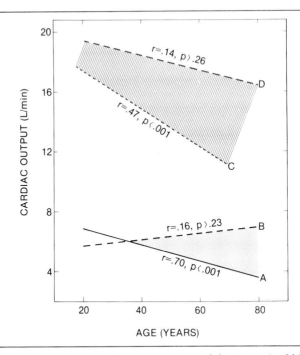

Figure 3-9. The effect of age on cardiac output at rest and during maximal bicycle exercise in different populations. In hospitalized patients recovering from noncardiac illnesses (line A), resting cardiac output was found to decline by approximately 50% between ages 20 and 90 [21]. Maximal cardiac output was found to decline significantly with age in a group of ambulatory volunteers not specifically screened to exclude occult coronary disease (line C) [41]. In contrast, cardiac output both at rest (line B) and during maximal upright bicycle exercise (line D) was not found to change significantly with age in a single group of healthy volunteers screened to exclude coronary disease by exercise ECG and thallium scintigraphy [24].

Circumferential fiber shortening

An index that may be more sensitive than ejection fraction for the assessment of intrinsic cardiac muscle function is the velocity of circumferential fiber shortening. Several studies have indicated that this variable is not age related at rest, again implying that resting cardiac muscle performance is not affected by age. Thus, although intrinsic muscle performance cannot be measured directly in intact man, the results presented strongly support the notion that no decline in cardiac function occurs at rest in healthy subjects. From estimates of volume from one- and two-dimensional echocardiograms and more directly calculated volumes from gated radionuclide scintigraphy, it is evident that resting stroke volume does not decline with age. Since resting heart rate is also not age related, it would follow that resting cardiac output as well probably does not decline with increasing age in healthy individuals.

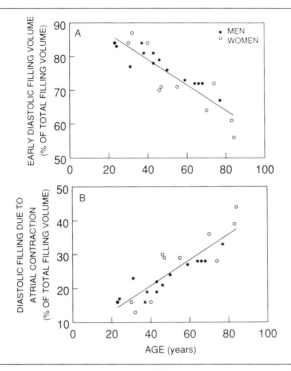

Figure 3-10. A. Reduction of early diastolic LV filling rate with age, measured by the Doppler peak E-wave flow velocity integral as a percentage of total diastolic filling, in healthy normotensive volunteers.
B. Augmentation of late diastolic filling with age, measured by the Doppler peak A-wave flow velocity integral as a percentage of total diastolic filling, in the same individuals shown in **A.** (Data from Swinne et al. [28].)

Such a result has been documented in the carefully screened Baltimore Longitudinal Study population (figure 3-9) [24].

Diastolic left ventricular filling rate

In contrast to systolic function, the early diastolic left ventricular filling rate, initially measured by the rate of closure of the mitral valve on M-mode echocardiography, is significantly reduced with increasing age in normal men [9,10]. Since these early observations, numerous studies using more sophisticated techniques such as Doppler echocardiography (figure 3-10) [26–28] and radionuclide ventriculography [29,30] have confirmed this age-related slowing of maximal early diastolic filling rate. This impairment of early left ventricular filling may derive at least in part from a diminished ventricular diastolic compliance, which in turn may be secondary to the aforementioned increase in ventricular wall thickness with age. In support of

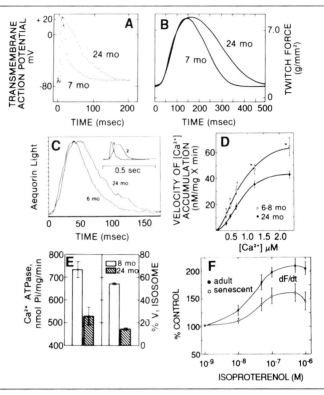

Figure 3-11. Representative data depicting differences in various aspects of excitation–contraction coupling mechanisms measured between young adult (6–9 months) and senescent (24–26 months) rats.
A. Transmembrane action potential.
B. Isometric contraction (from Wei et al. [33]).
C. Myoplasmic Ca^{2+} transient (from Orchard and Lakatta [32]).
D. Sarcoplasmic reticulum Ca^{2+} uptake (from Froehlich et al. [31]).
E. Myosin isoenzyme composition (50% of the heterodimer [V_2] is included in the total percentage of V_1) and Ca^{2+}-stimulated ATPase activity (from Effron et al. [34]).
F. Contractile performance in response to incremental doses of isoproterenol (from Guarnieri et al. [35]).

this hypothesis, animal studies in both intact hearts and isolated cardiac muscle have demonstrated prolongation of isovolumic relaxation and increased diastolic myocardial stiffness. At the cellular level, myocardial relaxation is effected by the removal of Ca^{2+} from the contractile proteins by the sarcoplasmic reticulum. Sarcoplasmic reticulum isolated from senescent animal hearts accumulates Ca^{2+} at a slower rate than that from young adult hearts (figure 3-11D) [31]. This is associated with a prolonged increase in cytosolic Ca^{2+} levels following excitation (figure 3-11C) [32]. The slower isometric relaxation observed in the cardiac muscle isolated from older animals (figure 3-11B) [33] may therefore be related to this diminished rate of Ca^{2+} accumulation by the sarcoplasmic reticulum.

Perhaps also as a result of this reduction of ventricular compliance, the left atrium has been found to enlarge with age in several human echocardiographic studies. Doppler echocardiography has further shown that the age-related slowing of maximal early diastolic mitral inflow is accompanied by a concomitant increase in mitral inflow velocity during atrial systole [26]. Since left ventricular end-diastolic volume is not diminished with age, this augmented late diastolic filling, as measured by the Doppler A-wave, can be construed as a successful adaptation to the reduced early filling rate in the thicker, stiffer senescent left ventricle. Thus, the relative importance of early and late diastolic filling phases is reversed with advancing age.

Although the reduced early diastolic filling rate of the senescent heart may not impair resting end-diastolic volume or stroke volume, the underlying impairment of ventricular compliance might cause a greater rise in left ventricular diastolic pressure at rest and especially during tachycardia associated with stressful situations in the elderly and thus lead to a lower threshold from dyspnea than in the young adult. Furthermore, it would not be surprising if the loss of the atrial contribution to left ventricular filling, as occurs during atrial fibrillation, would result in a greater impairment of diastolic function in older than in younger patients.

Physical findings

Given the structural and functional alterations in the cardiovascular system with age already described, what "abnormalities" in the cardiac physical examination might be expected in a healthy elderly individual? The apical impulse may be difficult to feel due to chest wall deformities and senile emphysema. Perhaps due to a decrease in the compliance of the pulmonary vasculature, inspiratory splitting of the second heart sound is audible in only approximately 30% to 40% of subjects older than 60 years. On the other hand, an S_4 gallop, which indicates a diminution of left ventricular compliance and is uncommon in normal individuals younger than 40, is heard in many normal geriatric subjects. A soft basal systolic ejection murmur has been found in 30% to 60% of subjects 60 years and older. The murmur probably arises from dilatation and decreased compliance of the aorta. Due to the increased stiffness of the peripheral vasculature, the carotid upstroke is usually brisk in the elderly and thus may mask significant aortic stenosis.

CARDIAC PERFORMANCE DURING STRESS

The preceding section has addressed those aging changes in cardiac performance evident at rest. In many organ systems, functional derangements may become manifest only under conditions that tax the capability of the system—that is, stress. The following discussion will center on the age-

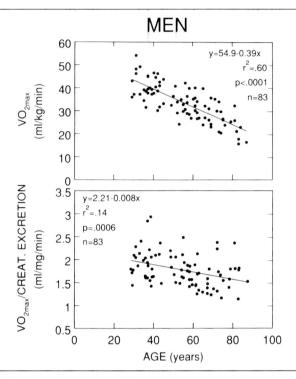

Figure 3-12. Maximal oxygen uptake (VO$_2$ max) as a function of age in healthy active men from the Baltimore Longitudinal Study.
A. When expressed per kilogram body weight, VO$_2$ max declines strikingly with age as shown by the solid line.
B. When VO$_2$ max is normalized for 24-hour urinary creatinine excretion, an index of muscle mass, the age-dependence of the variable is nearly abolished. (From Fleg and Lakatta [37].)

related changes in response to aerobic exercise, the best-studied cardiovascular stress.

Maximal oxygen uptake
In the laboratory setting, exercise performance is usually assessed by a multistage continuous treadmill or bicycle test, each successive stage of which requires greater energy expenditure than the preceding one. The cardiovascular system supports this effort by distributing increasing amounts of blood to the exercising muscles to enable them to obtain sufficient oxygen to satisfy their increased metabolic requirements. This ability to deliver oxygen is quantified by measuring the maximal oxygen consumption (VO$_2$max), which is the product of maximal cardiac output and maximal systemic arteriovenous oxygen (A-VO$_2$) difference. VO$_2$max is thus considered the best overall indicator of cardiovascular fitness. The value for a given

individual is not affected by adding other muscular work when more than 50% to 60% of the body's muscle mass is being exercised.

Over the last four decades, numerous investigators have found an age-related decline in VO_2max, which averages about 1% per year between the ages of 25 and 75 years [36]. This decline in VO_2max parallels the decline in maximal work capacity; thus, the lower oxygen uptake in elderly subjects does not reflect greater metabolic efficiency. In healthy men and women from the Baltimore Longitudinal Study population, the typical age-associated decline in VO_2max was nearly abolished when VO_2max was normalized for 24-hour urinary creatinine excretion, an index of muscle mass (figure 3-12) [37]. Thus, the decline in VO_2max with advancing age may be largely secondary to a diminished muscle mass.

The extent of the age-associated diminution of VO_2max is affected by physical conditioning, smoking, and degree of obesity. In one longitudinal study, for example, a 25% decline in VO_2max occurred over the ensuing 22 years in men initially aged 18 to 22 [38]. By cessation or reduction of cigarette smoking, entrance into long-term physical conditioning programs, and reduction in body weight, a subset of these individuals were able to increase their VO_2max an average of 11% over the next five-year period. Nevertheless, even champion athletes who continue to train after retirement from competition experience age-associated declines in VO_2max, although the degree of this decline may be attenuated [39].

Hemodynamic findings

The decline in VO_2max occurring with age has been attibuted to a decrease in both maximal cardiac output and maximal A-VO_2. A decrease in both maximum heart rate and maximum stroke volume contributed to the decrease in maximum cardiac output as determined by invasive methodology [40–42]. For example, when 17 clinically healthy Scandinavian men aged 61 to 83 years were compared with a group of young men (mean age of 23 years) studied previously, the following results were found: the older men had a lower maximal heart rate (130 versus 157 beats/min), lower stroke volume (101 versus 118 ml), lower maximal cardiac output (13.1 versus 18.5 l/min), and lower VO_2max (1.46 versus 2.06 l/min) than the younger men during recumbent bicycle exercise [40]. Systolic blood pressure was 39 mmHg greater than in young men at peak exercise. In addition, the pulmonary artery wedge pressure in the elderly individuals averaged 22 mmHg, 6.5 mmHg greater than in the younger men. Right ventricular end-diastolic pressure was also greater in the older men. Higher pulmonary wedge and left ventricular end-diastolic pressure in elderly subjects during exercise have been confirmed by other investigators. Detailed comparisons of blood pressure during exercise have usually shown no significant difference in systolic pressure at maximal exercise, although the values at rest and at given submaximal loads were greater in older than in younger individuals.

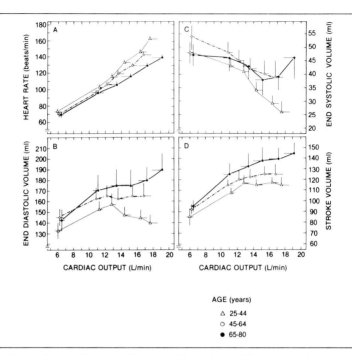

Figure 3-13. Cardiac performance determined by radionuclide angiography during upright bicycle ergometry in three age groups. Although age has no significant effect on exercise cardiac output in subjects carefully screened to exclude coronary artery disease, in the elderly a given cardiac output is achieved by greater cardiac dilatation, i.e., greater LV end-diastolic volume (**B**) and, in turn, greater stroke volume (**D**). The increase in stroke volume compensates for decreased cardio-acceleration (**A**) and less complete systolic emptying with advancing age (**C**). (Adapted from Rodeheffer et al. [24] by permission of the American Heart Association, Inc.)

In deriving conclusions regarding the effects of aging on cardiovascular performance during aerobic exercise, it is important to bear in mind that occult coronary artery disease was probably present in a significant number of the older individuals in these earlier studies, as suggested by the sizable proportion of these subjects with electrocardiographic abnormalities. Furthermore, maximum aerobic capacity may have been limited in these investigations by noncardiovascular factors such as physical activity status and respiratory function. The supine position and the invasive methodology employed in some of these studies may also limit their general applicability. Thus, conclusions based on these studies regarding the limits of cardiovascular performance imposed by aging per se must be tentative.

Gated cardiac blood pool scintigraphy and echocardiography

A better perspective for deriving conclusions about the age-related modifications of maximal cardiovascular performance can be achieved by studying

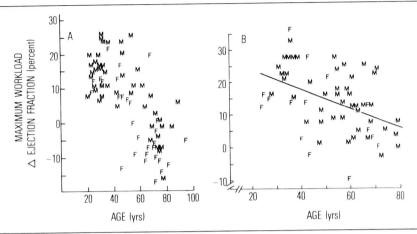

Figure 3-14. Changes in ejection fraction from rest to peak exercise (ΔEF) as a function of age in men (M) and women (F) from two apparently healthy populations. Although an age-associated decline in ΔEF occurred in both studies, note the large percentage of subjects in **A** who decreased their EF at peak exercise (ΔEF is negative) compared to the rarity of such a decline in EF in **B**. This difference between the two studies may relate to the presence of latent coronary heart disease in a high percentage of population A (as manifest by wall motion abnormalities during exercies), whereas population B, prescreened by thallium scintigraphy, had no exercise-induced wall motion abnormalities. (Adapted from Port et al. [43] by permission of the New England Journal of Medicine, and Rodeheffer et al. [24] by permission of the American Heart Association, Inc.)

physically active individuals who have been screened for the absence of latent ischemic heart disease by stress testing. In the Baltimore Longitudinal Study population, individuals thus screened by maximal exercise electrocardiography and thallium scanning have undergone gated radionuclide angiography during maximal upright bicycle exercise. This investigation confirmed the well-described decline in maximal heart rate with age, approximating 30% between ages 20 and 80 years. In contrast to the earlier studies, maximal cardiac output declined only 15% between these ages (figure 3-9) due to a compensatory rise in the stroke volume of older subjects at high work-loads (figure 3-13) [24]. This relative preservation of cardiac output was accomplished by a greater exercise-induced increment in end-diastolic left ventricular volume with advancing age; however, end-systolic volume at maximal loads did not decrease as much in the older individuals as in the young. Therefore, the normal exercise-induced increase in ejection fraction declined in magnitude with advancing age (figure 3-14B) [24]. Similar age changes in diastolic and systolic left ventricular volumes as assessed by two-dimensional echocardiography in carefully screened volunteers have been found during semisupine submaximal bicycle exercise [25]. Thus, increasing reliance on the Frank–Starling mechanism (increased ventricular preload) may be one adaptation that is employed by older individuals to maintain cardiac output during exercise. Clinically, it is important to realize that even though the exercise-induced augmentation of ejection fraction declined with increasing age, an absolute decline of ejection fraction during exercise was rarely observed in elderly subjects, in contrast to the response of patients with significant heart disease and to an earlier aging study in which rigorous prescreening for latent coronary artery disease was not employed (figure 3-14A) [43]. However, the specificity of a five-point rise in ejection fraction for the absence of coronary artery disease declines with age and is lower in older women than in older men [44].

Exercise response in animal models

The diminished heart rate response to beta-adrenergic stimuli observed in humans also occurs in both the rodent and canine models. The direct vasodilatory response of arteries and veins to beta-adrenergic stimulation decreases with age in humans and in isolated blood vessels in animal models. This diminished vasodilatation could affect vascular impedance during stress. Resting aortic input impedance has been shown to increase with age in humans [45]. No studies in humans have evaluated whether this age change is exacerbated during exercise. However, during exercise aortic impedance in young beagles has been shown to decline from resting values, and these animals demonstrated a stepwise increase in stroke volume with increasing workload [46]. In contrast, the aged beagles demonstrated a striking increase in characteristic aortic impedance during exercise, with minimal augmentation of stroke volume (figure 3-15). These age differences were abolished by beta-adrenergic blockade, which caused an increased impedance with exercise in the young beagles. If this age-associated increase in aortic impedance that occurs in the older beagle dog during exercise also occurs in humans, it could be a factor limiting the ejection fraction and stroke volume responses. Thus, the increased afterload in the elderly may reflect an impaired vasodilator response to catecholamines.

Beta-adrenergic responsiveness

Cardiovascular function is determined by a complex interaction of multiple hemodynamic variables (figure 3-16) [47]. Each of these is determined by basic cellular and extracellular biophysical mechanisms that are subject to autonomic modulation. Alterations in cardiovascular function due to aging (or disease) can be attributed to an effect of age on the basic (intrinsic) cellular mechanisms that determine the variables in figure 3-16, or on the autonomic modulation of these mechanisms. The autonomic modulation of these variables is not constant but shifts with the demands placed on the system at any given moment. For example, at rest, cholinergic modulation is dominant, and adrenergic influence is minimal. With changes in posture to the upright position, emotional stress, performance of routine daily activities, or exercise,

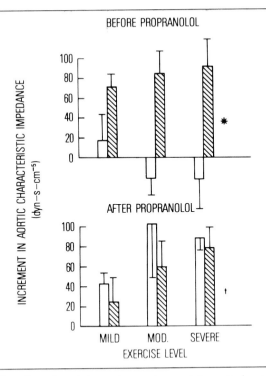

Figure 3-15. The effect of graded exercise on characteristic aortic input impedance in young adult (□) and senescent (⊠) beagles. Before propranolol, exercise caused a significant increase in aortic impedance in the old but not the young group. After propranolol, aortic impedance was increased by exercise in both groups to a similar extent. (From Yin et al. [46] by copyright permission of the American Society of Clinical Investigation.)

cholinergic modulation declines, and the influence of the adrenergic component in determining the level of cardiac function increases [48]. A given overall level of cardiovascular performance—for example, high cardiac output during exercise—can be achieved by different means, depending on the level and efficiency of adrenergic stimulation.

A most striking finding of the hemodynamic response to stress in highly motivated, volunteer, community-dwelling, normotensive subjects of a broad range who previously has been rigorously screened during exercise for signs of clinical and occult coronary artery disease [24] was that with advancing age, the hemodynamic profile during exercise took on the appearance of that seen with beta-adrenergic blockade. Specifically, as age increased, a high cardiac output during exercise was maintained by a slower heart rate, a greater stroke volume, and increased end-diastolic and end-systolic volumes. This finding and those of other studies that demonstrate a diminution of cardiovascular reflexes mediated by the adrenergic system [49] with

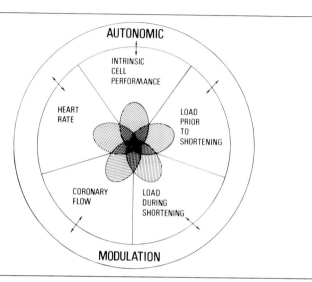

Figure 3-16. Factors that determine cardiovascular performance. The overlapping ovals denote the interaction among these variables. The bidirectional arrows indicate that each variable is modulated by, and in turn modulates, autonomic tone. (From Lakatta [47]. Reprinted with permission from Pergamon Press plc.)

aging suggest that a deficit in the effectiveness of adrenergic cardiovascular modulation occurs with advancing adult age.

The precise impact of beta-adrenergic modulation of heart rate and cardiac volumes during exercise can be determined when the exercise is performed in the presence of beta-adrenergic blockade. During exercise in the presence of beta-adrenergic blockade, the heart rate increase is blunted, and cardiac dilatation occurs at both end-diastole and end-systole compared to the unblocked state (when the beta-adrenergic system is intact). In fact, the hemodynamic profile of the exercising young subject during beta-adrenergic blockade closely resembles that of the older unblocked individual, adding credence to the concept of a "functional" beta-adrenergic blockade in the elderly. Thus, many of the age-associated findings noted in rigorously screened healthy older subjects during upright cycle ergometry, blunted heart rate with larger end-diastolic and end-systolic volumes, are similar to those caused by beta-blockade of younger people (table 3-2).

This altered hemodynamic profile seen with advancing age during exercise could be secondary to a decrease in the elaboration of catecholamines or a reduced end-organ responsiveness to their effects. Regarding the first possibility, plasma catecholamine levels measured during maximal treadmill exercise actually increased with age (figure 3-17A and B) [50]. In another study, catecholamine levels after five minutes of sustained handgrip behaved similarly [48]. Thus, the beta-blocked profile in elderly people occurs in

Table 3-2. Similarities between normal aging
and beta-adrenergic blockade during aerobic exercise

Variable	Aging	Beta-blockade
Maximal aerobic capacity	↓	↓
Maximal heart rate	↓	↓
Maximal end-diastolic volume	↑	↑
Maximal ejection fraction	↓	↓
Maximal cardiac output	↓ ↔	↓ ↔
Maximum plasma catecholamines	↑	↑

Note: ↓ = decrease; ↑ = increase; ↔ = no change.

the presence of higher rather than lower plasma levels of catecholamines. Although clearance of plasma catecholamines appears to be modestly reduced with age [51,52], spillover into the plasma increases with age, and this, rather than a diminished clearance rate, correlates with the increased plasma levels [52]. A diminution in beta-adrenergic modulation of cardiovascular function during stress in the presence of enhanced circulating catecholamines suggests a defect in the post-synaptic adrenergic response.

In humans, one approach to quantifying post-synaptic beta-adrenergic responsiveness has involved measuring the effects of infused adrenergic agonists. Bolus injection of isoproterenol caused a smaller increase in heart rate in elderly men than in the young (figure 3-18) [53]; a similar blunted response was found when cardiac index was monitored. However, no age difference in cardiac index was elicited by ergometer exercise at heart rates comparable to those evoked by isoproterenol, suggesting that some compensatory mechanism occurs during exercise to partially offset this age-related reduction in responsiveness to catecholamines. This compensation is likely due to the previously noted greater utilization of the Frank–Starling mechanism, i.e., ventricular dilatation. In older people, beta-adrenergic agonists also elicit a smaller decrease in the tonus of arteries and veins than they do in younger people [54–57].

The direct effect of beta-adrenergic stimuli to increase the strength of the myocardial contraction decreases with age [35,58]. In the senescent rat heart, force development and rate of force development measured over a wide range of resting muscle lengths are not age related. When Ca^{2+} in the muscle bath is increased, performance is augmented to a similar extent in adult and senescent cardiac muscle, secondary to enhanced Ca^{2+} activation of the contractile proteins [58]. Thus, maximal muscle performance is not limited by aging in this model. However, norepinephrine elicits a smaller increase in the rate of developed tension in senescent rat muscle than in young rat muscle at all doses prior to the onset of arrhythmias [35,38]. The diminution in the response of the senescent heart muscle to catecholamines therefore

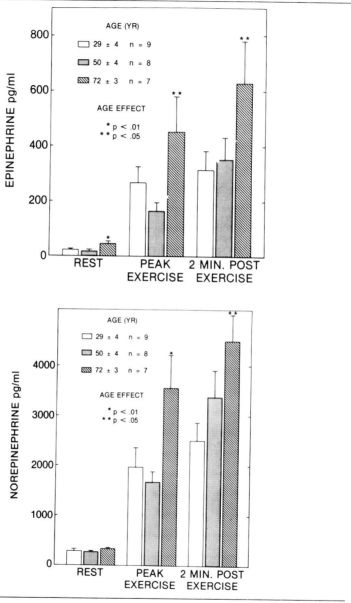

Figure 3-17. Plasma catecholamines at rest and during and after maximal treadmill exercise in 24 healthy men.
A. Plasma epinephrine is slightly increased in older men at rest. This increase is exaggerated both at peak exercise and two minutes after exercise.
B. Although resting plasma norepinephrine was not age related in this sample, the pattern during and after exercise was similar to that for epinephrine. (Redrawn from Fleg et al. [50].)

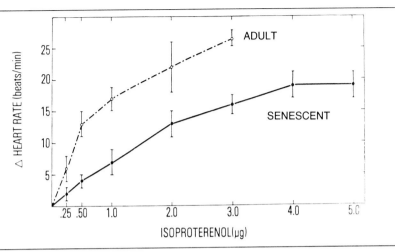

Figure 3-18. The increase in heart rate induced by incremental intravenous boluses of isoproterenol in healthy adult (18–24 years) and senescent men (62–80 years). A significantly greater increment in heart rate is observed in the younger men at all isoproterenol dosages greater than 0.25 µg. (From Lakatta [53].)

seems to be related to mechanisms mediating the catecholamine-induced augmentation of Ca^{2+} transport.

CONCLUSION

In the preceding discussion, we have attempted to summarize the effects of aging per se on cardiovascular structure and function. Although we have given priority to data obtained from healthy subjects who were carefully screened for the absence of latent coronary artery disease, it must be recognized that many of the important studies on cardiovascular aging were carried out before sophisticated noninvasive methods were available to screen for latent coronary disease. Similarly, the effects of physical deconditioning may have influenced the cardiovascular performance at rest and especially the performance during maximal exercise. Studies employing institutionalized populations are particularly suspect in this regard. Furthermore, the presence of disease in other organ systems may have affected the results in some investigations. Finally, the reader should realize that most of the available studies have been cross-sectional rather than longitudinal, thereby introducing the confounding effects of natural selection on their interpretation. For the optimal advancement of research in cardiovascular gerontology, it is important that future studies vigorously attempt to separate the effects of "pure" aging from those of such associated factors.

Practitioners in the real world, however, need not to be so concerned about the separation of aging from its confounding factors. Perhaps their most important realization is that *because* of these factors—i.e., deconditioning, latent coronary artery disease, and multiple organ system pathology acting on a substrate that has already been altered by time per se—the presentation of disease may be modified. Indeed, it is this multifaceted characteristic of human illness that requires the physician to treat the whole patient—not just the disease or the aging process.

REFERENCES

1. Elveback L and Lie JT. 1984. Continued high prevalence of coronary artery disease at autopsy in Olmstead County, Minnesota, 1950 to 1970. Circulation 70:345–349.
2. White NK, Edwards JE, and Dry TJ. 1950. The relationship of the degree of coronary atherosclerosis with age. Circulation 1:645–654.
3. Ackerman RF, Dry TJ, and Edwards JE. 1950. Relationship of various factors to the degree of coronary atherosclerosis in women. Circulation 1:1345–1354.
4. Kennedy RD, Andrevor GR, and Caird FI. 1977. Ischemic heart disease in the elderly. Br Heart J 39:1121–1127.
5. Fleg JL, Gerstenblith G, Zonderman AB, et al. 1990. Prevalence and prognostic significance of exercise-induced silent myocardial ischemia detected by thallium scintigraphy and electrocardiography in asymptomatic volunteers. Circulation 81:428–436.
6. Linzbach AJ and Kuamoa-Boateng E. 1973. Die Alternsveranderungen des menschlichen Herzens I. Das Herzgewicht im Alter. Klinische Wochenschrift 51:156–163.
7. Kitzman DW, Scholz DG, Hagen PT, et al. 1988. Age-related changes in normal human hearts during the first ten decades. Part II (Maturity). A quantitative anatomic study of 765 specimens from subjects 20 to 99 years old. Mayo Clinic Proc 63:137–146.
8. Sjogren AI. 1972. Left ventricular wall thickness in patients with circulatory overload of the left ventricle. Ann Clin Res 4:310–318.
9. Gerstenblith G, Frederiksen J, Yin FCP, et al. 1977. Echocardiographic assessment of a normal adult aging population. Circulation 56:273–278.
10. Gardin JM, Henry WL, Savage DD, et al. 1979. Echocardiographic measurements in normal subjects: Evaluation of an adult population without clinically apparent heart disease. J Clin Ultrasound 7:349–447.
11. Simonson E. 1972. The effect of age on the electrocardiogram. Am J Cardiol 29:64–73.
12. Fleg JL, Das DN, Wright J, and Lakatta EG. 1990. Age-associated changes in the components of atrioventricular conduction in apparently healthy volunteers. J Gerontol Med Sci 45:M95–100.
13. Fleg JL and Kennedy HL. 1982. Cardiac arrhythmias in a healthy elderly population. Detection by 24-hour ambulatory electrocardiography. Chest 81:302–307.
14. Kantelip JP, Sage E, and Duchene-Marullaz P. 1986. Findings on ambulatory electrocardiographic monitoring in subjects older than 80 years. Am J Cardiol 57:398–401.
15. Fleg JL and Lakatta EG. 1984. Prevalence and prognosis of exercise-induced nonsustained ventricular tachycardia in apparently healthy volunteers. Am J Cardiol 54:762–764.
16. Busby MJ, Shefrin EA, and Fleg JL. 1989. Prevalence and long-term significance of exercise-induced frequent or repetitive ventricular ectopic beats in apparently healthy volunteers. J Am Coll Cardiol 14:1659–1665.
17. Ensor RE, Fleg JL, Kim YC, et al. 1983. Longitudinal chest x-ray changes in normal men. J Gerontol 38:307–314.
18. Witteman JCM, Kannel WB, Wolf PA, et al. 1990. Aortic calcified plaques and cardiovascular disease (The Framingham Study). Am J Cardiol 66:1060–1064.
19. Gerstenblith G, Lakatta EG, and Weisfeldt ML. 1976. Age changes in myocardial function and exercise response. Prog Cardiovasc Dis 19:1–21.
20. Lakatta EG. 1986. Hemodynamic adaptation to stress with advancing age. Acta Med Scand 711(Suppl):39–52.
21. Brandfonbrener M, Landowne M, and Shock NW. 1955. Changes in cardiac output with age. Circulation 12:557–566.
22. Lakatta EG. 1988. Cardiovascular system. In B Kent and R Butler (eds), Aging, Vol. 34. Human Aging Research: Concepts and Techniques. New York: Raven Press, pp 199–219.

23. Avolio AP, Fa-Quan D, Wei-Qiang L, et al. 1985. Effects of aging on arterial distensibility in populations with high and low prevalence of hypertension, comparison between urban and rural communities. Circulation 71:202–210.
24. Rodeheffer RJ, Gerstenblith G, Becker LC, et al. 1984. Exercise cardiac output is maintained with advancing age in healthy human subjects: Cardiac dilatation and increased stroke volume compensate for a diminished heart rate. Circulation 69:203–213.
25. Van Tosh A, Lakatta EG, Fleg JL, et al. 1980. Ventricular dimension changes during submaximal exercise: Effect of aging on normal man (abstract). Circulation 62 (Suppl III): III-129.
26. Miyatake K, Okamoto J, Kimoshita N, et al. 1984. Augmentation of atrial contribution to left ventricular flow with aging as assessed by intracardiac Doppler flowmetry. Am J Cardiol 53:587–589.
27. Bryg RJ, Williams GA, and Labovitz AJ. 1987. Effect of aging on left ventricular diastolic filling in normal subjects. Am J Cardiol 59:971–974.
28. Swinne CJ, Shapiro EP, Lima SD, and Fleg JL. 1992. Age-related changes in left ventricular diastolic filling in normal subjects. Am J Cardiol 69:971–974.
29. Miller TR, Grossman SJ, Schechtman KB, et al. 1986. Left ventricular diastolic filling in the healthy elderly. Am J Cardiol 58:531–535.
30. Arora AA, Machac J, Goldman ME, et al. 1987. Atrial kinetics and left ventricular diastolic filling in the healthy elderly. J Am Coll Cardiol 9:1255–1260.
31. Froehlich JP, Lakatta EG, Beard E, et al. 1978. Studies of sarcoplasmic reticulum function and contraction duration in young and aged rat myocardium. J Mol Cell Cardiol 10: 427–438.
32. Orchard CH and Lakatta EG. 1985. Intracellular calcium transients and developed tensions in rat heart muscle. A mechanism for the negative interval-strength relationship. J Gen Physiol 86:637–651.
33. Wei JY, Spurgeon HA, and Lakatta EG. 1984. Excitation-contraction in rat myocardium: Alterations with adult aging. Am J Physiol 246 (Heart Circ Physiol 15):H784–H791.
34. Effron MB, Bhatnager GM, Spurgeon HA, et al. 1987. Changes in myosin isoenzymes, ATPase activity and contraction duration in rat cardiac muscle with aging can be modulated by thyroxine. Circ Res 60:238–245.
35. Guarnieri T, Filburn CR, Zitnik G, et al. 1980. Contractile and biochemical correlates of β-adrenergic stimulation of the aged heart. Am J Physiol 239 (Heart Circ Physiol 8): H501–H508.
36. Dehn MM and Bruce A. 1972. Longitudinal variations in maximal oxygen uptake with age and activity. J Appl Physiol 33:805–807.
37. Fleg JL and Lakatta EG. 1988. Role of muscle loss in the age-associated reduction in VO_{2max}. J Appl Physiol 65:1147–1151.
38. Robinson S, Dill DB, Ross JC, et al. 1973. Training and physiological aging in man. Fed Proc 32:1628–1634.
39. Heath GW, Hagberg JM, Ehsani AA, and Holloszy JO. 1981. A physiological comparison of young and older endurance athletes. J Appl Physiol 51:634–640.
40. Granath A, Jonsson B, and Strandell T. 1964., Circulation in healthy old men studied by right heart catheterization at rest and during exercise in supine and sitting position. Acta Med Scand 176:425–446.
41. Julius S, Amery A, Whitlock LS, and Conway J. 1967. Influence of age on the hemodynamic response to exercise. Circulation 36:222–230.
42. Conway J, Wheeler R, and Hammerstedt R. 1977. Sympathetic nervous activity during exercise in relation to age. Cardiovasc Res 5:577–581.
43. Port S, Cobb FR, Coleman RE, and Jones RH. 1980. Effect of age on the response of the left ventricular ejection fraction to exercise. N Engl J Med 303:1133–1137.
44. Fleg JL, Gerstenblith G, Becker LC, et al. 1990. Independent effects of age and gender on specificity of ejection fraction response to upright cycle exercise (abstract). Circulation 82 (Suppl III):III-137.
45. Nichols WW, O'Rourke MF, Avolio AP, et al. 1985. Effects of age on ventricular coupling. Am J Cardiol 55:1179–1184.
46. Yin FCP, Weisfeldt ML, and Milnor WR. 1981. Role of aortic input impedance in the decreased cardiovascular response to exercise with aging in dogs. J Clin Invest 68:28–38.

47. Lakatta EG. 1983. Determinants of cardiovascular performance: modification due to aging. J Chronic Dis 36:15–30.
48. Palmer GP, Ziegler MG, and Lake CR. 1978. Response of norepinephrine and blood pressure to stress increases with age. J Gerontol 33:482–487.
49. Lakatta EG. 1980. Age-related alterations in the cardiovascular response to adrenergic mediated stress. Fed Proc 39:3173–3177.
50. Fleg JL, Tzankoff SP, and Lakatta EG. 1985. Age-related augmentation of plasma catecholamines during dynamic exercise in healthy men. J Appl Physiol 59:1033–1039.
51. Esler M, Skews H, Leonard P, et al. 1986. Age-dependence of noradrenaline kinetics in normal subjects. Clin Sci 60:217–219.
52. Featherstone JA, Veith RC, and Halter JB. 1984. Effect of age and alpha 2 adrenergic stimulation on plasma norepinephrine kinetics in man (abstract). Clin Res 32:69A.
53. Lakatta EG. 1979. Alterations in the cardiovascular system that occur in advanced age. Fed Proc 38:163–167.
54. Godfraind T. 1979. Alternative mechanisms for the potentiation of the relaxation evoked by isoprenaline in aortae from young and aged rats. Eur J Pharmacol 53:273–279.
55. Fleisch JH. 1981. Age related decrease in beta adrenoceptor activity of the cardiovascular system. Trends Pharmacol Sci 2:337–339.
56. van Brummelin P, Buhler FR, Kiowski W, and Amann FW. 1981. Age-related decrease in cardiac and peripheral vascular responsiveness to isoprenaline: studies in normal subjects. Clin Sci 60:571–577.
57. Pan HY-M, Hoffman BB, Pershi RA, et al. 1986. Decline in beta adrenergic receptor-mediated vascular relaxation with aging in man. J Pharmacol Exp Ther 228:802–807.
58. Lakatta EG, Gerstenblith G, Angell CS, et al. 1975. Diminished inotropic response of aged myocardium to catecholamines. Circ Res 36:262–269.

SUGGESTED READING

Kitzman DW and Edwards WD. 1990. Age-related changes in the anatomy of the normal human heart. J Gerontol Med Sciences 45:M33–M39.
Lakatta EG. 1990. Changes in cardiovascular function with aging. Eur Heart J 11 (Suppl C) 22–29.
Weisfeldt ML, Lakatta EG, and Gerstenblith G. 1988. Aging and cardiac disease. In E Braunwald (ed), Heart Disease. A Textbook of Cardiovascular Medicine, 3rd ed. Philadelphia: W.B. Saunders, pp 1650–1662.

4. CLINICAL FINDINGS IN THE ELDERLY HEART PATIENT

JULES CONSTANT

The availability of the latest diagnostic technology, such as echocardiography, cardiac catheterization, and angiography, does not eliminate clinical skills, which are essential in planning the type and scope of investigations needed to establish the diagnosis. A thorough clinical evaluation is even more important in the elderly, in whom invasive diagnostic procedures are associated with significant morbidity and mortality.

CLINICAL CLUES FROM PHYSICAL APPEARANCE IN THE ELDERLY

Eyes

A corneal arcus, also known as gerontoxon in the ophthalmology literature, increases in incidence with age so that it is present in almost all people over age 80. The limbal vessels become increasingly permeable with age and allow high-density lipoproteins to pass into the cornea [1]. If the arcus reaches to the limbus, it has no known significance. However, if a patient is under age 60 and has an arcus that leaves iris pigment between the arcus and the limbus, it probably means that there is either significant coronary disease [2] or a high risk of lipid abnormality [3]. A thick arcus that begins inferiorly and has pigment peripheral to it is a sign of familial hypercholesterolemia; it is unlikely to be present after age 60 because most such patients have probably succumbed to an inevitable coronary event.

Franz H. Messerli (ed.), CARDIOVASCULAR DISEASE IN THE ELDERLY (Third Edition). Copyright © 1993 Kluwer Academic Publishers. ISBN 0-7923-1859-5. All rights reserved.

The term *arcus senilis* should be avoided, not only because an arcus may be seen in people younger than age 50—especially in blacks [4,5], in subjects with high alcohol intake [6], and in those with familial hypercholesterolemia— but also because the term may be read or overheard by the patient and be misunderstood to mean that it is a sign of senility.

The fundus or eye grounds can show both sclerotic and hypertensive changes. Some classifications mix the two, but they should be separated. The four degrees of fundal atherosclerosis are as follows:

Grade 1   Increased light reflex
Grade 2   Atrioventricular (A–V) nicking and right-angled crossings
Grade 3   Copper-wire arteries, because the light streak has widened to occupy the entire surface
Grade 4   Silver-wire arteries, i.e. no red color (Hollenhorst plaques are flakes of cholesterol emboli from carotid atheromas seen as sparkling spots at arteriolar bifurcations and often seeming larger than the vessels in which they reside)

Xanthelasma or xanthomas around the eyelids are often but not invariably associated with hypercholesterolemia.

Skin

One should look for xanthomas or cholesterol-filled nodules by palpating the Achilles tendon, the extensor tendons of the hands, and the patellar tendons. These usually indicate high cholesterol levels and premature coronary disease. In the palmar creases, they signify type III hyperlipidemia.

Skin temperature and color

If the hands and feet are warmer than expected and there is no fever, we may be dealing with hyperthyroidism, which may explain the patient's palpitations and atrial fibrillation. Recent findings of cold hands and feet suggest a low cardiac output. If only the feet are cold and this is also recent, suspect peripheral arterial obstruction.

If the patient is febrile, look for signs of infective endocarditis, such as clubbing and embolic splinter hemorrhages. Most splinter hemorrhages are not embolic and are in the nail substance. Therefore, they move with the nails as they grow and usually extend to the distal edge.

If the patient has a witnessed syncopal attack and the face is flushed on recovering consciousness, a cardiac arrest is suggested. The high CO_2 levels and reactive hyperemia cause marked postictal vasodilatation.

Look for livido reticularis. This is the marbling reticulation or "fishnet" type of mottling of the lower trunk, buttocks, and extremities, exaggerated by or only seen during cold temperatures or emotional upsets. In a patient over age 50, livido reticularis may suggest cholesterol embolization from an abdominal aneurysm.

Edema

Test for "fast" versus "slow" edema. Press edematous areas for 10 seconds. If the pitting disappears in less than 40 seconds, the cause is more likely low albumin than poor venous or lymphatic return due to congestive heart failure. If, however, ascites is marked, as in severe nephrotic syndromes, there may be enough obstruction to venous and lymphatic return from the legs to prolong the pitting beyond 40 seconds [7]. A normal jugular pressure is incompatible with a cardiac cause for the edema unless a diuretic has lowered venous pressure before getting rid of the edema. Face and hand edema helps to rule out a cardiac cause.

The extremities

If the patients has rheumatoid arthritis, remember that pericarditis and even occasionally pericardial constriction must be suspected if the patient has cardiac or chest symptoms or signs.

Head and neck

If the patient has cold intolerance and constipation, myxedema in the elderly should be suspected, and puffy eyelids, loss of the outer third of the eyebrows, scanty dry hair, coarse dry skin, expressionless face, and enlarged tongue should be looked for. These patients may have a cardiomyopathy due to interstitial fluid accumulation and infiltration. They may also have pericardial effusion.

Look for a diagonal ear crease that runs from the lower pole of the external meatus, diagonally backwards to the edge of the lobe at approximately 45°. The prevalence increases with age and the presence of diabetes. In one coroner's necropsy study, about 70% of those with and only 45% of those without diagonal creases had cardiovascular causes of death [8]. Ninety percent of patients over age 50 with significant triple-vessel disease have a deep crease. If unilateral, it suggests an intermediate degree of coronary obstruction. There is no strong correlation with blood lipids, blood pressure, or smoking. It should be considered an independent risk factor.

Chest and respiration

Cheyne–Stokes respiration in a patient with congestive heart failure is one of the common signs of severe low cardiac output.

ARTERIAL PULSES AND PRESSURE IN THE ELDERLY

Brachial pulses

The brachial artery in the elderly is medial to the biceps; in the young it is deep to the biceps. The brachials in the elderly will often undergo a snakelike motion known as locomotor brachialis, caused by tortuosity, lengthening, and hardening of the brachials due to medial sclerosis. These patients tend to have pure systolic hypertension, because they are pumping blood into a stiff system with poor elastic aortic recoil and no peripheral vasospasm or good aortic elastic recoil to raise the diastolic pressure.

Carotid pulses

Feel the carotids for evidence of aortic outflow tract obstruction or regurgitation. If the rate of rise is slow (i.e., a push rather than a tap), then aortic valve stenosis is likely. In the elderly, however, the patient with an aorta hardened by atherosclerosis may have a normal rate of rise in the peripheral pulses, despite significant valvular aortic stenosis. A rigid aorta apparently cannot expand slowly.

If the rate of rise of the carotid pulse is rapid or brisk, then there are three possibilities of mechanical problems:

1. The patient may have hypertrophic subaortic stenosis, which produces the fastest rate of rise. Hypertrophic subaortic stenosis, or hypertrophic obstructive cardiomyopathy, is not an uncommon finding in the elderly. (Its clinical recognition is elaborated later in the chapter.)
2. Another mechanical cause of a brisk rate of rise of a carotid pulse and a normal volume is mitral regurgitation.
3. If, however, the volume is larger than normal with a rapid rise, then aortic regurgitation is to be expected.

BLOOD PRESSURE AND THE HEART IN THE ELDERLY

Pseudohypertension refers to a misleadingly high systolic, diastolic, or mean blood pressure using a cuff and sphygmomanometer when compared to the pressure taken directly by intra-arterial needle. It is caused by medial sclerosis of the brachial arteries (Monckeberg's sclerosis), which may be severe enough to strongly resist compression by a blood pressure cuff (pipestem brachial arteries). This can give a falsely high systolic pressure of over 300 mmHg despite an intra-arterial-needle blood pressure of only about 160 mmHg. In a comparison of intra-arterial blood pressure with indirect cuff pressures in the elderly, the surprising finding in one study was that even the diastolic pressure was often higher with the cuff than with the intra-arterial needle, by as much as 30 mmHg [8]. In one study of blood pressure with simulated arteries, one investigator predicted that doubling of the thickness of the arterial wall would produce an auscultatory error of 30 mmHg [9]. Occasionally, only the diastolic pressure is falsely high, while the systolic pressure may be even lower than by the direct method. Therefore, mean blood pressure calculated from cuff measurements correlates better with mean direct pressures. Since about 85% of patients diagnosed as pseudohypertensive are actually hypertensive with their readings exaggerated by the stiff arteries

[10], the condition would be more accurately called *pseudo and exaggerated hypertension.*

A simple test for pseudohypertension due to excessive stiffness of the upper limb arteries consists of inflating a blood pressure cuff above systolic pressure and feeling for a palpable radial. This has been called Osler's maneuver because it is an improved variation of his method of occluding the radial with a proximal finger and feeling for a palpable radial with a distal finger. In one study it was found that if the radial remained clearly palpable despite being pulseless (Osler-positive), there was a likelihood that the cuff pressure could be from 10 to 55 mm higher than intra-arterial pressure [11].

The suspicion of pseudohypertension due to stiff or thick arteries is based on finding a diastolic pressure elevated disproportionately to the clinical findings, i.e. no left ventricular hypertrophy in the electrocardiogram, and no cardiomegaly, renal failure, or hypertensive retinopathy.

Elderly patients commonly have high systolic and normal diastolic pressures. It is not commonly understood that diastolic pressure depends not only on peripheral resistance but also on the elasticity or recoil energy imparted to the aortic wall by ventricular systole. Good elastic recoil is required to produce a high diastolic pressure. Therefore, an elderly patient may have a normal diastolic pressure despite a high peripheral resistance if the aortic wall is very stiff due to arteriosclerosis.

Thus it is possible for the elderly patient with *isolated systolic hypertension* to have a high peripheral resistance and to benefit from antihypertensive medications that lower peripheral resistance.

CARDIAC FUNCTION EVALUATION BY SPHYGMOMANOMETRY

In the elderly smoker who has dyspnea on exertion due to chronic obstructive pulmonary disease, it is often impossible to assess whether cardiac pump function is reduced enough to contribute to the dyspnea. The four readily available noninvasive methods of assessing cardiac pump function are (in order of decreasing cost) the radionuclide scan, the two-dimensimal echocardiogram, systolic time intervals, and the post-Valsalva blood pressure overshoot [12]. Since the latter is a cost-free office procedure, it should be the first method used [13]. With the patient supine, inflate a cuff to 25 mm above systolic pressure and hold it there during a 10-second Valsalva. Immediately on straining you will note the reappearance of Korotkoff sounds, which will disappear after a few beats due to a decrease in end-diastolic and stroke volume. If some Korotkoff sounds are heard within a few seconds after the Valsalva release, the ejection fraction is probably $70 \pm 10\%$. If there is no post-Valsalva overshoot of blood pressure, the ejection fraction is about $50 \pm 10\%$. If Korotkoff sounds are heard during the entire 10 seconds of Valsalva (square wave response), the ejection fraction is about $30 \pm 10\%$. This latter response is the result of a constant end-diastolic and stroke volume during straining [14]. (An atrial septal defect can cause a square wave response.)

The absence of such an overshoot, however, requires that no artifactual factors be present, such as the inability to perform a good Valsalva or the presence of drugs or abnormalities that affect the autonomic nervous system (e.g., beta-blockers or anxiety imparting a high catecholamine drive to the myocardium).

Soft Korotkoff sounds can usually be overcome by having the patient clench his fist 10 times in rapid succession before or during rapid inflation of the cuff. To help perform a Valsalva properly, have the patient push his abdomen against someone's compressing hand or attach a rubber tube to an aneroid manometer and have the patient blow it up to 40 mmHg.

JUGULAR PRESSURE AND PULSATIONS IN THE ELDERLY

To evaluate jugular venous pressure, note the top level of internal jugular pulsations. The upper normal level of internal jugular pulsations above the sternal angle is 4.5 cm with the chest raised to a 45° angle. A standard chest angle is necessary because the sternal angle is about 5 cm above the midright atrium supine, and about 10 cm above it with the chest elevated [15]. In the elderly, it is especially important not to use external jugulars to measure venous pressure, because the venous walls can be so sclerotic that they seem to be distended to higher levels than true venous pressure. The externals can also give a falsely low pressure reading because of the sharp angles through which the pressure waves must pass to be seen. Also, external jugulars may be absent because of congenitally small or aberrant veins, or because the high venous tone caused by heart failure may constrict small veins down to an invisible thread.

The carotids in the elderly may be pushed forward and laterally by a tortuous aorta so that the right internal jugular is compressed during each systole. This condition will suggest elevated internal jugular pressure falsely and produce a contour suggesting a dominant V-wave and Y-descent. Abdominal compression, however, will not raise the jugular top level of these pulsations as it would if the venous pressure were truly high. In some elderly patients with tortuous aortas, the left jugular, which is normally slightly lower in pressure than the right, may be higher than the right owing to compression of the left innominate vein between the sternum anteriorly and the large tortuous arteries arising from the high unfolded aortic arch posteriorly. Having the patient take a deep breath will decrease the manubrial compression against the innominate vein and help to exclude this left jugular artifact.

INSPECTION AND PALPATION OF THE CHEST IN THE ELDERLY

An apex beat is felt in the sitting position in about 1 of 5 patients over age 40, but in the elderly it is unusual to feel any apex beat at all in the sitting position. This is presumably due to the increased P-A diameter that occurs with increasing age, secondary to kyphosis. A palpable apical impulse in the sitting or supine position in the presence of an increased P-A diameter in the elderly is by itself suggestive of cardiomegaly.

AUSCULTATION OF THE HEART IN THE ELDERLY

The first heart sound (S_1)

A split S_1 is often more easily detected in the elderly than in the young because the second component of a widely split S_1 is usually due to aortic valve opening, i.e. an ejection sound. The aortic ejection sound is made louder by anything that stiffens the aortic root, such as atherosclerosis or hypertension. It will also be heard with slightly stiffened aortic valves due to fibrosis found in the elderly. The ejection sound will not be loud if the valve is stiff, because the loudness of the ejection click correlates with leaflet mobility and the distance of excursion. This split S_1 is best heard wherever aortic events are best heard, i.e. in a "sash area" from the second right interspace to the apex. If the ejection sound is loud, i.e. louder than the mitral closure sound or first component of the split, then we are probably listening to a bicuspid aortic valve (about 1% of the male population), and then we must search for trivial aortic regurgitation as well as a louder A_2 or aortic closure sound than normal.

A soft mitral component of the first heart sound is commonly found in the elderly [16]. Do not blame this on chest shape unless the increased PA diameter is obvious. The mitral closure loudness is controlled not only by contractility, which is reduced with aging, but also by the P-R interval, which tends to either prolong or at least be at upper limits of normal in the elderly. The longer the P-R interval, the softer is the mitral closure sound, because left ventricular events are delayed relative to left atrial events. A similar situation exists with left bundle branch block when left ventricular events are delayed relative to left atrial events due to a conduction defect in the bundle branch system.

The S_1 is especially important to note in complete A-V block, which is more common in the elderly than in the young for many reasons, one of which is the frequency of mitral annular calcification in the elderly. Autopsies performed in patients over age 60 show a prevalence of annular calcification as high as 13%; the prevalence increases linearly with age, so that by age 90 it is about 45%. Annular calcification is probably caused by the same degenerative process that causes fibrosis or calcification of the aortic valve, both of which are accelerated by hypertension. The close proximity of the calcification to the A-V node and bundle of His probably leads to the high incidence of complete A-V block. In one study, almost 90% of elderly patients with complete A-V block had mitral annular calcification [17]. The clinical diagnosis of complete A-V block is made mainly by finding a slow heart rate and a changing loudness of S_1 due to the changing P-R intervals. In the presence of atrial fibrillation or flutter, of course, only the slow heart rate will be the clue to complete A-V block, because the S_1 will not vary in loudness without P-waves.

The second heart sound (S_2)

The aortic component of the S_2 (A_2) usually is of normal loudness in the elderly with normal cardiac function. Although the systolic hypertension common in the elderly will tend to make the S_2 louder, any sclerosis of the aortic valves and any decrease in cardiac contractility will tend to decrease the loudness of the A_2. At the left sternal border the S_2 should be the same loudness as the S_1. Therefore, if it is softer than the S_1, and if there is no mitral stenosis or short P-R interval to make the first sound extra loud, we should consider that either the aortic valve is sclerotic or that contractility is reduced. The presence or absence of an aortic ejection murmur of aortic sclerosis should help solve the problem.

Splitting of the S_2 in the elderly is usually narrow or absent with respiration. This is thought to be because aging not only prolongs isovolumic contraction and the ejection time, thus delaying the A_2, but also causes a shortening of the Q-P_2 interval, thus bringing the P_2 earlier in the cycle. The earlier P_2 in the elderly is probably due to the increase in impedance in the pulmonary circuit with aging. Therefore, a normal split to the S_2 in the elderly should make us suspect a right bundle branch block.

A reversed split (widening with expiration) almost always means a left bundle branch block. However, reversed splits may occur without left bundle branch block if the patient is hypertensive and has had some myocardial damage such as that due to an old infarction. A reversed split can also cause a wide splitting of the second heart sound. Therefore, any widely split second sound in the elderly may be due to either a left or right bundle branch block.

In the elderly, the recognition of reversed splits may be difficult because of the increased distance between the heart and the stethoscope often found in these patients. This makes it difficult to hear the S_2 altogether at the left sternal border on inspiration. However, you can still tell if a split is reversed even without noting the effect of respiration by moving your stethoscope gradually to areas where the P_2 should disappear or become softer than the A_2, i.e. to the apex or second right interspace. If, as you move toward these areas, the first component of the split diminishes or disappears, then the order is P_2 A_2.

Another helpful way to determine the cause of a wide split in the elderly is to have the patient do a Valsalva strain. Immediately on release, more blood returns to the right side, and the P_2 occurs later. Therefore, if the split widens immediately on release, the patient has a right bundle branch block. If it narrows, the patient has a left bundle branch block.

The S_3 in the elderly

Since the physiologic S_3 disappears by about the fourth decade, any S_3 in the elderly is most likely pathological. The only situation for an S_3 in the elderly that is not necessarily pathological is the presence of a summation gallop. This implies that a long P-R interval in a patient with a tachycardia may cause the atrial contraction to coincide with the timing of a physiologic S_3 and produce a loud S_3-like sound. This is the physiologic summation gallop, which can be diagnosed by noting that the patient has a long P-R interval and a tachycardia that, when slowed by carotid sinus pressure, causes the disappearance of the summation sound because the P wave moves away from the previous QRS.

An S_3 in the elderly with heart failure simply tells us that the degree of failure is severe. In the presence of moderate to severe mitral regurgitation, the S_3 in the elderly correlates with the degree of mitral regurgitation. In the absence of failure, or moderate to severe mitral regurgitation, the S_3 implies the presence of a ventricular aneurysm, i.e. a past history of infarction. This assumes that the S_3 is not mistaken for the pericardial knock of constrictive pericarditis.

Ejection murmurs in the elderly

Aortic ejection murmurs without aortic stenosis occur in 50% of patients over age 50 and in even a higher percentage if the patients are hypertensive. These murmurs are caused by aortic sclerosis. Since they occur in 50% of patients over age 50, they have been called the 50/50 murmur. They have the characteristics of an ejection murmur in that they begin with the S_1, are crescendo–decrescendo, end before the S_2, become louder after long diastoles, and retain low and medium frequencies even when soft. The sclerosis murmur is probably due to fibrotic thickening and often some calcification involving the base of the cusps. Although they may not fully open because of stiffness, they do open enough to prevent a pressure gradient across the orifice. The aortic ejection murmur is not only more common in hypertensives but is twice as likely to be found in women as it is in men. It may be up to grade 4/6 in loudness, i.e. it may be associated with a thrill.

The murmur of aortic stenosis must be differentiated from the murmur of aortic sclerosis. A murmur is probably due to aortic sclerosis if palpation of the carotid shows a brisk rise, the S_2 is not soft, the murmur reaches its peak in the first third of systole, and the quality is slightly musical. The musical quality is probably due to a spray effect caused by the stiff cusp bases preventing commissural fusion, and the blood may then be ejected between the cusps rather than as a jet. This may make the murmur not only more musical but also less loud and harsh than the aortic stenosis murmur.

The valvular aortic ejection murmur must be distinguished from carotid murmurs. An aortic valvular murmur is usually amplified by the clavicle and is at least as loud over the clavicle as it is over the carotid. Therefore, any ejection murmur that is louder over the carotid than over the clavicle should be considered a murmur originating in the carotid. An ejection murmur that is disproportionately loud compared to the softness of the S_2 suggests a severe gradient across the valve, because a soft or absent S_2 implies heavy calcification of the aortic valve. The degree of calcification can be confirmed by echocardiography directly. Another reason why it is difficult to diagnose aortic stenosis in the elderly is because the murmur of severe aortic stenosis may be soft due to the common increase of anteroposterior chest diameter, especially at the base of the heart.

In the elderly the carotid pulse may have a normal rate of rise despite severe valvular aortic stenosis. This occurs presumably in those with a stiff arterial system due to atherosclerosis. A stiff arterial wall may not be able to expand slowly. Therefore, although a slow rate of rise of a carotid pulse in the elderly implies aortic stenosis (without telling you the severity), a normal rate of rise tells us little about the meaning of an ejection murmur if the patient has much arteriosclerosis. The appearance of the descending aorta on the lateral film of the chest x-ray will usually demonstrate the degree of aortic atherosclerosis and will warn us not to pay too much attention to the normal rate of rise of the carotids. The normal aorta is almost invisible distal to the arch on an x-ray.

A very brisk rate of rise of the carotids, together with an ejection murmur loudest near the lower left sternal border or apex, should alert us to the possibility of hypertrophic subaortic stenosis (HSS), or hypertrophic obstructive cardiomyopathy (HOCM), which should be suspected if there is a history of hypertension. If HSS is suspected, we must try to execute at least a few diagnostic maneuvers:

1. Increase the volume in the left ventricle, as when supine or squatting. This will make the murmur softer.
2. Decrease chamber volume as when sitting, standing, or during a Valsalva strain. This will make the murmur louder.
3. Increase the pressure against the mitral leaflet by raising systolic pressure. Squatting will cause an increase in both volume and pressure and will cause the murmur of HSS to become softer or disappear.
4. Decrease the pressure against the mitral leaflet by lowering aortic pressure by carotid sinus pressure [17] or amyl nitrite inhalation. This will make the murmur louder.

Mitral regurgitation in the elderly

The two common causes of mitral regurgitation that should be considered in the elderly are papillary muscle dysfunction and mitral annular calcification. The usual cause of papillary muscle dysfunction is myocardial infarction, recent or old, with or without a ventricular aneurysm, and with or without papillary muscle fibrosis. Infarction, or the acute ischemia of the ventricle at the base of the papillary muscle that may occur with angina, may cause marked mitral regurgitation even with a normal papillary muscle. The prevalence of mitral annular calcification increases with age so that it occurs in about 45% at age 90. It is more frequent in patients with aortic stenosis, hypertrophic obstructive cardiomyopathy, hypertension, and chronic renal failure. Clinically it not only may lead to mitral reguritation but also may extend into the conduction tissue, resulting in various degrees of A-V block. In elderly patients with atrial fibrillation, a slow ventricular response is often present due to mitral annular calcification extending into the conduction tissue between atria and ventricles.

The murmur of papillary muscle dysfunction is classically crescendo to the S_2, and like all mitral regurgitation murmurs is of maximal loudness about 1 cm lateral to the apex beat in the left lateral decubitus position. This site of maximal loudness is useful to know, because when a pansystolic murmur is heard loudest 1 to 2 cm medial to the apex beat during an acute myocardial infarction, it is probably not mitral regurgitation but a ventricular septal defect due to a ruptured septum.

The best clue that mitral regurgitation is not due to a primary valvular disorder, such as rheumatic disease or myxomatous transformation of the mitral valve, is to hear an S_4. An S_4 implies that the mitral regurgitation is secondary to a myocardial problem. An S_3, on the other hand, gives us a hint about the degree of mitral regurgitation (after the fourth decade when the physiologic S_3 disappears), and it implies that mitral regurgitation is at least moderate. If the patient is in failure, then the S_3 is only proportional to the degree of failure and not to the degree of mitral regurgitation. If the elderly patient is not in failure and has only slight mitral regurgitation (only a pure high-pitched murmur), then the S_3 implies the presence of a ventricular aneurysm.

In quantitating the degree of mitral regurgitation at the bedside, the same criteria are used for the elderly as for the young. That is, the mitral regurgitation is greater:

1. the larger the left ventricle is by palpation;
2. the greater and later is the left parasternal movement (this may represent the left atrium expanding with the regurgitant volume during systole);
3. the more palpable is the early filling wave at the apex (at the time of the S_3);
4. the louder and longer is the apical systolic murmur (with the exception of the decrescendo murmur caused by a very steep rise in left atrial pressure in acute mitral regurgitation secondary to ruptured chordae);
5. the louder is the S_3, since this is roughly proportional to the torrential early diastolic flow (the S_3 may disappear with the decrease in blood volume secondary to diuretics); and
6. the longer and louder is the diastolic flow murmur after the S_3.

Diastolic murmurs in the elderly
When the elderly patient develops complete A-V block, there will often be a middiastolic flow murmur due to excessive flow through the mitral valve.

This is because a very slow heart rate causes an increase in blood volume, just as in athletes with slow heart rates. The increase in blood volume drawn through the mitral valve in diastole by a healthy myocardium can produce a flow murmur.

Severe hypertension may cause aortic regurgitation in the elderly. The incidence of aortic regurgitation in hypertensives has ranged in different series from 6% to 60% [18]. The aortic regurgitation is usually trivial, and the cause is still to be determined. It may disappear when the diastolic pressure falls below 115 mmHg. A bicuspid valve should be suspected.

One of the inflammatory diseases of the elderly is giant-cell or temporal arteritis, and this is often associated with aortic regurgitation.

Usually when an aortic regurgitation murmur is heard better at the right sternal border than at the left, it is because of some unusual cause of the regurgitation, such as a dissecting aortic aneurysm, prolapsed aortic valve, or rupture of a sinus of Valsalva. But in the elderly with rheumatic aortic regurgitation, there may be such tortuosity of the aorta that the unfolded ascending aorta can go far to the right and displace the aortic regurgitation murmur to the right of the sternum.

A soft aortic regurgitationlike diastolic murmur may be heard at the second or third left intercostal space in some elderly patients with moderate obstruction of the anterior descending coronary artery. This usually means that the vessel is not more than 50% occluded. The murmur is best heard in diastole because maximum coronary flow occurs in diastole. It is most easily audible with the patient sitting and usually disappears after infarction.

Mitral diastolic murmurs in the elderly

Mitral stenosis diastolic rumbles are often missed in the elderly because they are likely to be silent or very soft. This occurs for two reasons. First, the elderly are more likely to be in atrial fibrillation due to the long-standing effect of their mitral stenosis, plus the development of coronary disease or additional cardiomyopathies of diverse etiology. When a mitral stenosis patient develops atrial fibrillation, the flow may decrease enough to eliminate the murmur. Second, the increased posterior–anterior thoracic diameter of the elderly patient separates the stethoscope too far from the apex. Soft mitral stenosis murmurs are very sensitive to auscultatory distance, so that even in the normal chest a soft murmur may disappear a few centimeters away from the apex.

Abdominal murmurs

Although almost one half of normal subjects under age 25 have midline or upper-quadrant systolic abdominal murmurs, they are found only in about 5% of subjects over age 50. Therefore, an abdominal murmur in an older subject should probably be considered abnormal. If the patient is hypertensive, a high-pitched continuous renal vascular murmur should be sought, but this is rare in the elderly because the kind of renal artery lesion that is most likely to have an arterial murmur is fibromuscular dysplasia, a condition usually found in the young (average age 36).

REFERENCES

1. Walton KW. 1974. Studies on the pathogenesis of corneal arcus. J Pathol 114:217.
2. Rifkind EM. 1965. Arcus senilis. Lancet 1:312.
3. Shanoff MH and Little JA. 1964. Studies of male survivors of myocardial infarction due to "essential" atherosclerosis. J Can Med Assoc 91:835.
4. Finley JK, Berkowitz D, and Croll MN. 1961. The physiological significance of gerontoxon. Arch Ophthalmol 66:211–213.
5. Macareag PVJ, Lasagna L, and Snyder D. 1968. Arcus not so senilis. Ann Intern Med 68:345.
6. Henry JA and Altmann P. 1978. Assessment of hypoproteinuric edema. Br Med J 1:890.
7. Kirkham N, Murrells T, Melcher DH, et al. 1989. Diagonal earlobe creases and fatal cardiovascular disease: a necropsy study. Br Heart J 61:361.
8. Spence JD, Sibbald WJ, and Cape RD. 1978. Pseudohypertension in the elderly. Clin Sci Mol Med 55:399.
9. Sacks AH, Raman KR, and Bwinell JA. 1963. A study of auscultatory blood pressure in simulated arteries. Report No. 119, Vidya Corporation, Palo Alto, CA.
10. Messerli FH, Ventura HO, and Amodeo C. 1985. Osler's maneuver and pseudo-hypertension. N Engl J Med 312:1545.
11. Zema MJ and Caccavano M. 1983. Detection of left ventricular dysfunction in ambulatory patients. Am J Med 75:241.
12. Constant J. 1985. Bedside Cardiology, 3rd ed. Boston: Little, Brown, p 73.
13. Little WC, Barr WK, Crawford MH. 1983. Altered effect of Valsalva maneuver on left ventricular volume in patients with cardiomyopathy. Circulation 71:227.
14. Saunders DE, Adcock DF, Head DS, et al. 1988. Relationship of sternal angle to right atrium in clinical measurement of jugular venous pressure. J Am Coll Cardiol 11:89A.
15. Reddy PS, Haidet K, and Meno F. 1985. Relation of intensity of cardiac sounds to age. Am J Cardiol 55:1383.
16. Klein HO, DiSegni E, Dean H, et al. 1988. Increased intensity of the murmur of hypertrophic obstructive cardiomyopathy with carotid sinus pressure. Chest 93:814.
17. Nair CK and Hibbard R. 1984. The association between mitral annular calcification and bradyarrhythmias. Pract Cardiol 10:77.
18. Luisada AA and Argano B. 1970. The phonocardiogram in systemic hypertension. Chest 58:598.

5. DIAGNOSTIC TESTING FOR CARDIOVASCULAR DISEASES

CARL J. LAVIE
FRANZ H. MESSERLI

Despite new statistics indicating declining mortality trends from cardio-vascular diseases in the United States, data from the American Heart Association (AHA) Task Force indicate that with aging of the population, the absolute incidence and prevalence of cardiovascular diseases will actually increase during the next two decades, total deaths will increase by nearly 20%, and total cost to society (adjusted for inflation) will increase by 30% [1,2]. Therefore, the diagnosis of cardiovascular diseases in the elderly will remain a major part of the clinical practice of general internists, family physicians, and cardiologists. Although invasive testing usually is the "gold standard" for identifying cardiovascular diseases, physicians often desire less invasive and less expensive procedures with fewer risks in order to diagnose disease and follow patients with known disease. Technological advances have made available a wider array of clinical studies which, if used appropriately, add to our ability to recognize and treat cardiovascular diseases in the elderly population.

CORONARY HEART DISEASE

Background

Epidemiologic and prognostic data regarding coronary heart disease (CHD) have been reviewed elsewhere in this text. Noninvasive assessment of CHD

Franz H. Messerli (ed.), CARDIOVASCULAR DISEASE IN THE ELDERLY (Third Edition). Copyright © 1993 Kluwer Academic Publishers. ISBN 0-7923-1859-5. All rights reserved.

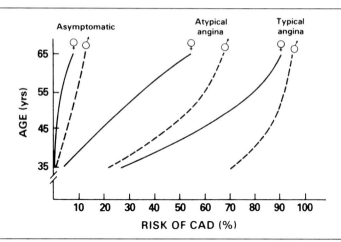

Figure 5-1. Effects of age, sex, and symptoms on the risk of coronary artery disease (CAD). Adapted with permission from Epstein SE: 1980. Implications of probability analysis on the strategy used for noninvasive detection of coronary artery disease: role of single or combined use of exercise electrocardiographic testing, radionuclide cineangiography and myocardial perfusion imaging. Am J Cardiol 46:491–499.

is extremely important to determine the presence and extent of disease. When screening patients with suspected disease, one must consider both the accuracy of a noninvasive test and the patient's pretest likelihood of significant disease [2,3]. A sensitive test has few false-negative results, whereas a specific test has few false-positive results. According to Bayes's theorem, the predictive value of any noninvasive test in estimating the probability of significant disease depends not only on the accuracy of the test but also, and equally importantly, on the prevalence of disease in the patient population or the pretest likelihood of disease. The latter factor depends on a number of variables, three of which are demonstrated in figure 5-1 [3], as well as on other well-known CHD risk factors [4–6]. Figure 5-1 demonstrates that coronary artery disease (CAD) is prevalent in elderly subjects with atypical angina, more so than in young females with typical angina. Any screening test is more useful in a patient population with intermediate pretest likelihood of disease (figure 5-2), and less useful in patients with a very high (e.g., elderly men with typical angina) or very low (e.g., young females with chest pain) pretest likelihood of disease [3].

For these reasons, there are no absolute indications for exercise testing in *asymptomatic* subjects, according to the AHA Task Force, although possible indications include older subjects with other risk factors and those planning to begin a vigorous exercise program (table 5-1) [7]. Other indications and contraindications of exercise assessment for the evaluation of CHD are listed in tables 5-1 and 5-2, respectively [2,7].

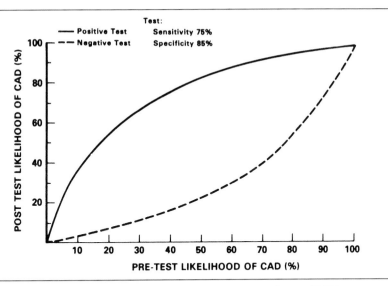

Figure 5-2. Influence of pretest likelihood of coronary artery disease (CAD) on posttest likelihood. Adapted with permission from Epstein SE: 1980. Implications of probability analysis on the strategy used for noninvasive detection of coronary artery disease: role of single or combined use of exercise electrocardiographic testing, radionuclide cineangiography and myocardial perfusion imaging. Am J Cardiol 46:491–499.

Exercise electrocardiogram (ECG)

The major noninvasive test in CHD is exercise ECG testing. At our institution, the Bruce protocol treadmill test is used in most young subjects and in very vigorous older patients. However, in most elderly patients we use either the Naughton–Bruce or Naughton protocol. Unlike the Bruce protocol, which starts at approximately 3 METS (metabolic equivalent), at 1.7 mph and 10% grade, and rapidly increases both the speed and incline (workload) in three-minute stages, the other protocols start at low workloads (1.5– 2.0 METS; 1–2 mph; 0% grade) and slowly increase the workload. The risks of exercise testing are extremely low, with a mortality rate of less than 1/10,000 and a major complication rate of less than 5/10,000. These complications do not seem to be increased in elderly patients.

Because of the ready availability, relatively low cost, and infrequent complications of routine treadmill ECG testing, it remains the most feasible noninvasive test for the workup of elderly patients with suspected CHD. However, one must appreciate the limitations of exercise testing in the elderly (table 5-3).

Although the hallmark of a positive test is usually considered to be 1 mm of horizontal or downward-sloping S-T-segment depression occurring 80 ms after the J point, the risk of CAD markedly increases with increasing S-T-

Table 5-1. Indications for exercise electrocardiographic testing

Asymptomatic subjects
  Definite indications
    None
  Possible indications
    Special occupations (e.g., pilots, police, fire fighters, bus drivers)
    Two or more risk factors in men ≥ 40 years of age
    Planned entry of sedentary men ≥ 40 years of age into a vigorous exercise program
Symptomatic subjects
  Definite indications
    Presence of atypical symptoms in men
    Assessment of prognosis in patients with known CAD
    Assessment of patients with exercise-induced dysrhythmias
  Possible indications
    Typical or atypical symptoms in women
    Assessment of response to various therapies
    Evaluation of variant angina
    Serial testing of patients with known CAD

Source: Adapted from Schlant RC, Blomquist CG, Brandenburg RO, et al. 1986. Guidelines for exercise testing: a report of the American College of Cardiology/American Heart Association on Assessment of Cardiovascular Procedures (Subcommittee on Exercise Testing). J Am Coll Cardiol 8:725–738. Used with permission of the American College of Cardiology.

Table 5-2. Contraindications to exercise electrocardiographic testing

Unstable angina
Severe uncontrolled hypertension
Recent or active cerebral ischemia
Aortic dissection
Uncompensated heart failure
Critical aortic stenosis
Critical left ventricular outflow tract obstruction
Inability to exercise

segment depression [2]. Recently, investigators have used various algorithms incorporating either an S-T-segment slope or S-T-segment index, in which the degree of S-T depression is corrected with the change in heart rate with exercise [8,9]. These techniques have been reported to improve the diagnostic accuracy of the exercise ECG and may be particularly applicable to elderly patients, who often fail to have significant increases in heart rate due to chronotropic insufficiency. Data from Okin and associates [9] have indicated that S-T-segment depression of 1.6 uV for every beat per minute best distinguishes patients with and without significant CHD. For example, a positive test would require 1.6 mm of S-T-segment depression if the exercise heart rate increased from 60 bpm to 160 bpm (100 bpm increase), whereas only 0.6 mm of S-T-segment depression would be required for a positive test if the heart rate increased from 80 bpm to only 120 bpm. Although S-T-

Table 5-3. Limitations of exercise testing in the elderly

I. ECG is nondiagnostic

II. ECG is uninterpretable for ischemia
   A. Drugs
      1. Digitalis
      2. Phenothiazines
      3. Antiarrhythmic agents
      4. Sensitivity impaired by anti-ischemic medications (nitrates, beta-blockers, calcium blockers)
   B. Resting ECG abnormalities
      1. Repolarization abnormalities
      2. LVH by ECG
      3. Left bundle-branch block
      4. Pacemaker

III. Patient is unable to perform adequate exercise
   A. Motivational
   B. Psychological
   C. Physical
      1. Poor conditioning
      2. Orthopedic and arthritic conditions
      3. Pulmonary disease (COPD, restrictive diseases)
      4. Obesity
      5. Peripheral vascular diseases
      6. Neuromuscular disease

Note: LVH = Left ventricular hypertrophy; COPD = Chronic obstructive pulmonary disease.

segment depression is generally required to indicate the diagnosis of ischemia using exercise ECG testing, other ECG findings with exercise are associated with ischemia, particularly U-wave inversion and T-wave pseudonormalization with exercise [2].

Unfortunately, many physicians place too much emphasis on the finding of either a "positive" or a "negative" exercise test result. Much more prognostic information is available from exercise ECG testing, as indicated in table 5-4 [2,7]. The prognosis is likely to be considerably better in a patient with 1.5-mm S-T-segment depression at 13 METS and a high exercise double product than in a patient with no S-T-segment depression who exercises only to 4 METS and has a low exercise double product.

Other tests may be helpful, however, when 1) routine exercise ECG testing is nondiagnostic; 2) factors are present that increase the likelihood of false ECG response to exercise or make the ECG uninterpretable for ischemia; and 3) the patient is unable or refuses to exercise long or hard enough to attain the target heart rate. Several alternative methods for detecting CAD that are particularly applicable to the elderly population are listed in table 5-5. Two radionuclide techniques, radionuclide angiography and thallium scintigraphy, are considered the best alternatives for identifying CHD in this population.

Table 5-4. Adverse prognostic signs on exercise assessment

Low workload (e.g., <6.5 METS or 5–6 min on Bruce protocol)
Low peak heart rate (e.g., <120 bpm without beta-blocker therapy)
Systolic pressure fall (e.g., >10 mmHg from baseline) or flat response (peak <130 mmHg)
Marked S-T-segment depression (e.g., >2 mm)
S-T-segment depression in multiple leads
Prolonged S-T-segment depression (e.g., >6 min) after exercise
S-T-segment elevation without pathologic Q-wave
Increase in complex ventricular ectopy (in association with S-T-segment shifts)
Exercise-induced typical angina[a]

[a] Probably only an adverse sign in screening tests, since most studies suggest that prognoses with symptomatic and silent ischemia are similar.
Note: MET, metabolic equivalent; 1 MET = resting oxygen consumption, or about 3.5 mL/kg/min; bpm, beats per minute.
Source: Adapted from Schlant RC, Blomquist CG, Brandenburg RO, et al. 1986. Guidelines for exercise testing: a report of the American College of Cardiology/American Heart Association on Assessment of Cardiovascular Procedures (Subcommittee on Exercise Testing). J Am Coll Cardiol 8:725–738. Used with permission of the American College of Cardiology.

Table 5-5. Alternatives to exercise ECG testing for diagnosis of coronary artery disease

  I. Myocardial perfusion imaging (thallium, technetium isonitriles)
     A. Exercise
     B. Pharmacologic (dipyridamole, adenosine, dobutamine)
 II. Ventricular function studies (radionuclide angiography, echocardiography)
     A. Exercise
     B. Pharmacologic (dipyridamole, adenosine, dobutamine)
III. Rapid atrial pacing (transthoracic or invasive)
 IV. Cold pressor testing
  V. Coronary angiography

Radionuclide angiography

One alternative is to analyze global and regional ventricular function during rest and exercise by using radionuclide angiography (RNA), which provides information about size, wall motion, and ejection fraction (EF) of both the right and left ventricles. This test is performed with technetium labeling of red blood cells. Although usually EF should increase by 5% or more with exercise, a decline of 5% or more, and particularly the development of new regional wall motion abnormalities, are more specific findings for CHD.

At our institution, RNA is usually performed with bicycle ergometry (most often supine) started at a workload of 150–300 kg·m/min (25–50 watts) and is gradually increased in three-minute stages by 150–300 kg·m/min per stage. Elderly patients are usually started at low workloads, and the workload is increased more slowly than in younger subjects. This technique requires gaiting by the R-R cycle on the ECG, and data are acquired during

Table 5-6. Advantages of radionuclide angiography and thallium scintigraphy

Radionuclide angiography	Thallium scintigraphy
Cost is lower than that of thallium scintigraphy	Wall-motion abnormalities detected by radionuclide angiography may occur without CAD in the following examples:
Ejection fraction (a major prognostic indicator) is determined	Severe valvular heart disease Severe hypertension
Allows timing of onset of ischemia	Hypertrophic cardiomyopathy[a] Left bundle branch block[a]
Potential advantages	Severe left ventricular hypertrophy
Volume can be determined	Varying R-R intervals (particularly atrial fibrillation)
Valvular regurgitation is quantifiable	Probably more sensitive and more specific with SPECT
Diastolic function can be assessed	Yields precise anatomic information desired

[a] Both radionuclide angiographic and thallium test results may be abnormal in the absence of macrovascular coronary disease.
Note: CAD, coronary artery disease; SPECT, single-photon emission computed tomography.
Source: From Lavie CJ, Ventura HO, and Murgo JP. 1991. Assessment of stable ischemic heart disease: which tests are best for which patients? Postgrad Med 89: 44–61.

the last two minutes of each exercise stage, with the final image representing the average for the time of acquisition.

Normal younger subjects respond to exercise with an increase in left ventricular EF of 5% or more. Although many elderly patients have a decrease in EF as well as a decreased response to exercise, data from the Baltimore Longitudinal Study [10] indicate that ventricular function remains preserved in elderly patients free of valvular, hypertensive, and coronary disease.

The advantages of RNA are listed in table 5-6, including the most important ones (relatively low cost compared to thallium scintigraphy and perhaps the most accurate determination of left ventricular EF, which provides major prognostic information in nearly all patients with CAD) [2]. As previously mentioned, when interpreting RNA data, clinicians should avoid neglecting other clinical, exercise hemodynamic, and ECG data, which still provide important information. In a study from the Mayo Clinic that utilized exercise RNA and cardiac catheterization [11], the three strongest predictors of severe CAD were peak left ventricular EF and two nonnuclear variables, exercise double product and degree of S-T-segment depression.

Myocardial perfusion imaging

Exercise

Thallium scintigraphy combined with exercise is the noninvasive test used most frequently to assess myocardial perfusion, with the myocardium absorbing thallium in proportion to its rate of delivery or regional blood flow. Usually thallium is injected during the last minute of exercise, scanning is performed 5–10 minutes after exercise, and delayed images are made 3–6 hours later. Left ventricular dilatation and increased pulmonary uptake of thallium after exercise are indicative of left ventricular dysfunction and a poor prognosis. If significant coronary stenosis limits the usual exercise-induced augmentation in coronary flow, the effect on the myocardium is detected as a "cold spot" on postexercise scanning. A reversible defect (present on the postexercise scan but not on the four-hour scan) usually indicates ischemia, whereas a fixed defect usually indicates an area of scar from prior myocardial infarction (MI). However, we now recognize that a fixed defect can indicate stunned or hibernating myocardium, particularly in patients with no history or ECG evidence of MI, often representing severely ischemic myocardium. Delayed scanning performed 24–48 hours after exercise, especially in conjunction with reinjection of thallium, often allows differentiation between scar tissue and severely ischemic but viable myocardium [2]. These data are particularly important for decisions regarding invasive revascularization techniques. Other adverse prognostic signs with exercise thallium include defects occurring in large areas of myocardium or in more than one vascular territory.

Although thallium studies are more costly than exercise ECG or exercise RNA, data with current tomographic techniques (single-photon emission computerized tomography (SPECT)) suggest that SPECT thallium is both more sensitive and more specific. RNA is more helpful in cases that require assessment of ventricular function, but there are several situations particularly applicable to the elderly in which thallium perfusion studies are preferred over RNA (table 5-6) [2].

It should be noted that the prevalence of severe hypertension, marked left ventricular hypertrophy (LVH), and left bundle branch block increases with age. In these cases, both RNA and thallium scintigraphy may be abnormal even in the absence of macrovascular CAD. Thallium scintigraphy is still considered the noninvasive procedure of choice for assessment of CHD in these patients, although coronary angiography is often needed to confirm significant macrovascular CAD.

Studies have demonstrated that exercise and radionuclide data, particularly when combined with thallium perfusion assessment, often provide prognostic information that is additive and superior to cardiac catheterization data alone [2,12,13]. These studies and others point out the limitations of cardiac catheterization data alone in determining the physiologic significance of any given coronary stenosis. Therefore, on many occasions, noninvasive data are extremely useful for assessing prognosis and determining the need for revascularization procedures even after invasive studies have delineated coronary anatomy. However, the applicability of these data and data from other noninvasive modalities to the assessment of prognosis in the 1990s is uncertain, and we have recently presented evidence [14] suggesting that further studies are needed to demonstrate that the prognostic ability of exercise assessment shown in the past is still applicable to patients currently referred for exercise testing.

New imaging agents

Technetium-99m (Tc-99m) hexakis methoxyisobutyl isonitril (RP-30A or sestamibi) has great promise for both evaluation of chronic ischemic heart disease and assessment of the amount of myocardium in jeopardy during acute ischemic syndromes, as well as the amount of myocardium salvaged by various acute reperfusion strategies [15]. Unlike thallium, sestamibi undergoes no significant redistribution after initial myocardial uptake. In acute ischemic syndromes, therefore, this agent can be injected before reperfusion, and then several hours later scanning can be performed that assesses the original area of myocardium at risk. After reinjection, the amount of myocardium salvaged can be measured.

In chronic ischemic heart disease, this imaging agent also appears very promising. The high quality of the sestamibi images is often superior to that of thallium images. In addition, a first-pass RNA can be obtained with this agent, which allows for the detection of LVEF and regional wall motion in addition to myocardial perfusion by planar or SPECT techniques [15,16].

Pharmacologic approaches

In patients unable to exercise adequately, often as a result of severe peripheral vascular disease or orthopedic or pulmonary limitation, several alternatives are available, including pharmacologic stimulation (e.g., dipyridamole, adenosine, or dobutamine) combined with either perfusion imaging or echocardiography. Among these approaches, dipyridamole thallium has emerged as the most commonly used alternative to exercise assessment. Dipyridamole acts in conjunction with adenosine and cyclic adenosine monophosphate to increase perfusion in myocardium, which is supplied by coronary arteries without significant stenoses but not in areas supplied by an obstructive coronary artery. The result is a relative imbalance in perfusion between areas with and without significant stenosis, producing defects ("cold spots") on perfusion scans. In some cases, dipyridamole induces a "steal syndrome" either from macrovascular or, more commonly, subendocardial steal. Because extensive safety data are readily available [17], this agent has recently been approved for intravenous use in conjunction with assessment of perfusion. Studies have demonstrated that high-dose oral (300–400 mg) or intravenous dipyridamole (0.56 mg/kg given over four minutes) is highly sensitive and specific for detection of CAD [2,17]. The intravenous drug is much easier to administer from the standpoint of scheduling, convenience, and management of side effects.

The major use of dipyridamole–thallium testing has been in the assessment of prognosis in patients before major noncardiac surgeries, particularly vascular, major orthopedic, and upper abdominal procedures.

Although several groups have reported the efficacy of dipyridamole–thallium testing in predicting prognosis in these patients, the largest study in over 200 patients was recently published by Eagle and colleagues [18]. They identified five major clinical variables (age over 70 years, diabetes, ECG evidence of pathologic Q-waves, ventricular arrhythmias requiring medications, and typical angina) and two dipyridamole–thallium variables (thallium redistribution and significant ECG changes) as predictive of poor prognosis.

Not surprisingly, dipyridamole–thallium testing was not very useful in patients at low risk (no clinical variables) or at high risk (three or more clinical variables), but was very useful for predicting prognosis in those at intermediate operative risk. Among patients with one or two of the major clinical variables listed above (including age greater than 70 years), cardiac events occurred in 16 (30%) of 54 with thallium redistribution, compared with only 2 (3%) of 62 without thallium redistribution. Others [2,19] have confirmed the significance of dipyridamole–thallium assessment in predicting cardiac events before major noncardiac procedures.

Adenosine has recently been released for the acute treatment of supraventricular arrhythmias. Compared to dipyridamole, adenosine produces more maximal coronary vasodilatation and is very short-acting, which is an advantage when the drug induces serious side effects, particularly severe myocardial ischemia or severe hypotension [20]. Although this agent appears to be extremely efficacious when combined with thallium for the assessment of ischemic heart disease, high cost is an obstacle to its routine use at present.

Stress echocardiography

Echocardiography has several advantages over other imaging techniques, including tremendous availability, absence of any adverse effects, and relatively low cost. With proper technician and physician training, stress echocardiography has been validated as an established method for assessment of CHD, with accuracy similar to that of the more established radionuclide techniques [21].

In the United States, most research regarding stress echocardiography has been associated with exercise assessment. Data from numerous laboratories now demonstrate that technically satisfactory exercise echocardiographic assessments can be obtained in the vast majority of patients (approximately 95%). Stress echocardiography has a high sensitivity and specificity for CHD and is useful for assessment of prognosis in patients known to have CHD.

Pharmacologic forms of stress echocardiography have technical advantages over exercise (it is often technically challenging to obtain high-quality images at peak exercise or immediately after exercise) and are applicable to patients who cannot exercise adequately. Data from Italy [22–26] have demonstrated the accuracy of dipyridamole echocardiography for the assessment of CHD, and this technique is also very useful for the short- and long-term assessment of prognosis. The recent data have suggested that a high-dose dipyridamole infusion is superior to the usual low-dose infusion (0.56 mg/kg over four minutes). After a four-minute infusion of dipyridamole, 0.56 mg/kg, and a four-minute waiting period, 0.28 mg/kg is infused over two minutes. This higher-dose protocol offers greater sensitivity than the low-dose protocol and is obtained without a significant increase in side effects.

Beta-adrenergic agonists increase heart rate, contractility, and myocardial oxygen consumption and, in the presence of coronary disease, may induce myocardial ischemia. Although dobutamine can be combined with thallium or RNA, dobutamine echocardiography seems particularly promising for the assessment of CHD [27]. Dobutamine is infused in three-minute stages (2.5–40 µg/kg/min), with the dose increasing by 2.5–5.0 µg/kg/min during each stage. As with dipyridamole, a positive test is development of a new regional wall motion abnormality. Dobutamine digital echocardiography is an excellent test for the assessment of CHD and should be particularly beneficial for patients who are unable to exercise. One advantage of dobutamine is that it enhances contractility in normal zones of myocardium, making it easier to recognize adjacent regions with wall motion abnormalities. In addition, the graded stress of dobutamine provides physiologic data (e.g., heart rate and blood pressure) unavailable with agents such as dipyridamole or adenosine. Dobutamine may also provide information regarding hibernating or stunned myocardium, which may develop enhanced contraction during testing. For this reason, dobutamine may become an ideal agent for pharmacologic stress testing in the 1990s. However, since the elderly may have a blunted response to stimulation with beta-agonists, the efficacy of this testing in older patients still must be established.

Rapid atrial pacing

This test increases heart rate and myocardial oxygen consumption in patients with coronary disease. Rapid atrial pacing induces ischemia manifested by angina, S-T-segment depression, increases in ventricular end-diastolic pressures, defects detected by myocardial perfusion scanning, and wall motion abnormalities and fall in EF detected by RNA or echocardiography [28]. Pacing is normally performed invasively with right heart catheterization and insertion of a pacing wire into the right atrium. However, noninvasive external transthoracic pacing is also safe and can effectively produce ischemia in patients with CAD [29]. Like several of the other tests discussed, atrial pacing with ECG and either perfusion scanning or wall motion assessment is particularly applicable for elderly patients who are unable to exercise, including patients in intensive care unit settings and particularly those who have programmable permanent pacemakers already implanted.

Upper-extremity exercise

Many elderly patients are unable to perform leg exercises because of arthritis, orthopedic conditions, or lower-extremity vascular disease. Dynamic exercise of the upper extremity and static isometric exercise (1/3 maximal handgrip for 3–5 minutes), or both, may be helpful in assessing myocardial ischemia. The combination of arm exercise with ECG and either myocardial perfusion testing or assessment of wall motion may be helpful in detecting CAD [30–32]. This type of assessment may be particularly applicable to the elderly patient who experiences symptoms more with upper-extremity exercise than with walking, although in most patients we prefer a form of pharmacologic stress assessment.

Catheterization and angiography

Left heart catheterization remains the definitive strategy for assessing ventricular function and coronary artery anatomy, but this test is invasive and involves some risk and considerable expense. At our institution, major complications occur in fewer than 1/1000 procedures; however, catheterization complications including thromboembolic events due to diffuse atherosclerotic disease and complications associated with radiocontrast material occur more frequently in the elderly [33].

In the past, it was often pointless to resort to coronary angiography if other medical problems made the elderly patient an unacceptable candidate for coronary artery bypass surgery. Cardiac and noncardiac risks of bypass surgery are three times greater in patients over age 70 than in younger patients [34]. Now, however, coronary revascularization can often be accomplished successfully with percutaneous transluminal coronary angioplasty (PTCA), a procedure suitable for many elderly patients with multiple medical problems [35]. Substantial data indicate that the primary success rate and complication rate of PTCA are similar in patients over age 65 years and in younger patients.

Definite indications for coronary arteriography include 1) angina refractory to maximal medical therapy; 2) severe ischemia by exercise ECG and nuclear assessment; 3) ischemia prior to major noncardiac surgery; 4) the need for valvular surgery; 5) unstable angina or other evidence of ongoing myocardial ischemia following MI; 6) ventricular septal defect following MI; 7) ventricular aneurysm associated with intractable heart failure or malignant ventricular arrhythmias; and 8) follow-up to cardiac arrest.

Elderly patients are known to have a decreased glomerular filtration rate and are particularly susceptible to renal dysfunction following any dye load [36–40]. Physical and laboratory evidence of adequate hydration and urine output is increasingly important in preventing renal dysfunction after cardiac catheterization. In elderly patients with renal impairment or insulin-dependent diabetes, the dosage of radiocontrast material can be reduced by noninvasive assessment of left ventricular function before cardiac catheterization using echocardiography or RNA.

VALVULAR HEART DISEASE

Doppler echocardiography has proved to be a major advance for the assessment of valvular heart disease, providing precise assessment of both valvular stenosis and regurgitation. In greater than 95% of patients, technically satisfactory studies are obtained for accurate determination of valve areas in both aortic and mitral stenosis. The prevalence and severity of mitral and tricuspid regurgitation can be assessed by a constellation of Doppler modalities, particularly color flow Doppler. Aortic regurgitation is assessed by continuous-wave, pulsed-wave, and color flow studies, including pulsed Doppler evaluation of descending aortic flow. Transesophageal echocardiography has added valuable diagnostic capabilities for the evaluation of valvular regurgitation, particularly mitral regurgitation and mitral prosthetic function and regurgitation. Using these noninvasive modalities, it is possible to determine the need for valvular surgery without invasive testing. In fact, some groups have suggested that valvular surgery can be safely undertaken without cardiac catheterization, particularly in young patients who lack significant CHD risk factors [41,42]. However, we believe that preoperative catheterization for coronary angiography is necessary because the elderly population has a high prevalence of silent CAD, and the need for concomitant revascularization should be determined. Although in the elderly the need for both coronary artery surgery and valvular surgery has been questioned, experience at our institution and elsewhere [43–48] has shown that both procedures can be performed safely and that patients who undergo both procedures do considerably better than those with significant CAD who have valvular surgery alone.

Recent data [49] have documented the increasing use of Doppler echocardiography, which is creating an apparent "epidemic" in valvular regurgitation. Using a constellation of Doppler modalities, including continuous-wave, pulsed-wave, and color flow Doppler, we recently demonstrated that mitral, tricuspid, and aortic regurgitation were detected by Doppler in 73%, 68%, and 12%, respectively, of patients with otherwise completely normal two-dimensional and M-mode echocardiograms [50]. In most cases, trivial and mild degrees of regurgitation were detected, although moderate to severe regurgitation was present in some patients (mitral 6%, tricuspid 5%, and aortic 2%). Although the prevalence of mitral and tricuspid regurgitation appears not to be related to age, severity of valvular regurgitation was strongly age related. Unlike mitral and tricuspid regurgitation, aortic regurgitation was 2 to 3 times more prevalent and more severe in our older patients.

These data suggest that trivial and mild mitral and tricuspid regurgitation are physiologically normal. Understanding this may be very important in

Table 5-7. Diagnostic tests for evaluating cerebrovascular disease

  I. Ultrasound and Doppler
 II. Oculoplethysmography
III. Nuclear cerebral imaging
 IV. Position emission tomographic (PET) scanning
  V. Intravenous digital subtraction angiography (DSA)
 VI. Cerebral angiography

the prevention of iatrogenic heart disease, since we have recently reported [51–53] that Doppler-detected valvular regurgitation strongly influences physicians' proscriptions of endocarditis prophylaxis recommendations in normal patients and in those with mitral valve prolapse. Although definitive data to provide guidelines for endocarditis prophylaxis in patients with Doppler-detected valvular regurgitation are unavailable, we believe that endocarditis prophylaxis should usually be administered to those with more than trivial–mild mitral and tricuspid regurgitation or any aortic regurgitation, particularly when valvular sclerosis is present. This information may also be important, since we recently reported a strong age bias for endocarditis prophylaxis recommendations [53]. Although the prevalence of infective endocarditis markedly increases with age, physicians' recommendations for endocarditis prophylaxis are inversely related to the patient's age. In fact, in Olmsted County studies, youth was the strongest independent factor for endocarditis prophylaxis recommendations in patients with Doppler-detected valvular regurgitation or mitral valve prolapse [51–53].

CEREBROVASCULAR DISEASE

A detailed discussion of cerebrovascular disease and diagnostic testing available for this disease is beyond the scope of this chapter. However, a number of diagnostic tests are now available for assessment of the severity of cerebrovascular disease (table 5-7). At our institution, most patients who have asymptomatic carotid bruits or who are at very high risk of cerebrovascular disease are screened with duplex ultrasound and Doppler techniques.

The indications for cerebral angiography continue to be controversial. Catheterization and angiography are definitely indicated before major elective surgery in patients with recent transient ischemic attacks in the carotid circulation or those with evidence by noninvasive studies of significant disease. At our institution and elsewhere, the severity of cerebrovascular disease is well determined by noninvasive studies. However, before carotid surgery, cerebral angiography is usually required to demonstrate the intra-cerebral vasculature and determine suitability for carotid artery surgery.

Previously, intravenous digital subtraction angiography (DSA) appeared to be a promising technique for noninvasive evaluation of atherosclerotic vascular disease, including cerebrovascular disease. However, this test requires

Table 5-8. Diagnostic tests for evaluating renal vascular disease

---

    I. Peripheral renin
   II. Captopril renin
  III. Nuclear renal scan
  IV. Captopril nuclear renal scan
   V. Renal artery ultrasound
  VI. Intravenous digital subtraction angiography (DSA)
 VII. Selective renal vein renin
VIII. Renal arteriography

---

a considerable dye load that may be nephrotoxic in elderly patients, thus raising concerns about its safety [54,55]. Data from our institution and elsewhere have also raised concern about the accuracy of DSA, indicating that it is not an effective surrogate for conventional catheter angiography and is a redundant test in patients with a high likelihood of significant cerebro-vascular disease [54,56–58]. Since an increased risk of contrast nephropathy is documented in patients undergoing several radiocontrast procedures, this redundancy should be avoided in the elderly population. Therefore, this procedure has only limited use in the 1990s, in patients who cannot tolerate or who refuse to undergo conventional catheter angiography.

RENAL VASCULAR DISEASE

As with cerebrovascular disease, a detailed discussion of renal hypertension and its assessment is beyond the scope of this review. The diagnostic tests available are listed in table 5-8. At our institution, the most frequently utilized techniques are the captopril nuclear renal scan and renal artery ultra-sound. Both techniques have excellent sensitivity and specificity for the detection of significant renal artery stenosis. The captopril renal scan has the advantage of assessing renal structure, and particularly renal function, as well as the likelihood of significant blood pressure reduction with renal artery revascularization (for example, percutaneous transluminal angioplasty or bypass surgery). The ultrasound technique has the advantage of more precisely assessing the location and severity of the arterial obstruction, including aneurysmal disease, which may help determine the suitability of revascularization strategies. The ultrasound technique also allows for deter-mination of renal structure and assessment of extrarenal causes of renal compromise.

REFERENCES

1. Frye RL, Higgins MW, Beller GA, et al. 1988. Task Force III: major demographic and epidemiologic trends affecting adult cardiology. J Am Coll Cardiol 12:840–846.
2. Lavie CJ, Ventura HO, and Murgo JP. 1991. Assessment of stable ischemic heart disease: which tests are best for which patients? Postgrad Med 89:44–61.
3. Epstein SE. 1980. Implications of probability analysis on the strategy used for noninvasive detection of coronary artery disease: role of single or combined use of exercise

electrocardiographic testing, radionuclide cineangiography and myocardial perfusion imaging. Am J Cardiol 46:491–499.

4. Lavie CJ, Squires RW, and Gau GT. 1987. Prevention of cardiovascular disease: of what value are risk factor modification, exercise, fish consumption, and aspirin therapy? Postgrad Med 81:52–72.
5. Lavie CJ, Gau GT, Squires RW, et al. 1988. Management of lipids in primary and secondary prevention of cardiovascular diseases. Mayo Clin Proc 63:605–621.
6. Lavie CJ, O'Keefe JH, Blonde L, et al. 1990. High-density lipoprotein cholesterol: recommendations for routine testing and treatment. Postgrad Med 87:36–51.
7. Schlant RC, Blomquist CG, Brandenburg RO, et al. 1986. Guidelines for exercise testing: a report of the American College of Cardiology/American Heart Association on Assessment of Cardiovascular Procedures (Subcommittee on Exercise Testing). J Am Coll Cardiol 8:725–738.
8. Kligfield P, Ameisen O, and Okin PM. 1989. Heart rate adjustment of ST segment depression for improved detection of coronary artery disease. Circulation 79:245–255.
9. Okin PM, Kligfield P, Milner MR, et al. 1988. Heart rate adjustment of ST-segment depression for reduction of false positive electrocardiographic responses to exercise in asymptomatic men screened for coronary artery disease. Am J Cardiol 62:1043–1047.
10. Rodeheffer RJ, Gerstenblith G, Becker LC, et al. 1984. Exercise cardiac output is maintained with advancing age in healthy human subjects. Cardiac dilatation and increased stroke volume compensate for a diminished heart rate. Circulation 69:203–213.
11. Gibbons RJ, Fyke FE 3d, Clements IP, et al. 1988. Noninvasive identification of severe coronary artery disease using exercise radionuclide angiography. J Am Coll Cardiol 11:28–34.
12. Kaul S, Lilly DR, Gascho JA, et al. 1988. Prognostic utility of the exercise thallium-201 test in ambulatory patients with chest pain: comparison with cardiac catheterization. Circulation 77:745–748.
13. Kaul S, Finkelstein DM, Homma S, et al. 1988. Superiority of quantitative exercise thallium-201 variables in determining long-term prognosis in ambulatory patients with chest pain: a comparison with cardiac catheterization. J Am Coll Cardiol 12:25–34.
14. Lavie CJ, Gibbons RJ, Zinsmiester, et al. 1991. Interpreting results of exercise studies after acute myocardial infarction altered by thrombolytic therapy, coronary angioplasty, or bypass. Am J Cardiol 67:116–120.
15. Sinusas AJ, Watson DD, Cannon JM Jr, et al. 1989. Effect of ischemia and postischemic dysfunction on myocardial uptake of technetium-99m-labeled methoxyisobutyl isonitrile and thallium-201. J Am Coll Cardiol 14:1785–1793.
16. Lavie CJ and Gersh BJ. 1990. Acute myocardial infarction: initial manifestations, management, and prognosis. Mayo Clin Proc 65:531–548.
17. Ranhosky A, Kempthorne-Rawson J, and the Intravenous Dipyridamole Thallium Imaging Study Group. 1990. The safety of intravenous dipyridamole thallium myocardial perfusion imaging. Circulation 81:1205–1209.
18. Eagle KA, Coley CM, Newell JB, et al. 1989. Combining clinical and thallium data optimizes preoperative assessment of cardiac risk before major vascular surgery. Ann Intern Med 110:859–866.
19. Lapeyre AC, Gibbons RJ, and Forstrom IA. 1988. Prediction of cardiac complications of non-cardiac surgery by intravenous dipyridamole thallium tomography (abstract). J Nucl Med 29:838.
20. Verani MS. 1991. Adenosine thallium 201 myocardial perfusion scintigraphy. Am Heart J 122:269–278.
21. Armstrong WF. 1988. Exercise echocardiography: ready, willing and able (editorial). J Am Coll Cardiol 11:1359–1361.
22. Pirelli S, Danzi GB, Alberti A, et al. 1991. Comparison of usefulness of high-dose dipyridamole echocardiography and exercise electrocardiography for detection of asymptomatic restenosis after coronary angioplasty. Am J Cardiol 67:1335–1338.
23. Picano E, Pirelli S, Marzilli M, et al. 1989. Usefulness of high-dose dipyridamole echocardiography test in coronary angioplasty. Circulation 80:807–815.
24. Picano E, Lattanzi F, Masini M, et al. 1986. High dose dipyridamole echocardiography test in effort angina pectoris. J Am Coll Cardiol 8:848–854.

25. Picano E, Pirelli S, Orlandini A, et al. in press. The safety of high dose intravenous dipyridamole-echocardiography test. J Am Coll Cardiol.

26. Picano E, Lattanzi F, Orlandini A, et al. 1991. Stress echocardiography and the human factor: the importance of being expert. J Am Coll Cardiol 17:666–669.

27. Cohen JL, Greene TO, Ottenweller J, et al. 1991. Dobutamine digital echocardiography for detecting coronary artery disease. Am J Cardiol 67:1311–1318.

28. Slutsky R, Watkins J, Peterson K, et al. 1981. The response of left ventricular function and size to atrial pacing, volume loading, and afterload stress in patients with coronary artery disease. Circulation 63:864–870.

29. Feldman MD, McKay RG, Gervin EV, et al. 1985. The noninvasive thoracic pacing tachycardia test: hemodynamic responses (abstract). Circulation 72:20.

30. Brown BG, Josephson MA, Peterson MA, et al. 1981. Intravenous dipyridamole combined with isometric handgrip for near maximal acute increase in coronary flow in patients with coronary artery disease. Am J Cardiol 48:1077–1085.

31. Bodenheimer MM, Banka VA, Fooshie CM, et al. 1978. Detection of coronary heart disease using radionuclide determined regional ejection fraction at rest and during handgrip: correlation with coronary angiography. Circulation 58:640–648.

32. Peter CA, and Jones RH. 1980. Effect of isometric handgrip and dynamic exercise in left ventricular function. J Nucl Med 21:1131–1138.

33. Kennedy JW. 1982. Complications associated with cardiac catheterization and angiography. Cathet Cardiovasc Diagn 8:5–11.

34. Rose DM, Gelbfish J, Jocobowitz IJ, et al. 1985. Analysis of morbidity and mortality in patients 70 years of age and over undergoing isolated coronary artery bypass surgery. Am Heart J 110:341–346.

35. Raizner AE, Hust RG, Lewis JM, et al. 1986. Transluminal coronary angioplasty in the elderly. Am J Cardiol 57:29–32.

36. Goldman R. 1979. Decline in organ functioning with aging. In I Rossman (ed), Clinical Geriatrics, 2nd ed. Philadelphia: J.B. Lippincott, pp 23–59.

37. Krumlovsky FA, Simon N, Santhanam S, et al. 1978. Acute renal failure: association with administration of radiographic contrast material. JAMA 239:125–127.

38. Bryd L and Sherman RL. 1979. Radiocontrast-induced acute renal failure. A clinical and pathophysiologic review. Medicine 58:270–279.

39. Cochran ST, Wong WS, and Roe DJ. 1983. Predicting angiography-induced acute renal impairment: a clinical risk model. AJR 141:1027–1033.

40. Taliercio CP, Vliestra RE, Fisher LD, et al. 1986. Risks for renal dysfunction with cardiac angiography. Ann Intern Med 104:501–504.

41. Brandenbury RO. 1981. No more routine catheterization for valvular heart disease? N Engl J Med 305:1277–1288.

42. St John Sutton MG, St John Sutton M, Oldershaw P, et al. 1981. Valve replacement without preoperative cardiac catheterization. N Engl J Med 305:1233–1238.

43. Richardson JV, Kouchoukos NT, Wright JO III, et al. 1979. Combined aortic valve replacement and myocardial revascularization: result in 220 patients. Circulation 59:75–81.

44. Kirblen JW and Kouchoukos NT. 1981. Aortic valve replacement without myocardial revascularization. Circulation 63:252–253.

45. Borow RO, Kent KM, Roseng DR, et al. 1981. Aortic valve replacement without myocardial revascularization in patients with combined aortic valvular and coronary artery disease. Circulation 63:243–251.

46. Teply JF, Grunkemeier GL, and Starr A. 1981. A cardiac valve replacement in patients over 75 years of age. Thorac Cardiovasc Surg 29:47–50.

47. Murphy ES, Lawson RM, Starr A, et al. 1981. Severe aortic stenosis in patients 60 years of age and older: left ventricular function and 10-year survival after valve replacement. Circulation 2 (Suppl II):II-184–II-188.

48. Jamieson WR, Dooner J, Munro AI, et al. 1981. Cardiac valve replacement in the elderly: a review of 320 cases. Circulation 2 (Suppl II):II-177–II-183.

49. Ballard DJ, Khandheria BK, Tajik AJ, et al. 1989. A population–based study of echocardiography: time trends in utilization and diagnostic profile of an evolving technology, 1975–1987. Int J Technol Assess Health Care 5:249–261.

50. Lavie CJ, Hebert K, and Cassidy M. in press. Prevalence and severity of Doppler-detected

valvular regurgitation and estimation of right sided cardiac pressures in patients with normal 2-dimensional echocardiograms. Chest.

51. Lavie CJ, Khandheria BK, Seward JB, et al. 1989. Factors associated with the recommendation for endocarditis prophylaxis in mitral valve prolapse. JAMA 262:3308–3312.

52. Ballard DJ, Lavie CJ, Taylor CL, et al. 1988. Impact of Doppler echocardiography detected mitral regurgitation on endocarditis prophylaxis recommendations: a population-based study (abstract). Circulation 78 (Suppl II):II-585.

53. Lavie CJ, Khandheria B, Taylor C, et al. 1990. Age bias in endocarditis prophylaxis recommendations: a review of population-based studies (abstract). J Am Geriatr Soc 38:11A.

54. Cebal RD and Paulus RA. 1986. The failure of intravenous digital subtraction angiography in replacing carotid anteriography. Ann Intern Med 104:572–574.

55. Aaron JO, Hesselink JR, Oot R, et al. 1984. Complication of intravenous DSA performed for carotid artery disease: a prospective study. Radiology 155:675–678.

56. Crocker EF Jr, Tutton RH, and Bowen JC. 1986. The role of intravenous digital subtraction angiography in the evaluation of extracranial carotid artery disease: can the decision for carotid artery surgery be made solely on the basis of its findings? J Vasc Surg 4:157–163.

57. Hoffman MG, Gomes AS, and Pais SO. 1984. Limitations in the interpretation of intravenous carotid digital subtraction angiography. AJR 142:261–264.

58. Glover JL, Bendick PJ, Jackson VP, et al. 1984. Duplex sonography, digital subtraction angiography, and conventional angiography in assessing carotid atherosclerosis. Arch Surg 119:664–669.

6. HEART FAILURE

BARRY M. MASSIE
CHRISTOPHER L. WOLFE

Congestive heart failure is a common problem in the elderly [1,2]. Although the causes of heart failure in older patients are generally the same as those in the general adult population, the clinical presentation and required diagnostic evaluation often differ. Age-related changes in cardiac function and in the peripheral vasculature and the more sedentary life-style of the older patient may mask or, conversely, mimic the usual signs of heart failure. Physicians must be suspicious of vague symptoms, as well as the sometimes unimpressive physical signs of heart failure. At the same time, they must be aware that complaints and physicial signs, which in younger patients suggest cardiac decompensation, may in the elderly be nonspecific. Most importantly, as in other groups of patients, confirmation of the diagnosis of heart failure should be the starting point in a search for reversible or specifically treatable underlying causes.

In this chapter we discuss the causes and pathophysiology of heart failure in the elderly, the diagnostic evaluation of these patients, and their therapy.

EPIDEMIOLOGY

Congestive heart failure is a major and growing problem in the United States. Two to three million patients carry this diagnosis, and approximately

Franz H. Messerli (ed.), CARDIOVASCULAR DISEASE IN THE ELDERLY (Third Edition). Copyright © 1993 Kluwer Academic Publishers. ISBN 0-7923-1859-5. All rights reserved.

400,000 new cases occur yearly. Heart failure is the discharge diagnosis in over 900,000 hospitalizations each year and is the most common reason for hospitalization in patients over 65 years. To a large extent, heart failure is a disease of the elderly. In the Framingham Heart Study [2], the prevalence of heart failure rises progressively with age, from approximately 1% in 50- to 59-year-olds to 10% in persons over age 80. Similarly, the incidence of new cases approximately doubles with each decade from age 45 to age 84, from an annual rate of 1 to 2 per 1000 patients in women and men age 45 to 54 to 13 to 14 cases per year per 1000 patients between ages 75 and 84. After age 85, the incidence of new cases of heart failure increases four- to sixfold.

PATHOPHYSIOLOGY

Changes in cardiac function with aging

Aging is associated with a number of changes in the heart and the peripheral vasculature that may cause or exacerbate congestive heart failure [3–5]. Left ventricular weight increases by an average of 1 g per year in men and 1.5 g per year in women [6], primarily as a result of an increase in left ventricular wall thickness [7]. This may be caused primarily by the progressive rise in systolic blood pressure with aging, but may occur even in persons in whom hypertension is carefully excluded. At the microscopic level, aging is associated with lipofuscin deposits and basophilic degeneration [3,4]. The clinical significance of these changes is unclear, but they are associated with reduction in the number of mitochondria and in the activity of mitochondrial enzymes. Focal deposits of amyloid material are quite common, particularly in patients over age 80.

There are also changes in myocardial function with aging. Several investigators have reported a decrease in maximal cardiac output with aging, primarily associated with a decrease in maximum heart rate [8]. There is also a decline in exercise capacity and ejection fraction response to exercise [9–11]. However, some studies in which coexisting atherosclerotic disease has been carefully excluded have found that these changes in systolic function are rather small [10,12]. In contrast, aging is associated with quite dramatic changes in indices of diastolic filling and function [10,13,14]. The proportion of diastolic filling that occurs passively in early diastole decreases, while that which occurs due to atrial contraction in late diastole increases. These changes in diastolic function probably reflect a combination of impaired chamber compliance (due to both hypertrophy and interstitial changes) and impaired myocardial relaxation. These may have important clinical relevance, since it has become increasingly recognized that many cases of congestive heart failure in the elderly are due to predominant diastolic dysfunction.

Aging is also associated with significant changes in the properties of the peripheral vasculature, which alter left ventricular loading conditions [15]. The medium and larger arteries become thickened or calcified and less compliant. Peripheral vascular resistance rises, as does vascular impedance, which reflects the distensibility of the vasculature, These changes are responsible for the rising systolic blood pressure and, indirectly, for increasing left ventricular mass in many older patients. This increasing vascular load, while insufficient to cause heart failure by itself, lowers the threshold for decompensation in patients with significantly impaired left ventricular systolic function.

Other changes associated with aging that can lead to congestive heart failure include degeneration of the heart valves and dilatation of the ascending aorta, which can lead to mitral and aortic regurgitation. Aortic valve calcification is also a common cause of aortic stenosis, which is the most common, clinically significant valvular pathology in the elderly.

Regulation of left ventricular function in the failing heart

Clinical congestive heart failure primarily reflects the body's compensatory mechanisms in response to chronically impaired left ventricular function [16]. Left ventricular performance is determined by the interaction of four variables: 1) the inotropic state of the myocardium; 2) left ventricular afterload (a combination of systemic vascular resistance and myocardial systolic wall stress); 3) left ventricular preload (the end-diastolic volume or wall stress); and 4) heart rate. As long as myocardial contractile reserve remains normal, changes in left ventricular loading conditions or in cardiac output requirements can be accommodated either by the Frank–Starling mechanism or reflex autonomic responses. Thus, a requirement for increased cardiac output is met by a rise in heart rate and contractility mediated by the sympathetic nervous system, and by a further increment in stroke volume in response to an augmented end-diastolic volume. An increase in afterload— for example, a rise in blood pressure—is similarly compensated for by an increase in contractility and by the added stroke volume produced by the Frank–Starling mechanism in response to left ventricular dilatation. In addition, chronic pressure and volume overloading stimulate left ventricular hypertrophy with a consequent reduction in systolic wall stress and an added capability to maintain normal stroke volume. This may be the basis for the increase in left ventricular mass with aging, which can have important consequences for left ventricular diastolic function (see below).

The pathophysiology of congestive heart failure is illustrated schematically in figure 6-1. When cardiac contractility is reduced as a result of myocardial disease, loss of myocardium, or chronic pressure or volume overload, the compensatory mechanisms described above may be inadequate. If the depression is severe, stroke volume and cardiac output fall. The immediate effect of the decrease in cardiac output is a fall in arterial blood pressure. Sympathetic tone to the heart and peripheral circulation increase as a result of the decrease in carotid sinus and aortic arch-baroreceptor stretch. This has several important effects. Heart rate rises to maintain cardiac output in the

PATHOPHYSIOLOGY OF CHF

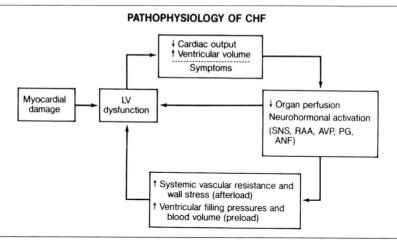

Figure 6-1. The pathophysiology of heart failure is shown schematically. The damage, which results in left ventricular pump dysfunction, is characterized by a diminished cardiac output and left ventricular dilatation. These hemodynamic changes result in the characteristic symptoms of dyspnea, edema, exercise intolerance, and fatigue. As a result of the impaired cardiac output, perfusion of vital organs, such as the kidneys and exercising muscle, is reduced. Furthermore, important homeostatic reflex systems such as high- and low-pressure baroceptors become dysfunctional. These changes lead to activation of a number of neurohormonal systems, which themselves increase left ventricular afterload and preload and cause progressive left ventricular dysfunction. In addition, neurohormonal activation may directly affect the heart, causing progressive left ventricular damage, dysfunction, and arrhythmias.

presence of a reduced stroke volume. Neurally mediated catecholamine release enhances myocardial performance. Arterial venoconstriction increases blood pressure by increasing systemic vascular resistance. Since vasoconstriction is regionally selective, blood flow is redistributed away from the renal, hepatic, and splanchnic circulations to maintain central aortic blood pressure and sufficient coronary and cerebral blood flow. Vasoconstriction also decreases venous capacitance and promotes blood return to the heart to produce ventricular high filling volumes and to take advantage of the Frank–Starling effect.

While these mechanisms help to maintain cardiac output and arterial pressure, they also increase myocardial metabolic requirements and potentially further depress ventricular function. Thus, the tachycardia, increased inotropy, elevated wall stress resulting from left ventricular dilatation, and increased systemic vascular resistance all augment myocardial oxygen demand. The higher systemic vascular resistance, especially, increases the work of the failing myocardium and may further impair left ventricular systolic function.

Table 6-1. Pathophysiology of chronic heart failure

Left heart failure
   Secondary to systolic dysfunction
   Secondary to mechanical defects
Diastolic heart failure
High-output heart failure
Right heart failure

Renal and neuroendocrine responses

The decrease in cardiac output also precipitates sodium and water retention by the kidney [17]. Renal perfusion pressure decreases, and this deficit is intensified by the compensatory redistribution of blood flow away from the renal circulation. As renal blood flow decreases, the glomerular filtration rate falls, the filtration fraction increases, and the net result is an increase in proximal tubule sodium and water reabsorption. Sodium retention and extracellular fluid volume expansion are also enhanced by increasing circulating levels of aldosterone. The decrease in renal blood flow, as well as increased sympathetic nervous system activity, stimulates renin release from the juxtaglomerular apparatus, resulting in increased levels of angiotensin II, which in turn stimulates adrenal aldosterone secretion. Angiotensin II itself probably contributes to both the arterial and venous vasoconstriction that increase peripheral vascular resistance, and may also inhibit both renal blood flow and the glomerular filtration rate in heart failure. It also may stimulate thirst and, together with elevated circulating levels of antidiuretic horomone, may further decrease renal water excretion.

MECHANISMS OF CHRONIC HEART FAILURE

Table 6-1 lists the differing pathophysiologic types of chronic heart failure. Left heart failure, defined by elevated pulmonary venous pressures, pulmonary congestion, and a low cardiac output, is usually due to loss of muscle (as in ischemic heart disease) or a generalized cardiomyopathy. However, it may occur in the absence of left ventricular systolic dysfunction by a variety of mechanisms. Mechanical abnormalities, such as obstructive and regurgitant valvular disease or left-to-right intracardiac shunts, may be the initial finding in elderly patients. In addition, high-output states and impaired left ventricular diastolic function as well as isolated right ventricular overload or dysfunction may lead to clinical presentations similar to the more usual forms of systolic dysfunction, but with very different underlying pathophysiology requiring different therapeutic approaches.

High-output heart failure

High-output heart failure, though unusual in the elderly, is an important syndrome to recognize, since it is often amenable to specific therapy. The primary abnormality is an excessive demand for cardiac output caused by extracardiac factors, superimposed on a ventricle with either normal systolic function or impaired cardiac reserve. The onset of heart failure in conditions of high-output demand, such as hyperthryoidism, beriberi, severe anemia, arteriovenous fistulas, and Paget's disease, is marked by a rise in intracardiac pressures with pulmonary and circulatory congestion resulting from the inability of the heart to meet the elevated demand for systemic blood flow, even though cardiac output may remain normal or above normal.

Diastolic heart failure

With the advent of routine noninvasive testing in patients with symptoms of congestive heart failure, it has become apparent that 20% or more of patients presenting with symptoms and signs of heart failure have preserved left ventricular systolic function [18–21]. While some of these patients may have pulmonary disease or other conditions causing these symptoms, the majority probably have underlying left ventricular diastolic dysfunction secondary to decreased left ventricular compliance or increased myocardial stiffness. Hemodynamically, this is characterized by an upward shift in the pressure–volume relationship, so that at normal left ventricular volumes, left ventricular diastolic pressures are elevated. This elevated pressure is transmitted backward to the atria and the pulmonary and systemic veins. Thus, the patient may have symptoms of pulmonary congestion and systemic edema without impairment of left ventricular contractility.

A variety of conditions can lead to diastolic dysfunction. As mentioned earlier, aging is associated with diminished left ventricular compliance and impaired diastolic filling. Chronic hypertension and left ventricular hypertrophy are probably the most common causes of diastolic dysfunction [20,22], but it also may occur in patients with diabetes or many of the infiltrative cardiomyopathies (amyloidosis is the most common type in elderly patients). Diastolic dysfunction is also the most frequent presentation of hypertrophic cardiomyopathy, whether it be obstructive or nonobstructive. The occurrence of a variant of the hypertrophic cardiomyopathy syndrome has been described in hypertensive elderly patients [23,24]. These patients, as well as many others with diastolic dysfunction, are often thought to have systolic dysfunction and are treated accordingly. As a result, it is essential that most older patients with heart failure symptoms undergo noninvasive assessment of cardiac function by echocardiography or nuclear techniques.

Right heart failure

Right heart failure is usually secondary to left heart failure and may mask the clinical presentation of the latter. Right heart failure can also result from chronic pulmonary disease, from pulmonary emboli, or rarely in adults from congenital heart diseases such as atrial septal defect, ventricular septal defect,

Ebstein's anomaly, or pulmonic stenosis. Elevated pulmonary artery pressure and arterial resistance impose an increasing afterload on the right ventricle. As contractility begins to fail, both right ventricular and right atrial volumes and pressure rise. The patient develops hepatic and splanchnic congestion and peripheral edema. Generally, stroke volume is maintained so that cardiac output is normal until the process is far advanced.

CLINICAL PRESENTATION

Left heart failure

Early in the progression of heart failure, cardiac output at rest is usually maintained in the normal range by the previously discussed compensatory mechanisms. Therefore, patients with left ventricular failure commonly first notice symptoms related to pulmonary congestion. Often, dyspnea is initially precipitated by unusual exertion and then later by normal activities. In the elderly patient, exertional breathlessness may be confused with an age-related reduction in exercise capacity. Easy fatiguability and a feeling of weakness or loss of energy are common complaints. The patient may feel anxious due to increased sympathetic activity, or may complain of cold extremities and feeling chilled as a result of peripheral vasoconstriction. Appetite may decrease due to reduced splanchnic blood flow or venous congestion. In the extreme, malnutrition may occur, producing *cardiac cachexia*. Reduced cerebral perfusion, particularly in the presence of cerebrovascular disease, may lead to altered mental status or confusion. Cheynes–Stokes respirations may be sensed by the patient as acute episodes of shortness of breath. Renal blood flow is also reduced in patients with heart failure, but this rarely leads to clinical evidence of renal dysfunction until heart failure is far advanced. Then, particularly when intravascular volume is depleted by diuretic therapy, severe azotemia and oliguria may appear.

As the reader has probably already appreciated, these symptoms of chronic heart failure are often common complaints in elderly patients who do not have cardiac disease. Thus, physicians must be attuned to the subtle manifestations of chronic heart failure, but, conversely, must also be cautious in making this diagnosis. The availability of reliable noninvasive techniques for evaluating cardiac function has removed much of this difficulty, as will be discussed later.

Right heart failure

The onset of right heart failure may be more insidious, and the patient may not be aware of an abnormality until signs of peripheral edema appear. As systemic and splanchnic venous congestion increase, the patient may become aware of increasing girth and complain of early satiety, epigastric or right upper-quadrant abdominal discomfort or pain, and nausea. Hepatic and gastrointestinal congestion may cause anorexia, increased borborygmi, flatulence, and constipation. The first indication of peripheral edema may be a change in the way a patient's shoes fit between morning and night. In later stages, edema may be extreme and associated with ascites. In spite of the previously mentioned fact that right heart failure in adults is most frequently secondary to left heart failure, elderly patients with biventricular failure may present with these right-sided signs and symptoms with few complaints referable to pulmonary congestion. In particular, this may be the case after tricuspid insufficiency develops secondary to right ventricular failure. At that point, pulmonary artery pressure falls because of the low right ventricular foward output, producing a syndrome characterized by manifestations of low cardiac output and severe right heart failure.

Acute heart failure

Acute heart failure generally involves the abrupt onset of dyspnea with concomitant signs of pulmonary edema. Not infrequently in the elderly, this may actually represent an exacerbation of previously undetected chronic heart failure; therefore, the picture may be a mixture of acute and chronic manifestations. When the precipitating cause is an acute myocardial infarction or acute valvular insufficiency, signs of low output, including hypotension and shock, may be present.

ETIOLOGY

The causes of acute and chronic heart failure in the elderly are essentially the same as in the general adult population. Most patients have underlying coronary artery disease, chronic hypertension, or both. Chronic hypertension is particularly common in older patients and is the most common etiology of diastolic dysfunction. Diabetes (which also often causes diastolic dysfunction), valvular heart disease, and various cardiomyopathies are also fairly commonly involved. However, other etiologies amenable to specific, possibly even curative, therapy must be carefully searched for.

Acute heart failure

The first group of etiologies to be considered are those that produce acute heart failure. They are listed in table 6-2.

Acute myocardial infarction

Acute myocardial infarction is the most likely cause of sudden cardiac decompensation. "Silent" myocardial infarctions presenting as acute heart failure are more common in elderly patients [25,26]. When myocardial infarction is complicated by either pulmonary edema or a low-output state, the prognosis is grave, particularly in the elderly patient. Mechanical defects such as mitral insufficiency from papillary muscle rupture or dysfunction and ventricular septal defect may be present in some patients with acute postinfarction decompensation. In appropriately selected individuals, surgical

Table 6-2. Causes of acute heart failure

Acute myocardial infarction
    Pump failure due to extensive myocardial necrosis
    Acquired mitral regurgitation
    Acquired ventricular septal defect
Ischemic left ventricular paralysis
Acute valvular insufficiency
    Bacterial endocarditis
    Aortic dissection
    Ruptured chordae tendinae
    Trauma
Arrhythmias
    Complete heart block
    Sick sinus syndrome
    Supraventricular tachycardia
    Ventricular tachycardia
Hypertensive crisis
Acute right heart failure
    Pulmonary embolus
    Right ventricular infarction
Pericardial tamponade

intervention may be successful, even with advanced age. Acute left ventricular failure due to ischemia (often called *left ventricular paralysis*) may occur in patients with severe coronary artery disease and cause little or no myocardial necrosis. This syndrome may be more common in elderly patients and is an indication for early revascularization, if feasible.

Valvular incompetence

When acute heart failure results from acute incompetence of either the aortic or mitral valves, bacterial endocarditis should be the primary consideration. The presentation of endocarditis may be initially overlooked due to the fact that elderly patients commonly have heart murmurs and may remain afebrile when infected. Other potential causes of acute valvular regurgitation include ruptured chordae tendineae, aortic dissection, and trauma.

Arrhythmias

Arrhythmias are another important cause of acute cardiac decompensation, particularly in the elderly patient with reduced cardiac reserve. Both bradyarrhythmias—for example, complete heart block or even sinus bradycardia—and tachyarrhythmias—for example, rapid atrial fibrillation or other supraventricular or ventricular tachycardias—may precipitate heart failure. In general, such patients will have underlying cardiac disease. Two classic examples of arrhythmia-induced decompensation are the patient with mitral stenosis and the patient with hyperthyroidism, who intermittently develop rapid atrial fibrillation. Atrial fibrillation may also precipitate

Table 6-3. Causes of chronic left ventricular systolic failure

Coronary artery disease with healed myocardial infarction
Chronic hypertension
Valvular heart disease
  Aortic stenosis
  Aortic or mitral regurgitation
  Mitral stenosis
Congestive cardiomyopathy
  Idiopathic
  Infectious
  Toxic (alcoholic)
  Infiltrative (amyloidosis, others)
  Miscellaneous
Myocardial dysfunction following heart surgery

pulmonary edema in patients with impaired left ventricular diastolic function, such as those with chronic hypertension or diabetes.

Acute right heart failure

If it is not secondary to left-sided decompensation, acute right heart failure is most likely due to either pulmonary emboli or right ventricular infarction. Pericardial tamponade is another, generally easily recognized cause of acute heart failure. The etiologies and clinical manifestations of pericardial disease are discussed in another chapter.

Lastly, the existence of previously unrecognized cardiac disease or an exacerbation of previously compensated failure should always be considered in evaluating a patient with acute heart failure. Infections such as pneumonia or relatively mild viral illnesses are poorly tolerated in older patients with heart disease. Dietary indiscretion, discontinuation of medicines, or a change in therapy that promotes sodium retention may also produce sudden decompensation.

Chronic left heart failure

Most patients with chronic congestive heart failure have the syndrome of left heart failure, generally due to impaired left ventricular function. The major entities producing this picture are listed in table 6-3.

Coronary artery disease

The most common cause of left ventricular dysfunction is coronary artery disease with extensive myocardial infarction. Heart failure may occur after a single large infarction (almost invariably one that involves the anterior wall), or it may have a gradual onset because of several small or moderate episodes of necrosis. In general, the diagnosis of ischemic heart disease can be made from the history and electrocardiogram. However, autopsy studies reveal that unrecognized, perhaps asymptomatic, coronary artery disease has a higher prevalence in the aged population than is clinically apparent [27,28]. Additionally, multiple small scars may be present at postmortem in patients with extensive coronary artery disease who do not have clinical histories of infarction.

Arterial hypertension

Arterial hypertension is another major etiology of heart failure. In the Framingham study, hypertension was present as either the primary cause or as an exacerbating factor in approximately 75% of patients who developed congestive heart failure [29]. As a result of the current aggressive approach to detection and treatment of hypertension, its etiologic role has diminished. Nonetheless, "burnt-out" hypertension is probably responsible for left ventricular failure in some elderly patients who exhibit normal blood pressure. Perhaps more commonly, heart failure in the elderly hypertensive patient is due to diastolic dysfunction.

Valvular heart disease

Valvular heart disease remains an important cause of left heart failure in the elderly, although acute rheumatic fever and rheumatic heart disease are rare in younger native-born Americans. Aortic stenosis, most frequently secondary to calcific degenerative changes in normal valves, is the most common valvular pathology. Because of the growing prevalence of calcific aortic stenosis, the mean age at presentation with this lesion has risen from 48 to 61 years [30,31]. Rheumatic disease or congenitally bicuspid valves may also progress to severe stenosis. The clinical presentation of aortic stenosis in the elderly may be insidious, and the physical signs are often difficult to evaluate. Nevertheless, the diagnosis should be diligently pursued, to the point of cardiac catheterization in many patients, since valve replacement may dramatically improve cardiac function.

The volume overload that accompanies chronic aortic or mitral insufficiency may ultimately cause a deterioration in left ventricular function and consequent left heart failure. At that point, surgery entails added risk and, even if successful, may not improve left ventricular function. Unfortunately, no reliable method exists for determining the optimum timing for valve replacement in order to preserve myocardial function, but progression to irreversible left ventricular dysfunction is rare in isolated aortic insufficiency if the patient is followed carefully to detect the onset of symptoms and declining ejection fraction. Prophylactic surgery in asymptomatic or mildly symptomatic patients can be justified in younger patients; it is, however, more problematic in the elderly. Mitral stenosis has become uncommon in the elderly, but an occasional case of "silent" mitral stenosis may appear, particularly in immigrant groups. These persons may have signs of predominant right heart failure, in spite of their high left atrial pressures. Left atrial myxoma may mimic mitral stenosis and present with acute or chronic dyspnea.

Congenital abnormalities

It is unusual for congenital abnormalities to present initially in older patients. The one exception is atrial septal defect, which may be first recognized in the seventh or even eighth decade of life. These patients usually have secundum defects with moderate-size shunts, characterized by a pulmonic to systemic flow ratio of approximately 2. They present with dyspnea and often atrial fibrillation. If pulmonary hypertension is not severe, surgery is usually successful in eliminating heart failure. In the future, more patients with corrected congenital heart disease will live to old age. These patients will require management by physicians with expertise in this area.

Primary cardiomyopathy

The final category of entities producing left heart failure is that of primary myocardial disease with associated congestive cardiomyopathy [32,33]. These patients usually are first seen in biventricular congestive heart failure of insidious onset. Because no etiology is immediately apparent, they are often given the diagnosis of idiopathic cardiomyopathy. Although a number of etiologies are discussed below, most causes of primary cardiomyopathy are not amenable to specific therapy, and consequently, extensive diagnostic workup is not warranted in most older patients.

VIRAL MYOCARDITIS. Viral myocarditis is usually diagnosed clinically when cardiac decompensation follows the acute manifestations of a viral illness by several weeks. However, since a comprehensive history in patients with heart failure of recent onset often reveals signs and symptoms suggestive of a nonspecific viral illness in the recent past, the diagnosis must be confirmed by a rise in antibody titers to a virus known to produce myocarditis. Although many viruses can involve the heart, coxsackie viruses and echovirus are the principal causes of viral myocarditis. Nonviral infectious myocarditis is extremely rare. Some workers advocate myocardial biopsy followed by corticosteroid or immunosuppressive therapy in patients with myocarditis with ongoing acute immune responses. At this time, this approach should be considered experimental and is best avoided in the elderly, who are less likely to have histologic evidence of active myocarditis.

ALCOHOLIC CARDIOMYOPATHY. The only important toxic myopathy, alcoholic cardiomyopathy, is uncommon in the elderly, occurring mainly in young or middle-aged men. The diagnosis is based on a history of heavy ethanol intake, a picture of left-sided or biventricular heart failure, and the exclusion of other etiologies. Unlike in most cardiomyopathies, myocardial function may recover dramatically following a period of abstinence, especially if the onset of failure has been acute.

INFILTRATIVE CARDIOMYOPATHIES. Infiltrative cardiomyopathies comprise a heterogeneous group of entities, some of which are of relevance to the elderly. Amyloidosis, in particular, has been considered a disease of the elderly, and some believe it to be a part of the aging process [32–34]. Amyloidosis is characterized by the deposition in various tissues of eosinophilic fibrous protein, which is related to antibody light chains. There are four recognized forms, with some degree of overlap. *Familial amyloidosis* is an uncommon disorder typified by little cardiac involvement. *Primary amyloidosis* is characterized by involvement of the heart, gastrointestinal tract, nerves, skin, and tongue, and is not preceded or accompanied by other systemic diseases. It appears to be a primary disorder of antibody formation or metabolism related to multiple myeloma. Cardiac involvement is a common and often the predominant manifestation. *Secondary amyloidosis* occurs as a late complication of chronic inflammatory disease and is characterized by protein deposition in the reticuloendothelial system, including the liver, spleen, and kidney. Cardiac involvement is uncommon and seldom clinically apparent. *Senile amyloidosis* is the most perplexing in terms of its pathophysiologic and clinical significance. The prevalence and extent of cardiac amyloid deposition on pathologic examination increases with age and exceeds 10% for persons older than 75 years. The composition of the fibrillar protein differs from that in other forms of amyloidosis. However, clinical cardiac disease is uncommon, even in persons with prominent amyloid deposition in the left ventricular myocardium.

The most common manifestation of cardiac amyloidosis is a congestive cardiomyopathy with biventricular failure. Less frequently, the presentation is one of a restrictive cardiomyopathy with predominant right-sided findings and normal heart size. Conduction-system involvement is common in either form and may be the only clinical manifestation of cardiac involvement. The diagnosis can be made by rectal or gingival biopsy, as well as by right ventricular endocardial biopsy, but no specific treatment is available.

Other infiltrative cardiomyopathies that may affect the elderly include hemochromatosis, sarcoidosis, and Loeffler's endocarditis, although all are unusual. Many other processes may produce left heart failure in rare instances, including hypothyroidism, acromegaly, oxalosis, metastatic calcification in uremia, porphyria, Whipple's disease, endomyocardial fibrosis, and hematologic malignancies. Usually, the underlying disorder is apparent in these cases.

High-output heart failure

Manifestations of congestive heart failure may occur in the absence of primary cardiac pathology in the presence of increased metabolic or hemodynamic demands. Most often in the elderly, decompensation occurs when excessive demand is superimposed on existing left ventricular dysfunction or valvular abnormalities. A number of entities associated with high-output states are listed in table 6-4.

Table 6-4. High-output states
that produce or exacerbate heart failure

Thyrotoxicosis
Anemia
Infection
Renal disease
Systemic arteriovenous fistulas
Paget's disease
Kaposi's sarcoma
Beriberi heart disease

Thyrotoxicosis

Thyrotoxicosis is the most common of these disorders [35,36]. Since it may be difficult to recognize and is easily treated, is should be carefully excluded in elderly patients with heart failure. Thyrotoxicosis produces a high-output state because of increased metabolic demands, increased requirements for heat dissipation, direct effects of thyroid hormone on peripheral vessels producing vasodilatation, direct effects on the myocardium augmenting myocardial contractility, and a facilitating effect of thyroid hormone on adrenergic stimuli. Excessive thyroid hormone does not appear to produce any direct toxic effects on the heart. Cardiovascular decompensation occurs predominantly in patients with underlying heart disease or when rapid atrial fibrillation supervenes. Although the classic presentation of hyperthyroidism is easy to recognize, many of the usual clinical manifestations may be absent in elderly patients, particularly in those with autonomous hyperfunctioning adenomas. The descriptive phrase *apathetic hyperthyroidism* is often applied to the elderly patient who presents with unexplained heart failure, usually with rapid atrial fibrillation and few other clues to thyrotoxicosis.

Chronic anemia

Severe chronic anemia, usually with a hematocrit below 20%, may produce high-output heart failure. This commonly occurs with hemoglobinopathies in younger patients and with pernicious anemia, chronic blood loss, or blood dyscrasias in older patients. Cardiac decompensation probably occurs both because of the excessive peripheral demand for blood flow and because of impaired cardiac reserve resulting from limitation of myocardial oxygen supply. In the elderly, anemia is most frequently an exacerbating factor. Especially in patients with obstructive coronary artery disease, the reduced oxygen-carrying capacity in the presence of limited coronary blood flow may produce ischemia and left ventricular dysfunction.

Other causes of high-output failure

Increased cardiac output may occur in hepatic disease as a result of arteriovenous shunting and in renal failure as a result of hypervolemia and anemia. Similarly, systemic arteriovenous fistulas may markedly reduce peripheral resistance and lead to high-output states. These fistulas may be hereditary, as in hereditary hemorrhagic telangiectasia (Osler–Weber–Rendu syndrome), or acquired, as with hemodialysis shunts. A more subtle cause of increased peripheral blood flow may occur in Paget's disease, which is fairly common in patients older than 65 years. Involved bone is extremely vascular, with flow increasing as much as nine times normal. Invariably, alkaline phosphatase levels will be high in persons with high cardiac output states secondary to Paget's disease. Extremely high flows can also occur through the skin in dermatologic diseases such as Kaposi's sarcoma and psoriasis.

The classic syndrome of high-output heart failure is beriberi heart disease, which results from chronic thiamine deficiency. Patients with this entity have extremely low peripheral vascular resistance and correspondingly high cardiac outputs. The cardiac pathology in this disease is unremarkable, strongly suggesting that the primary abnormality is the excessively high cardiac output requirement. Fulminant beriberi heart disease has become an arcane diagnosis in the United States, but latent thiamine deficiency may be present in some malnourished elderly persons.

Chronic right heart failure

In most cases, right heart failure in the elderly is a late manifestation of left-sided failure. Chronic left atrial hypertension leads to pulmonary hypertension and ultimately to right ventricular failure in response to this pressure overload. Manifestations of right-sided failure may occur earlier when the underlying disease affects the right ventricle directly, as in some patients with coronary artery disease or cardiomyopathies. Tricuspid regurgitation may develop as a result of right ventricular dilatation. The combination of pulmonary hypertension and tricuspid incompetence usually results in a low cardiac output, with a consequent reduction in left-sided pressures. In such patients, symptoms of dyspnea and signs of left heart failure may abate, giving the appearance of isolated right heart dysfunction. So-called silent mitral stenosis may present in this manner. Thus, it is important to evaluate the left ventricle and the mitral valve in patients with unexplained right-sided failure.

Other causes of chronic right heart failure are listed in table 6-5. Cor pulmonale secondary to pulmonary parenchymal disease is the most common etiology. In the elderly, chronic obstructive pulmonary disease, particularly the bronchitic form, is the most frequent underlying pathology. The various entities producing hypoventilation and chronic or intermittent hypoxemia may also lead to right heart failure. These include neuromuscular disorders, chest wall abnormalities, the obesity-hypoventilation syndrome, the sleep-apnea syndrome, and upper airway obstruction. A number of these diagnoses should be considered in elderly patients.

Although primary pulmonary vascular disease is uncommon in older

Table 6-5. Causes of chronic right heart failure

Left heart failure
Pulmonary parenchymal disease
Hypoventilation syndromes
Pulmonary vascular disease
   Pulmonary embolic disease
   Eisenmenger's syndrome
Right ventricular dysfunction
   Right ventricular infarction
   Cardiomyopathy
Valvular abnormalities

Table 6-6. Diastolic dysfunction of the heart

Restrictive cardiomyopathy
   Amyloid heart disease
   Postoperative left ventricular dysfunction
   Postradiation myocarditis
   Miscellaneous infiltrative processes
Excessive left ventricular hypertrophy
   Hypertrophic cardiomyopathy
   Chronic hypertension
Pericardial disease
   Tamponade
   Constrictive pericarditis

patients, recurrent pulmonary emboli may lead to right-sided failure. Occasionally, patients with congenital left-to-right shunts and resultant pulmonary vascular disease will develop symptoms at an older age.

Most diseases that affect the left ventricle can involve the right ventricle as well, and sometimes right-sided signs predominate. This may be the case in rare patients with coronary disease who experience right ventricular infarction. It also may occur in the infiltrative cardiomyopathies. The pulmonary and tricuspid valves may also be affected by pathologic processes, such as infectious endocarditis or carcinoid heart disease. The latter syndrome has a predilection for the right side of the heart, since the circulating serotonin released by bowel tumors and hepatic metastases is inactivated by the lung. The major clinical manifestations of cardiac involvement are tricuspid regurgitation and pulmonic stenosis.

Diastolic dysfunction of the heart

This category includes a number of entities whose common feature is impaired filling or abnormally high diastolic pressure in either side of the heart (table 6-6).

Restrictive cardiomyopathy

The term *restrictive cardiomyopathy* is used to describe patients whose primary derangement is impairment of diastolic filling resulting from increased ventricular stiffness. While patients with these syndromes may have concomitant systolic dysfunction, it is not the major abnormality. Generally, the underlying pathology is an infiltrative cardiomyopathy or extensive left ventricular fibrosis. The characteristic hemodynamic feature of restrictive cardiomyopathy is the deep and rapid decline in the ventricular pressure in early diastole, followed by a rapid rise to a high plateau (the "square root sign"). Correspondingly, the jugular venous pulse reveals a prominent atrial wave and Y-descent. The clinical presentation may involve predominantly the right or left side of the heart.

Amyloid heart disease

Amyloid heart disease is the most common cause of restrictive cardiomyopathy, although it more frequently presents as a congestive cardiomyopathy (see above). Occasionally, patients who have undergone open heart surgery may develop a picture of restriction months or years later. Similarly, patients who have undergone extensive mediastinal radiation may exhibit a restrictive cardiomyopathy. Since both of these latter processes also cause constrictive pericarditis, the differential diagnosis is problematic; sometimes, exploratory surgery is required. Indeed, pericardial and myocardial abnormalities may coexist.

Diabetic cardiomyopathy

Some patients with diabetic cardiomyopathy also have a restrictive picture, with small hearts and high filling pressures. The underlying pathology in these patients appears to be patchy fibrosis of the left ventricle, especially in the subendocardium, probably a result of multiple small infarcts.

Hypertrophic cardiomyopathy

Another cause of left heart failure that has been noted with increased frequency in the elderly is hypertrophic cardiomyopathy [23,24]. Approximately one third of the patients with this entity are older than 60 years of age. Two types of hypertrophic cardiomyopathy are recognized: the obstructive and the nonobstructive forms. In the former, a variable pressure gradient is produced during systole by encroachment of the hypertrophied septum and the mitral valve apparatus into the aortic outflow tract. However, even when signs of obstruction are present, it is now thought that most symptoms relate to increased chamber stiffness from the hypertrophy. Dyspnea is usually the primary symptom. Patients may also experience syncope, angina, and less frequently, over congestive heart failure. Those with obstruction have a systolic murmur, which may be confused with valvular heart disease. Echocardiography provides the most reliable means of diagnosis.

Other processes that impair cardiac diastolic performance involve the pericardium (see chapter 14). Briefly, they can be categorized into those that cause collection of fluid in the pericardial sac, leading to tamponade, and those that lead to pericardial fibrosis, contraction, and calcification, producing constriction of the heart.

In either case, atrial and ventricular diastolic pressures are elevated. In tamponade, the clinical presentation is dominated by the reduced stroke volume and cardiac output resulting from impaired cardiac filling, leading ultimately to hypotension and vascular collapse. In constrictive pericarditis, the clinical picture is predominantly one of high filling pressures. As mentioned previously, differentiation of constrictive pericarditis and restrictive cardiomyopathy can be difficult or impossible without surgical exploration.

DIAGNOSTIC EVALUATION

In evaluating a patient with suspected heart failure, the physician should follow the usual procedures of history taking, physical examination, and diagnostic testing [37]. In this process, three major questions must be addressed: 1) Are the patient's symptoms due to heart failure? 2) If so, what is the likely cause? 3) Is the underlying pathology reversible, and is specific therapy available?

Medical history

The classic symptomatology of left heart failure consists of progressive exertional dyspnea, paroxysmal nocturnal dyspnea, and orthopnea. Nocturia is usually a concurrent symptom, and dependent edema may later develop. In advanced heart failure, fatigue, loss of appetite, and dysfunction of other organ systems may be noted. If this picture is present, the diagnosis is apparent.

Elderly patients, however, may not experience exertional dyspnea if their activity is limited. Orthopnea and paroxysmal nocturnal dyspnea may not occur because of compensatory pulmonary vascular changes in response to chronically elevated pulmonary venous volume and pressure. Instead, the elderly patient may complain of a chronic dry cough and easy fatiguability. In fact, it is not uncommon to see patients who have a few nonspecific complaints with physical findings of advanced heart failure. Conversely, shortness of breath, fatigue, and nocturia are not pathognomonic for heart failure and can be common complaints in the elderly. The patient may have pulmonary disease, diabetes, a lingering viral illness, or no specific diagnosis. In such cases, the physical examination and special diagnostic tests are critical.

If the diagnosis of heart failure is made, it is important to establish its duration and whether any acute exacerbating factors are present. Has the patient had a recent myocardial infarction, infection, or other illness? Has there been a change in the diet or medications? Often, an elderly patient's cardiac status will improve with the restoration of other medical problems.

Physical examination

The elderly patient with possible heart failure should be examined thoroughly, to detect subtle cardiovascular abnormalities, as well as accompanying or alternative disorders. Unfortunately, some physical findings may be difficult to interpret in the elderly. In chronic heart failure, some of the expected signs are obscure, and other signs that are remarkable in younger patients may go unnoticed in older patients.

In general, the patient with mild or moderate heart failure has normal vital signs and is comfortable at rest. Even patients with severe cardiac dysfunction may adapt to chronically elevated pulmonary venous pressure at rest. Patients who have resting tachycardia or hypotension and those who are dyspneic at rest are either acutely ill, poorly compensated, or have other diagnoses. Resting tachycardia should raise the question of thyrotoxicosis. Severe bradycardia may itself be the cause of failure. A narrow pulse pressure may be evidence of pericardial tamponade as well as myocardial or valvular disease, and pulsus paradoxus should be sought. Dyspnea at rest should always raise the question of pulmonary disease. Cheynes–Stokes respiration may be a sign of low cardiac output or may signify central nervous system disease. Cachexia may be the result of severe heart failure, or it may indicate other serious pathology.

Age-related arteriosclerotic changes in the aorta and peripheral arteries may make pulse palpation difficult. The carotid pulse, in particular, may be misleading, since the stiffness of the arterial wall amplifies the pressure wave and obscures abnormalities in the pulse contour. Thus, in aortic stenosis the characteristic slow upstroke and anacrotic shoulder may be replaced by an apparently normal pulse. Conversely, the decreased pulse amplitude sometimes noted in low-output states may be produced by atherosclerotic involvement of the carotids. Nonetheless, findings such as pulsus alternans or the *pulsus tardus et parvus* in aortic stenosis retain their diagnostic value.

Inspection of the jugular venous pulse provides useful information concerning right atrial pressure. Elevated pressure suggests right heart failure, although it provides little insight into left-sided filling pressure. A prominent A-wave may indicate pulmonary hypertension, while a dominant V-wave suggests tricuspid regurgitation. Kussmaul's sign or an exaggerated Y-descent should raise the question of a restrictive cardiomyopathy or constrictive pericarditis.

Pulmonary rales are a common but nonspecific finding in congestive heart failure, although their absence does not exclude chronic left ventricular failure. Wheezing may be a sign of heart failure, but it should alert the examiner to the possibility of lung disease. Pleural effusions are also common in heart failure, but again are nonspecific for diagnosis.

The location and size of the apical impulse can provide useful information about left ventricular size and function. A parasternal lift is a valuable sign of significant pulmonary hypertension. Often, a second left ventricular impulse alerts the examiner to the presence of a segmental wall motion abnormality. A systolic thrill felt at the base of the heart or over the sternum supports the significance of an aortic stenosis murmur. A soft S_1 suggests myocardial dysfunction, while a loud S_1 may be the only indication of silent mitral stenosis. A single or paradoxically split S_2 may indicate significant aortic stenosis, long-standing hypertension, or other left ventricular dysfunction. A P_2 that is louder than A_2 strongly suggests pulmonary hypertension. An S_3 gallop is always abnormal in the older patient and suggests left ventricular failure or abnormal early diastolic filling of the left ventricle, as occurs with mitral insufficiency or with very slow heart rates. However, an S_3 may be absent, even with severe left ventricular dysfunction. An S_4 gallop is relatively nonspecific in the older patient. Heart murmurs in the elderly carry much the same significance as those in other age groups. However, aortic flow murmurs are quite common in elderly patients, especially in those with chronic hypertension, and may simply indicate degenerative changes in the valve. Similarly, mitral systolic murmurs may be caused by calcification of the mitral annulus. Also, there is a tendency for aortic stenosis murmurs to radiate to the apex where, in fact, the murmur is most prominent in nearly 50% of patients.

Hepatosplenomegaly and ascites may be signs of right-sided failure. A pulsatile liver during quiet, held expiration suggests tricuspid regurgitation, even if not auscultated. Splenomegaly, particularly in patients without right heart failure, may be a sign of subacute bacterial endocarditis. Peripheral edema is a common, though nonspecific, finding in heart failure.

Routine laboratory testing

Routine laboratory testing should include a complete blood count, chemistry battery, and urinalysis. The blood count may reveal anemia or polycythemia, and the white count will alert the physician to hematologic or infectious disease. The serum electrolytes, urea nitrogen, and creatinine will characterize the patient's renal function, which may be important for both diagnosis and therapy. Similarly, it will help to characterize hepatic function and detect diabetes, Paget's disease, and severe hypercalcemia. Thyroid function should be evaluated in most elderly patients with heart failure, especially if they are in atrial fibrillation, in order to detect the occasional unsuspected case of thyrotoxicosis or myxedema.

ECG

An electrocardiogram may establish the diagnosis of coronary artery disease by revealing acute or old myocardial infarction. Left ventricular hypertrophy is a nonspecific finding, since it is present in hypertrophic cardiomyopathy, aortic stenosis, and chronic hypertension, and in many patients with congestive cardiomyopathy. However, the absence of any evidence of left ventricular hypertrophy is strong evidence against the first two of these etiologies. The simultaneous occurrence of a variety of conduction abnormalities raises the possibility of an infiltrative process. Right ventricular hypertrophy is an important finding in patients with right heart failure. The cardiac rhythm is also important. Not only are supraventricular tachycardias a frequent precipitating factor in heart failure, but they should raise suspicion that thyrotoxicosis or silent mitral stenosis is the underlying cause.

Chest x-ray

Although the chest x-ray is no longer the method of choice to measure chamber size and function, it provides much useful data. Coexisting pulmonary disease can be detected, and the pulmonary vasculature can be assessed. The presence of valvular calcification may be helpful, and a globular configuration of the cardiac silhouette raises the possibility of pericardial effusion.

Special diagnostic tests

The availability of new methods for noninvasively evaluating the heart has markedly affected the evaluation of heart failure. Now the presence or absence of heart failure can be established with near certainty without invasive measurements. Furthermore, many of the causes of heart failure that are amenable to specific therapy can be detected.

Echocardiography

Echocardiography is the most useful technique in this setting and should be considered a routine test in most older patients with heart failure unless the diagnosis and etiology are readily apparent. Because echocardiography can reveal the size of the various cardiac chambers and the function of the two ventricles, it can help determine whether the clinical picture is one of left heart or isolated right heart failure. If contractility is apparently normal or even hyperkinetic, high-output failure should be considered. Echocardiography is diagnostic in hypertrophic cardiomyopathy and in pericardial effusion, and it can point the physician toward the diagnosis of restrictive cardiomyopathy. It can also help the physician recognize a number of treatable forms of left heart failure, including valvular disease and hypertrophic cardiomyopathy. Doppler echocardiography provides a rough assessment of left ventricular *diastolic filling*, but delayed filling is common in the elderly and is not necessarily evidence for *clinically significant diastolic dysfunction*.

Radionuclide studies

Radionuclide ventriculography is another technique that is useful in assessing global and segmental left ventricular function, both at rest and during exercise.

This technique is especially helpful in patients with chronic pulmonary disease, where it may be technically difficult to obtain echocardiographic studies of suitable quality. Radionuclide ventriculography can also assess right ventricular function.

Stress testing

Various approaches to stress testing may be very helpful in evaluating the elderly patient with heart failure. Ischemic left ventricular dysfunction is an important, potentially treatable cause of left ventricular failure. Typical angina pectoris may not be present in these patients. Thus, when symptoms are episodic and baseline left ventricular function is relatively preserved (ejection fraction above 30% to 35%), further diagnostic testing is warranted. Exercise electrocardiography may be adequate if the patient has been relatively active and has a relatively normal resting electrocardiogram. In many cases, associated myocardial perfusion scintigraphy with thallium[201] or the newer technetium-based tracers will provide additional information about the location and extent of ischemia. An assessment of left ventricular function with exercise, by either radionuclide angiography or echocardiography, may be particularly helpful. Since many elderly patients will be unable to exercise adequately, if at all, pharmacologic stress testing may be required. The most common approaches are to perform thallium[201] scintigraphy following the infusion of either intravenous dipyridamole or adenosine. In some patients, particularly those with valvular heart disease, quantitation of exercise tolerance may be helpful in objectively quantifying symptoms and in determining therapy. Thus, poor exercise tolerance or a progressive decline in exercise capacity may be an indication for valve replacement. Serial measurements of exercise tolerance may also be helpful in assessing the response to therapy.

Catheterization

With the availability of noninvasive tests, cardiac catheterization should generally be reserved for patients being considered for cardiac surgery. Especially in elderly patients, the risk of catheterization must be weighed against the benefits of the procedure. Right heart catheterization may be necessary to establish the diagnosis of heart failure in patients with pulmonary disease and to identify high-output states. Right heart catheterization is often essential in the management of acute heart failure, since therapy is generally guided by serial measurements of cardiac output and left ventricular filling pressure.

Left heart catheterization is usually performed primarily to evaluate the significance of valvular lesions or to exclude coronary disease. The patient with aortic valve disease and left ventricular failure, even if severe, is usually a candidate for hemodynamic evaluation and valve replacement. Mitral insufficiency, if associated with symptoms of heart failure or progressive left ventricular dilatation or dysfunction, should also be considered an indication for surgery, although the risk becomes high when left ventricular dysfunction is severe. With the availability of percutaneous coronary angioplasty, revascularization has become more feasible in the elderly patient in whom ischemia may be playing a role. Coronary artery bypass grafting should also be considered in the elderly when episodic ischemic heart failure is thought to be occurring. Results of aneurysmectomy for intractable heart failure have been disappointing, and this procedure should be considered a therapy of last resort.

THERAPY

The goals of therapy in patients with heart failure are threefold: 1) correction of the underlying abnormality; 2) reversal of precipitating or exacerbating factors; and 3) achievement of hemodynamic and symptomatic improvement.

Identification of reversible causes

As has been noted previously, most elderly patients have heart failure secondary to chronic left ventricular dysfunction for which there is no curative treatment. Nonetheless, the minority with correctable lesions, such as valvular disease, thyrotoxicosis and other high-output states, and pericardial disease, should be diligently sought using the approach discussed in the previous section. The question as to whether cardiac surgery is feasible in the elderly must be approached on an individual basis and is often affected more by the patient's general state of health and life-style than by the cardiac pathology itself. Certainly, the risks of surgery are increased in patients above 70 years of age, but the risk-to-benefit ratio must be considered [38]. Aortic stenosis is one entity in which valve replacement has proven feasible and relatively successful in the elderly, even in the presence of severe left ventricular dysfunction. The results are less optimal in patients with valvular regurgitation once ventricular function has begun to deteriorate.

Heart failure secondary to left ventricular diastolic dysfunction may be reversible in some cases, but for the most part treatment is also symptomatic. In patients with hypertensive left ventricular hypertrophy, therapy should be directed toward regression of left ventricular mass. Blood pressure control is the first priority, but some data indicate that certain classes of agents may be more successful in reversing left ventricular hypertrophy, at least in the short run. These include the nondihydropyridine calcium-channel blockers and the angiotensin-converting enzyme inhibitors. One study has shown an improvement in symptoms and exercise capacity in patients with heart failure secondary to diastolic dysfunction treated with verapamil [39].

The second goal, removal of precipitating factors, is especially important in the elderly, since their cardiac reserve is often marginal. Thus, the patient should be questioned about dietary or medication changes and about changes in activity or living environment. Infectious processes, such as bronchitis or urinary tract infections, should be sought. Increases in blood pressure, even if modest, and either bradyarrhythmias or tachyarrhythmias may also exacerbate cardiac dysfunction.

Pharmacologic therapy

Once it has been established that the cause of heart failure is not curable, therapy must be directed toward achieving hemodynamic and functional improvement, preventing progressive cardiac dysfunction, and prolonging survival. The management of congestive heart failure has recently been extensively reviewed [37]. Three avenues of medical therapy are available: 1) medications or dietary changes that reduce fluid and salt retention; 2) medications that improve the heart's contractile performance; and 3) medications and activity restriction that reduce the workload of the heart. A series of large trials has clearly demonstrated that treatment with angiotensin-converting enzyme inhibitors prolongs survival in patients with both severe and mild-to-moderate congestive heart failure. Even patients with asymptomatic left ventricular dysfunction, or minimal symptoms, have a lesser rate of progression to more severe degrees of heart failure when they are treated with these agents. Other vasodilators may have the same beneficial effects, but probably not to the degree of a converting enzyme inhibitor. The use of other therapeutic approaches should be guided by the severity of the hemodynamic derangement and the needs of the individual patient. The patient who is symptomatic only with moderate or strenuous exertion may be treated by dietary sodium restriction or a thiazide diuretic if he or she is comfortable with a more limited life-style. If the patient desires to return to more vigorous activity, more aggressive therapy may be needed. On the other hand, the patient with a severe low-output syndrome may require monitoring in the intensive care unit and intravenous medications.

While the modalities of therapy used in the elderly are the same as those used in younger patients, they are employed somewhat differently. When possible within the clinical context, therapy should be undertaken more gradually and judiciously in the elderly patient, since it may not be necessary to achieve the same degree of hemodynamic normalization in older persons with more limited activity levels, and they may be considerably less able to tolerate iatrogenic complications. In addition, age-related decreases in renal and hepatic function may require downward adjustment of drug dosages.

Diuretics

Diuretics have become the mainstay of therapy in patients with symptomatic heart failure. While sodium restriction is helpful in preventing or reducing fluid retention, compliance is often poor, and the diuretics now available can generally compensate for excessive salt intake. Since most patients with heart failure are symptomatic predominantly because of their high ventricular filling pressures, diuretics are usually the most efficacious therapeutic modality. Those with mild heart failure can often be managed with a thiazide agent alone. Patients with more advanced disease and those with renal dysfunction often require more potent "loop" diuretics, such as furosemide or bumetanide. Patients with severe decompensation may respond only to a combined regimen of a loop diuretic and metolazone, a long-acting agent that acts primarily on the proximal tubule, although this approach must be undertaken very cautiously. With the agents currently available, adequate diuresis can be induced in almost all patients with heart failure. As a result, more patients now demonstrate signs of low cardiac output and depleted intravascular volume, such as prerenal azotemia, and fewer complaints of dyspnea. Serial measurements of body weight may be invaluable in managing patients with severe heart failure on potent diuretics. It is also essential to monitor serum potassium and sodium closely in all elderly patients on diuretics, since these patients are predisposed to diuretic-induced hypokalemia and hyponatremia.

Although the idea of substituting the converting enzyme inhibitor for maintenance diuretic therapy is attractive, it is rarely successful in patients with documented left ventricular systolic dysfunction and signs and symptoms of fluid retention [40,41]. However, even in elderly patients, it is often desirable to add converting enzyme inhibitors to diuretics in order to minimize the diuretic dosage, prevent electrolyte imbalance, and accomplish the additional goals of preventing progressive left ventricular dysfunction and mortality.

Digitalis

The only medication currently available that improves cardiac contractility is digitalis and its derivatives. Digoxin is the most widely employed preparation. In most patients with left ventricular dysfunction, digoxin has a positive inotropic effect, which results in an increase in stroke volume and a reduction in left ventricular filling pressure.

The efficacy of digoxin in patients with chronic heart failure has been questioned, but recent data confirm its long-term beneficial effects in individuals with well-documented left ventricular dilitation and dysfunction [42]. In a comparison trial of captopril and digoxin in patients with mild and moderate heart failure, digoxin reduced the need for additional diuretic therapy and prevented hospitalizations and emergency room visits for heart failure [43]. If anything, digoxin was better tolerated than the angiotensin-converting enzyme inhibitor. In a second trial, in which the efficacy of digoxin and a new inotropic agent, milrinone, were compared, the group of patients in whom digoxin was withdrawn experienced a three-fold greater rate of clinical deterioration than those in whom digoxin was continued [44]. The effect of digoxin on survival has not been assessed, but a large multicenter trial is ongoing that should answer this question. In the meantime, digoxin should be utilized in patients who remain symptomatic on diuretics and angiotensin-converting enzyme inhibitors, and should be considered an alternative to the latter agents when they are contra-indicated.

The dosage of digoxin must be adjusted for body size and renal function. The patient who weighs 60 to 90 kg and has a serum creatinine below 1.3 mg/dl or a creatinine clearance greater than 50 cc per hour usually can be treated with 0.25 mg a day. A steady-state serum drug level will be achieved after about a week when renal function is normal. The serum digoxin level should be checked at that point, particularly in the elderly, who more often exhibit digoxin toxicity. Some writers have thought that advanced age itself predisposes patients to digitalis toxicity, but this propensity probably reflects reduced renal function, severe cardiac disease, or the multiple drug regimens that characterize many elderly patients. It is important to note that elderly patients may have significantly reduced renal function in the face of normal serum creatinine levels due to the reduction in lean body (muscle) mass. If the initial dosage is kept low, the digoxin level is checked, and serum potassium is maintained in the high-normal range, digitalis toxicity can usually be avoided.

Angiotensin-converting enzyme inhibitors

Over the past decade, the angiotensin-converting enzyme (ACE) inhibitors have been evaluated in a number of clinical trials, and as a result of their favorable outcome, the use of these agents has increased markedly. The CONSENSUS Trial [45] demonstrated that enalapril significantly reduced mortality and improved symptomatology in patients with severe heart failure, which remained refractory despite treatment with diuretics, digoxin, and other vasodilators. It is noteworthy that despite their mean age of over 70 years, these patients tolerated average dosages of nearly 20 mg per day. An earlier trial with captopril [46] also showed that ACE inhibition improved symptoms, increased exercise tolerance, and tended to prolong life in more ambulatory patients who continued to have moderate to severe symptoms despite treatment with diuretics and digitalis.

More recently, studies have indicated an important role for ACE inhibitors in patients with less severe heart failure. The Captopril–Digoxin Multicenter Study [43] showed that addition of captopril to a diuretic in patients with mild-to-moderate heart failure symptoms improved exercise capacity, reduced symptoms, and prevented episodes of deterioration when compared to a diuretic-only regimen. The SOLVD study [47] provided the strongest justification for the early and almost universal use of ACE inhibitors in patients with heart failure. This trial consisted of two arms: a treatment arm, in which over 2000 patients with symptomatic heart failure were randomly assigned to enalapril or placebo with a mortality endpoint, and a prevention arm, in which over 4000 patients with confirmed left ventricular dysfunction but no or only few symptoms of heart failure were randomized to the same treatments, with the endpoints of mortality and progression to clinically manifest heart failure. The treatment arm confirmed previous studies, demonstrating a significant reduction in mortality, as well as marked reductions in the hospitalizations for worsening heart failure. These benefits were seen across virtually all predefined subsets of patients, including those in both NYHA class II and III CHF (class IV was excluded), those with ejection fraction less than 30%, and those with ischemic as well as nonischemic cardiomyopathies. This benefit was present in older, as well as younger, patients. At this time, the results of the prevention arm have been presented but not published. A reduction in the rate of progression to heart failure, as judged by hospitalizations, was found in patients with asymptomatic left ventricular dysfunction, as determined by ejection fractions less than 35%. There was also a strong trend toward a reduction in mortality in this group, but this became apparent only after the first 18 months of follow-up. Taken together, the earlier studies and the SOLVD Trial strongly support the use of ACE inhibitors in virtually all patients with symptomatic left ventricular systolic dysfunction and also in persons with ejection fractions less than 30–35% who are not currently symptomatic.

However, as is the case with any drug, these agents must be used with caution in older patients. The major limiting side effect and adverse reactions to the ACE inhibitors are hypotension and its most common manifestations: episodic dizziness, light-headedness, and renal dysfunction. Hypotension is most common in patients who begin with relatively low systolic blood pressures (<110 mmHg), especially if they appear to have intravascular volume depletion as manifested by low jugular venous pressures, hyponatremia (serum sodium <135 mEq/L), or prerenal azotemia. In such patients, it may be helpful to hold or reduce diuretic dosing prior to initiation of ACE inhibitors. The patient should be observed for symptomatic hypotension after the initial dosage, and therefore it is most convenient to initiate captopril therapy (6.25 mg or 12.5 mg p.o.), since its peak effect will occur within 30 to 90 minutes. Renal dysfunction is most commonly associated with hypotension, since it reflects functional renal insufficiency due to inadequate renal perfusion pressure or altered intrarenal hemodynamics. Since older patients, as well as diabetics and patients taking nonsteroidal anti-inflammatory agents, are particularly predisposed to this problem, renal function should be evaluated within days to at most one week after the initiation of ACE inhibitors. Older patients also are predisposed to hyperkalemia, so care must be taken to discontinue potassium-sparing agents and potassium supplements, as least until after subsequent measurement. Despite these cautions, most older patients can tolerate the chronic use of ACE inhibitors. Indeed, given the relatively high doses of the agents utilized in the clinical studies (10 to 20 mg of enalapril daily and 25 to 50 mg of captopril three times daily), it is likely that many patients are being undertreated. In contrast, there are no studies showing that lower dosages are beneficial.

It is also important to note that while the beneficial effects of ACE inhibitors are well documented and widely advocated, these agents often cannot replace other drugs and cannot be tolerated in perhaps 10% of potential patients. Patients who have significant symptoms of heart failure and evidence of fluid retention, as manifested by peripheral edema and pulmonary congestion, usually cannot be managed by ACE inhibitors alone. In these patients, diuretic therapy should be maintained and ACE inhibition should be considered adjunctive therapy. The major trials have also made the role of digoxin somewhat unclear. While the addition of ACE inhibitors has produced clinical benefit, the use of digoxin in these studies has been variable. Since digoxin also improves symptoms and prevents clinical deterioration, it should be used in persons who remain symptomatic despite therapy with diuretics and converting enzyme inhibitors. Future studies will also be necessary to determine the specific patient subsets in which digoxin may have a beneficial effect on prognosis that is additive to that of ACE inhibitors.

Direct-acting vasodilators

With all the attention that has been directed toward the ACE inhibitors, the role of other vasodilating agents is sometimes neglected. These agents have similar favorable effects on cardiac loading conditions but lack the ability of ACE inhibitors to inhibit neurohormonal activation, which may play an important role in the pathophysiology of heart failure. Nonetheless, the first Veterans Administration Cooperative Heart Failure Trial (V–HeFT I) showed that a combination of hydralazine and isosorbide dinitrate reduced mortality in patients with NYHA class II and III heart failure who were treated with diuretics and digoxin [48]. V–HeFT II compared this combination to enalapril; although mortality was significantly reduced at the two-year follow-up point by enalapril, hydralazine and nitrates produced greater improvement in symptoms and exercise capacity [49]. A newer, direct-acting vasodilator, flosequinan, is likely to become available in the near future. Thus, these agents should be considered as alternatives to converting enzyme inhibitors when the latter are not tolerated. A future study will determine whether the combination of enalapril and a direct-acting vasodilator produces added benefit, but it seems likely that such a multidrug regimen will not be feasible in many older patients.

CONCLUSION

This chapter has emphasized several key points. Heart failure is to a large extent a disease of the elderly patient. While heart failure in the elderly is usually caused by the same processes as in other adult groups, its presentation may be more insidious and may be clouded by the presence of concomitant illnesses. Most patients will have underlying ischemic heart disease or other cardiomyopathies that impair left ventricular systolic function, but heart failure due to diastolic dysfunction is not uncommon, especially in older patients with a history of hypertension or diabetes. Therefore, noninvasive assessment of left ventricular function should usually be carried out before initiation of treatment. Although extensive further diagnostic evaluation is usually unnecessary, curable processes and exacerbating factors should be diligently sought. In particular, thyroid dysfunction, recurrent myocardial ischemia, and valvular abnormalities should be excluded. Lastly, therapy of congestive heart failure due to left ventricular systolic or diastolic dysfunction is also similar to that in younger patients, but added caution and a less aggressive approach are warranted.

REFERENCES

1. Klainer LM, Gibson TC, and White KC. 1965. The epidemiology of cardiac failure. J Chronic Dis 18:797–814.
2. Kannel WB and Belanger AJ. 1991. Epidemiology of heart failure. Am Heart J 121:951–957.
3. Waller BF and Roberts WC. 1983. Cardiovascular disease in the very elderly: Analysis of 40 necropsy patients aged 90 years or over. Am J Cardiol 51:403–422.
4. Pomerance A. 1981. Cardiac pathology in the elderly. Cardiovasc Clin 12:9–54.
5. Morley JE and Reese SS. 1989. Clinical implications of the aging heart. Am J Med 86:77–86.
6. Linzbach AJ and Akuamoa-Boateng E. 1973. The alterations of the aging human heart. I. Heart weight with progressing age. Klin Wochenschar 51:156–159.
7. Gerstenblith G, Frederiksen J, Yin FCP, et al. 1977. Echocardiographic assessment of a normal adult aging population. Circulation 56:273–278.
8. Brandfonbrener M, Landowne M, and Shock NW. 1955. Changes in cardiac output with age. Circulation 12:557–577.
9. Posner JD, Gorman KM, Klein HS, et al. 1986. Exercise capacity in the elderly. Am J Cardiol 57:52C–58C.
10. Fleg JL. 1986. Alterations in cardiovascular structure and function with advancing age. Am J Cardiol 57:33C–44C.
11. Port S, Cobb FR, Coleman RG, et al. 1980. Effect of age on the response of the left ventricular ejection fraction to exercise. N Engl J Med 303:1133–1137.
12. Rodeheffer RJ, Gerstenblith G, Becker L, et al. 1984. Exercise cardiac output is maintained in healthy human subjects: Cardiac dilation and increased stroke volume compensate for a diminished heart rate. Circulation 69:203–213.
13. Bryg RJ, Williams GA, and Labovitz AG. 1987. Effect of aging on left ventricular diastolic filling in normal subjects. Am J Cardiol 59:971–974.
14. Pearson AC, Gudipati CV, and Labovitz AJ. 1991. Effects of aging on left ventricular structure and function. Am Heart J 121:871–875.
15. Nichols WW, O'Rourke MF, Avoalio AP, et al. 1985. Effects of age on ventricular-vascular coupling. Am J Cardiol 55:1179–1184.
16. Weber KT and Janicki JS. 1989. Pathogenesis of heart failure. Cardiol Clin 7:11–24.
17. Cody RJ, Covilt AB, Schaer GL, et al. 1986. Sodium and water balance in chronic congestive heart failure. J Clin Invest 77:1441–1452.
18. Dougherty AH, Naccarelli GV, Grey EL, et al. 1984. Congestive heart failure with normal systolic function. Am J Cardiol 54:778–782.
19. Soufer R, Wohlgelernter D, Vita NA, et al. 1985. Intact systolic left ventricular function in clinical congestive heart failure. Am J Cardiol 55:1032–1036.
20. Grossman W. 1991. Diastolic dysfunction in congestive heart failure. N Engl J Med 325:1557–1564.
21. Papadakis MA and Massie BM. 1988. Appropriateness of digoxin use in medical outpatients. Am J Med 85:365–368.

22. Inouye I, Massie BM, Loge D, et al. 1984. Diastolic left ventricular dysfunction: An early finding in mild to moderate systemic hypertension. Am J Cardiol 53:120–126.
23. Krasnow N and Stein RA. 1978. Hypertrophic cardiomyopathy in the aged. Am Heart J 96:326–336.
24. Topol EJ, Traill TA, and Fortuin NJ. 1985. Hypertensive hypertrophic cardiomyopathy of the elderly. N Engl J Med 312:277–283.
25. Bayer AS, Chandha JLS, Farag RR, et al. 1986. Changing presentation of myocardial infarction with increasing old age. J Am Geriatr Soc 34:263–266.
26. Kannel WB and Abbott RD. 1984. Incidence and prognosis of unrecognized myocardial infarction: An update on the Framingham Study. N Engl J Med 311:1144–1147.
27. Rose GA and Wilson RR. 1959. Unexplained heart failure in the aged. Br Heart J 21: 511–517.
28. Pomerance A. 1965. The pathology of the heart with and without heart failure in the aged. Br Heart J 27:697–710.
29. Kannel WB. 1974. Role of blood pressure in cardiovascular morbidity and mortality. Prog Cardiovasc Dis 17:5–24.
30. Selzer A. 1987. Changing aspects of the natural history of aortic stenosis. N Engl J Med 317:91–98.
31. Lombard JT and Selzer A. 1987. Valvular aortic stenosis: clinical and hemodynamic profile of patients. Ann Intern Med 106:292–298.
32. Shaver JA (ed). 1988. Cardiomyopathies: Clinical presentation, differential diagnosis, and management. Cardiovasc Clin 19:1.
33. Perloff JK (ed). 1988. The cardiomyopathies. Cardiol Clin 6.
34. Wright JR and Calkins E. 1981. Clinical-pathologic differentiation of common amyloid syndromes. Medicine (Balt) 60:429–448.
35. Davis PJ and Davis FB. 1974. Hyperthyroidism in patients over the age of 60 years. Medicine 53:161–181.
36. Levey GS. 1975. The heart and hyperthyroidism. Med Clin North Am 59:1193–1202.
37. Christoph I, Minotti J, and Massie BM. 1991. Current status of the treatment of congestive heart failure. Prog Cardiol 4:3–42.
38. Jolly WW, Isch JH, and Shumaker HB. 1981. Cardiac surgery in the elderly. Cardiovasc Clin 12:195–210.
39. Setaro JF, Zaret BL, Schulman DS, et al. 1990. Usefulness of verapamil for congestive heart failure associated with abnormal left ventricular diastolic filling and normal left ventricular systolic performance. Am J Cardiol 66:981–986.
40. Richardson A, Bayliss J, Scriven A, et al. 1987. Double-blind comparison of captopril alone against furosemide plus amiloride in mild heart failure. Lancet 2:709–711.
41. Cowley AJ, Stainer K, Wynne RD, et al. 1986. Symptomatic assessment of patients with heart failure: double-blind comparison of diuretics and captopril in moderate heart failure. Lancet 2:770–772.
42. Jaeschke ER, Oxman AD, and Guyatt GH. 1990. To what extent do congestive heart failure patients in sinus rhythm benefit from digoxin therapy? A systematic overview and meta-analysis. Am J Med 88:279–286.
43. Captopril-Digoxin Multicenter Research Group. 1988. Comparative effects of therapy with captopril and digoxin in patients with mild to moderate heart failure. JAMA 259:539–544.
44. DiBianco R, Shabatai R, Rostuk WV, et al. 1989. A comparison of oral milrinone, digoxin, and their combination in the treatment of patients with chronic heart failure. N Engl J Med 320:677–683.
45. The CONSENSUS Trial Study Group. 1987. Effect of enalapril on mortality in severe congestive heart failure. N Engl J Med 316:1429–1435.
46. Captopril Multicenter Research Group. 1983. A placebo-controlled trial of captopril in refractory chronic congestive heart failure. J Am Coll Cardiol 2:755–763.
47. The SOLVD Investigators. 1991. Effect of enalapril on survival in patients with reduced left ventricular ejection fractions and congestive heart failure. N Engl J Med 325:293–302.
48. Cohn JN, Archibald PF, Ziesche S, et al. 1986. Effect of vasodilator therapy on mortality in chronic congestive heart failure. N Engl J Med 314:547–552.
49. Cohn JN, Johnson G, Ziesche S, et al. 1991. A comparison of enalapril with hydralazine-isosorbide dinitrate in the treatment of chronic congestive heart failure. N Engl J Med 325:303–310.

7. HYPERTENSION AND HYPERTENSIVE EMERGENCIES

HYPERTENSION

FRANZ H. MESSERLI
TOMASZ GRODZICKI

Despite several recent review articles [2–7], there is still widespread confusion regarding the definition, evaluation, treatment, and prognosis of essential hypertension in patients older than age 65. Several misconceptions may contribute to this disarray. First, arterial pressure increases with age in Westernized populations, and therefore an elevated pressure is believed to be a normal finding in the elderly population. Second, function and perfusion of vital organs diminish with age, and an elevated pressure is regarded as a physiologic compensatory process serving to restore or maintain adequate blood flow. Third, elderly patients with essential hypertension have predominantly systolic hypertension, and many physicians believe that only diastolic hypertension is a harbinger of heart attack, stroke, and death. Fourth, little has been published indicating that the mechanisms of pressure elevation differ in older and younger patients with established essential hypertension.

In an elderly patient with established essential hypertension, two distinctly different pathogenetic processes should be considered. On one side, progressive aging per se affects the cardiovascular system and can result in age-specific changes; on the other side, the cardiovascular system of an elderly hypertensive patient has been exposed to long-standing hypertension

Franz H. Messerli (ed.), CARDIOVASCULAR DISEASE IN THE ELDERLY (Third Edition). Copyright © 1993 Kluwer Academic Publishers. ISBN 0-7923-1859-5. All rights reserved.

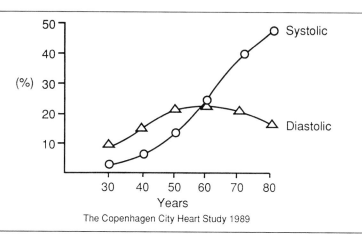

The Copenhagen City Heart Study 1989

Figure 7-1. Percentage of population with hypertension (blood pressure ≥160/95 mmHg), from the Copenhagen City Heart Study, 1989. (Adapted from T. Hilden, personal communication, with permission.)

that by itself damages various target organs. Thus, distinguishing the two pathogenetic factors—age and hypertension—becomes increasingly difficult.

In an attempt to untangle these two pathogenetic factors, we matched 30 patients older than age 65 with essential hypertension to an equal number of patients younger than age 42 with regard to mean arterial pressure, race, and sex [8]. We assessed cardiovascular hemodynamics, fluid volume, and endocrine aspects in these two groups, which have an average age difference of more than 40 years. This chapter is based partially on this comparison as well as on epidemiologic, pathophysiologic, clinical, and therapeutic aspects of geriatric hypertension. Hypertension is arbitrarily defined as a blood pressure exceeding 160/90 mmHg. The term *elderly* refers to patients age 65 and older.

EPIDEMIOLOGY

Arterial pressure increases with age in Westernized populations, and each year an increasing number of elderly patients fulfill (arbitrarily set) criteria of hypertension (figure 7-1). The National Health Survey in the United States has shown that the prevalence of hypertension may reach 50% in patients older than age 65 [9,10]. Since life expectancy has increased from approximately 47 years at the turn of the century to 73 years today [11] and continues to increase, in the near future we can expect up to 25 million hypertensive elderly patients in this country (more than 10% of the total population).

Despite such impressive numbers, there is nothing benign about hypertension in the elderly. The Veterans Administration Cooperative Study

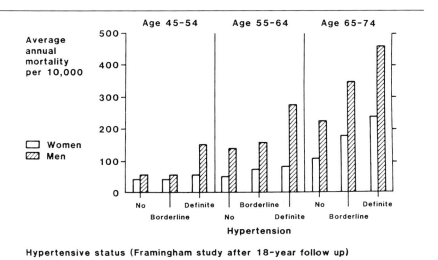

Figure 7-2. Mortality increases with the presence of hypertension in all age groups. (Reproduced from Kannel WB and Gordon T. 1978. Evaluation of cardiovascular risk in the elderly: the Framingham study. Bull NY Acad Med 54:573–591.)

[12] has shown that 63% of those over age 60 with untreated hypertension will suffer a cerebral vascular accident, congestive heart failure, myocardial infarction (MI), or dissecting aneurysm within five years. Further studies from the Framingham cohort (figure 7-2) [13], the United States [14], Belgium [15], and Scandinavia [16] corroborate these findings. Even patients with purely systolic hypertension have a much higher mortality from all cardiovascular and renal diseases than patients without hypertension [17].

Can we therefore expect that correction of hypertension would improve both the length and quality of life in our senior citizens? Findings from early studies were contradictory in this regard and did not allow definite conclusions [18–27]. However, the European Working Party for Hypertension in the Elderly [18] and, most recently, the Systolic Hypertension in the Elderly Program (SHEP) [28] and the Swedish Trial in Old Patients with Hypertension (STOP) study [29] showed distinct improvements in morbidity and mortality in patients receiving antihypertensive therapy. The SHEP study has documented that, even in patients with isolated systolic hypertension, lowering of blood pressure distinctly reduces stroke and heart attack rates.

PATHOPHYSIOLOGY

Hemodynamics

In contrast to the young patient with borderline and early established essential hypertension, in whom cardiac output is often elevated, the elderly patient is characterized by a low cardiac output (figure 7-3) [1] secondary to a

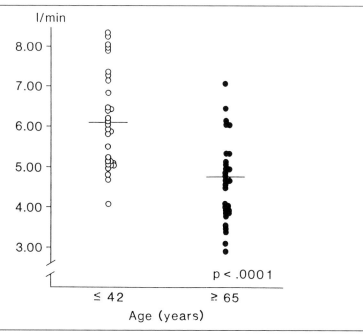

Figure 7-3. Cardiac output was found to be lower in elderly hypertensive patients when compared with younger patients having similar levels of arterial pressure. (Reproduced with permission from Messerli FH. 1985. Hypertension Update II Symposium, Health Learning Systems, Washington, DC.)

decreased stroke volume and relative bradycardia [8]. Cardiac output has been found to be 20% to 30% lower in senescence than in comparable youth among patients with similar blood pressure levels (figure 7-3), even in the absence of congestive heart failure. At the same time, elderly patients have higher systolic and lower diastolic pressures (figure 7-4) [8,30,31], elevated left ventricular stroke work, and a distinctly increased total peripheral resistance (figure 7-5) when compared with younger patients [8,31]. The only long-term follow-up study available was done by Lund-Johansen [32] in mildly hypertensive patients who were left untreated for as long as 17 years. He documented a distinct fall in cardiac output, mostly because of a reduction in stroke volume and an increase in total peripheral resistance, both during rest and after treadmill exercise. A fall in cardiac output with age has been observed in normotensive populations, too, although to a lesser degree [29,33–37]. In contrast, a recent study [38,39] indicated that normotensive subjects who were free of coronary artery disease and hypertension exhibited no decline in cardiac output either at rest or during exercise. Aging per se did not limit cardiac output in normal subjects, but it seemed to change the

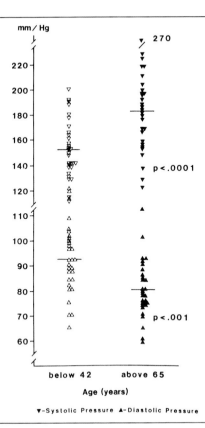

Figure 7-4. Systolic pressure was found to be higher and diastolic pressure to be lower in elderly hypertensive patients than in younger patients having similar levels of mean arterial pressure. Thus, systolic hypertension merely reflects decreased arterial compliance. (Reproduced with permission from Messerli FH. 1985. Essential hypertension in the elderly. Triangle 24:35–47. Copyright Sandoz Pharma Ltd., Basel, Switzerland.)

mechanism by which cardiac output was increased during exercise: whereas young patients respond to exercise with a catecholamine-mediated increase in heart rate and a reduction in end-systolic volume, older patients compensate for the less dramatic response in heart rate with an increase in end-systolic and stroke volume (the Frank–Starling mechanism) [39].

Unlike the situation in normal subjects, the hypertensive patient's heart bears the hemodynamic burden of an excessive afterload that accelerates the decline in cardiac function that occurs with advancing age. The main hemodynamic abnormality in established essential hypertension (in the middle-aged and older patient) is an elevated total peripheral resistance. As cardiac output declines with advancing age, total peripheral resistance becomes further elevated (figure 7-6) [40]. Freis [41] indicated 30 years ago

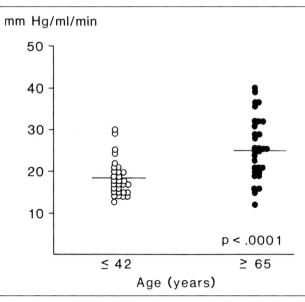

Figure 7-5. Total peripheral resistance was found to be elevated in elderly hypertensive patients when compared with younger patients having similar levels of mean arterial pressure. (Reproduced with permission from Messerli FH. 1985. Essential hypertension in the elderly. Triangle 24:35–47. Copyright Sandoz Pharma Ltd., Basel, Switzerland.)

that an increase in total peripheral resistance reflects either a constriction of arteriolar smooth muscle or a restriction of the arteriolar vascular bed by arteriosclerotic structural changes. Therefore, total peripheral resistance closely parallels systemic hypertensive vascular disease [41]. Elderly patients can thus be expected to be at high risk for hypertensive vascular disease and/or end-organ damage such as nephrosclerosis, cerebral vascular lesions, and hypertensive heart disease.

Cardiac adaptations

Unlike other organs, the heart does not atrophy with age; in fact, left ventricular mass progressively increases throughout life, reaching its greatest magnitude in senescence (figure 7-7) [42]. Various studies have documented an increase in wall thickness with age in the presence of unchanged chamber volume [43–45]. In a stepwise multiple regression analysis of a very heterogeneous population of 171 patients, we demonstrated that age was an independent determinant of posterior and septal wall thickness as well as of left ventricular mass [46]. Posterior wall thickness increased by about 25% between the second and the seventh decade of life, and the ratio of radius to wall thickness declined (figure 7–8) [31], indicating left ventricular hypertrophy (LVH) of the concentric type. The fact that left ventricular wall

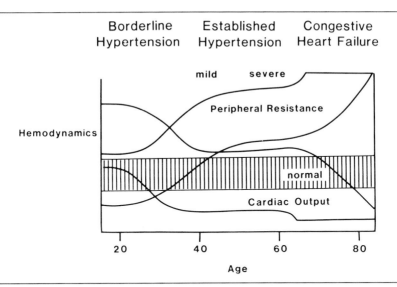

Figure 7-6. Hemodynamic change with age and as hypertension becomes more severe. The young patient is characterized by an elevated cardiac output and a normal total peripheral resistance. As hypertension becomes established, cardiac output reverts to normal and resistance becomes elevated. In the elderly and in the patient with congestive heart failure, cardiac output declines and total peripheral resistance becomes even more elevated. (Reproduced with permission from Messerli FH. 1981. Individualization of antihypertensive therapy: an approach based on hemodynamics and age. J Clin Pharmacol 21:517–528.)

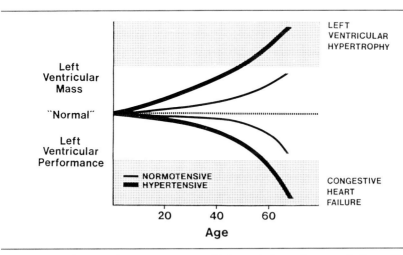

Figure 7-7. Left ventricular mass increases and left ventricular performance declines with age in normotensive subjects. Hypertension acts as a time accelerator, producing a steeper increase in left ventricular mass and a steeper decline in left ventricular performance. (Reproduced with permission from Messerli FH. 1983. Clinical determinants and consequences of left ventricular hypertrophy. Am J Med 75:51–63.)

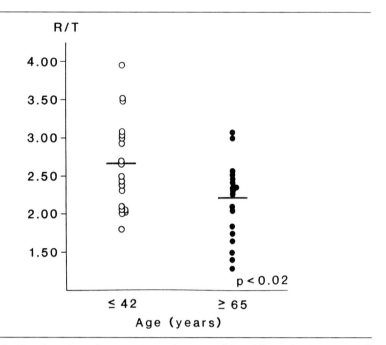

Figure 7-8. Cardiac adaptation to hypertension is characterized by a fall in radius/posterior wall thickness (R/T) indicating concentric left ventricular hypertrophy in the elderly hypertensive patient. (Reproduced with permission from Messerli FH. 1985. Essential hypertension in the elderly. Triangle 24:35–47. Copyright Sandoz Pharma Ltd., Basel, Switzerland.)

stress is normal in the elderly hypertensive patients [5] is an argument against the occurrence of so-called pseudohypertrophy (replacement of contractile myocytes by fat or other noncontractile tissue).

The greater the afterload is to the left ventricle (i.e., the more severe is arterial hypertension), the faster the increase is in relative posterior wall thickness. Thus, arbitrarily set echocardiographic or electrocardiographic criteria of LVH will be reached considerably earlier in life when arterial hypertension is present [8]. By the same token, an increase in afterload will accelerate the decline in cardiac function because of additional hemodynamic load burdening the left ventricle. Hypertension therefore accelerates physiologic changes of aging in the heart, thereby resetting the biological clock at a faster pace.

LVH usually is considered an adaptive physiologic process of the myocardium that compensates for increased afterload. However, data from the Framingham cohort [47,48] indicate that patients with LVH are at greater risk for sudden death (and other cardiovascular morbidity and mortality) than subjects with normal hearts. If, indeed, LVH is a risk factor for sudden death, is it possible to identify the patients at highest risk in this population?

Table 7-1. Increased ventricular ectopy
in patients with left ventricular hypertrophy

Maximal Lown's Class	Normotensive	Hypertensive	
		Without LVH	With LVH[a]
0	10	6	2
1	4	4	4
2	0	0	5
3	0	0	3
4	0	0	2

[a] p, 0.004 vs. both other groups.
Reproduced with permission from Messerli FH, Ventura HO, Elizardi DJ, et al. 1984. Hypertension and sudden death: increased ventricular ectopic activity in left ventricular hypertrophy. Am J Med 77:18–22.

We recently demonstrated [49] that patients with LVH had more complex ventricular ectopy more frequently than those with a normal or less hypertrophied myocardium. In the group with LVH, not only were premature ventricular contractions 40 to 50 times more prevalent but so were Lown's class III and class IV ectopies such as coupled and multifocal beats (table 7-1) [49].

LVH by echocardiographic criteria can be found in up to 50% of elderly patients with essential hypertension (figure 7-6) [8,40]. At any given level of arterial pressure, these subjects have a far more serious prognosis than those without LVH. The appearance of premature ventricular contractions in asymptomatic patients with LVH becomes an ominous electrocardiographic sign. Holter monitoring of these patients allows identification of those who are at the highest risk and therefore require the most aggressive and specific antihypertensive treatment.

Dysfunction of the autonomic nervous system

Reactivity of the baroreceptor reflex decreases with progressing age. The heart rate response to upright tilt, a reduction in heart rate produced by bolus injection of phenylephrine (a common way to estimate baroreceptor sensitivity), and cardioacceleration evoked by hypoxia or carbon dioxide retention were found to be diminished in normal elderly subjects when compared with 20-year-old patients. Hence, both baroreceptor and chemoreceptor reflexes become blunted with aging, although the exact underlying mechanism remains unknown. Since hypertension per se impairs baroreceptor function, its presence will accelerate the deteriorating effects of aging. As a consequence, elderly hypertensive patients become predisposed to orthostatic hypotension and syncope. This propensity to orthostatic hypotension can be unmasked by diuretic therapy. Shannon et al. [50] demonstrated a 24-mm drop in systolic pressure during upright tilt associated

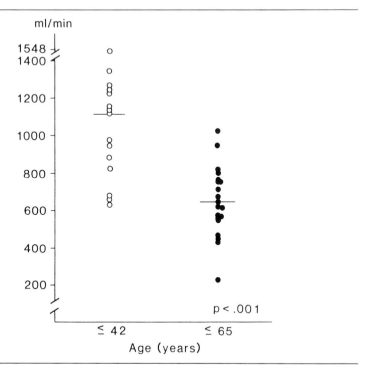

Figure 7-9. Renal blood flow was found to be lower in elderly hypertensive patients when compared with younger patients having similar levels of arterial pressure. (Reproduced with permission from Hollenberg NK, Epstein M, Basch RI, et al. 1969. "No man's land" of the renal vasculature. An arteriographic and hemodynamic assessment of the interlobar and arcuate arteries in essential and accelerated hypertension. Am J Med 47:845–854.)

with orthostatic symptoms in elderly subjects receiving hydrochlorothiazide, whereas no change in blood pressure occurred in the pretreatment phase or in younger subjects on the same dose of diuretics.

Renal adaptations

Renal blood flow has been shown to decline progressively with advancing age in normal subjects but declines even more dramatically in patients with essential hypertension. Studies [7,51] have shown that renal blood flow was disproportionately more reduced than cardiac output in senescence (39% versus 24%, respectively), indicating a redistribution of systemic flow (figure 7-9). Accordingly, renal vascular resistance was distinctly elevated in elderly hypertensive patients, reflecting diffuse nephrosclerosis resulting from long-standing essential hypertension. A decrease in renal blood flow has been shown to occur early in mild essential hypertension [52,53], and this should be suspected whenever an unexplained mild increase in plasma uric acid

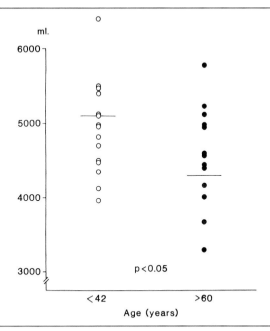

Figure 7-10. Total blood volume was found to be contracted in elderly hypertensive patients when compared with younger patients having similar levels of mean arterial pressure. (Reproduced with permission from Messerli FH. 1985. Essential hypertension in the elderly. Triangle 24:35–47. Copyright Sandoz Pharma Ltd., Basel, Switzerland.)

occurs [54]. In contrast, glomerular filtration rate usually remains well preserved throughout life and falls only after age 65. Thus, filtration fraction and renal vascular resistance become elevated even in an early phase of hypertensive renal involvement [53].

Intravascular volume

Intravascular volume seems not to change very much with advancing age in normotensive subjects [55]. However, our study [8,31] in hypertensive subjects revealed a significantly lower intravascular volume in elderly patients than in younger patients with similar arterial pressures (figure 7-10) [31]. As in younger patients, intravascular volume correlated inversely with total peripheral resistance in the elderly. If arterial hypertension in senescence were more volume-dependent, a direct (and not inverse) correlation between intravascular volume and total peripheral resistance would be expected. Clearly, hypertension in the elderly is no more or less volume dependent than in younger counterparts, despite plasma renin activity that is often low and unresponsive. Elderly hypertensive patients with decreased intravascular volume are susceptible to orthostatic hypotension. This is another reason

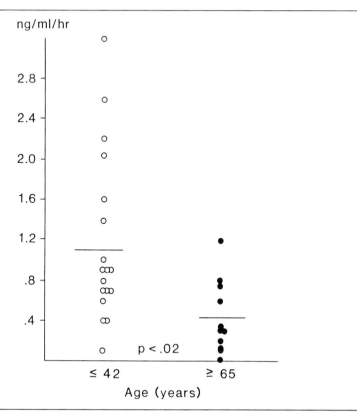

Figure 7-11. Plasma renin activity (ng/ml/hr, after one hour of recumbency and free sodium intake) was found to be lower in elderly hypertensive patients when compared with younger patients with similar levels of mean arterial pressure. (Reproduced with permission from Messerli FH. 1985. Essential hypertension in the elderly. Triangle 24:35–47. Copyright Sandoz Pharma Ltd., Basel, Switzerland.)

why diuretics should be used with great caution, if at all, in the management of these patients.

Endocrine changes

Plasma renin activity has been shown to decrease with advancing age [56–61]. This relationship has been established in patients with essential hypertension but not always in normotensive subjects. Similarly, in our study [8,31], plasma renin activity was significantly lower in elderly hypertensive patients than in the younger group with similar arterial pressure levels (figure 7-11) [31]. The inverse association between plasma renin activity and age has been attributed to progressive nephrosclerosis, which could impair both basal renin secretion and its response to stimulation.

Once frank congestive heart failure ensues, the renin–angiotensin–

aldosterone system becomes activated and, with elevated norepinephrine concentration, maintains arterial pressure at a level that permits perfusion of vital organs. Plasma renin activity has been reported to be highest in patients with congestive heart failure without peripheral edema, somewhat lower in those with accumulated edema, and within normal limits in those who are in a relatively stable state of congestive heart failure [62].

In contrast to plasma renin activity, norepinephrine levels have been shown to increase progressively with advancing age more in normotensive than in hypertensive subjects [35,63–65]. That high circulating norepinephrine levels indicate a poor prognosis in patients with congestive heart failure was suggested by Cohn et al. [66]. In their study, plasma norepinephrine levels proved to be a more powerful determinant of the prognosis than any of the hemodynamic parameters.

In asymptomatic, mildly hypertensive elderly patients, elevated norepinephrine values probably reflect a mechanism that compensates for the relative insensitivity of beta-adrenoreceptors. Clinical and experimental evidence from isolated animal tissue and isolated human cells [67–69] indicates that, with age, the responsiveness of the beta-adrenoreceptors diminishes in ways not associated with changes in beta-adrenoreceptor density [70]. Whether or not alpha-adrenoreceptor sensitivity changes with aging is less clear at present [70].

CLINICAL FINDINGS

Systolic blood pressure elevation and arterial compliance

When a given stroke volume is ejected into a stiff arterial system, a higher systolic and a lower diastolic pressure will result than when the same volume is ejected into a more elastic system. Since arterial compliance decreases with age because of progressive atheromatosis and medial hypertrophy, systolic hypertension becomes a common entity in elderly population [71]. Accordingly, elderly hypertensive patients will have a higher systolic pressure and lower diastolic pressure than comparable younger subjects with the same mean arterial pressure (figure 7-4). Therefore, although systolic hypertension reflects merely decreased arterial compliance [72–75], systolic pressure is still an important determinant of left ventricular wall stress and thus remains a powerful risk factor for the development of hypertensive heart disease.

Pseudohypertension

It may be difficult to estimate how much of the hardness and firmness is due to the blood within the vessel and how much to the thickening of the wall. If, for example, when the radial is compressed with the index finger, the artery can be felt beyond the point of compression, its walls are sclerosed (p. 485).

—Sir William Osler [76]

These sentences were written more than a quarter of a century before blood pressure was routinely measured in clinical practice. Osler not only described an entity known today as pseudohypertension but also suggested an elegant clinical maneuver for its identification. Spence et al. [77] reported that cuff pressures do not always accurately reflect intra-arterial pressures, particularly in the elderly population, and that discrepancies of up to 80 mmHg can be found between cuff and intra-arterial readings secondary to arteriosclerosis and medial hypertrophy. Pseudohypertension should be suspected in all hypertensive elderly patients in whom cuff pressure is found to be inappropriately elevated, with regard to the extent of target-organ disease such as nephrosclerosis or LVH.

We recently evaluated "Osler's maneuver" in a population of elderly hypertensive patients [78] and found an inverse relationship between arterial compliance and the degree of pseudohypertension (difference between intra-arterial and cuff pressure); in other words, the stiffer the arterial system was, the more likely was the presence of pseudohypertension. To perform Osler's maneuver, the brachial artery is occluded by inflation of a cuff above systolic pressure levels and the radial or brachial artery is carefully palpated. The patient was described as *Osler-positive* if the sclerotic wall of the pulseless artery remained palpable and *Osler-negative* if the artery could no longer be palpated. All patients found to be Osler-positive had falsely elevated cuff blood pressure readings that exceeded intra-arterial values by 10 to 54 mmHg (figure 7-12) [78].

Clinical consequences arising from such spurious elevation of arterial pressure are most important. Patients misdiagnosed as having essential hypertension may be subjected needlessly to the inconvenience, cost, risk, and adverse effects of antihypertensive treatment. This becomes particularly important in the elderly, who are more susceptible to the adverse effects of antihypertensive therapy than middle-aged or younger patients. Could part of this susceptibility be due to the fact that arterial pressure is often overestimated and therefore overtreated in this age group because of the concomitant or sole presence of pseudohypertension? Not surprisingly, inappropriate antihypertensive therapy in the elderly has been shown to lead to transient ischemic episodes as well as to more severe, even fatal, neurologic events.

Secondary hypertension

Because of the higher prevalence of arteriosclerosis in elderly hypertensive patients, renal arterial disease is frequently seen in this population. Renovascular hypertension or other secondary forms should be strongly suspected if high blood pressure develops de novo in an older patient in whom previously normal values have been documented. However, identification of renal arterial stenosis does not always imply renovascular

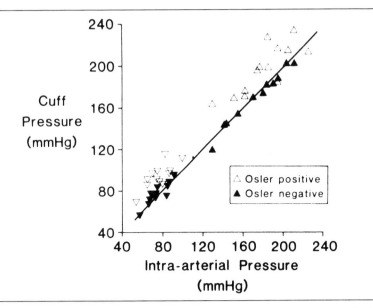

Figure 7-12. Discrepancy between cuff blood pressure measurements and intra-arterial values in Osler-positive (and Osler-negative) patients. (Reproduced from Messerli FH, Ventura HO, Amodeo C. 1985. Osler's maneuver and pseudohypertension. N Engl J Med 312:1548–1551.)

hypertension. Distinct narrowing of renal arteries by arteriosclerotic plaques can also be found in normotensive subjects. The presence of a significant stenosis of the renal artery should therefore be carefully evaluated in the elderly patient. Despite a lateralizing renal venous/renin ratio (>2.0), surgical correction may not always be beneficial in the elderly because of the distinctly elevated risk of the intervention. Clearly, however, age per se should not be considered a contraindication to surgery, since the majority of elderly subjects operated on for renovascular hypertension seem to benefit from this treatment. If renal filtration function in the affected kidney is minimal, a simple nephrectomy will facilitate antihypertensive treatment or even allow arterial pressure to return to normal values. Transluminal angioplasty may be helpful in a few selected cases, but patients with arteriosclerotic lesions (common in the elderly) usually do worse than those with fibromuscular dysplasia (uncommon in the elderly). Patients with bilateral arteriosclerotic lesions almost invariably do poorly after transluminal angioplasty. Other secondary forms of hypertension, such as primary aldosteronism and pheochromocytoma, occur in young patients as well as in the elderly and should be dealt with similarly.

Post-transplant hypertension has become more common in the geriatric population as well. Although the exact pathogenetic mechanism remains to be identified, the increase in arterial pressure occurs commonly after prolonged medication with cyclosporine. Calcium antagonists of the dihydro-pyridine type are particularly useful in the management of post-transplant hypertension. In this group, isradipine and nifedipine have the advantage of having no interaction with cyclosporine.

THERAPEUTIC APPROACH

Nonpharmacologic modalities

Nonspecific measures such as salt restriction, weight loss, and perhaps mild exercise should be enforced in the overweight, inactive, elderly patient. An excess of adipose tissue expands intravascular volume and additionally burdens the left ventricle with a high preload [79]. This may further impair left ventricular function and thereby accelerate the decline of its performance. The Framingham Study [80] has indicated that obese hypertensive patients are at particularly high risk for congestive heart failure. Similarly, elderly patients are more susceptible to the effects of fluid and salt overload; an excessive salt load (particularly when combined with alcohol, as often happens at birthday parties, etc.) may temporarily overload the extracellular fluid volume space by more than 2000 ml and thereby give rise to congestive heart failure and acute pulmonary edema. Such a dismal course of events is particularly likely to occur in an elderly patient whose heart had a poorly compensated contractile function to start with.

However, for various reasons, the elderly patient's compliance with dietary measures is notoriously poor. First, the elderly person tends to have a very established rigid daily schedule and life-style, and may be reluctant to consider any changes. Second, it is cumbersome, time-consuming, and expensive to prepare fresh (unprocessed and therefore low-salt) meals three times a day, whereas canned food and TV dinners (high in salt) are much more convenient to prepare. Third, because the taste buds of elderly persons lack sensitivity, they tend to use more salt to overcome lack of taste. Fourth, dietary salt restrictions in the elderly usually have little antihypertensive effect (and thus impress neither patient nor physician), although to some extent these restrictions prevent diuretic-induced hypokalemia. Finally, to follow a daily exercise program may be next to impossible because of concomitant problems such as osteoarthritis, peripheral vascular disease, parkinsonism, lack of appropriate facilities, or even fear of being assaulted. Although it is tedious to motivate elderly patients to change their life-style and dietary habits and to encourage them to participate in a regular physical fitness program, the benefits from such nonspecific measures often outweigh the frustration created by the hindrances.

Selection of antihypertensive agents

As outlined above, the elderly hypertensive patient is characterized by a distinct hemodynamic, endocrine, and fluid-volume profile that gradually evolves with advancing age. Based on this profile, one can compose a "wish list" that enumerates all the desirable properties of an ideal hypertensive drug

Table 7-2. The "ideal" antihypertensive agent in the elderly

1. It should not further depress cardiac performance or systemic blood flow
2. It should lower vascular resistance systemically and predominantly in the renal vascular bed
3. It should improve cardiac and vascular compliance
4. It should reduce or prevent left ventricular hypertrophy
5. It should not further contract intravascular volume or impede sodium and water handling of the kidney
6. It should not adversely affect other cardiovascular risk factors
7. It should have a smooth onset of action and a receptor half-life of more than 12 hours, allowing once-daily dosage
8. It should not be contraindicated because of concomitant disorders or medications
9. It should be inexpensive

in this age group (table 7-2). Although no single drug is available at present that would completely fulfill all requirements, despite equal antihypertensive properties some agents are immediately preferable to others.

Diuretics

Diuretics are efficacious antihypertensive agents in elderly patients with essential hypertension. In most studies in which diuretics were used as first-line therapy, a marked reduction of strokes has been reported. In the British Medical Research Council study [81], patients receiving diuretics had an even lower stroke rate than patients with similar blood pressures receiving a placebo. Thus, diuretics may well have a "cerebroprotective" effect. In contrast, the effects of diuretics on the prevention of coronary artery disease and acute MI have been less impressive. Findings from the European Working Party on High Blood Pressure in the Elderly [18] showed a significant reduction in total cardiac mortality but not in the occurrence of acute MI. In isolated systolic hypertension, the efficacy of diuretics as step-1 medication was documented by the SHEP study [28]. Most recently, the STOP trial [29] showed a significant reduction of primary endpoints (94 versus 58; $p = 0.0031$) and stroke morbidity and mortality (53 versus 29; $p = 0.0081$). This thorough, placebo-controlled, double-blinded study documented a distinct reduction in cardiovascular morbidity in patients who were treated with chlorthalidone (as step 1) and atenolol (as step 2) when compared with the placebo group. However, as in many previous studies, no significant reduction in endpoints of coronary artery disease was achieved.

Of note, long-term therapy with thiazide diuretics has been documented to reduce osteoporosis and consequently the incidence of hip fractures [82,83]. The antiosteoporotic effect of diuretics clearly becomes an important consideration in women at risk for this disease, particularly in view of the fact that hip fractures are still one of the most deadly complications in elderly patients.

Despite these favorable attributes, diuretics should be used with diligence only for antihypertensive therapy in the geriatric population (table 7-3) [42]. We consider them (in low doses) excellent step-2 agents in patients receiving angiotensin-converting enzyme (ACE) inhibitors; furthermore, in elderly

Table 7-3. Why not a diuretic?

Pathophysiologic findings in elderly hypertensive patients	Pharmacologic effects of thiazide diuretics
− High prevalence of left ventricular hypertrophy predisposing to ventricular ectopy and possibly sudden death	− Produces hypokalemia and hypomagnesemia, thereby increasing ventricular ectopic activity
− Contracted intravascular volume, impaired baroreflexes	− Sodium and water depletion, orthostatic hypotension
− Low renal blood flow and glomerular filtration rate	− Decrease in glomerular filtration rate and renal blood flow
− Impaired sodium- and water-conserving capacity	− Increased sodium excretion, decrease in free-water clearance
− Tendency to hyperuricemia, glucose intolerance, and hyperlipidemia	− Increase in uric acid plasma lipids and impaired glucose tolerance

Reproduced with permission from Messerli FH. 1983. Clinical determinants and consequences of left ventricular hypertrophy. Am J Med 75:51–63.

Table 7-4. Indications for diuretics in elderly patients with essential hypertension

1. High risk of cerebrovascular disease and stroke
2. Congestive heart failure with predominantly systolic dysfunction
3. Osteoporosis?
4. States involving fluid volume overload
5. Combination therapy

patients with congestive heart failure secondary to systolic dysfunction, diuretics remain a cornerstone of management (table 7-4).

Beta-blockers

Most beta-blockers lower arterial pressure by decreasing cardiac output secondary to a fall in heart rate without affecting or even increasing total peripheral resistance. This hemodynamic pattern clearly makes them a poor choice for treatment of elderly hypertensive patients characterized by a low cardiac output with a slow heart rate and a high peripheral resistance. Beta-blockers should also be avoided in patients with isolated systolic hypertension, since the negative chronotropic effect of these agents tends to elevate systolic pressure and lower diastolic pressure (table 7-5) [42]. It must be emphasized, however, that the hemodynamic effects of beta-blockers are not all alike. Latetalol and carvedilol (alpha- and beta-blockers), pindolol, bopindolol (a beta-blocker with high sympathomimetic activity), and celiprolol have been shown to maintain cardiac output and dilate the peripheral vasculature [84–87]. Celiprolol, by exerting its antihypertensive effect through beta$_2$-stimulation (which produces vasodilation) and beta$_1$-

Table 7-5. Why not a beta-blocker?

Pathophysiologic findings in elderly hypertensive patients	Pharmacologic effects of beta-adrenoeceptor blockade
– Low cardiac output, bradycardia	– Negative inotropic and chronotropic effects
– High total peripheral resistance	– Increase (or at best no change) in total peripheral resistance
– Low renal blood flow and glomerular filtration rate	– Decrease in renal blood flow and (less) in glomerular filtration rate
– Low plasma renin activity	– Decrease in plasma renin activity

Note: Concomitant disorders such as chronic obstructive pulmonary disease, glucose intolerance, and peripheral vascular disease are common in elderly patients and provide a relative contraindication to beta-adrenoreceptor blockade.
Reproduced with permission from Messeril FH. 1983. Clinical determinants and consequences of left ventricular hypertrophy. Am J Med 75:51–63.

Table 7-6. Clinical indications for use of beta-blockers in elderly patients with hypertension

1. After acute myocardial infarction, to prevent reinfarction
2. Hyperkinetic heart syndrome
3. Combination therapy with dihydropyridine calcium antagonists
4. Angina pectoris
5. Certain tachyarrhythmias

blockade, seems to have a particularly attractive hemodynamic profile. Apart from these considerations, beta-blockers remain an excellent choice for patients concomitantly suffering from a hyperkinetic heart syndrome, which is not uncommon in elderly hypertensive patients. Beta-blockers have also been clearly documented to reduce reinfarction rate and mortality in post-MI patients and therefore remain a good choice in this clinical situation (table 7-6).

Centrally acting antiadrenergic drugs
Low doses of centrally acting antiadrenergic agents (methyldopa, clonidine, guanabenz, etc.) have been used in the past to treat hypertension in the elderly. However, with the advent of more modern antihypertensive modalities with a purer side-effect profile, these drugs have been abandoned. Centrally acting antiadrenergic drugs should be used in combination therapy only as third- and fourth-step agents.

Peripherally acting antiadrenergic drugs
These agents exert their antihypertensive effect by reducing total peripheral resistance while maintaining or increasing cardiac output. Since they also dilate capacitance vessels, orthostatic hypotension has been known to occur.

This was particularly a problem with the first dose of prazosin and inappropriate escalation of the dose. Pretreatment with a diuretic (which was standard practice in the past) made patients much more susceptible to this first-dose effect. Orthostatic hypotension is very uncommon with the more modern agents such as trimazosin and doxazapin. The postsynaptic alpha$_1$-blockers have been shown to favorably affect dyslipoproteinemia; they lower total cholesterol and increase high-density lipoprotein cholesterol. Although the long-term benefits of these lipid effects remain to be determined (particularly in the elderly), postsynaptic alpha$_1$-blockers should be considered first-line agents in hypertensive patients with dyslipoproteinemias.

Calcium antagonists

Calcium antagonists inhibit calcium entry into vascular smooth muscle and therefor lower arterial pressure by reducing total peripheral resistance [88]. Their effect on the capacitance vessels is minimal, and orthostatic hypotension is therefore an uncommon adverse effect of calcium-channel blockade. Inhibition of calcium entry into the cell is the common property that all calcium antagonists share. However, apart from this property, calcium antagonists exhibit a variety of pharmacologic effects. For practical purposes, it is useful to divide them into the dihydropyridine and nondihydropyridine derivatives.

DIHYDROPYRIDINE CALCIUM ANTAGONISTS (NIFEDIPINE, NICARDIPINE, ISRADIPINE, FELODIPINE, AND AMLODIPINE). When given acutely, all dihydropyridine calcium antagonists produce a reflexive increase in heart rate and cardiac output and a marked reduction in total peripheral resistance. With chronic administration, this cardioacceleration diminishes somewhat (nifedipine and nicardipine) and seems to disappear completely with the newer agents (isradipine, felodipine, and amlodipine). Dihydropyridine calcium antagonists decrease left ventricular mass to a lesser extent than the nondihydropyridine derivatives. In general, an increase in renal blood flow and glomerular filtration rate can be observed. Dihydropyridine calcium antagonists are excellent antihypertensive agents in elderly hypertensive patients with concomitant bradycardia. Acute-release formulations, such as nifedipine, should be strictly avoided in elderly patients, since they can precipitate an inappropriate reduction in arterial pressure with profound cardioacceleration leading to myocardial ischemia and even acute MI. This sequence of events has not been documented with the sustained-release formulation (Procardia XL^R or Adalat SR^R). The newer calcium antagonists (isradipine, felodipine, and amlodipine) seem to have little if any negative inotropic or chronotropic effects. Thus, they do not slow sinus-node activity and atrioventricular (A-V) conduction or diminish contractility. The term *vasoselective* has been coined to describe their mechanism of action. Of note, these agents do not stimulate the activity of the sympathetic nervous system or the renin–angiotensin–aldosterone system. In contrast to other calcium antagonists, they have been shown to have a favorable effect on systemic and regional hemodynamics in patients with congestive heart failure. Isradipine, felodipine, and amlodipine can therefore be considered agents of choice in hypertensive elderly patients with coronary artery disease and systolic dysfunction. The safety, efficacy, and tolerability of isradipine in the geriatric population have been well documented. Unlike other calcium antagonists, isradipine does not affect digoxin levels and therefore no adjustment of dose is needed.

NONDIHYDROPYRIDINE CALCIUM ANTAGONISTS (VERAPAMIL, DILTIAZEM, AND GALLAPAMIL). As with the dihydropyridine calcium antagonists, the acute administration of verapamil, diltiazem, or gallapamil results in cardio-acceleration. With prolonged administration, however, heart rate falls below pretreatment levels. All three of these agents have negative chronotropic and inotropic effects; that is, they slow sinus-node activity and A-V-node conduction. They therefore should be avoided in patients with second-degree heart block or congestive failure from systolic dysfunction. In contrast, nondihydropyridine calcium antagonists, particularly verapamil, are excellent agents in patients with congestive heart failure secondary to impaired filling. Impaired left ventricular filling or diastolic dysfunction is a common sequela of long-standing hypertension and LVH. A recent study has documented that verapamil given one week after acute MI diminishes reinfarction rate and increases survival [89]. The decrease in reinfarction rate induced by verapamil was in excess of 20%, that is, similar to that documented with beta-blockers. In patients with non-Q-wave infarction, diltiazem has been documented to reduce reinfarction rates [90]. Although beta-blockers remain the agents of choice in the management of post-MI patients, calcium antagonists that slow heart rate should be considered when beta-blockers are contraindicated or when patients cannot tolerate them [91].

The nondihydropyridine calcium antagonists have been shown to markedly reduce LVH. Concomitantly, these agents improve left ventricular filling, reduce ventricular ectopy associated with LVH, improve myocardial ischemia, and preserve contractile function. Given that LVH has been identified as one of the most powerful cardiovascular risk factors, this effect can hardly be ignored. However, whether or not reduction of LVH, as induced by calcium antagonists, will diminish the morbidity and mortality of a given patient remains to be determined.

ANTIATHEROMATOUS EFFECTS. Calcium antagonists have been shown to exert antiatheromatous effects in certain experimental models [92]. Some recent clinical studies have documented that calcium antagonists inhibit the development of new atheromatous lesions in the coronary circulation. No effect on existing atheromatous plaque was observed. These recent findings make calcium antagonists a very attractive choice in elderly hypertensive patients at risk of or suffering from atheromatosis.

Angiotensin-converting enzyme inhibitors

Angiotensin-converting enzyme (ACE) inhibitors lower arterial pressure by decreasing total peripheral resistance while maintaining or enhancing systemic and regional blood flow [93,94]. ACE inhibitors affect capacitance vessels, thereby diminishing preload to the left ventricle, and also have the potential to produce orthostatic hypotension. Despite the fact that plasma renin activity is often low and unresponsive in elderly hypertensive patients, ACE inhibitors have been shown to lower blood pressure effectively and safely in the geriatric population. This clearly demonstrates that the antihypertensive effect of ACE inhibition is not solely dependent on circulating plasma renin activity. Since ACE inhibitors lower both preload and afterload to the left ventricle, they are the agents of choice in hypertensive patients with congestive heart failure of systolic dysfunction. ACE inhibitors are the only agents that have been shown to prolong life in patients with severe congestive heart failure (class III, class IV, New York Heart Association). ACE inhibitors also reduce LVH and increase renal blood flow without affecting glomerular filtration rate. In fact, with acute administration of an ACE inhibitor, often a transient decrease in glomerular filtration rate is observed. ACE inhibitors should be used with caution, if at all, in elderly patients with significant renal impairment. In this situation, high doses of ACE inhibitors have been shown to deteriorate renal function and lead to life-threatening hyperkalemia. Milder degrees of hyperkalemia are not uncommonly seen with ACE inhibition, since in elderly patients the mechanism of potassium excretion is often disturbed because of hyporeninemic hypoaldosteronism, renal failure, or both.

ACE inhibitors, when given after acute MI, have been shown to prevent progressive dilatation of the left chamber (remodeling). A multicenter study evaluating the effect of ACE inhibitors on morbidity and mortality in the post-MI patient is currently in progress.

Much ink has been wasted regarding differences in efficacy and safety among various ACE inhibitors. From a practical standpoint, blood-pressure-lowering properties are rather similar for all ACE inhibitors, provided that an adequate dose is given. Clearly, in unstable hemodynamic situations, short-acting agents are preferable to long-acting ACE inhibitors. With prolonged administration, and in stable hemodynamic situations, the once-a-day formulations (enalapril, lisinopril, ramipril, fosinopril, monapril, and trandolapril) are more convenient than the b.i.d. or t.i.d. ACE inhibitors.

Combination therapy

Table 7-7 provides information regarding good, acceptable, and poor combinations of antihypertensive drug classes in the elderly hypertensive patient. The combination of an ACE inhibitor with a calcium antagonist has been particularly useful in our hands. Hypertensive heart disease in the

Table 7-7. Combinations of antihypertensive drug classes in the elderly

	Diuretic	ACE-inhibitor	Beta-blocker	Dihydropyridine calcium antagonist	Nondihydropyridine calcium antagonist	Alpha-blocker	Central blocker
Diuretic		A	P	A	A	A	A
ACE-inhibitor	A		A	G	G	A	P
Beta-blocker	P	A		A	P	A	P
Dihydropyridine calcium antagonist	A	G	A		?	P	A
Nondihydropyridine calcium antagonist	A	G	P	?		A	A
Alpha-blocker	A	A	A	P	A		P
Central blocker	A	P	P	A	A	P	

Note: G = good; A = acceptable; P = poor combination.

elderly is commonly associated with both systolic and diastolic dysfunction. Combining an ACE inhibitor with a calcium antagonist will exert a favorable effect on both pathogenetic components. A nondihdropyridine calcium antagonist should be chosen in patients with predominantly diastolic dysfunction, whereas a dihydropyridine derivative such as isradipine, felodipine, or amlodipine is the combination agent of choice in patients with predominantly systolic dysfunction. In all patients with congestive heart failure, a loop or thiazide diuretic is most often needed to prevent fluid accumulation.

The combination of an ACE inhibitor with low doses of a thiazide diuretic will enhance antihypertensive efficacy. This combination is usually well tolerated in the elderly, although occasionally orthostatic hypotension is observed. Potassium-sparing diuretics should not be combined with ACE inhibitors in the geriatric population because of the danger of hyperkalemia.

In the post-MI patient with or without hypertension, it is tempting to combine two "cardioprotective" strategies—for example, beta-blockers and a calcium antagonist that slows heart rate. No study has shown that this combination is more efficacious than either drug alone. Since both drugs have negative inotropic and negative chronotropic effects, their combination may result in exacerbation of congestive failure or heart block.

CONCLUSION

Hypertension in the elderly is an asymptomatic disease and should remain so when treated. Although it clearly puts the patient at a higher risk of stroke, sudden death, congestive heart failure, and acute MI, the benefits of antihypertensive treatment remain less well proven in the geriatric population than among other patient groups. However, hemodynamics, fluid volume, and endocrine mechanisms of blood pressure elevation in elderly patients are very different from these mechanisms in young people with similar blood pressure elevations. Individualized treatment should aim not only to lower arterial pressure but at the same time to reduce target-organ damage such as nephrosclerosis, cerebrovascular disease, and LVH. Elderly patients are particularly susceptible to the adverse effects of drugs. Therefore, it becomes even more important to follow the advice of Aristotle:

Even in medicine, though it is easy to know what honey, wine, hellebore, cautery and surgery are, to know how and to whom and when to apply them so as to effect a cure, is no less an undertaking than to be a physician.

—Aristotle, 384–322, B.C.

SECTION TWO OF CHAPTER 7
HYPERTENSIVE EMERGENCIES

DWIGHT DAVIS
K. DANNER CLOUSER
ROBERT ZELIS

Medical advances in the care of patients with life-threatening and previously terminal illness have raised significant ethical issues regarding appropriate care of the elderly in certain emergency situations, and physicians are being questioned about their "lifesaving" decisions by patients, families, ancillary health personnel, other health care workers, and society.

Common cardiovascular emergencies in the elderly include unstable anginal syndromes, acute MI associated with hemodynamically significant arrhythmias or mechanical complications, severe left ventricular dysfunction associated with pulmonary edema, dissecting aortic aneurysm, and hypertensive emergencies. The former disorders are discussed in other sections of this book.

Over the past two decades, awareness has been heightened and increasing attention paid to the preventive aspects of medical care, with a significant focus on early detection and simplified management of blood pressure in all age groups, including the elderly. Correspondingly, the number of patients with uncontrolled hypertension has declined [95]. This has also led to a decrease in the number of patients presenting with hypertensive emergencies. Despite these changes, elderly patients with hypertensive emergencies continue to present a significant and challenging clinical problem. The treatment of these patients is often more difficult than treatment of younger patients because of the higher prevalence of coexisting disorders that adds to the complexity of management decisions and the potential for morbidity and mortality. Early recognition and aggressive management can often prevent complications and improve clinical outcome. There is now a strong emphasis on early, aggressive treatment of hypertensive emergencies in the elderly [96].

DEFINITIONS

Although *elderly* is a relative term, is is used here to refer to patients who are 65 years of age and older. A hypertensive emergency is a diastolic blood pressure greater than 120 mmHg in an elderly patient who was previously normotensive or who has one of the following associated conditions: acute left ventricular failure, hypertensive encephalopathy, high-grade retinopathy, acute cerebrovascular syndromes, acute ischemic syndromes, progressive renal insufficiency, or acute aortic dissection [97]. Under these circumstances, the blood pressure must be controlled within a short period to avoid death or permanent end-organ damage such as blindness, stroke, MI, or renal damage.

GENERAL GUIDELINES FOR INITIAL EVALUATION AND MANAGEMENT

In a clinically stable elderly patient presenting with a hypertensive emergency, the physician should perform an expeditious and organ–specific evaluation to determine the immediacy and aggressiveness of initial management. When possible, this initial evaluation should attempt to distinguish patients with hypertensive emergencies from those with hypertensive urgencies based on the severity of hypertension and the presence or absence of target organ dysfunction [98]. A brief history regarding prior illnesses, medications, and events leading to the current problem is helpful. A history of long-standing hypertension and the degree of previous blood pressure control have a significant bearing on management decisions. Elderly patients with a history of poorly controlled hypertension may be less sensitive to severe hypertension but more sensitive to rapid decreases in blood pressure than previously normotensive patients, and vice versa. A listing of prior medications is important and should include both physician-prescribed and over-the-counter preparations.

The findings on the physical examination should be compared with findings from the patient's baseline examination when possible. It is important to identify underlying medical problems that may complicate antihypertensive therapy, such as prior neurologic events, existing heart disease, evidence of congestive heart failure, retinopathy, the presence of aortic dissection, or evidence of significant peripheral vascular disease. The initial laboratory evaluation should include an electrocardiogram, a chest x-ray, urine analysis, a complete blood count, serum electrolytes, and determination of renal and liver function. More specialized tests such as computed tomography (CT) scans, angiograms, or echocardiograms, if necessary, may be indicated by preliminary findings.

Elderly patients with hypertensive emergencies should have immediate intravenous access established for drug administration and an arterial line placed for continuous monitoring of blood pressure. Continuous electrocardiographic monitoring should also be performed. Arrangements should be made for admission to an intensive care unit where high-level nursing supervision can be provided. Antihypertensive therapy should be started as soon as possible and without major delay. Often, the underlying cause for the hypertensive emergency will be established during treatment of the blood pressure.

The initial goals of therapy in elderly patients with severe hypertension are to gain control of blood pressure, limit or reverse target organ dysfunction, and avoid overaggressive treatment that can lead to hypoperfusion to vital organs, thereby compromising clinical outcome [99]. It is often helpful to decide on an initial target blood pressure and the time within which it should be achieved. In most circumstances this will involve rapidly lowering the diastolic blood pressure to less than 120 mmHg within the first few hours of therapy. Previously normotensive patients may require a lower initial target diastolic blood pressure. *An essential principle of therapy of hypertensive emergencies in the elderly is to avoid overzealous treatment.* Elderly patients are often very sensitive to the hypotensive effects of overaggressive therapy, which may result in periods of hypoperfusion to vital organs. Thus, strokes, MIs, and renal failure are not uncommonly caused by excessive blood pressure reduction in the geriatric population.

Another important aspect of therapy is tailoring treatment to fit the clinical situation. Elderly patients commonly have other complicating medical problems that require concurrent consideration while the blood pressure is being treated. In certain situations, the agent(s) selected can provide control of the blood pressure and, in addition, ameliorate complicating disorders such as coronary artery disease or congestive heart failure.

The preliminary evaluation of elderly patients with hypertensive emergencies occasionally indicates the need for consultative medical or surgical specialty services. Consultants should be contacted early in the clinical course so that they can become familiar with the patient and provide regular follow-up. This will often improve care of elderly patients if the clinical course deteriorates and urgent specialized care becomes necessary. In these situations, the primary physician should be responsible for coordinating total care of the patient.

Another important consideration in the initial evaluation of elderly patients with hypertensive emergencies is poor compliance with the prescribed regimen as a precipitating factor. Elderly patients caring for themselves with (or without) previously unrecognized senility are particularly predisposed to inadvertent drug withdrawal as an etiology for severe hypertension. Severe hypertension developing in this setting can either represent the loss of blood pressure control or exaggeration of hypertension through a drug withdrawal syndrome. The antihypertensive drugs most often implicated in withdrawal syndromes are the centrally acting agents such as clonidine or beta-blockers. In addition to severe hypertension, other clinical findings such as inappropriate tachycardia, abdominal pain, nausea, anxiety, and diaphoresis may suggest the diagnosis of a withdrawal syndrome. Multidrug, complex antihypertensive regimens may also play an important role in compliance problems in the elderly. Accordingly, it is important to design effective and convenient regimens when making the transition from acute to chronic therapy.

SELECTED AGENTS FOR THE TREATMENT OF HYPERTENSIVE EMERGENCIES

In elderly patients, drug selection should be individualized with careful consideration of underlying illnesses. Ideally, the agent selected should be given parenterally and have a rapid onset and a short half-life so that effects can be quickly reversed. It is also helpful if the agent is titratable over a wide range of blood pressures, allowing precise control. An ideal agent would also be effective for a variety of hypertensive syndromes and be easy to administer and monitor.

A large number of drugs have been used to treat hypertensive emergencies. Some continue to be efficacious, while others have become obsolete for various reasons. The following list of drugs is not intended to be exhaustive but may provide an overview of agents suited for primary or adjunctive therapy. Most of the drugs currently used for the management of hypertensive emergencies can be categorized into two groups: direct vasodilators and antiadrenergic agents.

Direct vasodilators

Sodium nitroprusside

This agent is the most commonly used and effective drug for the treatment of hypertensive emergencies. It is a potent arteriolar and venous vasodilator. It is administered as an intravenous infusion with very rapid onset of action, and the vasodilation dissipates almost immediately with termination of the infusion. With careful monitoring, it can be used to titrate blood pressure smoothy to any preselected level [100,101]. This agent should be administered to elderly patients only in an acute care setting with close nursing supervision and continuous direct blood pressure monitoring because of its potent vasodilatory effects. The potent arterial vasodilating property of nitroprusside may cause a dose-dependent increase in heart rate, which can be controlled with the simultaneous administration of a beta-blocker.

A major side effect of nitroprusside is hypotension, which can have an adverse effect on clinical outcome in elderly patients. Hypotension can usually be avoided by close clinical observation and by setting initial limits on the degree of blood pressure reduction. Thiocyanate toxicity represents another potential side effect. Nitroprusside degradation produces cyanide, which is metabolized by the liver to thiocyanate and excreted by the kidney. Elderly patients, particularly those with liver and kidney dysfunction, are at increased risk of cyanate toxicity. In general, nitroprusside infusions should be limited to 1 to 2 days. When the drug is administered for more than two days in the elderly, serum thiocyanate levels should be measured and the patient monitored closely for symptoms of toxicity. These symptoms are nonspecific and can include fatigue, weakness, nausea, vomiting, confusion, hallucinations, and in extreme cases convulsions, coma, and death. To avoid thiocyanate toxicity in the elderly, nitroprusside administration should be tapered and discontinued with concomitant initiation of oral or alternate therapy as early as is clinically feasible.

Nitroglycerine

In elderly patients with hypertensive emergencies, intravenous nitroglycerine is primarily used to treat accompanying myocardial ischemia or to protect potentially ischemic myocardium in patients with acute MI [102]. In low doses, nitroglycerine dilates venous capacitance vessels, which decreases ventricular preload. In higher doses it also dilates arterioles. The major pharmacodynamic advantage of nitroglycerine is that it can decrease blood pressure while maintaining or improving coronary blood flow. This property can be beneficial as primary or adjunctive therapy in elderly patients with severe hypertension associated with ischemic syndromes. Reflex tachycardia can be a problem with the use of nitroglycerine. Another drawback to the use of intravenous nitroglycerine is the rapid development of tolerance, which occurs within the first 24 hours [103]. If adjunctive anti-ischemic therapy is anticipated beyond the first 24 hours, other agents such as beta-blockers, calcium antagonists, or oral nitrates should be started as soon as possible. The clinical use of nitroglycerine as a first-line agent for severe hypertension is also limited by the fact that it is a less potent vasodilator than nitroprusside.

Calcium antagonists

These agents are increasingly being used to treat patients with severe hypertensive episodes [104]. Although a number of second-generation calcium antagonists have been used, nifedipine is the agent with the greatest clinical experience [105]. It is formulated as a liquid in a capsule which, when administered with the "puncture, bite, and swallow" method, has an onset of action within 15 minutes and antihypertensive effects lasting for 3 to 4 hours. Since the drug is absorbed by the stomach and not the buccal mucosa, it is important that the contents of the capsule be swallowed. Typically the degree of blood pressure reduction is related to the severity of pretreatment hypertension. In certain clinical situations, nifedipine offers the advantage of relatively rapid onset of action and ease of administration [106].

Nifedipine also possesses a number of properties that pose significant problems for its use in the elderly. Under most situations of severe hypertension in elderly patients, it is important not only to lower blood pressure rapidly but also to titrate predictably the blood pressure response and avoid prolonged episodes of hypotension. The drug's relatively long duration of action and the fact that it cannot be given parenterally make titration of blood pressure difficult. In addition, patients with decreased vascular compliance because of peripheral atherosclerotic disease may have unpredictable blood pressure responses. Nifedipine can also produce reflex tachycardia, which can aggravate myocardial ischemia in patients with underlying ischemic heart disease. Because of these problems, the use of nifedipine in elderly patients should be avoided completely or reserved for selected situations in which the blood pressure must be lowered rapidly in a conscious patient who does not have intravenous access.

Diazoxide

This potent direct arteriolar dilator has little effect on the venous system [107]. It was once the mainstay of initial therapy for hypertensive emergencies because blood pressure could be rapidly decreased with a single bolus injection [108,109]. In addition, it caused no central nervous system depressive effects. With single-bolus administration, titration of blood pressure is limited by the relatively long half-life. The use of repeated small doses or constant infusion has been shown in some studies to be effective in lowering blood pressure while providing better control. However, a number of other properties of diazoxide suggest that its use in elderly patients should be limited [110,111]. Although diazoxide-induced hypotension is uncommon, it can occur, with long-lasting effects. Diazoxide can also be responsible for sodium and water retention, which may require diuretic therapy to restore the antihypertensive effect. Other side effects of diazoxide include flushing, weakness, nausea, and vomiting [112]. Considering the potential problems associated with the use of diazoxide in elderly patients, this agent is best avoided in most clinical settings.

Hydralazine

This direct arterial vasodilator has little effect on the venous system [113]. It has a number of drawbacks that limit its usefulness in hypertensive emergencies in the elderly. When administered intravenously, the onset of action of hydralazine is unpredictable and may be delayed for 15 to 20 minutes. The antihypertensive effect is variable. Hydralazine can produce reflex tachycardia and an increase in myocardial oxygen consumption leading to myocardial ischemia in elderly patients with coronary artery disease. It is therefore not a recommended agent for primary management of hypertensive emergencies.

Antiadrenergic agents

Labetalol

This agent has combined peripheral alpha-blocking and nonselective beta-blocking activity with proven efficacy in the treatment of hypertensive emergencies. When administered intravenously, it can be given as a single bolus, as repeated miniboluses, or as a constant infusion [114–116]. The predominant hemodynamic effect is a decrease in the systemic vascular resistance characteristic of its peripheral alpha-blocking activity. The drug's beta-blocking activity protects against reflex tachycardia and causes a mild decrease in heart rate, with little or no change in cardiac output. These effects are advantageous in the treatment of elderly patients with hypertensive emergencies who have underlying coronary artery disease. The beta-blocking properties warrant caution in the treatment of elderly patients with certain underlying conditions such as impaired ventricular systolic function, bradycardia, bronchospasm, and atrioventricular conduction abnormalities. The oral form of labetalol simplifies the transition from parenteral therapy.

Propranolol

This beta-antagonist is primarily used as adjunctive therapy in patients with hypertensive emergencies. It is commonly used with nitroprusside in the management of aortic dissection to protect against increases in heart rate, cardiac output, and aortic shear stress (ratio of change in pressure to change in time). As with labetalol, it should be avoided in clinical situations in which beta-blockade may aggrevate an underlying condition.

Esmolol

This ultra-short-acting cardioselective beta-blocker [117] has a half-life of nine minutes and a duration of action of less than 25 to 30 minutes, allowing for smooth control of desired beta-blocking effects. Esmolol has demonstrated efficacy in the management of perioperative hypertension and fine control of the ventricular response to atrial fibrillation [118]. It is rapidly metabolized by tissue, liver, and blood esterases to inactive metabolites that are cleared by the kidney. Thus it can be safely used in elderly patients with renal insufficiency.

Trimethaphan camsylate

This ganglionic blocking agent inhibits both sympathetic and parasympathetic autonomic activities. It is a potent antihypertensive agent with a short onset and duration of action. Since trimethaphan is administered by constant intravenous infusion, constant monitoring of the blood pressure is necessary to prevent hypotensive episodes [119]. The short half-life of this agent, coupled with both sympathetic and parasympathetic ganglionic blockade, once made trimethaphan a useful agent for treatment of aortic dissection [120] because blood pressure could be smoothly controlled, and it produced a decrease in cardiac output, heart rate, and left ventricular ejection rate.

Despite the beneficial antihypertensive properties of trimethaphan, a number of drawbacks significantly limit its use, particularly in the elderly. Elderly patients may be especially bothered by its many side effects, which include blurred vision, constipation, paralytic ileus, exacerbation of glaucoma due to mydriasis, urinary retention, and azotemia from decreased renal blood flow. In addition, tachyphylaxis often develops within 42 hours, so transition to other antihypertensive agents is advisable during this period. Thus, trimethaphan is best avoided in hypertensive emergencies in the elderly because of its side-effect profile.

SPECIAL CLINICAL SITUATIONS

Acute left ventricular failure

Elderly patients have a high prevalence of underlying cardiovascular conditions that can cause abnormal systolic or diastolic function such as ischemic heart disease, long-standing hypertension with LVH, and valvular heart disease. Under these circumstances, an acute and severe elevation in mean systemic blood pressure can lead to deterioration in left ventricular function and elevation in end-diastolic pressure to levels that can produce pulmonary edema.

Nitroprusside is the agent of choice because of its ability rapidly and finely to control blood pressure and to decrease preload, which in turn relieves pulmonary congestion and reduces ventricular volume. Morphine and supplemental oxygen are typically given in conjunction with a loop diuretic [121]. In elderly patients with underlying myocardial ischemia, nitrates may also play an important therapeutic role. After the acute episode has been treated, it is important to plan chronic antihypertensive therapy carefully in the elderly in order to prevent recurrent episodes.

Acute cerebrovascular syndromes

There is a well-established relationship between hypertension and cerebrovascular disease in the elderly [122]. Severe hypertension can be both a cause and a result of cerebrovascular disease in the elderly. It is therefore not uncommon for elderly patients to present with severe hypertension and a variety of concomitant cerebrovascular events, including thrombotic or embolic events or intracerebral hemorrhage.

Management of these syndromes in the elderly is based on the physiology of cerebral blood flow. Under normal circumstances, the cerebrovascular bed is autoregulated by changes in resistance within the bed to maintain a relatively constant blood flow. This process is complex and involves many levels of control such as the perfusing oxygen and carbon dioxide tensions, tissue acidosis, the renin–angiotensin system, and alpha sympathetic tone in perivascular nerves. These mechanisms collectively maintain constant cerebral blood flow for mean arterial blood pressures within a range of approximately 50 to 150 mmHg. In patients with chronic hypertension, cerebrovascular autoregulation adapts over time by shifting this range to higher values of mean arterial pressure [123].

Following a cerebrovascular insult that results in a decrease in regional blood flow to the brain, autoregulation may be lost or significantly compromised. In this setting, cerebral blood flow becomes a function of perfusion pressure that, in turn, depends on mean arteriolar pressure. The release of hemoglobin from red blood cells inhibits the basal dilatory effects of the endothelium-derived relaxing factor (EDRF) and precipates vasoconstriction. Local cerebral vasospasm can further impair regional blood flow, and interventions that abruptly decrease blood pressure can lead to ischemic damage.

The reduction in blood pressure must be guided by the clinical picture. Blood pressure tends to be labile during the early days following a stroke, and minor manupulations can cause rapid decreases to hypotensive levels [124]. If the blood pressure is severely elevated (diastolic >130 mmHg), blood pressure reduction must be accomplished carefully to avoid worsening cerebral ischemia. Some investigators argue that blood pressure should be treated only when it is extremely elevated, with reduction in the mean pressure by no more than 20% to 25% during the first 24 hours [98]. Others recommend decreasing the diastolic blood pressure to the 110 to 120 mmHg range within the first hour [125].

In patients with severe hypertension and intracerebral hemorrhage, similar arguments can be made regarding the aggressiveness of blood pressure reduction. Rapid reductions in blood pressure may prevent rebleeding, but they also place the patient at risk for cerebral hypoperfusion [126]. Again, if the blood pressure is lowered it must be done so cautiously, with close monitoring of the patient's clinical status. If the neurologic picture worsens as the blood pressure is lowered, the blood pressure should be allowed to rise, but not to pretreatment levels. The physician should bear in mind that under normal conditions of upright posture, the intracerebral blood pressure is much lower than the blood pressure at heart level. By changing the patient's position in bed (head–up vs. Trendelenburg), gravity can be an ally or a foe, and the effects on intracerebral blood pressure are instantaneous.

Nitroprusside is the agent of choice. Neither diazoxide nor labetalol offers the same degree of control as nitroprusside, and either one may be associated with prolonged episodes of cerebral hypoperfusion. Agents with central nervous system depressing effects must be avoided because of the importance of monitoring the patient's mental status.

Table 7-8. Diseases that may mimic hypertensive encephalopathy in the elderly

1. Cerebrovascular accident
2. Intracranial mass lesion
3. Metabolic encephalopathy
4. Drug overdose
5. Postictal state
6. Central nervous system infection

Hypertensive encephalopathy

Hypertensive encephalopathy is a clinical syndrome characterized by extreme elevation of blood pressure (diastolic blood pressure often > 130 mmHg), neurologic dysfunction, and associated retinopathy. This syndrome is frequently seen in elderly patients, probably because it represents a progressive phase of chronic hypertension [127].

The clinical presentation develops over a 1- or 2-day period following acute elevation of blood pressure. Elderly patients have variable and changing symptoms that are often nonspecific, including headache, nausea, and vomiting. Visual symptoms are common and include blurred vision, scotomata, diplopia, or blindness. Neurologic abnormalities take the form of focal deficits, seizures, or altered levels of consciousness. Eye examination may demonstrate arteriolar spasm, hemorrhages, exudates, or papilledema. A characteristic feature of the syndrome is rapid resolution of neurologic abnormalities with treatment of hypertension [128]. Before this diagnosis is entertained in the elderly, other processes should be excluded (table 7-8).

Neurologic abnormalities in the syndrome are due to alterations in cerebrovascular autoregulation. The result is an alteration in cerebral capillary permeability with translation of plasma, cerebral edema, and development of petechial hemorrhages [123]. The goal of therapy is to reduce the diastolic blood pressure to approximately 100 mmHg or the mean blood pressure by 20% to 25% (whichever is higher) gradually within the first hour [129].

Nitroprusside is the agent of choice in this syndrome because of its potent vasodilating property and very short half-life. Labetalol and diazoxide have been used but are less desirable because of their longer half-lives and the fact that blood pressure cannot be finely titrated with these agents.

Acute myocardial ischemic syndromes

Hypertension and age are both significant risk factors for coronary artery disease. Consequently, it is not surprising that elderly patients with severe hypertension often have associated acute ischemic syndromes, including unstable angina or MI. Both situations warrant rapid control of blood pressure to improve the clinical outcome. The elevated afterload on the left ventricle induced by severe hypertension increases ventricular wall tension and myocardial oxygen consumption. Patients with unstable angina are at risk of developing an MI, and patients in the process of an acute infarction can extend the area of necrosis to surrounding ischemic zones if hypertension is not rapidly controlled [130].

Elderly patients with a past history of hypertension and LVH are also susceptible to myocardial ischemia with acute and severe elevations in blood pressure. Here the heightened myocardial oxygen demand of a thickened ventricle can exceed oxygen supply (sometimes with normal coronary vasculature). Ischemia in this setting can manifest itself as compromised ventricular systolic and diastolic function and occasionally pulmonary edema [131,132].

The initial goals of therapy are to decrease the blood pressure rapidly to below the ischemic threshold for the left ventricle and to improve the balance between myocardial oxygen supply and demand. Several classes of drugs can concomitantly lower the blood pressure and treat myocardial ischemia, including nitrates, beta-blockers, and calcium antagonists. In addition, the preload- and afterload-reducing properties of nitroprusside allow this drug to decrease myocardial oxygen demand while effectively controlling blood pressure.

Selection of the first-line antihypertensive agent for elderly patients depends on the clinical situation. In patients with extreme elevations in blood pressure, cautious use of nitroprusside may allow rapid control of blood pressure, with the addition of other agents as indicated for adjunctive therapy. On the other hand, in certain clinical situations, intravenous nitroglycerine may be adequate to control blood pressure and treat ischemia.

Esmolol, because of its short-acting beta-blocking property, may be useful as adjunctive therapy in patients with normal ventricular function to decrease myocardial oxygen consumption and to increase coronary blood flow by slowing heart rate and prolonging diastole. In general, hydralazine and diazoxide should not be used because of their potential to induce reflex tachycardia and worsen ischemia. In elderly patients who have experienced an MI, ACE inhibitors should be considered for chronic therapy to decrease blood pressure, since they favorably affect left ventricular remodeling and may prevent development of left ventricular dilation later [133].

Acute aortic dissection

Two important risk factors for the development of aortic dissection include chronic hypertension and atherosclerotic vascular disease, making aortic dissection a common disease in the elderly. Acute dissection is often associated with severe hypertension. The typical presentation is severe, abrupt, and persistent chest or abdominal pain that radiates to the back. These symptoms may mimic acute ischemia, which should be considered in the evaluation. Elderly patients with acute aortic dissection may also have nonspecific symptoms including anxiety, headache, altered mental status, syncope, loss of vision, hemoptysis, and vague gastrointestinal symptoms.

In hypertensive elderly patients, particularly those with nonspecific symptoms, physical findings and laboratory results may suggest the diagnosis of acute aortic dissection and may guide definitive diagnostic evaluation. A number of physical findings support the diagnosis. Deficits in pulses and blood pressures between the upper extremities or between the upper and lower extremities are part of the clinical syndrome. The finding of new aortic regurgitation may suggest a proximal aortic dissection with involvement of the aortic valve apparatus. The chest x-ray may demonstate widening of the mediastinum caused by proximal aortic root dilatation. Aortography is the definitive procedure for determining the location and extent of aortic dissection. However, the increasing use of CT scans and transcsophageal echocardiography may make aortography unnecessary in a large number of cases as more experience is gained.

While the diagnosis is being established, the goal of therapy is to control blood pressure rapidly, decrease aortic wall shear stress, and avoid aortic rupture, which can lead to cardiovascular collapse and death. In general, the diastolic pressure should be lowered to 10 mmHg or less with protection of vital organ perfusion [128,129]. The preferred antihypertensive regimen in elderly patients is nitroprusside in combination with a beta-blocker. Short-acting esmolol may work well in this setting. Labetalol has also proven efficacious [134]. The use of trimethaphan in elderly patients is decreasing because of its significant side effects [135]. Therapy with diazoxide, sublingual nifedipine, and hydralazine should be avoided because of the potential for reflex tachycardia and augmentation of ventricular contractility, which can combine to worsen the dissection.

The decision to use chronic therapy for aortic dissection in the elderly depends on a number of factors. The first is location of the dissection. Patients with involvement distal to the left subclavian artery generally require chronic medical therapy. Here therapy must be selected carefully because of the continued need to control blood pressure while maintaining low shear stress on the aortic wall. Elderly patients with proximal aortic dissections have a higher incidence of complications from extension and often require surgery after the blood pressure is controlled and the patient is clinically stable. Emergency surgery is associated with a high mortality. For a very old patient who is severely disabled by coexisting diseases, it is difficult to recommend surgery. This is a typical situation in which one has to consider ethical as well as medical issues.

NOTES

[1] Portions of this section and the figures were taken from a publication from the Hypertension Update II Symposium, Washington, DC, June 1984, with permission from Health Learning Systems, Inc. [1].

REFERENCES

1. Messerli FH. 1985. Hypertension Update II Symposium, Health Learning Systems, June 1984, Washington, DC.
2. Gavras H and Gavras I (eds). 1983. Hypertension in the Elderly. Boston: John Wright Publishers.
3. Kaplan NN. 1980. Hypertension in patients over 65. Consultant (May):210–217.
4. Kirkendall WM and Hammond JJ. 1980. Hypertension in the elderly. Arch Intern Med 140:1155–1161.
5. Messerli FH. 1984. Hypertension in the elderly. In FH Messerli (ed), Cardiovascular Disease in the Elderly. Boston: Martinus Nijhoff, pp 65–81.
6. Niarchos A and Laragh JH. 1980. Hypertension in the elderly. Mod Concepts Cardiovasc Dis 49:43–48.
7. Ostfeld AM. 1978. Elderly hypertensive patient: epidemiologic review. NY State J Med 78:1125–1129.
8. Messerli FH, Ventura HO, Glade LB, et al. 1983. Essential hypertension in the elderly: Haemodynamics, intravascular volume, plasma renin activity, and circulating catecholamine levels. Lancet 2:983–986.
9. National Health Survey. 1964. Vital and Health Statistics USA: Blood Pressure of Adults by Age and Sex. Washington, DC: U.S. Government Printing Office, p 9.
10. National Health Survey. 1975. Vital and Health Statistics Series 11, No. 150. Blood pressure of persons 18 to 74 years, United States, 1971–72. Bethesda, MD: U.S. Department of Health, Education and Welfare.
11. Fries JF. 1980. Aging, natural death, and the compression of morbidity. N Engl J Med 303:130–135.
12. Veterans Administration Cooperative Study on Antihypertensive Agents. 1962. Double blind control study of antihypertensive agents. III. Chlorothiazide alone and in combination with other agents; preliminary results. Arch Intern Med 110:230–236.
13. Kannel WB and Gordon T. 1978. Evaluation of cardiovascular risk in the elderly: the Framingham study. Bull NY Acad Med 54:573–591.
14. Shekelle RB, Ostfeld AM and Klawans HL Jr. 1974. Hypertension and risk of stroke in an elderly population. Stroke 5:71–75.
15. Forette F, Henry JF, Forette B, et al. 1975. Hypertension arterielle du sujet age prevalence en milieu long sejour. Nouv Presse Med 4:2997–2998.
16. Svärdsudd K and Tibblin G. 1979. Mortality and morbidity during 13.5 years' follow up in relation to blood pressure. The study of men born in 1913. Acta Med Scand 205:483–492.
17. Kannel WB, Wolf PA, McGee DL, et al. 1981. Systolic blood pressure, arterial rigidity, and risk of stroke: the Framingham Study. JAMA 245:1225–1229.
18. Amery A, Birkenhäger W, Brixko P, et al. 1985. Mortality and morbidity results from the European Working Party on High Blood Pressure in the Elderly trial. Lancet 1:1349–1354.
19. Report by the Management Committee. 1980. The Australian Therapeutic Trial in Mild Hypertension. Lancet 1:1261–1269.
20. Hypertension Detection and Follow-up Program Cooperative Group. 1979. Five-year findings of the Hypertension Detection and Follow-up Program: II. Mortality by race-sex and age. JAMA 242:2572–2577.
21. Hypertension-Stroke Cooperative Study Group. 1974. Effect of antihypertensive treatment on stroke recurrence. JAMA 229:409–418.
22. Kuramoto K, Matsushita S, Kuwajima I, et al. 1981. Prospective study on the treatment of mild hypertension in the aged. Jpn Heart J 22:75–85.
23. Veterans Administration Cooperative Study Group on Antihypertensive Agents. 1972. Effects of treatment on morbidity in hypertension: III. Influence of age, diastolic pressure, and prior cardiovascular disease; further analysis of side effects. Circulation 45:991–1004.
24. Hollifield JW, Moore LC, Winn SP, et al. 1983. The role of magnesium, potassium, and beta adrenergic agonists in ventricular arrhythmias associated with hydrochlorothiazide therapy in hypertensives (abstract). Circulation 68 (Suppl III):III-92.
25. Lund-Johansen P. 1983. Hemodynamic response: decrease in cardiac output vs reduction in vascular resistance. Hypertension 5 (Suppl III):III-49–III-57.
26. Multiple Risk Factor Intervention Trial Research Group. 1982. Multiple risk factor intervention trial: risk factor changes and mortality results. JAMA 248:1465–1477.

27. Weidmann P, Gerber A and Mordasini R. 1983. Effects of antihypertensive therapy on serum lipoproteins. Hypertension 5 (Suppl III):III-120–III-131.
28. SHEP Cooperative Research Group. 1991. Prevention of stroke by antihypertensive drug treatment in older persons with isolated systolic hypertension: final results of the Systolic Hypertension in the Elderly Program (SHEP). JAMA 265:3255–3264.
29. Dahlöf B, Lindholm LH, Hansson L, et al. 1991. Morbidity and mortality in the Swedish Trials in Old Patients with Hypertension (STOP-Hypertension). Lancet 338:1281–1285.
30. Terasawa F, Kuramoto K. 1973. The study on the hemodynamics in old hypertensive subjects. Jpn Circ J 37:723–729.
31. Messerli FH. 1985. Essential hypertension in the elderly. Triangle 24:35–47.
32. Lund-Johansen P. 1985. Heart pump function and total peripheral resistance in mild essential hypertension: A 17-year follow-up study. In B Folkow, M Nordlander, BE Strauer, et al. (eds), Hypertension: Pathophysiology and Clinical Implications of Early Structural Changes. Molndal, Sweden: Hassle, pp 392–407.
33. Brandfonbrener M, Landowne M and Shock NW. 1955. Changes in cardiac output with age. Circulation 12:557–566.
34. Conway J, Wheeler R and Sannerstedt R. 1971. Sympathetic nervous activity during exercise in relation to age. Cardiovasc Res 5:577–581.
35. Julius S, Amery A, Whitlock LS, et al. 1967. Influence of age on the hemodynamic response to exercise. Circulation 36:222–230.
36. Messerli FH, Frohlich ED, Suarez DH, et al. 1981. Borderline hypertension: relationship between age, hemodynamics and circulating catecholamines. Circulation 64:760–764.
37. Standell T. 1964. Circulatory studies on healthy old men. Acta Med Scand 175 (Suppl 414):1–44.
38. Fleg JL, Gerstenblith G and Lakatta EG. 1984. Pathophysiology of the aging heart and circulation. In FH Messerli (ed), Cardiovascular Disease in the Elderly. Boston: Martinus Nijhoff, pp 11–34.
39. Rodeheffer RJ, Gerstenblith G, Becker LC, et al. 1984. Exercise cardiac output is maintained in advancing age of healthy human subjects: cardiac dilatation and increased stroke volume compensate for a diminished heart rate. Circulation 69:203–213.
40. Messerli FH. 1981. Individualization of antihypertensive therapy: an approach based on hemodynamics and age. J Clin Pharmacol 21:517–528.
41. Freis ED. 1960. Hemodynamics of hypertension. Physiol Rev 40:27–53.
42. Messerli FH. 1983. Clinical determinants and consequences of left ventricular hypertrophy. Proceedings of a symposium: left ventricular hypertrophy in essential hypertension—mechanisms and therapy. Am J Med 75:51–63.
43. Gardin JM, Henry WL, Savage DD, et al. 1977. Echocardiographic evaluation of an older population without clinically apparent heart disease (abstract). Am J Cardiol 39:277.
44. Gerstenblith G, Lakatta EG and Weisfeldt ML. 1976. Age changes in myocardial function and exercise response. Prog Cardiovasc Dis 19:1–21.
45. Sjögren A-L. 1971. Left ventricular wall thickness determined by ultrasound in 100 subjects without heart disease. Chest 60:341–346.
46. Messerli FH, Sundgaard-Riise K, Ventura HO, et al. 1984. Clinical and hemodynamic determinants of left ventricular dimensions. Arch Intern Med 144:477–481.
47. Kannel WB. 1983. Prevalence and natural history of electrocardiographic left ventricular hypertrophy. Am J Med 75:4–11.
48. Kannel WB, Gordon T and Offutt D. 1969. Left ventricular hypertrophy by electrocardiogram: prevalence, incidence and mortality in the Framingham study. Ann Intern Med 71:89–105.
49. Messerli FH, Ventura HO, Elizardi DJ, et al. 1984. Hypertension and sudden death: increased ventricular ectopic activity in left ventricular hypertrophy. Am J Med 77:18–22.
50. Shannon RP, Wei JY, Rosa RM, et al. 1986. The effect of age and sodium depletion on cardiovascular response to orthostasis. Hypertension 8:438–443.
51. Hollenberg NK, Epstein M, Basch RI, et al. 1969. "No man's land" of the renal vasculature. An arteriographic and hemodynamic assessment of the interlobar and arcuate arteries in essential and accelerated hypertension. Am J Med 47:845–854.
52. Hollenberg NK and Adams DF. 1976. The renal circulation in hypertensive disease. Am J Med 60:773–784.

53. Reubi FC, Weidmann P, Hodler J, et al. 1978. Changes in renal function in essential hypertension. Am J Med 64:556–563.
54. Messerli FH, Frohlich ED, Dreslinski GR, et al. 1980. Serum uric acid in essential hypertension: an indicator of renal vascular involvement. Ann Intern Med 93:817–821.
55. Chien S, Usami S, Simmons RL, et al. 1966. Blood volume and age: repeated measurements on normal men after 17 years. J Appl Physiol 21:583–588.
56. Crane MG, Harris JJ and Johns VJ Jr. 1972. Hyporeninemic hypertension. Am J Med 52:457–466.
57. Flood C, Gherondache C, Pincus C, et al. 1967. The metabolism and secretion of aldosterone in elderly subjects. J Clin Invest 46:960–966.
58. Jose A, Crout R and Kaplan NM. 1970. Suppressed plasma renin activity in essential hypertension: roles of plasma volume, blood pressure, and sympathetic nervous system. Ann Intern Med 72:9–16.
59. Lijnen PJ, Amery AK, Fagard RH, et al. 1978. Relative significance of plasma renin activity and concentration in physiologic and pathophysiologic conditions. Angiology 29:354–366.
60. Meade TW, Imeson JD, Gordon D, et al. 1983. The epidemiology of plasma renin. Clin Sci 64:273–280.
61. Weidmann P, De Myttenaere-Bursztein S, Maxwell MH, et al. 1975. Effect of aging on plasma renin and aldosterone in normal man. Kidney Int 8:325–333.
62. Dzau VJ, Colucci WS, Hollenberg NK, et al. 1981. Relation of renin-angiotensin-aldosterone system to clinical state in congestive heart failure. Circulation 63:645–651.
63. Franco-Morselli R, Elghozi JL, Joly E, et al. 1977. Increased plasma adrenaline concentrations in benign essential hypertension. Br Med J 2:1251–1254.
64. Goldstein DS. 1983. Plasma catecholamines and essential hypertension: an analytical review. Hypertension 5:86–99.
65. Lake CR, Ziehler MG, Coleman MD, et al. 1977. Age-adjusted plasma norepinephrine levels are similar in normotensive and hypertensive subjects. N Engl J Med 296:208–209.
66. Cohn JN, Levine TB, Olivari MT, et al. 1984. Plasma norepinephrine as a guide to prognosis in patients with chronic congestive heart failure. N Engl J Med 311:819–823.
67. Bertel O, Buhler FR, Kiowski W, et al. 1980. Decreased beta-adrenoreceptor responsiveness as related to age, blood pressure, and plasma catecholamines in patients with essential hypertension. Hypertension 2:130–138.
68. van Brummelen P, Bühler FR, Kiowski W, et al. 1981. Age-related decrease in cardiac and peripheral vascular responsiveness to isoprenaline: studies in normal subjects. Clin Sci 60:571–577.
69. Vestal RE, Wood AJJ and Shand DG. 1979. Reduced β-adrenoceptor sensitivity in the elderly. Clin Pharmacol Ther 26:181–186.
70. Kelly J and O'Malley K. 1984. Adrenoreceptor function and ageing. Clin Science 66:509–515.
71. Colandrea MA, Friedman GD, Nichaman MD, et al. 1970. Systolic hypertension in the elderly: an epidemiologic assessement. Circulation 41:239–245.
72. Messerli FH, Ventura HO, Aristimuno GG, et al. 1982. Arterial compliance in systolic hypertension. Clin Exp Hypertens A4:1037–1044.
73. van den Bos GC, Randall OS and Westerhof N. 1981. Blood pressure and cardiac output during decreased arterial compliance. J Physiol 317:68P–69P.
74. Vardan S, Mookherjee S, Warner R, et al. 1983. Systolic hypertension: direct and indirect BP measurements. Arch Intern Med 143:935–938.
75. Simon AC, Safar MA, Levenson JA, et al. 1979. Systolic hypertension: hemodynamic mechanisms and choice of antihypertensive treatment. Am J Cardiol 44:505–511.
76. Osler W. 1892. Principles and Practice of Medicine. New York: Appleton, Century & Croft.
77. Spence JD, Sibbald WJ and Cape RD. 1978. Pseudohypertension in the elderly. Clin Sci Mol Med 55 (Suppl 4):399s–402s.
78. Messerli FH, Ventura HO and Amodeo C. 1985. Osler's maneuver and pseudohypertension. N Engl J Med 312:1548–1551.
79. Messerli FH. 1982. Cardiovascular effects of obesity and hypertension. Lancet 1:1165–1168.
80. Hubert HB, Feinleib M, Menamacre PM, et al. 1983. Obesity as an independent risk factor

for cardiovascular disease: a 26-year follow-up of participants in the Framingham Heart Study. Circulation 67:968–977.

81. Medical Research Council Working Party. 1985. MRC trial of treatment of mild hypertension: principal results. Br Med J 291:97–104.

82. Wasnich RD, Benfante RJ, Yano K, et al. 1983. Thiazide effect on the mineral content of bone. N Engl J Med 309:344–347.

83. Ray WA, Griffin MR, Downey W, et al. 1989. Long-term use of thiazide diuretics and risk of hip fracture. Lancet 1:687–690.

84. Flamenbaum W and Dubrow A. 1990. Labetalol. In FH Messerli (ed), Cardiovascular Drug Therapy. Philadelphia: W. B. Saunders, pp 573–591.

85. Carlson WD. 1990. Carvedilol. In FH Messerli (ed), Cardiovascular Drug Therapy. Philadelphia: W. B. Saunders, pp 603–622.

86. Reid JL. 1990. Celiprolol. In FH Messerli (ed), Cardiovascular Drug Therapy. Philadelphia: W. B. Saunders, pp 554–560.

87. Man in't Veld AJ and Schalekamp MADH. 1982. How intrinsic sympathomimetic activity modulates the haemodynamic responses to beta-adrenoreceptor antagonists: a clue to the nature of their antihypertensive mechanism. Br J Clin Pharmacol 13 (Suppl 2):245S–248S.

88. Bühler FR and Hulthen L. 1982. Calcium channel blockers: A pathophysiologically based antihypertensive treatment concept for the future? Eur J Clin Invest 12:1–3.

89. The Danish Study Group on Verapamil in Myocardial Infarction. 1990. Effect of verapamil on mortality and major events after acute myocardial infarction (The Danish Verapamil Infarction Trial II—DAVIT II). Am J Cardiol 66:779–785.

90. The Multicenter Diltiazem Postinfarction Trial Research Group. 1988. The effect of diltiazem on mortality and reinfarction after myocardial infarction. N Engl J Med 319:385–392.

91. Bühler FR, Hulthén UL, Kiowski W, et al. 1984. Beta blockers and calcium antagonists: Cornerstones of antihypertensive therapy in the 1980's. Drugs 6 (Suppl 6):9888–9894.

92. Henry PD. 1985. Atherosclerosis, calcium and calcium antagonists. Circulation 72:456–459.

93. Dunn FG, Oigman W, Ventura HO, et al. 1984. Enalapril improves systemic and renal hemodynamics and allows regression of left ventricular mass in essential hypertension. Am J Cardiol 53:105–108.

94. Tarazi RC, Bravo EL, Fouad FM, et al. 1980. Hemodynamic and volume changes associated with captopril. Hypertension 2:576–585.

95. Gudbrandsson T. 1981. Malignant hypertension. A clinical follow-up study with special reference to renal and cardiovascular function and immunogenetic factors. Acta Med Scand Suppl 650:1–62.

96. Moser M. 1989. Physiologic changes in the elderly: are they clinically important in the management of hypertension? Geriatrics 44 (Suppl B):4–9.

97. Koch-Weser J. 1974. Hypertensive emergencies. N Engl J Med 290:211–214.

98. Calhoun DA and Oporil S. 1990. Treatment of hypertensive crisis. N Engl J Med 323:1177–1183.

99. Ferguson RK and Vlasses PH. 1986. Hypertensive emergencies and urgencies. JAMA 255:1607–1613.

100. Tinker JH, Michenfelder JD. 1976. Sodium nitroprusside: pharmacology, toxicity and therapeutics. Anesthesiology 45:340–354.

101. Palmer RF and Lasseter KC. 1975. Sodium nitroprusside. N Engl J Med 292:294–297.

102. Chatterjee K and Parmley WW. 1983. Vasodilator therapy for acute myocardial infarction and chronic congestive heart failure. J Am Coll Cardiol 1:133–153.

103. Packer M, Lee WH, Kesler PD, et al. 1987. Prevention and reversal of nitrate tolerance in patients with congestive heart failure. N Engl J Med 317:799–804.

104. DeVault GA Jr. 1991. Therapy in hypertensive emergencies, Part 2: calcium antagonists, ACE inhibitors. J Crit Illness 6:388–394.

105. Sorkin EM, Clissold SP and Brogden RN. 1985. Nifedipine: a review of its pharmacodynamic and pharmacokinetic properties, and therapeutic efficacy, in ischemic heart disease, hypertension and related cardiovascular disorders. Drugs 30:182–274.

106. Houston MC. 1988. The comparative effects of clonidine and nifedipine in the treatment of hypertensive crisis. Am Heart J 115:152–159.

107. Koch-Weser J. 1976. Diazoxide. N Engl J Med 294:1271–1273.
108. Miller WE, Gifford RW Jr, Humphry DC, et al. 1969. Management of severe hypertension with intravenous injections of diazoxide. Am J Cardiol 24:870–875.
109. Mroczek WJ, Leibel BA, Davidov M, et al. 1971. The importance of the rapid administration of diazoxide in accelerated hypertension. N Engl J Med 285:603–606.
110. Thiem TA, Huysmans FT, Gerlad PG, et al. 1979. Diazoxide infusion in severe hypertension and hypertensive crisis. Clin Pharmacol Ther 25:795–799.
111. McDonald WJ, Smith G, Woods JW, et al. 1977. Intravenous diazoxide therapy in hypertensive crisis. Am J Cardiol 40:409–415.
112. Kumar GK, Dastoor FC, Robayo JR, et al. 1976. Side effects of diazoxide. JAMA 235:275–276.
113. Koch-Weser J. 1976. Hydralazine. N Engl J Med 295:320–323.
114. Cumming AM, Brown JJ, Lever AF, et al. 1979. Treatment of severe hypertension by repeated bolus injections of labetalol. Br J Clin Pharmacol 8:199S–204S.
115. Wilson DJ, Wallin JD, Vlachakis ND, et al. 1983. Intravenous labetalol in the treatment of severe hypertension and hypertensive emergencies. Am J Med 75:95–102.
116. Cumming AM, Brown JJ, Lever AF, et al. 1982. Intravenous labetalol in the treatment of severe hypertension. Br J Clin Pharmacol 13:93S–96S.
117. Frishman WH, Murthy VS and Strom JA. 1988. Ultrashort acting beta-adrenergic blockers. Med Clin North Am 72:359–372.
118. Schwartz M, Michelson EL, Sawin HS, et al. 1988. Esmolol: safety and efficacy in post-operative cardiothoracic patients with supraventricular tachyarrhythmias. Chest 93:705–711.
119. Segal JL. 1980. Hypertensive emergencies: practical approach to treatment. Postgrad Med 68:107–125.
120. Finnerty FA. 1981. Treatment of hypertensive emergencies. Heart Lung 10:275–284.
121. McRae RP Jr and Liebson PR. 1986. Hypertensive crisis. Med Clin North Am 70:749–767.
122. Spence JD and del Maestro RF. 1985. Hypertension in acute ischemic stroke. Arch Neurol 42:1000–1002.
123. Strandgaard S, Olesen J, Skinhoj E, et al. 1973. Autoregulation of brain circulation in severe arterial hypertension. Br Med J 1:507–510.
124. Britton M, deFaire U and Helmars C. 1980. Hazards of therapy for excessive hypertension in acute stroke. Acta Med Scand 207:253–257.
125. DeVault GA Jr. 1990. Therapy in hypertensive emergencies: a disease-specific approach. J Crit Illness 6:477–484.
126. Clinical Management Study Group. 1973. Medical and surgical management of stroke. Stroke 4:273–320.
127. Gifford RW Jr and Westbrook E. 1974. Hypertensive encephalopathy: mechanisms, clinical features, and treatment. Prog Cardiovasc Dis 17:115–124.
128. Houston MC. 1986. Hypertensive urgencies and emergencies: pathophysiology, clinical aspects and treatment. Crit Care Med 7:151–246.
129. Garcia JY Jr and Vidt DG. 1987. Current management of hypertensive emergencies. Drugs 34:263–278.
130. Ram CV. 1983. Hypertensive crisis. Primary Care 10:41–61.
131. Strauer BE. 1987. Left ventricular wall stress and hypertrophy. In FH Messerli (ed), The Heart and Hypertension. New York: Yorke Medical Books, pp 154–165.
132. Marcus ML, Koyanagi S, Harrison DG, et al. 1987. Abnormalities in the coronary circulation that occur as a consequence of cardiac hypertrophy. In FH Messerli (ed), The Heart and Hypertension. New York: Yorke Medical Books, pp 231–293.
133. Pfeffer MA, Lamas GA, Vaughan DE, et al. 1988. Effect of captopril on progressive ventricular dilatation after anterior myocardial infarction. N Engl J Med 319:80–86.
134. Grubb BP, Sirio C and Zelis R. 1987. Intravenous labetalol in acute aortic dissection. JAMA 258:78–79.
135. Kaplan NM. 1986. Hypertensive crises. In NM Kaplan (ed), Clinical Hypertension, 4th ed. Baltimore: Williams & Wilkins, pp 273–291.

8. DISTURBANCES OF CARDIAC RHYTHM

KELLY ANNE SPRATT
ERIC L. MICHELSON
LEONARD S. DREIFUS

A 102-year-old man complained to his physician about pain in his right knee. The physician dismissed it. "What can you expect at 102?" But the patient retorted, "My left knee is 102 years old too, and it doesn't hurt." [1]

DEFINING THE ISSUES

Embarking on a discussion of cardiac arrhythmias in the elderly presents a special challenge. Over the past decade, criteria for characterizing both *elderly* and *arrhythmias* have changed considerably. At one time, the term *elderly* merely referred to persons over 65 years of age. Today the elderly are often subclassified into young-old, old-old, and oldest-old. The criteria for these subdivisions alternatively emphasize the functional, social, and health status of the patient or the actual age. Young-old are those persons over age 65 years who are vigorous, competent, and functionally independent, while old-old are those elderly individuals who have suffered progressively major physical, mental, and social losses and consequently require considerable supportive care. Others use the terms young-old, old-old, and oldest-old strictly to divide the elderly by age: 65–75 years, 75–85 years, and over 85 years, respectively. These distinctions have obvious potential clinical implications.

Franz H. Messerli (ed.), CARDIOVASCULAR DISEASE IN THE ELDERLY (Third Edition). Copyright © 1993 Kluwer Academic Publishers. ISBN 0-7923-1859-5. All rights reserved.

In a similar manner, criteria for defining clinically significant arrhythmias have evolved. Analogous to the quote above, it is necessary to view cardiac arrhythmias in light of expected as well as pathologic changes associated with aging.

Unfortunately, many clinical trials have purposely excluded the elderly in the belief that this population is too frail to be placed in experimental protocols. Therefore, accurate data regarding the cardiovascular responses to various interventions in the elderly are scant. With the realization that this is the very population that often stands to benefit most from more aggressive therapeutic modalities, more emphasis will be focused on studies assessing this special population.

This chapter will address the following questions regarding rhythm disturbances peculiar to the elderly and to the senescent heart:

1. What factors associated with the aging process predispose to the development of arrhythmias?
2. Which arrhythmias are especially prevalent in the elderly?
3. Which arrhythmias in the elderly should be treated and which should *not*?
4. What diagnostic modalities and therapeutic strategies are most efficacious in the elderly?

THE DIAGNOSTIC AND THERAPEUTIC CHALLENGE

Advances in diagnosis and therapy

The prevalence of cardiac arrhythmias in the elderly and the impact of these arrhythmias on quality of life and longevity demand closer scrutiny as diagnostic and therapeutic options continue to expand.

The spectrum of pharmacologic agents to treat arrhythmias has recently broadened considerably. Newer additions to the armamentarium include tocainide, mexiletine, amiodarone, propafenone, encainide, flecainide, adenosine (intravenous), and moricizine, as well as a vast array of beta-blockers and calcium antagonists. Established drugs such as quinidine, procainamide, disopyramide, lidocaine (intravenous), bretylium (intravenous), and digoxin are also still available. This variety of pharmacologic agents is evidence that clinicians are aware of the limits of these agents, and, to date, the antiarrhythmic "wonder drug" has yet to be discovered. The bothersome systemic, cardiac, and potentially lethal proarrhythmic side effects of these drugs warrant that patients with non-life-threatening arrhythmias only be exposed to them with clear indications and considerable caution. Subjective clinical outcomes must be documented and assessed in light of objective data regarding functional status, morbidity, and mortality.

Another area of major clinical advance that also has had considerable impact on the management of arrhythmias in the elderly is the burgeoning field of invasive cardiac electrophysiology. Unquestionably, there will be an ever-increasing reliance upon invasive diagnostic clinical electrophysiologic testing and upon the utilization of invasive therapeutic interventions such as pacemakers, antitachycardia devices, and implantable cardioverter defibrillators, as well as catheter-ablative procedures and antiarrhythmic surgery. The potential use of these procedures seems limited only by allocation of resources and severity of concomitant medical conditions.

Current diagnostic limitations

Questions of arrhythmia detection, quantitation, variability, risk stratification, and therapeutic endpoints are also highly relevant in the elderly. For example, day-to-day variability in ambient ectopy, as detected by 24-hour ambulatory electrocardiographic monitoring, can be so marked that using one algorithm [2], an almost 85% reduction in ventricular ectopy would be needed to attribute the improvement to the antiarrhythmic agent rather than to spontaneous variability. Extended or repeated 24-hour monitoring for long periods to minimize this variability is impractical and expensive. In addition, elderly patients are often unable to accurately document episodic symptoms because of incomplete instruction or impaired cognitive functioning, and the obtained information is often inconclusive or incomplete. Unfortunately, event recorders, which are best suited for documentation of less frequent but more prolonged bouts of arrhythmias, may also prove unreliable in the elderly for similar reasons; impaired agility or psychomotor functioning in the elderly population may also adversely affect event recorder reliability.

Historically, investigators utilizing only conventional 12-lead electrocardiograms noted a high prevalence of cardiac arrhythmias with advancing age [3]. However, since the presence of cardiovascular disease also increases with age, it has been difficult to define the prevalence of cardiac arrhythmias in a "normal" aging population. Most reports reflect evaluations of asymptomatic persons, but only a few address the magnitude of occult heart disease in the elderly. The investigation of cardiac arrhythmias in this population therefore would require meticulous, extensive invasive and noninvasive testing, which has generally been impractical. Furthermore, difficulties in the collection of both initial and follow-up data in this population may challenge the accuracy of any subsequent results. The elderly may be intimidated by long-term monitoring devices and, not infrequently, may fail to keep accurate diaries that provide clinical correlation with electrocardiographic findings [3,4]. Even more confounding is the inability to adequately follow these individuals over long periods due to comorbid disease processes independent of the patient's cardiac or arrhythmic status. Therefore, detailed and accurate longitudinal evaluations of this population are not readily attainable [5].

Recognition of the limitations of ambulatory electrocardiographic monitoring and recording has led to heightened interest in pursuing alternative noninvasive testing strategies. Recently, the technique of signal-averaged electrocardiography has shown promise as a means to identify in particular patients at risk for life-threatening ventricular tachyarrhythmias after myocardial infarction [6]. Finally, the use of invasive intracardiac programmed electrophysiologic studies to guide therapy is an option being applied more widely. At present, it is the procedure of choice for guiding definitive therapy in most patients, including the elderly, with life-threatening, hemodynamically intolerable arrhythmias.

CHARACTERISTICS OF THE ELDERLY PATIENT

While a departure from normal sinus rhythm will affect cardiac performance at any age, certain conditions render the elderly especially vulnerable to development of various rhythm abnormalities, further predispose them to be less tolerant of such arrhythmias, and, unfortunately, also complicate therapy. Autopsy studies conducted in the 1950s and 1970s [7] revealed that a substantial proportion of the elderly have significant coronary artery disease, including the 25% to 55% in whom coronary artery disease is "silent."

As detailed elsewhere, the elderly are particularly likely to be afflicted with a cumulative burden of progressive degenerative diseases and processes that may either directly or indirectly render them susceptible to develop and suffer consequences from rhythm and conduction disorders. These include coronary artery obstructive lesions resulting in myocardial ischemia (whether occult or manifest) and myocardial infarction; myocardial hypertrophy, dilatation, fibrosis, and infiltrative lesions (e.g., amyloid); systolic and diastolic dysfunction; valvular stenosis (e.g., aortic) and incompetence; and diminution of vascular compliance, elasticity, and relaxation properties. In addition, changes in neurohumoral responsiveness and alterations in autonomic tone affect cardiac pacemaker cells, the specialized conduction tissues, and myocardial mechanical function, thereby influencing arrhythmogenesis. Also important is the milieu engendered by the effects of other systemic disorders and medications affecting such diverse factors as electrolytes, glucose, lipids, acid–base balance, and arterial blood gases, as well as less common contributing factors attributable to abnormal function of other organs, infection, tumors, intracranial processes, etc. In particular, decreased hepatic and renal function, decreased serum albumin levels, and electrolyte abnormalities are likely to affect the choice, dosing, efficacy, safety, and monitoring of antiarrhythmic drug therapy.

Another important factor is the potential effect of impaired cognition on therapeutic compliance. Up to 70% of patients reporting good compliance with antiarrhythmic medications were found to have subtherapeutic serum drug levels [8]. Finally, other issues impact on the elderly. As health care costs spiral upward, many elderly persons on fixed incomes will be faced with the financial reality of the considerable costs of antiarrhythmic (and other) medications. The treatment of any elderly patient necessitates examination of his or her living arrangement. Any decrease in quality of life for the patient usually translates into a tremendous emotional and financial burden for the family as well.

HEART RATE

Anecdotal evidence that the resting heart rate decreases with advancing age has not been consistently confirmed by objective evaluation. Camm et al. [4] noted only a 10% incidence of sinus bradycardia in 106 ambulatory persons older than age 75, most of whom had no cardiovascular history. This conclusion was reinforced by the results of another study of subjects older than age 80 during sleeping and waking periods; heart rates of 40 to 50 beats per minute occurred in only 14% of 50 healthy subjects [9]. Marked bradycardias of less than 40 beats per minute did not occur in any subject. On the other hand, Camm et al. [4] found a number of persons whose sinus rates varied only by 10 beats per minute or less throughout a 24-hour period; such decreased heart rate variability is a potential marker of advanced cardiac disease and poor prognosis.

While the resting heart rate falls little with age, there is a progressive decrease in the maximum heart rate response to exercise. This decline in maximum heart rate may be due, in part, to reduced adrenergic sensitivity in aging sinus-node pacemaker cells [10]. In addition, fat may accumulate around the sinoatrial node at times, producing partial or complete separation of the node from the atrial musculature. Hinkle et al. [11] evaluated a group of middle-aged men to determine their risk for acute cardiac death and found that a heart rate that did not rise during the day's activities indicated greater risk than the resting rate itself. Kostis et al. [12] documented that the reduction in maximum heart rate achieved with daily activity was associated with lower exercise tolerance in older persons. While in young, conditioned persons a decreased heart rate may reflect physical fitness, from middle age onward this cannot be reliably concluded. Rather, instead of accepting the notion that slowing of the resting heart rate is a normal aging phenomenon, the available data seem to indicate that sustained marked bradycardia in an older adult may be a pathologic finding warranting attention if it is associated with symptoms. On the other hand, a number of patients with syncope, structural heart disease, and bradyarrhythmias are also found to have inducible sustained ventricular tachyarrhythmias when evaluated by invasive electrophysiologic testing. In these cases, management of tachyarrhythmia is usually associated with improved clinical outcome.

Typical heart rates at rest in men have been shown to be slightly lower than in women, approximately 70 beats per minute and 76 beats per minute, respectively [4,13]. Another influence on heart rate is diurnal variation. Normally, peak heart rate occurs from 2:00 to 5:00 p.m. and the nadir from 4:00 to 6:00 a.m., with an abrupt increase shortly after awakening. These fluctuations reflect changes in activity and are in part mediated by the neurohumoral axis [9]. No specific drug is yet available that is effective, safe, and well tolerated for the treatment of persistent inappropriate sinus bradycardia. (The use of antibradycardia pacemakers is discussed in chapter 9.) Somewhat paradoxically, some patients with paroxysmal bradycardia may be candidates for beta-blockers. These include patients who on provocative tilt testing initially manifest relative tachycardia and catechol discharge before demonstrating subsequent bradycardia and hypotension.

SICK SINUS SYNDROME

Definition

The term *sick sinus syndrome* was initially used by Lown [14] to describe patients with abnormally prolonged sinus-node recovery times after cardioversion of atrial tachyarrhythmias. The term has since evolved to include a constellation of cardiac electrophysiologic derangements manifesting as pathologic bradyarrhythmias and alternating supraventricular tachyarrhythmias interrupting sinus rhythm (the *brady-tachy* syndrome). This entity accounts for up to 50% of permanent pacemaker implants [15]. Although coexisting diseases may be seen in the elderly, the most common etiology for sick sinus syndrome is an idiopathic sclerodegenerative process [16] that leads to an increase in fibrous tissue in the conduction system. The development of sick sinus syndrome in the setting of an acute myocardial infarction, usually transient, is due to the combination of sinus-node ischemia, local autonomic neural effects, and inflammation. Abnormal sinus-node function and several manifestations of sick sinus syndrome are also relatively common transiently following open-heart surgery, during which sinoatrial tissue may be traumatized. Recently, atherosclerotic occlusive disease of the sinus-nodal artery has been recognized as a specific etiologic factor in some cases [17].

Diagnosis

The diagnosis of sinus-node dysfunction is often made by 12-lead electro-cardiography or cardiac monitoring (figure 8-1). Classic manifestations of sick sinus syndrome are listed in table 8-1. However, if noninvasive testing, including tilt testing, fails to document the disorder and if the index of suspicion is high in a symptomatic patient, invasive electrophysiologic testing may be warranted [18]. Intracardiac electrophysiologic testing may reveal derangements of sinus-node automaticity, conduction, or both, and may confirm abnormal responses to autonomic and pharmacologic perturbations. Provocative testing often reveals derangements other than sinus-node dysfunction, such as unsuspected ventricular tachycardia [19]. Because the clinical relevance of invasive testing of sinus-node function is not always clear, the diagnostic standard continues to be ambulatory electrocardiographic

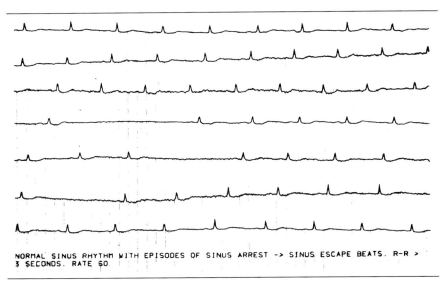

NORMAL SINUS RHYTHM WITH EPISODES OF SINUS ARREST -> SINUS ESCAPE BEATS. R-R > 3 SECONDS. RATE 60.

Figure 8-1. Continuous electrocardiographic monitoring in a 75-year-old man evaluated for episodic lightheadedness and dizziness revealed frequent spontaneous sinus pauses of two to longer than three seconds' duration. The baseline rhythm was sinus with rate approximately 60 beats/min.

Table 8-1. Manifestations of sick sinus syndrome

- Inappropriate sinus bradycardia
- Paroxysmal atrial tachyarrhythmias and atrial fibrillation culminating in chronic atrial fibrillation
- Paroxysmal supraventricular tachyarrhythmias and bradyarrhythmias, the "tachy-brady" syndrome (including atrial fibrillation and atrial flutter)
- Prolonged long pauses following cardioversion of atrial tachyarrhythmias
- Prolonged pauses (e.g., greater than three seconds) following carotid sinus massage
- Sinus pauses, arrest, or exit block
- Atrial fibrillation with slow ventricular response in the absence of drugs
- Failure of subsidiary escape junctional or idioventricular pacemakers during sinus pauses resulting in profound bradycardia or marked asystolic pauses
- Altered sensitivity of the sinus node to autonomic perturbations, including vagomimetic interventions and sympatholytic drugs
- Enhanced depression of sinus-node function by cardiotonic drugs including antiarrhythmics and calcium antagonists

monitoring correlated with patient symptomatology. This modality often reveals alternating tachyarrhythmias and bradyarrhythmias as well as bursts of atrial fibrillation or flutter (figure 8-2). These paroxysms are often preceded by atrial premature depolarizations, default of sinus-node activity, or both [20]. Symptoms such as lightheadedness and syncope often occur during

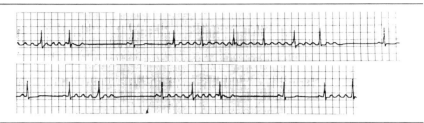

Figure 8-2. A 71-year-old woman was evaluated for palpitations and dizziness. Ambulatory electrocardiographic monitoring revealed recurrent paroxysms of atrial flutter terminating with pauses.

a prolonged pause following tachycardia, and therefore are also due to failure of escape pacemakers and not merely sinus-node dysfunction. On the other hand, palpitations, exacerbations of angina, shortness of breath, and paroxysmal heart failure including episodes of "flash pulmonary edema" are usually attributable to paroxysmal tachycardias [16].

Therapy

Drugs used to suppress tachyarrhythmias and to control the ventricular rate, such as digitalis, beta-blockers, or calcium antagonists, may further depress sinus-node automaticity or sinoatrial conduction and consequently aggravate bradycardias associated with this syndrome. Often a combination of these drugs (to control tachyarrhythmias) and pacemaker therapy (to prevent resultant bradyarrhythmias) is required for treatment of this challenging and multifaceted entity.

Acutely, in attempting to terminate the supraventricular tachycardias in patients with sick sinus syndrome, clinicians using vagomimetic maneuvers or other cardioversion techniques must be careful to have electrocardiographic monitoring, external pacing, and resuscitative measures available. The elderly are extremely sensitive to these procedures and may be likely to develop prolonged sinus pauses or atrioventricular conduction block (figure 8-3) [20].

SUPRAVENTRICULAR TACHYARRHYTHMIAS

Epidemiology

Supraventricular tachyarrhythmias appear to be more frequent in older populations even after careful screening for latent coronary artery disease. Twenty-four hour ambulatory electrocardiographic monitoring of 98 active healthy elderly patients aged 60 to 85 years who were noninvasively screened for the presence of cardiac disease revealed the presence of isolated supraventricular ectopic beats in 88%, with 26% having more than 100 supraventricular ectopic beats in 24 hours [13]. Most of the patients with

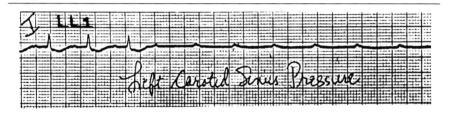

Figure 8-3. A 68-year-old man was referred after a syncopal episode. Baseline electrocardiogram revealed first-degree A-V block. Left carotid sinus massage caused prolonged complete A-V block, presumably at the level of the A-V node, and asystole. For this reason, carotid sinus massage should not be performed routinely in the elderly unless preparations have been made for resuscitation if necessary.

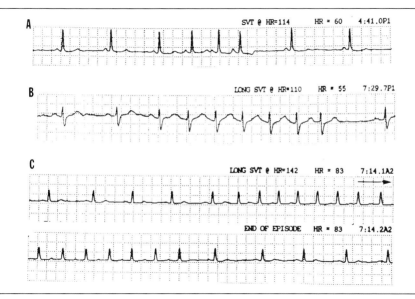

Figure 8-4. Ambulatory electrocardiographic recordings in three elderly patients (rhythm strips on panels **A**, **B**, and **C**) revealed typical runs of nonsustained supraventricular tachyarrhythmias (SVTs). These SVTs occur at different heart rates (HRs) and may last from a few beats to several seconds. In many cases, no symptoms are reported by patients in association with these paroxysms. Not uncommonly, patients may report "palpitations," but there is no evidence of hemodynamic compromise, and reassurance is preferable to prescribing drug therapy.

more complex ectopy were older than 70 years of age. Over 13% had asymptomatic paroxysmal supraventricular tachycardia (figure 8-4). Of interest, only one case of atrial flutter was documented, and there were no cases of atrial fibrillation. It can be concluded that the appearance of either of these arrhythmias in an elderly patient is abnormal. In this series, no apparent

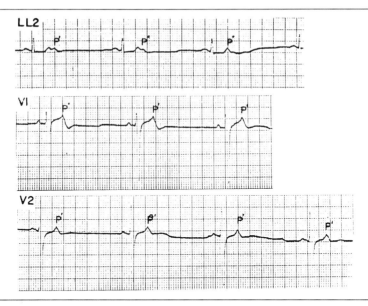

Figure 8-5. Recordings from various electrocardiographic leads in a 79-year-old woman noted on examination to have marked bradycardia. She had complaints of easy fatigability, dyspnea on exertion, and mild chest pain and was referred for pacemaker evaluation. Electrocardiographic monitoring revealed sinus bradycardia with frequent nonconducted premature atrial contractions. These were readily suppressed by the use of a class IA antiarrhythmic agent, and the patient did not require a pacemaker.

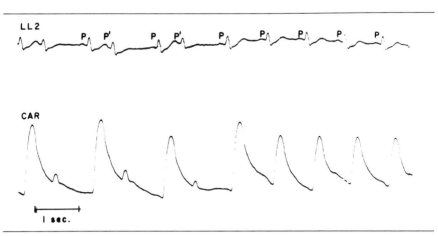

Figure 8-6. A 72-year-old man was evaluated for complaints of episodic palpitations and associated generalized weakness. In the upper tracing, the patient demonstrated frequent premature atrial beats on the electrocardiogram. On the lower tracing, the carotid pressure tracing revealed that these premature contractions were ineffective hemodynamically. An empiric trial of antiarrhythmic therapy resulted in suppression of atrial ectopy and resolution of symptoms.

differences were found between men and women, smokers and nonsmokers, or hypertensive and normotensive subjects with respect to prevalence of supraventricular tachycardia. Occasionally, even seemingly benign atrial arrhythmias may cause hemodynamic compromise and require therapy (figures 8-5 and 8-6).

Supraventricular arrhythmias, in particular paroxysmal atrial fibrillation and atrial flutter, have been associated with ingestion of alcohol, especially with binge-type drinking, the so-called "holiday heart syndrome" [21]. This was further substantiated by Engel et al., who were able to induce atrial fibrillation or flutter in 10 of 14 patients following ingestion of 60 to 120 ml of whiskey. The blood alcohol level in these patients ranged from 49 to 101 mg/dl and thus was below the usual level causing intoxication [22]. Examination of patients who rarely used alcohol but occasionally binged socially revealed the same increased vulnerability to rhythm disturbances [23]. Explanations for this phenomenon have included the acute toxic-metabolic effects of alcohol; subclinical cardiomyopathy; malnutrition and associated electrolyte abnormalities such as hypokalemia or hypomagnesemia; the increased release of catecholamines that is promoted by alcohol; or the rise in free fatty acids, thought to be arrhythmogenic, in response to alcohol ingestion [24]. In addition, controversy exists regarding the role of the principal metabolite of alcohol, acetaldehyde, in arrhythmogenesis [25]. It is therefore of utmost importance when evaluating an elderly patient to obtain an accurate social history including use of alcohol.

Definition

Supraventricular tachyarrhythmias (SVTs) include

1. arrhythmias primarily of atrial origin, such as atrial premature beats, ectopic atrial rhythms, multifocal atrial tachycardia, intra- and interatrial reentrant rhythms (including atrial flutter), and atrial fibrillation;
2. arrhythmias arising primarily within the atrioventricular (A-V) node, such as A-V nodal reentrant tachycardia, junctional premature beats, and nonparoxysmal junctional tachycardias (often associated with digitalis toxicity); and
3. arrhythmias that are partially supraventricular in origin, involving reentry utilizing accessory A-V connections as well as both supraventricular and ventricular tissue. These are designated *A-V reciprocating tachycardias*, to which patients with preexcitation syndromes, the prototype of which is Wolff–Parkinson–White (WPW) syndrome, are more prone.

ATRIAL FIBRILLATION

Etiology

Clinical and experimental observations indicate that atrial fibrillation is often the result of wavelets of intraatrial reentry encountering areas of varying refractoriness resulting in "chaotic" fibrillatory waves. The fibrillating atria discharge impulses at approximately 300 to 600 depolarizations/minute. These impulses arrive at the A-V junction in a disorganized manner, resulting in the characteristic irregular ventricular response, typically at rates of 130 to 200 beats per minute in the absence of A-V nodal blocking drugs.

Atrial fibrillation occurs in as many as 10% to 20% of hospitalized or institutionalized elderly patients and is more likely to occur in the setting of underlying organic heart disease. However, other contributory causes of atrial fibrillation include alcoholic binges (the "holiday heart syndrome"), hypoxemia, hypokalemia, autonomic surges and thyrotoxicosis, and excesses of other stimulants, which may include nonprescription medication.

Atrial fibrillation in the absence of heart disease or metabolic aberration has been termed *lone atrial fibrillation*. The incidence of thromboembolic events in the setting of lone atrial fibrillation is controversial. A study at the Mayo Clinic using a younger population (mean age of diagnosis 44 years) evaluated 97 patients, all initially under age 60, and found only eight embolic events during a mean follow-up of 14.8 years, for a yearly risk of 0.55% [26]. The Framingham study reported a 30-year follow-up of 5209 patients regarding the development of atrial fibrillation. Of the 376 patients who developed atrial fibrillation, 43 or 0.8% were felt to have lone atrial fibrillation [27]. This study noted a marked increase in embolic stroke occurrence in patients with lone atrial fibrillation when compared with the control population (28% versus 7%, respectively) [27]. The patients in this study were much older (mean age 70 years) than those in the Mayo Clinic study, and almost one third had preexisting hypertension. The annual risk of stroke in this cohort was 2.6%. The low risk of thromboembolism in the younger population suggests that atrial fibrillation may potentiate the thromboembolic risk of other cardiovascular abnormalities. Thus, even this entity, once presumed to be a benign form of atrial fibrillation, also mandates consideration of long-term anticoagulation. However, through advanced echocardiography techniques, including transesophageal echocardiography, it has become apparent that true lone atrial fibrillation is even less common; in the setting of a negative history of thromboembolism and absent spontaneous left atrial contrast echoes or thrombus, thromboembolic risk is quite low. Of note, the presence of atrial fibrillation may itself engender abnormalities detected by echocardiography, such as atrial enlargement, that may resolve after resumption of normal sinus rhythm.

The prognosis of patients with atrial fibrillation depends upon the etiology of the arrhythmia. In a study of over 3700 patients over age 50, chronic atrial fibrillation without identifiable structural heart disease was associated with a seven-fold increase in mortality, while atrial fibrillation associated with valvular disease had a 17-fold increase in mortality [28].

Complications of atrial fibrillation

The elderly are least able to tolerate the hemodynamic insults associated with atrial fibrillation; these include the loss of atrial contraction (which in the elderly may account for 20% to 40% of cardiac output) and inadequate ventricular filling time associated with rapid ventricular rates, particularly with short R-R intervals. The onset of atrial fibrillation can precipitate pulmonary congestion as well as decreased cardiac output, occasionally causing acute cardiopulmonary collapse.

The situation is made even worse if there is critical stenosis in any of the major vascular beds, since the decreased cardiac output can lead to ischemic compromise. Similarly, even mild-to-moderate valvular stenosis or ventricular hypertrophy may be poorly tolerated if atrial fibrillation is superimposed. In this regard, the elderly are particularly vulnerable, since calcific aortic valvular sclerosis is common in the geriatric population.

An additional consideration is that 36% of all ischemic strokes in persons older than age 80 are associated with atrial fibrillation, and 50% of these strokes result in disability or death [29]. Thus there has been renewed interest in the issue of anticoagulation. The benefits and risks of long-term anticoagulation in the elderly must be carefully considered, with screening to identify patients with bleeding conditions and other potential contraindications. Currently recommended to receive long-term anticoagulation are patients with atrial fibrillation and a history of previous cardioembolic event, cardiomyopathy, valvular heart disease, coronary artery disease, or hypertensive heart disease [30–34]. Even patients over 60 years old with lone atrial fibrillation should be considered for anticoagulation. In a study of over 1000 patients (mean age of 74 years) with nonrheumatic chronic atrial fibrillation, warfarin therapy (approximate prothrombin time ratio: 1.5 to 2.0 times control) for two years significantly reduced mortality, decreasing the incidence of thromboembolism from 5.5% to 2.0% [30] when compared with low-dose aspirin (75 mg) and placebo. Although coagulation is currently an area of controversy, an American College of Chest Physicians/ National Heart, Lung and Blood Institute panel [34] has recommended low-dose anticoagulation (prothrombin time ratio: 1.5 times control) for three weeks prior to elective cardioversion to decrease the possibility of embolic complications. Anticoagulation should be continued for three weeks after cardioversion, since a thrombus can still remain due to a delay in resumption of mechanical atrial contraction. Not all patients are candidates for warfarin, and aspirin may be considered as an alternative in some cases [31].

Management—acute therapy

Depending on the clinical status of the patient, the acute management of atrial fibrillation may involve attempts either to simply control the ventricular rate or to convert the rhythm to sinus using direct-current cardioversion or drug therapy. Once the patient is more stable, the feasibility of restoring sinus rhythm can be determined. If the patient's hemodynamic stability is critically dependent on preservation of the atrial kick despite rate control, direct-current cardioversion with or without prior administration of an antiarrhythmic agent is the treatment of choice.

In the acute treatment of atrial fibrillation where the initial goal is control of a rapid ventricular rate, digoxin traditionally was the cornerstone of therapy. This was thought to be especially effective if there was associated heart failure. Recently, the role of digoxin in the treatment of atrial fibrillation has come into question. The relatively delayed onset of action (20 to 30 minutes), delayed peak effect (two hours), and long half-life (≥ 36 hours) make it a less than ideal agent in the acute setting. Both intravenous verapamil and esmolol have better pharmacokinetic profiles in this regard (and beta-blockers facilitate reversion to sinus rhythm), although each may depress cardiovascular function. Digoxin also has significant toxicity, particularly in sick elderly patients with decreased creatinine clearance. Unfortunately, the effectiveness of digoxin in certain clinical settings is also limited. A principal therapeutic effect of digoxin is mediated via its ability to enhance vagal tone. However, in situations in which catecholamine levels are quite high, such as thyrotoxicosis, exercise, or even early morning awakening, digoxin is relatively ineffective.

A recent study of ambulatory patients with recurrent atrial fibrillation [35] revealed that patients on digoxin had nearly the same number of paroxysms of atrial fibrillation as those not taking the drug. In addition, digoxin did not control the ventricular response at the onset of a paroxysm. Patients receiving digoxin had substantially more numerous episodes of fibrillation lasting 30 minutes or more. Consequently, rather than additional and possibly excessive doses of digoxin, primary or adjunctive therapy with other drugs such as beta-blockers or verapamil is an option. Not only do these agents slow A-V conduction but also there may be a synergistic effect with digoxin. Attempts to restore and maintain sinus rhythm, if indicated, can then be undertaken with conventional antiarrhythmic agents.

However, the need for caution when using conventional antiarrhythmic drugs such as quinidine must be emphasized. It has recently been noted [36] that while quinidine is efficacious in suppressing recurrent atrial fibrillation, its use may be associated with an increased overall mortality. Notwithstanding the limitations of that recent meta-analysis, the potential for proarrhythmia (particularly *torsade de pointes*), as well as exacerbation of conduction abnormalities and depression of cardiac function, particularly in patients with more advanced cardiac disease, must be balanced with the possible benefits. Atrial fibrillation with an inappropriately slow ventricular rate in the absence of drugs such as digoxin, beta-blockers, or verapamil may be a manifestation of sick sinus syndrome [37]. Cardioversion in this situation may precipitate prolonged pauses if the sinus node or subsidiary pacemaker fails to emerge in the usual fashion.

The duration of atrial fibrillation prior to emergent or elective cardioversion is an issue that often arises. While atrial fibrillation with a duration of less than 48 hours, and particularly of 24 hours, appears to have a low incidence of thromboembolic complications, this risk is not zero. The margin of safety is enhanced by a negative echocardiogram that reveals no thrombus and no left atrial spontaneous contrast echoes. Unless intravenous heparin is contraindicated, the safest course for elective cardioversion may be to initiate it immediately until warfarin therapy can be started, followed by cardioversion three weeks later if still indicated.

Chronic atrial fibrillation—therapeutic options

Options for chronic treatment of atrial fibrillation include pharmacologic therapy or recently developed procedures involving catheter ablation or surgery. While quinidine has been utilized in the past for maintenance of sinus rhythm, other options such as the class IC antiarrhythmic agents (flecainide, propafenone) may prove to be even more effective [38]. Additionally, amiodarone and sotalol (a beta-blocker with potent class III amiodaronelike activity) have been used in other countries for the treatment of atrial fibrillation. However, further data regarding toxicity, especially that of amiodarone, should be elucidated before this agent is approved for use in the United States.

Various studies have suggested the relative importance of factors such as atrial dimensions, etiology of cardiac disease, characteristics of the atrial fibrillatory waves, extent of cardiac dysfunction, duration of atrial fibrillation, and even patient age, among others, as possible predictors of the restoration and maintenance of sinus rhythm. However, none of these precludes a successful outcome in an individual patient.

For patients who cannot tolerate drug therapy or in whom ventricular rates cannot be adequately controlled, catheter ablation of the A-V junction or His bundle to create complete A-V block eliminates the need for antiarrhythmic therapy. However, it does require placement of a permanent pacemaker. More recent investigation has focused on catheter ablative techniques using a radiofrequency that merely modifies conduction across the A-V node, resulting in a more readily controlled ventricular rate.

Finally, surgical treatment of atrial fibrillation presents new horizons for patients who have failed drug therapy. The two most successful approaches, applied in only a relatively small number of patients to date, are the "corridor" procedure and the "maze" procedure. In the corridor procedure, a strip of tissue from the sinus node to the A-V node is isolated from the remainder of the atrium [39]. Although the atria continue to fibrillate, the sinus node fires and thus activates the ventricles. However, the patient does not regain atrial kick and hence is also still vulnerable to thromboembolism after this investigational procedure. The maze procedure involves creation of multiple blind alleys of electrical conduction over the entire atrial myocardium. Sinus rhythm with partially effective atrial contraction typically resumes within weeks of surgery. In follow-up electrophysiologic testing, atrial fibrillation has not been inducible even using aggressive protocols [40].

ATRIAL FLUTTER

Diagnosis

Atrial flutter is characterized by coarse, regular "sawtooth" undulations of the baseline, referred to as flutter waves. The atrial rate is between 240 and 400 beats/min, most often 280 to 320 beats/min. In atrial flutter, the most common ventricular rate is 140 to 160 beats/min with a 2:1 A-V conduction ratio. Maneuvers that slow A-V nodal conduction usually have no effect on the perpetuation of atrial flutter, but they may be helpful in making the recognition of flutter waves more obvious and in excluding as the arrhythmia mechanism paroxysmal A-V nodal supraventricular tachyarrhythmias (SVTs) (which may abruptly terminate).

In typical atrial flutter, the flutter waves are regular and negative in polarity in the inferior leads, at a rate of 280 to 320 beats/min. The underlying mechanism appears to be reentry involving the low right atrium near the coronary sinus. In the atypical form, the flutter waves have other morphologies and rates, various sites of origin of the ectopic depolarizations, and in some cases may result from mechanisms other than reentry. The distinction between atypical atrial flutter and coarse atrial fibrillation may not be readily apparent with limited electrocardiographic recordings.

Atrial flutter often indicates significant structural heart disease, but occasionally it is virtually an isolated finding. This rhythm may be paroxysmal or chronic, may degenerate to paroxysmal or chronic atrial fibrillation, or may present as part of the spectrum of sick sinus syndrome.

Acute therapy

Therapy to convert atrial flutter to sinus rhythm may involve antiarrhythmic drugs, direct-current cardioversion, or rapid atrial pacing, with the latter two being the preferred treatment options. Drug therapy (for example, with a class IA or IC agent) may be adjunctively beneficial to slow the ventricular response, enhance the efficacy of rapid atrial pacing, or increase the likelihood that sinus rhythm will be maintained after direct-current cardioversion. However, it should be emphasized that antiarrhythmic drugs that reliably convert atrial flutter to sinus rhythm do not currently exist and therefore cannot be recommended [41].

Atrial pacing techniques in which the atria are paced at 120% to 130% of the spontaneous atrial rate for durations of 10 to 15 seconds have been shown to be effective in terminating atrial flutter, particularly the more typical form.

Inevitably, in a few patients, rapid atrial pacing will precipitate atrial fibrillation, which is usually transient and associated with a more readily slowed ventricular response. Even if this atrial fibrillation does not convert spontaneously to sinus rhythm within a few minutes, it is usually amenable to standard medications or cardioversion, if indicated.

Another alternative for acute treatment of atrial flutter is the initial use of direct-current cardioversion. One caveat is that the need for an anesthetic agent mandates that the patient *not* have eaten prior to the procedure. Energy requirements may be as low as 25 joules or less, but usually 50 to 100 joules are used to terminate the flutter and minimize the likelihood of atrial fibrillation.

Chronic therapy

Therapy for chronic paroxysmal atrial flutter, rarely life-threatening, is usually initiated to preserve quality of life; therefore, the treatment plan must be designed accordingly. While class IA, class IC, beta-blockers (class II), and class III antiarrhythmic agents have been used to attempt to suppress paroxysmal atrial flutter, none has proven consistently successful with an acceptable side-effect profile.

Implantable devices such as permanent atrial antitachycardia pacemakers have been shown in a small number of carefully selected patients to be capable of promptly interrupting recurrent atrial flutter [42]. However, these devices do not prevent the onset of atrial flutter, and patients may still require drugs to slow the ventricular rate if atrial fibrillation follows the termination of atrial flutter. In some patients, antibradycardia dual-chamber A-V pacing may reduce the frequency of recurrent atrial flutter and fibrillation.

Recently, catheter ablative techniqes have been investigated for the management of atrial flutter. A general approach involves A-V junctional or His bundle ablation, creating complete A-V conduction block. This obviates the need for concurrent antiarrhythmic drug therapy but necessitates placement of a permanent pacemaker [43].

A more specific technique of catheter ablation involves mapping the atria to identify an area of slow conduction within the flutter reentry circuit. A shock or radiofrequency pulse is then delivered to this area to destroy a critical region and thus eliminate the reentry loop [44]. Investigations currently in progress [45] are also exploring the potential of surgery and cryoablation to control recurrent atrial flutter.

In the treatment of atrial flutter with a rapid ventricular response, it is paramount that the ventricular rate be controlled with an A-V nodal blocking agent prior to initiation of class I antiarrhythmic agents such as quinidine, procainamide, or disopyramide, or even an IC agent such as propafenone [46]. These latter agents can slow the flutter rate to 200 to 240 beats/min and also have vagolytic effects on the A-V node; consequently, 1:1 A-V conduction can ensue with paradoxical acceleration of the ventricular rate.

Before elective cardioversion of atrial flutter or atrial fibrillation, it is probably prudent to obtain an echocardiogram to evaluate ventricular dimensions and function, atrial size, and particularly the presence of left atrial or ventricular thrombus. Long-term maintenance of sinus rhythm is less likely in patients with a significantly decreased left ventricular ejection fraction, poor functional status, underlying rheumatic valvular heart disease, or prolonged duration of atrial fibrillation. Recent data [47] suggest that the likelihood of maintaining sinus rhythm after cardioversion of atrial flutter is relatively high.

MULTIFOCAL ATRIAL TACHYCARDIA

Multifocal atrial tachycardia (MAT) is defined as a tachyarrhythmia in which 1) the atrial rate is greater than 100 beats/min; 2) there is evidence of discrete P-waves of at least three separate morphologies superimposed on an isoelectric baseline; and 3) there is an irregular variation in the P-P interval. Clinically, this rhythm must be distinguished from atrial fibrillation. Etiologically, MAT is presumably due to altered automaticity of the atria. This arrhythmia often occurs in elderly patients; the average age of 315 patients described in eight series was 70 years old [48]. Often these patients are quite ill with underlying cardiac and pulmonary disease and metabolic derangements such as hypokalemia, hypomagnesemia, and hypoxemia. Digoxin is usually ineffective in controlling these tachycardias, while verapamil may be efficacious for rate control because it reduces the number of atrial beats [49]. Treatment should be focused on management of underlying disorders. Acutely, adjunctive use of intravenous procainamide may also be useful. However, most antiarrhythmic agents have failed to achieve long-term successful maintenance of sinus rhythm.

A similar but less disabling disorder is known as *chaotic atrial rhythm* or *wandering atrial pacemaker*. Typically, premature atrial beats with varying morphologies interrupt sinus rhythm but with a heart rate within the normal range of 60 to 100 beats per minute.

A-V NODAL REENTRANT TACHYCARDIA

A-V nodal reentrant tachycardia is presumably the most common form of sustained paroxysmal SVT seen in nonelderly adults; however, its incidence in the elderly is not well defined. Typically, there is near synchronous activation of the ventricles and atria at rates of 140 to 160 beats/min involving a reentrant circuit confined to the A-V nodal region.

Acute therapy

While A-V nodal reentrant tachycardia itself is rarely life-threatening, if coupled with the underlying heart disease or comorbid medical conditions so often seen in the elderly it may result in hemodynamic compromise or myocardial ischemia. The rapid rates, inadequate diastolic filling times, loss of atrial kick, and occurrence of a negative atrial kick related to atrial contraction after the onset of ventricular systole all contribute to hemodynamic compromise. Patients often complain of palpitations, lightheadedness, chest discomfort, or shortness of breath and may develop frank syncope, ischemia, or pulmonary congestion.

In the presence of hemodynamic collapse, the treatment for A-V nodal reentrant tachycardia is direct current cardioversion. If the clinical situation is more stable, vagal maneuvers such as Valsalva or gagging may be effective in terminating the tachycardia by blocking the anterograde limb of the reentrant circuit. Of note, given the increased prevalence of both carotid sinus hypersensitivity and carotid atherosclerotic disease in the elderly, the use of carotid sinus massage should be approached cautiously.

Acutely, intravenous verapamil terminates approximately 90% of these tachycardias via interference of the anterograde loop [50]. However, elderly patients with impaired left ventricular function will be especially susceptible to the drug's adverse negative inotropic effects and marked vasodilating and hypotensive properties. Beta-blockers such as propranolol also act on the anterograde limb of the circuit. The short-acting beta-blocker, esmolol, may eventually be incorporated in the acute management of A-V nodal reentrant tachycardia, but it is not currently approved for use in this situation. It may also depress cardiac function and cause transient hypotension [51].

Adenosine, recently introduced for the conversion of paroxysmal supraventricular tachycardias, including A-V nodal reentrant tachycardia, has demonstrated greater than 90% successful conversion to sinus rhythm after a bolus of 12 mg or less intravenously [52]. The extremely brief half-life of <10 seconds minimizes the potential for side effects of any significant duration [53], although transient symptoms such as chest discomfort and flushing are relatively common and, in a number of cases, the SVT may reemerge. Vagomimetic agents, pressors, and/or digoxin are now rarely used in acute situations, although digoxin may be appropriate subacutely. Occasionally, patients can be managed with rapid atrial pacing to induce transient atrial fibrillation as a means of terminating A-V nodal SVT reentrant tachycardia, which usually rapidly and spontaneously converts to sinus rhythm.

For patients with infrequent and mildly symptomatic episodes of documented A-V nodal reentrant tachycardia, intermittent administration of antiarrhythmic agents on an outpatient basis—the so-called cocktail approach—has been described [54]. Although this has not been specifically evaluated in the elderly, it would seem to be a relatively restricted therapeutic option for this cohort given the decreased cognitive functioning, decreased psychomotor ability, and increased potential for drug mix-ups given the usual polypharmacy in the elderly. In addition, the relatively prolonged lapse of time (1 to 2 hours) from administration of the cocktail to termination of arrhythmia may not be tolerated by elderly patients, many of whom already have a degree of myocardial or cerebrovascular compromise.

Chronic therapy

Chronic therapy for A-V nodal reentrant tachycardia is usually empiric and often includes daily digoxin and possibly a once-daily beta-blocker or calcium-antagonist. In patients incapacitated by the arrhythmia or intolerant of their drugs, treatment is often best guided by a complete electrophysiologic evaluation. Decisions regarding treatment must be based on several factors, including the frequency, severity, and duration of episodes, ease of termination, associated sequelae, and efficacy and tolerability of therapeutic interventions. Occasionally, one of the class IA or IC agents may be efficacious as adjunctive or primary therapy; however, these drugs have a higher incidence of proarrhythmia as well as the potential for other noncardiac side effects.

The nonpharmacologic armamentarium for the therapy of A-V nodal reentrant tachycardias has expanded considerably over the past few years. For example, antitachycardia pacemakers can be used to prevent or terminate A-V nodal reentrant tachycardia [55]. Prevention currently is achieved by overdrive pacing or multisite stimulation. More sophisticated pacers can be programmed to terminate reentrant tachycardias by introducing multiple extrastimuli, burst pacing, or both.

Perhaps the most promising advance is the use of catheter ablation, particularly using radiofrequency, to modify one limb of the reentrant circuit. Although initial studies are promising [56,57] and clearly demonstrate the feasibility and remarkable short-term efficacy of this approach, long-term studies of a large number of patients are required to assess the ultimate safety and efficacy of this procedure for A-V nodal reentrant tachycardia.

Finally, surgical approaches have recently been described [58] that utilize techniques that modify or partially isolate the A-V node from the perinodal tissue. These initial series report relatively high short-term success rates in relatively small numbers of patients with only modest morbidity, including complete A-V block and pacemaker dependency; however, catheter ablative techniques may drastically reduce the number of candidates for such operations.

A-V RECIPROCATING TACHYCARDIAS

A-V reciprocating tachycardias involve a reentrant circuit loop composed of the atrium, A-V node, His–Purkinje system, ventricular myocardium, and accessory A-V connections. These connections, or bypass tracts, are congenital anomalies that provide abnormal electrical pathways between the atria and ventricles. During a bout of reentrant tachycardia, the accessory pathway most often conducts in a retrograde manner (orthodromic). Alternatively, it may conduct in an anterograde fashion (antidromic), with the A–V nodal pathway forming the retrograde limb of the circuit. Although A–V reciprocating tachycardias require a bypass tract as part of the reentrant circuit, patients with bypass tracts fall into two distinct clinical categories. Patients with anterograde A–V conduction that bypasses the A–V node have so-called ventricular preexcitation. Some of these persons have paroxysmal A–V reciprocating tachycardias or paroxysmal atrial fibrillation, and Wolff–Parkinson–White (WPW) syndrome is the diagnosis. However, another group of patients have bypass tracts incapable of anterograde conduction, and only conduct in a retrograde fashion from ventricle to atrium. These "concealed" bypass tracts pose no threat of rapid A–V conduction and are only evident clinically during paroxysms of tachycardia. Thus, while A–V reciprocating rhythms have a narrow QRS and are usually classified as a form of supraventricular tachycardia, the ventricular component is clearly an integral part of the circuit.

Effect of aging on accessory pathways

The incidence of WPW syndrome appears to decrease with age. It has been suggested that accessory pathways may undergo the same fibrotic degenerative changes as other conduction tissue. It is speculated that, over time, these fibrotic changes cause a progressive decrease in the ability of the accessory pathway to sustain rapid anterograde conduction. Klein et al. [59] noted that 30% of 29 patients studied lost the ability to conduct in an anterograde fashion over accessory pathways, as shown by two electrophysiologic studies completed at least three years apart. They postulated that an asymptomatic older patient with electrocardiographic evidence of WPW syndrome would be less likely to develop serious arrhythmias, even if atrial fibrillation were to occur. Another study [60], in which the anterograde effective refractory period of the accessory pathway was measured, also concluded that the risk of rapid ventricular rates during atrial fibrillation was reduced with increasing patient age. Nonetheless, since atrial fibrillation is common in the elderly, the possibility of an accessory pathway should be considered in the emergency-room assessment of an older patient with atrial fibrillation and an irregular, rapid ventricular response, particularly if there is evidence of wide QRS beats that appear preexcited in addition to those that may represent aberrancy. The distinction between preexcited beats and ventricular tachycardia may also be difficult, but in either case electrical cardioversion can be used in restoring sinus rhythm. Early recognition is particularly important, in that atrial fibrillation can deteriorate to ventricular fibrillation when drugs such as digoxin or verapamil, which are commonly administered for other paroxysmal tachycardias, are used in this setting [61,62]. In a patient known to have preexcitation or WPW syndrome, it is presumed that there is a potentially increased propensity to develop atrial fibrillation with potentially rapid rates and bizarre QRS complexes, as well as a predisposition to A–V reciprocating tachycardias. Patients with concealed bypass tracts are predisposed only to the latter.

Diagnosis

Several clues from the surface electrocardiogram can be helpful in the diagnosis of a tachycardia involving an accessory pathway. Recognition of preexcitation on a routine electrocardiogram is based on eccentric A-V conduction occurring simultaneously with conduction over the usual A-V nodal pathway. Typically, the electrocardiogram shows a short P-R interval (≤0.12 seconds), a wide QRS interval (≥0.12 seconds), slurring of the initial upstroke of the QRS complex (delta wave), and repolarization abnormalities. The ECG may mimic or mask bundle branch or infarct patterns. These electrocardiographic findings, in association with paroxysmal arrhythmias, constitute the WPW syndrome.

A-V reciprocating tachycardias can occur in patients with (preexcitation) or without (concealed bypass tract) anterograde A-V conduction over an accessory pathway. Most commonly, the patient presents emergently with a paroxysmal narrow QRS complex tachycardia. The rate of the tachycardia is often 160 to 180 beats/min. The P-wave, if discernible, follows the QRS complex, signifying atrial depolarization following ventricular depolarization. At more rapid rates, QRS alternans may occur. Retrograde P-waves will be negative in polarity in leads overlying the atrial insertion site of the bypass tract (e.g., I, AVL if left-sided; AVR if right-sided).

Therapy

Since the tachycardia involves a macroreentrant circuit, therapy can be directed at several potentially critical points, including the bypass tract, the A-V node, or both. Although in some cases this can be achieved pharmacologically, definitive catheter ablative therapy directed at the accessory pathway is evolving rapidly.

In acute management of a hemodynamically unstable patient with A-V reciprocating tachycardia, direct-current cardioversion is a first-line option unless the patient has recently eaten, since administration of anesthesia is required. Several other options are available for most patients, including interventions that affect the A-V node (e.g., vagomimetic, adenosine, beta-blockers, calcium antagonists) or other parts of the circuit (e.g., procainamide affecting the accessory pathway). In patients with no preexcitation the choice of therapies is rather broad, whereas in patients with known ability to conduct anterogradely down a bypass tract, drugs that block the A-V node (particularly verapamil and occasionally digoxin) may inadvertently facilitate more rapid A-V bypass tract conduction if atrial fibrillation occurs, and generally should be avoided. To date, this potential untoward effect has not limited more frequent use of adenosine, both therapeutically and diagnostically, in acute management of SVTs [53].

Adenosine has potent A-V nodal blocking effects. Its advantages include a rapid onset of action (within seconds of an intravenous bolus) and rapid elimination (half-life of <10 seconds) that limits the duration of any adverse effects.

Long-term management of A-V reciprocating tachycardias historically has included drugs that slow conduction and/or prolong refractoriness at various points along the circuit, particularly the A-V node or accessory pathway. Therapy can either be empiric or guided by invasive electrophysiologic testing. Catheter ablative techniques are evolving so rapidly that algorithms are being updated regularly. Most promising is the use of radiofrequency current for definitive therapy in A-V reciprocating tachycardias. In a recent study [63], a median of three applications of radiofrequency current eliminated accessory-pathway conduction in 164 or 166 patients, with a complication rate of only 1.8%. In addition, it appears that it is feasible to confirm the diagnosis and carry out therapeutic radiofrequency ablation in a single electrophysiologic test [64]. Unfortunately, the most rapidly conducting bypass tracts are generally least responsive to antiarrhythmic drugs [65], and therefore these patients are the best candidates for definitive ablative procedures, particularly if they are capable of rapid anterograde A-V conduction over a bypass tract during atrial fibrillation.

Of further interest, a recent cost analysis of electroshock catheter ablation versus surgical ablation [66] revealed that catheter ablation was substantially less expensive and had a much shorter recuperation period than surgical ablation. Thus the tendency in the future may be to attempt ablation initially with catheters, reserving surgery for catheter-ablation failures. Presumably, using more refined radiofrequency techniques, the costs and risks of catheter ablation will be further reduced.

VENTRICULAR ARRHYTHMIAS

Epidemiology

Pooled data from several studies, including the Baltimore Longitudinal Study of Aging, indicate an age-related increase in the prevalence, frequency, and complexity of ventricular arrhythmias. The etiology for this increase is multifaceted as a result of the changes associated with the aging process. For example, it has been documented [67] that the elderly have an increased incidence of ventricular hypertrophy, often the result of systemic hypertension, and this has been shown to potentiate both the complexity and frequency of ventricular arrhythmias. Asymptomatic isolated ventricular ectopic beats in the absence of significant structural heart disease are generally of little clinical consequence. However, even the presence of simple ventricular ectopy has been shown to increase mortality in patients with coronary heart disease. Hinkle et al. [68] documented this in a 2.5-year follow-up of men in which an increased incidence of coronary death was seen in those patients with greater than 10 ventricular ectopic beats per 1000 QRS complexes. However, this only applied to patients with underlying coronary artery disease. From currently available data [69], the increase in ventricular arrhythmias seen in healthy asymptomatic patients does not enhance the risk of coronary death.

Increased awareness of the influence of age on the complexity and prevalence of ventricular ectopy is necessary to establish stratification guidelines when determining which patients require intensive investigation and, more importantly, which do *not* require therapy.

These issues deserve particular consideration in light of the results to date of the double-blind, randomized, placebo-controlled Cardiac Arrhythmia Suppression Trial (CAST) [70]. These data suggest that even the essentially complete eradication of asymptomatic ventricular ectopy resulted in a several-fold increase rather than a decrease in mortality in post-myocardial infarction patients treated with encainide or flecainide. Pending further substantial data, it is not possible to recommend either routine monitoring or treatment of ventricular arrhythmias in most otherwise stable elderly patients.

Classification

Chronic ventricular arrhythmias have traditionally been classified according to various hierarchical schema that relate prognostically to either immediate or long-term arrhythmic risk of sudden cardiac death. Developed in the setting of managing patients with acute myocardial infarction in coronary care units, the Lown classification [71] has been widely applied as a means of characterizing ventricular ectopy based on frequency of beats, multiformity, couplets, salvos, and so-called "R on T" phenomena. Refinements of this system have considered other quantitative aspects, such as the number of hours with various grades of arrhythmias present or the lengths or rates of runs of salvos. Other classifications have been more qualitative—for example, one that categorized ventricular ectopy as either benign, prognostically important, or malignant [72]. In general, patients with more severe cardiac disease (whether acute or chronic), more cardiac dysfunction, greater decompensation, more ongoing ischemia, and more advanced concomitant disorders are most likely to have and suffer the consequences of more malignant arrhythmias, but arrhythmias are of independent and additional prognostic significance [73,74].

Malignant ventricular arrhythmias

Malignant and ventricular arrhythmias are immediately and potentially life-threatening and include various hemodynamically embarrassing prolonged or sustained (>30 seconds) ventricular fibrillation. Patients with malignant ventricular arrhythmias usually have severe organic heart disease and need both effective therapy to survive their initial episode and aggressive prophylactic antiarrhythmic therapy, if possible, to prevent any initial or subsequent episodes, since there is a 20% to 40% rate of recurrence of arrhythmia within 1 to 2 years [75,76]. In patients with sustained ventricular tachyarrhythmias, therapy should be designed to be as fail-safe as feasible, and this almost always requires a thorough evaluation of every aspect of cardiac function and anatomy. Usual diagnostic studies include cardiac catheterization and angiography, as well as an assessment of all contributing factors including reversible ischemia and metabolic derangements. Ideally, therapy should be based on electrophysiologic testing and often includes aggressive use of antiarrhythmic drugs, implantation of a cardioverter-defibrillator, or both. Admittedly, the dianostic and therapeutic algorithm involves considerable expense and some risk, but it is justified by tremendous potential benefit in well-selected patients. Empiric therapy or therapy based on eradication of ambient ectopy or monitoring is less frequently successful. Occasionally, patients are candidates for primary antiarrhythmic surgery (e.g., aneurysmectomy with bypass grafting and endocardial resection); rarely, patients may be candidates for cardiac transplantation.

Benign ventricular arrhythmias

Patients are often classified as having benign arrhythmias on the basis of having only isolated ectopy and minimal organic heart disease. If patients in this category become severely symptomatic, related to the frequency of beats, cautious use of a beta-blocker or possibly a class IA agent (such as procainamide or quinidine) may be justified. However, the risk of proarrhythmic effects must be weighed against the benefit of symptomatic relief. Recently, the effect of quinidine or procainamide compared to no antiarrhythmic therapy was assessed in an elderly population with asymptomatic complex ventricular arrhythmias but no evidence of sustained ventricular tachycardia or ambulatory monitoring. The 406 patients studied included those with and those without structural heart disease. A high incidence of side effects was noted with both quinidine (48%) and procainamide (55%), necessitating cessation of therapy. More noteworthy, however, is that neither of these agents caused a reduction in sudden cardiac death, total cardiac death, or total death compared with no antiarrhythmic therapy [77]. Therapy is directed solely at relief of burdensome or incapacitating symptoms and restoration of optimal function without severe cardiac or systemic adverse effects.

Prognostically important ventricular arrhythmias

The most controversial area concerns patients with so-called prognostically important ventricular arrhythmias. These are patients with either frequent or high-grade ectopy (e.g., salvos) (figure 8-7), usually seen in the setting of ischemic heart disease. While these patients are often essentially asymptomatic and their condition is not immediately life-threatening, they

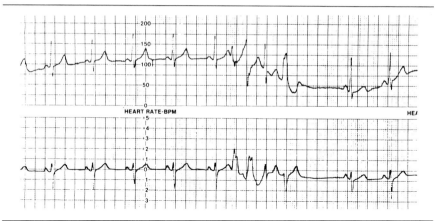

Figure 8-7. Simultaneous ambulatory monitoring of two electrocardiographic leads in an 80-year-old hypertensive woman who recently began to experience palpitations. The tracing revealed periods of nonsustained ventricular tachycardia that temporally correlated with her symptoms.

are at increased risk for sudden death. A common but controversial clinical situation is congestive heart failure. Approximately one half of deaths in this population are sudden and are presumably due to ventricular tachycardia or fibrillation. Most patients with heart failure have complex ventricular premature beats, and the majority have nonsustained ventricular tachycardia. However, no cause-and-effect relationship with sudden cardiac death has been demonstrated. In addition, treatment regimens for heart failure can serve to worsen the ventricular arrhythmia. Diuretics may induce hypokalemia and hypomagnesemia, inotropic support may increase circulating catecholamines, and digitalis may exacerbate ventricular arrhythmias.

Although empiric therapy for prognostically important ventricular arrhythmias was commonplace in the past, this approach needs reassessment now that preliminary results of the CAST indicate the excessive proarrhythmic effects with the agents encainide and flecainide [70]. While this study is still in progress with the drug moricizine, the resounding message to the cardiology community is that treatment of these ventricular arrhythmias in the postinfarct period cannot be undertaken in a cavalier fashion. Data for heart failure patients regarding the relative risks and benefits of various antiarrhythmic regimens, especially in the elderly, are rather limited; therefore, no specific recommendations can be made for empiric therapy. Of further interest, a recent retrospective review [78] of exercise-induced ventricular tachycardia in 3551 patients aged 21 to 88 years indicated that this relatively uncommon occurrence (1.5%) was also not a particularly useful marker of poor prognosis. Importantly, several trials now in progress are evaluating algorithms for risk stratification and therapy that variously include patients with recent myocardial infarction or advanced cardiac dysfunction. The investigators hope to assess the prognostic accuracy of such diagnostic modalities as ambulatory electrocardiographic monitoring, signal-averaged electrocardiography, and clinical electrophysiologic testing. Therapeutically aggressive interventions including amiodarone [79] and implantable defibrillators are under evaluation, and early results are promising. Recently, recommendations for these antitachyarrhythmia devices have been reevaluated in light of data supporting their efficacy in patients at risk for sudden death [80]. Empirically, in patients who either have seemingly benign ectopy but advanced cardiac disease or have prognostically important ectopy and even mild cardiac disease, it is probably prudent to initiate therapy in the hospital with electrocardiographic monitoring for the first several days. This affords the opportunity to identify at least a significant number of such persons who might be predisposed to more severe adverse effects, including potentially malignant proarrhythmia. Data from CAST [70], however, indicate that the risk of proarrhythmia with the class IC agents flecainide and encainide is considerable even after one year of drug therapy in the post-myocardial infarction population.

In following and assessing therapy, it is necessary to keep in mind the goals of therapy (e.g., eradication of symptoms and improvement of quality of life without shortening longevity) and the vagaries of "spontaneous" variations in arrhythmia frequency, as well as either occult or overt changes in the patient's underlying clinical status that may affect either the occurrence or consequences of arrhythmias. Unfortunately, virtually every antiarrhythmic drug has the potential to further depress many aspects of cardiac function in a susceptible individual, including sinus-node automaticity, A-V conduction, and contractility.

The use of intracardiac programmed electrophysiologic studies to assess the efficacy of specific agents for ventricular tachycardia or fibrillation results in more directed therapy. Although initially electrophysiologic testing is more invasive, empiric treatment tends to result in a higher incidence of side effects, complications, and drug failures.

The combination of a systematic approach to the evaluation of the lethal potential of ventricular arrhythmia, an organized collection of baseline data, and a closely monitored therapeutic regimen yield the greatest potential for successful management of these patients. In most instances of managing arrhythmias in the elderly, an expert in the field should be consulted, given the relatively narrow windows of risks and benefits in many cases and the general complexities not only of managing these difficult issues but also of integrating so many evolving diagnostic therapeutic options into effective patient-management strategies.

Acute management of ventricular arrhythmias

Arguably, the single greatest impetus to advances in the recognition and management of ventricular arrhythmias was the development of coronary care units with electrocardiographic monitoring. Associated with coronary care was the aggressive deployment of lidocaine as a first-line agent to prevent ventricular fibrillation, with the adjunctive use of other drugs. It is therefore particularly noteworthy that a recent meta-analysis indicated that, in the prethrombolytic era, prophylactic lidocaine either in the prehospital or early hospital setting of acute myocardial infarction did not reduce mortality. Although there was a minor reduction in ventricular fibrillation, there was a suggestion of excess mortality, particularly in higher-risk patients such as those with heart failure [81]. Moreover, lidocaine is only infrequently successful in terminating ventricular tachycardia when it occurs outside the setting of acute ischemia; procainamide is a more effective first-line agent, and electrical cardioversion is the definitive option. The first-line use of lidocaine appears to be restricted to eradication of ongoing malignant and possibly hemodynamically compromising arrhythmias in the setting of acute ischemia; aggressive anti-ischemic measures are probably of greater importance.

In patients with recurrent ventricular arrhythmias refractory to other measures, those occurring in the setting of a long Q-T interval on the electrocardiogram, or those induced by antiarrhythmic agents, the administration of magnesium (e.g., 2 g magnesium sulfate intravenously) can be useful to facilitate stabilization while other offending drugs are stopped, electrolytes (potassium, magnesium) are repleted, or ischemia is reversed [82].

CONCLUSION

The elderly are susceptible to a wide variety of arrhythmias, the clinical significance of which must often be assessed in the complex setting of other comorbid illnesses and concomitant drug therapy. The rapid evolution of both diagnostic and therapeutic modalities challenges even the most astute and experienced practitioners and requires fluency in the management of these arrhythmias, as well as an understanding of the special issues particular to the elderly patient. As a larger percentage of the population is defined as elderly, these issues will become increasingly important on a societal level as well. Undoubtedly, optimal patient management will involve the collaboration of primary caretakers and subspecialists to formulate effective, safe, and tolerable therapeutic regimes.

ACKNOWLEDGMENTS

We thank Carolyn Siwinski, Donna Thompson, Russil Tamsen, and Robyn Brown for their diligent assistance in the preparation of this chapter.

REFERENCES

1. Butler R. 1975. Why Survive? Being Old in America. New York: Harper and Row.
2. Michelson EL and Morganroth J. 1980. Spontaneous variability of complex ventricular arrhythmias detected by long-term electrocardiographic recordings. Circulation 61:690–695.
3. Mihalick MJ and Fisch C. 1974. Electrocardiographic findings in the aged. Am Heart J 87:117–121.
4. Camm AJ, Evans KE, Ward DE, et al. 1980. The rhythm of the heart in active elderly subjects. Am Heart J 99:598–603.
5. Martin A, Benbow LJ, Butrous GS, et al. 1984. Five year follow-up of 101 elderly subjects by means of long term ambulatory monitoring. Eur Heart J 5:592–596.
6. Gomes JA, Winters SL, Stewart D, et al. 1987. A new non-invasive index to predict sustained ventricular tachycardia and sudden death in the first year after myocardial infarction: based on signal-averaged electrocardiogram, radionuclide ejection fraction and holter monitoring. J Am Coll Cardiol 1:349–357.
7. Elveback L and Lie JT. 1984. Continued high prevalence of coronary artery disease at autopsy in Olmstead County, Minnesota 1950–1970. Circulation 70:345–349.
8. Squire A, Goldman ME, Kupersmith J, et al. 1984. Long-term antiarrhythmic therapy: problem of low drug levels and patient compliance. Am J Med 77:1035–1038.
9. Kantelip JP, Sage E and Duchenne-Marullary P. 1986. Findings on ambulatory electrocardiographic monitoring in subjects older than 80 years. Am J Cardiol 57:398–401.
10. Jones J, Srodulski ZM and Romisher S. 1990. The aging electrocardiogram. Am J Emerg Med 80:240–245.
11. Hinkle LE, Jr, Carrer ST and Plakun I. 1972. Slow heart rate and increased risk of cardiac death in middle-aged men. Arch Intern Med 129:732–748.
12. Kostis JB, Moreyna AE, Amendo MT, et al. 1982. The effects of age on heart rate in subjects free of heart disease. Circulation 65:141–145.
13. Fleg JL and Kennedy HL. 1982. Cardiac arrhythmias in a healthy elderly population: detection by 24-hour ambulatory electrocardiography. Chest 81:302–307.
14. Lown B. 1967. Electrical reversion of cardiac arrhythmias. Br Heart J 29:469–489.
15. World Survey on Cardiac Pacing (1981). 1983. PACE 6:A157–A172.
16. Rodriquez RD and Schocken DD. 1990. Update on sick sinus syndrome: a cardiac disorder of aging. Geriatrics 45:26–36.
17. Alboni P, Baggioni GF, Scarfo S, et al. 1991. Role of sinus node artery disease in sick sinus syndrome in inferior wall myocardial infarction. Am J Cardiol 67:1180–1184.
18. Reiffel JA, Ferrick K, Simmerman J, et al. 1985. Electrophysiologic studies of the sinus node and atria. In LS Dreifus (ed), Cardiovascular Clinics. Philadelphia: F.A. Davis, pp. 37–61.
19. Engel TR, Kowey PR and Wetstein L. 1985. Electrophysiologic studies of the ventricle. In LS Dreifus (ed), Cardiovascular Clinics. Philadelphia: F.A. Davis, pp. 83–96.
20. Dreifus LS, Michelson EL and Kaplinsky E. 1983. Bradyarrhythmias: clinical significance. J Am Coll Cardiol 1:327–338.
21. Ettinger PO, Wu CF, DeLa Cruz D Jr, et al. 1978. Arrhythmias and the holiday heart: alcohol-associated cardiac rhythm disorders. Am Heart J 95:555–562.
22. Engel TR and Luck JC. 1983. Effect of whiskey on atrial vulnerability and the "holiday heart." J Am Coll Cardiol 1:816–818.
23. Thornton JR. 1984. Atrial fibrillation in healthy non-alcoholic people after an alcoholic binge. Lancet 2:1013–1014.
24. Tansey MJB and Opie LH. 1983. Relation between plasma free fatty acids and arrhythmias within the first twelve hours of acute myocardial infarction. Lancet 2:419–420.
25. James TN and Bear ES. 1967. Effects of ethanol and acetaldehyde on the heart. Am Heart J 74:243–255.
26. Kopecky SL, Gersh BJ, McGoon MD, et al. 1987. The natural history of lone atrial fibrillation: a population-based study over three decades. N Engl J Med 317:669–674.
27. Brand FN, Abbott RD, Kannel WB, et al. 1985. Characteristics and prognosis of lone atrial fibrillation: 30 year follow-up in the Framingham study. JAMA 254:3449–3453.
28. Gajewski J. 1981. Mortality in an insured population with atrial fibrillation. JAMA 245:1540–1544.
29. Stults BM, Dere WH and Caine TH. 1989. Long-term anticoagulation: indications and management. West J Med 151:414–429.

30. Petersen P, Boysen G, Godtfredsen J, et al. 1989. Placebo-conrolled, randomized trial of warfarin and aspirin for prevention of thromboembolic complications in chronic atrial fibrillation: the Copenhagen AFASAK Study. Lancet 1:175–179.
31. Stroke Prevention in Atrial Fibrillation Study Group Investigators. 1990. Preliminary report of the Stroke Prevention Atrial Fibrillation Study. N Engl J Med 322:863–868.
32. Anderson DC, for the SPAF Investigators. 1990. Progress report of the Stroke Prevention in Atrial Fibrillation study. Stroke 21 (Suppl III):III-12–III-17.
33. The Boston Area Anticoagulation Trial for Atrial Fibrillation Investigators. 1990. The effect of low-dose warfarin on the risk of stroke in patients with non-rheumatic atrial fibrillation. N Engl J Med 323:1505–1511.
34. Dalen JE and Hirsh J (eds). 1989. Second ACCP conference on antithrombotic therapy. Chest 95:1S–169S.
35. Rawles JM, Metcalfe MJ and Jennings K. 1990. Time of occurrence, duration and ventricular rate of paroxysmal atrial fibrillation: the effect of digoxin. Br Heart J 63: 225–227.
36. Coplen SE, Antman EM, Berlin JA, et al. 1990. Efficacy and safety of quinidine therapy for maintenance of sinus rhythm after cardioversion. Circulation 82:1106–1116.
37. Shugoll WM and Silverman ME. 1986. Successful cardioversion of atrial fibrillation. Cardiol Illustr 1:3–8.
38. Anderson JL, Gilbert EM, Alpert BL, et al. 1989. Prevention of symptomatic recurrences of paroxysmal atrial fibrillation in patients initially tolerating antiarrhythmia therapy: a multi-center, double-blind, crossover study of flecainide and placebo using transtelephonic monitoring. Circulation 80:1557–1570.
39. Leitch JW, Guiraudon GM, Klein GJ, et al. 1990. The corridor operation for atrial fibrillation: initial results and long term follow-up. Circulation 82:III–470.
40. Cox JL. 1987. Surgical management of cardiac arrhythmias. Cardiovasc Clin 17:381–413.
41. Waldo AL. 1990. Clinical evaluation in therapy of patients with atrial fibrillation or flutter. Cardiol Clin 8:479–490.
42. Barold SS, Wyndham CRC, Kappenberger LL, et al. 1987. Implanted atrial pacemakers for paroxysmal atrial flutter: long term efficacy. Ann Intern Med 107:144–149.
43. Scheinmann MM. 1989. Catheter techniques for ablation of supraventricular tachycardia. N Engl J Med 320:460–461.
44. Saoudi N, Atallah G, Kirkorian G, et al. 1990. Catheter ablation of the atrial myocardium in human type I atrial flutter. Circulation 81:762–772.
45. Guiraudon GM, Klein GJ, Sharma AD, et al. 1989. Surgical alternatives for supraventricular tachycardias. Am J Cardiol 64:925–930.
46. Marcus FI. 1990. The hazards of using type IC antiarrhythmic drugs for the treatment of paroxysmal atrial fibrillation. Am J Cardiol 66:366–367.
47. Van Gelder IC, Crijns HJ, Van Gilst WH, et al. 1991. Prediction of uneventful cardioversion and maintenance of sinus rhythm from direct-current electrical cardioversion of chronic atrial fibrillation and flutter. Am J Cardiol 68:41–46.
48. Kastor JA. 1990. Multifocal atrial tachycardia. N Engl J Med 322:1713–1717.
49. Salerno DM, Anderson B, Sharkey PJ, et al. 1987. Intraveneous verapamil for treatment of multifocal atrial tachycardia with and without calcium pre-treatment. Ann Intern Med 107:623–628.
50. Sung RJ, Elser B and McAllister RG Jr. 1980. Intravenous verapamil for termination of reentrant supraventricular tachycardias. Ann Intern Med 93:682–689.
51. Greer GS, Ramirez NM, Fananapazin L, et al. 1987. Bolus esmolol in the treatment of supraventricular tachycardias (abstract). Circulation 76 (Suppl IV):IV-67.
52. Caruso AC, Miles WM, Klein LS, et al. 1989. Double-blind, placebo-controlled, dose-ranging study of adenosine in patients with supraventricular tachycardia (abstract). Circulation 80 (Suppl II):II-632.
53. DiMarco JP, Sellers TD, Lerman BB, et al. 1985. Diagnostic and therapeutic use of adenosine in patients with supraventricular tachycardia. J Am Coll Cardiol 6:417–425.
54. Margolis B, DeSilva RA, Lown B. 1980. Episodic drug treatment in the management of paroxysmal arrhythmias. Am J Cardiol 45:621–626.
55. Fisher JD, Kim SG and Mercando AD. 1988. Electrical devices for treatment of arrhythmias. Am J Cardiol 61:45A–57A.

56. Iinuma H, Dreifus LS and Mazgalev T. 1983. Role of the perinodal region in atrioventricular re-entry. J Am Coll Cardiol 2:465–473.
57. Haissaguerre M, Warin JF, Lemetayer P, et al. 1989. Closed chest ablation of retrograde conduction in patients with AV nodal re-entry tachycardia. N Engl J Med 320:426–433.
58. Ross DL, Johnson DC, Koo CC, et al. 1987. Surgical treatment of supraventricular tachycardia without the Wolff–Parkinson–White syndrome: current medications, techniques and results. In P Brigada and HJJ Wellens (eds), Cardiac Arrhythmias: Where to Go from Here? Mt. Kisco, NY: Futura, p 591.
59. Klein GJ, Yee R and Sharma AD. 1989. Longitudinal electrophysiologic assessment of asymptomatic patients with the Wolff–Parkinson–White electrocardiographic pattern. N Engl J Med 320:1229–1233.
60. Michelucci A, Padeletti L, Mezzani A, et al. 1989. Relationship between age and anterograde refractoriness of the accessory pathway in Wolff–Parkinson–White patients. Cardiology 76:270–273.
61. McGovern B, Garan H and Ruskin JN. 1986. Precipitation of cardiac arrest by verapamil in patients with Wolff–Parkinson–White syndrome. Ann Intern Med 104:791–794.
62. Sellers TD, Bashore TM and Gallagher JJ. 1977. Digitalis in the preexcitation syndrome. Circulation 56:260–267.
63. Jackman WM, Wang X, Friday KJ, et al. 1991. Catheter ablation of accessory atrioventricular pathways (Wolff–Parkinson–White syndrome) by radiofrequency current. N Engl J Med 324:1605–1611.
64. Calkins H, Sousa J, El-Atassi R, et al. 1991. Diagnosis and cure of the Wolff–Parkinson–White syndrome or paroxysmal supraventricular tachycardias during a single electrophysiologic test. N Engl J Med 324:1612–1618.
65. Wellens HJJ, Bar FW, Dassen WRM, et al. 1980. Effect of drugs in the Wolff–Parkinson–White syndrome: importance of initial length of effective refractory period of accessory pathway. Am J Cardiol 46:665–669.
66. DeBuitleir M, Bove EL, Schmaltz S, et al. 1990. Cost of catheter versus surgical ablation in the Wolff–Parkinson–White syndrome. Am J Cardiol 66:189–192.
67. McLenachan JM, Henderson E, Morris KI, et al. 1987. Ventricular arrhythmias in patients with hypertensive left ventricular hypertrophy. N Engl J Med 3117:787–792.
68. Hinkle LE, Carver T, Stevens M. 1969. The frequency of asymptomatic disturbances of cardiac rhythm and conduction in middle-aged men. Am J Cardiol 24:629–650.
69. Kennedy HL, Whitlock JA, Sprague MK, et al. 1987. Long-term follow-up of asymptomatic healthy subjects with frequent and complex ventricular ectopy. N Engl J Med 312:193–197.
70. Cardiac Arrhythmia Suppression Trial (CAST) Investigators. 1991. Mortality and morbidity in patients receiving encainide, flecainide, or placebo. N Engl J Med 324:781–788.
71. Lown B and Wolf M. 1971. Approaches to sudden death from coronary heart disease. Circulation 44:130–137.
72. Bigger JT Jr. 1983. Definition of benign versus malignant arrhythmias: target for treatment. Am J Cardiol 52:47C–54C.
73. Mujharji K, Rude RE, Poole WK, et al. 1984. Risk factors for sudden death after acute myocardial infarction: two year follow-up. Am J Cardiol 54:31–36.
74. Bigger JT Jr. 1986. Relation between left ventricular dysfunction and ventricular arrhythmias after myocardial infarct. Am J Cardiol 57:8B–14B.
75. Lown B. 1979. Sudden cardiac death: the major challenge confronting contemporary cardiology. Am J Cardiol 43:313–328.
76. DeMarco JP, Garan H and Hawthorne JW. 1981. Intracardiac electrophysiological techniques in recurrent syncope of unknown cause. Ann Intern Med 95:542–550.
77. Aronow WS, Mercando AD, Epstein S, et al. 1990. Effect of quinidine or procainamide versus no antiarrhythmic drug on sudden cardiac death, total cardiac death, and total death in elderly patients with heart disease and complex ventricular arrhythmias. Am J Cardiol 66:423–428.
78. Yang JC, Wesley RC Jr and Froelicher VF. 1991. Ventricular tachyardia during routine treadmill testing. Arch Intern Med 151:349–353.
79. Burkart F, Pfisterer M, Kiowski W, et al. 1990. Effect of antiarrhythmic therapy on mortality in survivors of myocardial infarction with asymptomatic complex ventricular

arrhythmias: Basel Antiarrhythmic Study of Infarct Survival (BASIS). J Am Coll Cardiol 16:1711–1718.

80. Dreifus LS, Fisch C, Griffin JC, et al. 1991. Guidelines for implantation of cardiac pacemakers and antiarrhythmia devices. J Am Coll Cardiol 18:1–13.
81. Hine LK, Laird N, Hewitt P, et al. 1989. Meta-analytic evidence against prophylactic use of lidocaine in acute myocardial infarction. Arch Intern Med 149:2694–2698.
82. Tzivoni D, Keren A, Cohen AM, et al. 1984. Magnesium therapy for torsades de pointes. Am J Cardiol 53:528–530.

9. HEART BLOCK/CARDIAC PACING

SETH J. RIALS
ROGER A. MARINCHAK
PETER R. KOWEY

Bradyarrhythmias frequently cause symptoms in the elderly and may result from impaired conduction from the atria to the ventricles. In this chapter, we will discuss the etiology, diagnosis, and management of heart block in the elderly with special emphasis on permanent pacing. Included in this discussion will be information regarding pacing for sick sinus syndrome, although a more complete review of sinus-node dysfunction in the elderly is provided elsewhere in this text.

HEART BLOCK IN THE ELDERLY

The term *heart block* generally implies abnormal atrioventricular conduction. However, it is a nonspecific term that indicates neither the precise location nor the severity of the conduction abnormality. In its most common usage, the term refers to complete atrioventricular (A-V) block, in which there is failure of any atrial impulses to conduct to the ventricles. As a result, atrial and ventricular activity are completely independent. Heart block is a common indication for permanent pacing in adults and is probably the most common indication in elderly patients. Levander-Lindgren and Lantz [1] found that of 1265 patients receiving permanent pacemakers, 38% had complete A-V block. Almost 85% of the patients in their study were age 60 years or older.

Franz H. Messerli (ed.), CARDIOVASCULAR DISEASE IN THE ELDERLY (Third Edition). Copyright © 1993 Kluwer Academic Publishers. ISBN 0-7923-1859-5. All rights reserved.

The diagnosis of complete A-V block is made electrocardiographically by the complete independence of atrial and ventricular activity. The atrial rate in the majority of cases is faster than the ventricular rate, although this is not an absolute requirement. The site of block can be located in the A-V node, the proximal His bundle, or in the distal conduction system. The ventricular escape rhythm often arises from a site just distal to the site of block. If the escape rhythm originates from tissue proximal to the bifurcation of the His bundle, the QRS complex duration will be normal (assuming no other conduction abnormality exists); if the escape rhythm originates below the bifurcation, the duration of the QRS complex will be prolonged.

Differentiation of complete A-V block from simple A-V dissociation is essential. The latter may occur when the sinus rate is exceeded by the rate of a subsidiary focus located in the A-V junction or His–Purkinje system. Conduction of an atrial (sinus or ectopic) depolarization into the ventricle will still occur if an atrial depolarization arrives at a time when the A-V node and His–Purkinje system are not refractory. Thus, A-V dissociation is a necessary but insufficient condition for the diagnosis of complete A-V block. Some irregularity of a ventricular "escape" rhythm occurring at a rate greater than the dissociated atrial rate should therefore alert the clinician to the possibility that the A-V block is incomplete. In these cases, causes for sinus rate slowing and/or acceleration of subsidiary rhythms should be sought.

Etiology

Complete A-V block can be congenital or acquired. The congenital variety most commonly occurs without structural heart disease, is usually asymptomatic, is recognized early in life, and will not be considered further here. Acquired complete A-V block is not unusual in the elderly and can result from coronary artery disease, degenerative A-V conduction disease, nonischemic myocardial diseases, valvular disease, drugs, vagal stimulation, and trauma. Accurate diagnosis of the etiology is critical because some of these causes are reversible and others require early consideration for permanent pacing.

A common cause of acquired complete A-V block in the elderly is idiopathic degenerative disease of the cardiac conduction system. Various series have reported a prevalence of 20% to 40% at autopsy [1–4]. Two forms of this disease have been described: Lenegre's disease [5] and Lev's disease [6].

Lenegre's disease

Lenegre's disease is characterized by diffuse fibrosis or "sclerodegenerative destruction" of the bundle branches distal to the bifurcation of the His bundle [5]. It usually is first manifest as typical bundle branch block and then slowly progresses to complete A-V block. Histologic study reveals fibrotic replacement of the conduction fibers. In patients without concomitant coronary disease or other identifiable heart disease, the myocardium surrounding the ventricular conduction system is normal. Of 28 cases of complete heart block described by Lenegre, 18 were thought to be idiopathic [5].

Lev's disease

Degeneration of the proximal portion of the His bundle is characteristic of Lev's disease [6]. This form of idiopathic degenerative disease appears to be less common than Lenegre's disease and results from fibrocalcific changes involving the central fibrous body, membranous septum, aortic valve annulus, and mitral valve annulus [7,8]. Lev considered an exaggerated focal sclerosis and fibrocalcification of the upper interventricular septum that occurs with aging as likely etiologies of this form of conduction disease [6,9]. A contributing factor may also be mechanical strain, especially left ventricular hypertrophy due to hypertension [6,9].

Coronary artery disease

Coronary artery disease can produce complete A-V block either acutely during an infarction or chronically via fibrosis from a healed infarct. Various degrees of A-V block can occur during acute infarction, but complete A-V block occurs in only 2% to 8% [10,11]. Inferior infarcts are most likely to produce complete A-V block, although it is usually transient. The escape rhythm is characterized by a narrow QRS complex because inferior infarcts are usually caused by occlusion of the right coronary artery. Although this vessel often gives rise to the A-V node artery, it provides very little blood supply to the distal A-V node or His bundle. Inferior infarcts are also associated with reflex hypervagotonia that may contribute to A-V block independent of ischemia involving the conduction system. Conversely, anterior infarctions must involve a significant portion of the interventricular septum to produce complete A-V block. This, in turn, requires a proximal occlusion of the left anterior descending artery that usually produces a large infarction. Not surprisingly, the prognosis for patients with complete A-V block due to an anterior infarction is significantly worse than for patients with inferior infarctions [12]. Complete A-V block in patients with acute anterior infarct usually follows the sudden development of right bundle branch block, especially if there is a Q-wave in lead V1 [11]. The escape rhythm usually is located in the distal His–Purkinje system, resulting in a wide QRS complex at a slow, unreliable rate; prolonged periods of asystole are not uncommon. Unrecognized healed infarction is also a common cause of complete A-V block. Various autopsy studies suggest that fibrosis due to healed infarction may be associated with complete A-V block in 10% to 17% of cases [5,8,13].

Table 9-1. Classification system of indications for permanent pacemaker implantation

Class I:	Conditions for which there is general agreement that permanent pacemakers should be implanted
Class II:	Conditions for which permanent pacemakers are frequently used but for which there is divergence of opinion regarding the necessity of their insertion
Class III:	Conditions for which there is general agreement that pacemakers are unnecessary

Adapted and reprinted with permission of Elsevier Science Publishing Company, Inc. from Joint American College of Cardiology/American Heart Association Task Force on Assessment of Cardiovascular Procedures (1991). Guidelines for implantation of cardiac pacemakers and antiarrhythmic devices. J Am Coll Cardiol 18: 1–13.

Other causes

Less common causes of acquired complete A-V block in the elderly include collagen vascular disease such as ankylosing spondylitis [14,15], cardiac amyloidosis [16,17], Lyme disease [18], myxedema [19,20], hemochromatosis, and surgical trauma at the time of aortic or mitral valve replacement.

Evaluation

When evaluating a patient with acquired complete A-V block, it is necessary to determine whether a reversible etiology such as acute ischemia or drug effect is present. The elderly are particularly susceptible to drug-induced A-V block. The very drugs most likely to cause A-V block (digoxin, beta-blockers, and calcium-channel blockers) are used to treat illnesses that are especially prevalent in the elderly, such as hypertension, coronary artery disease, and atrial fibrillation. In addition, the absorption, metabolism, and elimination of these drugs are likely to be altered by changes in vital organ function resulting from concomitant disease and aging. Impaired perceptive and cognitive abilities increase the likelihood of dosing errors. Finally, many elderly patients are on multiple medications and are therefore at risk for drug interactions. Therefore it is imperative that a careful drug history be obtained during evaluation of a patient with acquired complete A-V block. Treatment should be aimed at supporting the ventricular rate until the offending drug is eliminated.

CARDIAC PACING IN THE ELDERLY

Permanent cardiac pacing has been used to treat symptomatic bradyarrhythmias for more than 30 years. The majority of pacemakers are implanted in patients who are over age 65 [1,21], most often for A-V block or for sinus-node dysfunction [1]. Detailed reviews of the general aspects of cardiac pacing [22,23] are beyond the scope of this discussion. We will focus on aspects of pacing particularly relevant to the elderly.

Guidelines for implanting permanent pacemakers, outlined by a joint task force of the American College of Cardiology and the American Heart

Table 9-2. Additional factors to consider when evaluating a patient for pacemaker implantation

1. Overall physical and mental state of the patient, including the presence of associated diseases that may result in limited life expectancy
2. Presence of associated underlying cardiac disease(s) that may be adversely affected by bradycardia
3. Desire of the patient to drive a motor vehicle
4. Remoteness of medical care, including patients who travel widely or live alone and therefore might be unable to seek medical help if serious symptoms arise
5. Need for administering medication(s) that may depress escape heart rhythms or aggravate atrioventricular (A-V) block
6. Slowing of the basic escape rhythm
7. Significant cerebrovascular disease that might result in symptomatic cerebral ischemia if cerebral perfusion were to suddenly decrease
8. Desires of the patient and family

Adapted and reprinted with permission of Elsevier Science Publishing Company, Inc. from Joint American College of Cardiology/American Heart Association Task Force on Assessment of Cardiovascular Procedures (1991). Guidelines for implantation of cardiac pacemakers and antiarrhythmic devices. J Am Coll Cardiol 18: 1–13.

Association, are not age specific [24]. Indications for permanent pacemakers are classified as shown in table 9-1. Class I indications are those for which there is general agreement that a pacemaker should be implanted; class II indications are those for which there is a divergence of opinion about the appropriateness of pacing; and class III indications are those for which pacemakers are considered unnecessary. Table 9-2 also summarizes additional factors to consider when evaluating a patient for permanent pacing.

A-V block

Specific indications for permanent pacemaker implantation in patients with A-V block are summarized in table 9-3. Syncope or other symptoms due to documented, acquired, complete A-V block are a class I indication for permanent pacing, and pacing improves survival in these patients [25,26]. However, many patients with symptoms due to bradyarrhythmia do not fall into this category because their symptoms are transient and occur in an unmonitored setting. Since episodes of complete A-V block may be episodic, the clinician must therefore identify patients at risk for transient complete A-V block. These patients are usually identified using either the 12-lead ECG and/or electrophysiologic testing.

Patients at high risk for episodic complete A-V block include those with ECG evidence of type II second-degree A-V block, defined as the presence of intermittently blocked P-waves with no change in the P-R interval of conducted beats. Because the site of conduction block during Mobitz II block is within or below the His bundle, the prognosis for these patients is worse when complete A-V block develops. This relates to the fact that a distal site of conduction block produces a more distal escape rhythm that will likely be slow and unreliable. Therefore, these patients are often symptomatic from

Table 9-3A. Indications for permanent pacing in acquired A-V block in adults

Class I

A. Complete heart block, permanent or intermittent, at any anatomic level, associated with any one of the following complications:
1. Symptomatic bradycardia (discussed in the introduction). In patients with these symptoms in the presence of complete heart block, the symptoms must be presumed to be due to the heart block unless proven to be otherwise
2. Congestive heart failure
3. Ventricular ectopy and other conditions that require treatment with drugs that suppress the automaticity of escape foci
4. Documented periods of asystole of 3.0 seconds or longer, or any escape rate of less than 40 beats/min in symptom-free patients
5. Confusion states that clear with temporary pacing
6. Post-A-V junction ablation, myotonic dystrophy
B. Second-degree A-V block, permanent or intermittent, regardless of the type or the site of the block, with symptomatic bradycardia
C. Atrial fibrillation, atrial flutter, or rare cases of supraventricular tachycardia with complete heart block or advanced A-V block, bradycardia, and any of the conditions described under I-A. The bradycardia must be unrelated to digitalis or drugs known to impair A-V conduction

Class II

A. Asymptomatic complete heart block, permanent or intermittent, at any anatomic site, with ventricular rates of 40 beats/min or faster
B. Asymptomatic type II second-degree A-V block, permanent or intermittent
C. Asymptomatic type I second-degree A-V block at intra-His or infra-His levels

Class III

A. First-degree A-V block (see section on bi-trifascicular block)
B. Asymptomatic type I second-degree A-V block at the supra-His (A-V nodal) level

---

Table 9-3B. Indications for permanent pacing in bifascicular and trifascicular block

Class I

A. Bifascicular block with intermittent complete heart block associated with symptomatic bradycardia (as defined)
B. Bifascicular or trifascicular block with intermittent type II second-degree A-V block with symptoms attributable to the heart block

Class II

A. Bifascicular or trifascicular block with syncope that is not proved to be due to complete heart block, but other possible causes for syncope are not identifiable
B. Markedly prolonged H-V ($>100\,\text{ms}$)
C. Pacing-induced infra-His block

Class III

A. Fascicular block without A-V block or symptoms
B. Fascicular block with first-degree A-V block without symptoms

---

Adapted and reprinted with permission of Elsevier Science Publishing Company, Inc. from Joint American College of Cardiology/American Heart Association Task Force on Assessment of Cardiovascular Procedures (1991). Guidelines for implantation of cardiac pacemakers and antiarrhythmic devices. J Am Coll Cardiol 18: 1–13.

severe bradycardia when complete A-V block occurs [27–29]. Type II second-degree A-V block is an indication for permanent pacing in the presence of symptoms (class I indication) and is a class II indication in the absence of symptoms.

Electrophysiologic (EP) testing may be useful for evaluating patients with ECG evidence of conduction disease and symptoms that may be due to intermittent bradyarrhythmia, in order to assess the likelihood of episodic progression to complete A-V block. EP testing is of little use in patients without ECG evidence of conduction disease, since the likelihood of finding a significant abnormality is low [30,31]. Similarly, EP testing is not helpful in asymptomatic patients with bifascicular block on ECG, since the test fails to accurately identify the small percentage of patients who ultimately progress to complete A-V block [32]. However, when patients with both symptoms and bifascicular block are evaluated, the results have prognostic utility. Specifically, the finding of abnormally prolonged conduction through the distal His–Purkinje system (H-V interval) identified patients at high risk of progressing to complete A-V block [33,34].

Once the indication for permanent pacing is established, some physicians may still hesitate to recommend the procedure to elderly patients because of a perceived higher risk or lower likelihood of symptom relief. However, numerous studies have specifically examined permanent pacing in elderly patients and have documented both its efficacy and lack of excess morbidity and mortality [21,35,36].

Selection of pacemaker system

After the need for a pacemaker has been established, the next decision to be made is the selection of a pacemaker system. Specifically, should a dual-chamber system be implanted, should it be rate responsive, and if so, what parameter should determine the rate response? For patients with complete A-V block, pacing systems that increase ventricular rate on demand are superior to systems with fixed ventricular rates. It is less clear whether dual-chamber pacing is superior to rate-responsive single-chamber pacing. For review purposes, the pacemaker code is summarized in table 9-4 [37].

Dual-chamber pacing is purported to have significant benefits compared to single-chamber pacing. These benefits include restoration of A-V synchrony, increase in ventricular rate when appropriate, and prevention of pacemaker syndrome. The disadvantages include increased complexity, susceptibility to pacemaker-mediated tachycardias, decreased generator longevity, and higher cost. These issues will be examined with special consideration of the needs of elderly patients.

One of the primary benefits of dual-chamber pacemakers is preservation of A-V synchrony. Atrial systole serves to complete ventricular filling. The importance of this function may increase with age, especially when there is diminished ventricular compliance resulting from hypertension, ischemia, or

Table 9-4. The NASPE/BPEG generic (NBG) pacemaker code

Category	Position				
	I	II	III	IV	V
	Chamber(s) paced	Chamber(s) sensed	Response to sensing	Programmability, rate modulation	Antitachyarrhythmia function(s)
	O = None	O = None	O = None	O = None	O = None
	A = Atrium	A = Atrium	T = Triggered	P = Simple programmable	P = Pacing (antitachyarrhythmia)
	V = Ventricle	V = Ventricle	I = Inhibited	M = Multiprogrammable	S = Shock
	D = Dual (A + V)	D = Dual (A + V)	D = Dual (D + I)	C = Communicating	D = Dual (P + S)
				R = Rate modulation	
Manufacturer's designation only	S = Single (A or V)	S = Single (A or V)		Comma optional here	

Note: Positions I through III are used exclusively for antibradyarrhythmia function.
From Bernstein et al. (1987). The NASPE/BPEG generic pacemaker code for antibradyarrhythmia and adaptive-rate pacing and antitachyarrhythmia devices. PACE 10:794–799.

cardiomyopathy [38,39]. The absolute contribution that atrial contraction makes to ventricular systolic performance, however, is dependent on a number of factors, including body position, heart rate, atrial and ventricular chamber volumes, and A-V conduction time, to name a few. The majority of studies examining the importance of A-V synchrony have compared dual-chamber pacemakers (DDDs) to fixed-rate ventricular pacemakers (VVIs). These studies found that patients with dual-chamber pacemakers have better exercise tolerance and hemodynamic profiles [40–43]. A small study of elderly patients has shown the same benefit [44]. For the most part, however, these studies did not determine whether the benefit of dual-chamber pacing resulted from the ability to increase ventricular rate or from the maintenance of A-V synchrony.

Direct comparisons between DDDs and single-chamber, rate-responsive ventricular pacemakers (VVIRs) have been limited. Fananapazir et al. [41] studied 14 patients with idiopathic complete A-V block (mean age 69 years) and found no significant difference between the two modes of ventricular pacing in terms of exercise time, arterial blood pressure, or symptoms. However, both modes were superior to fixed-rate ventricular pacing [41]. A similar small study [45] of 16 patients (mean age 60) with a variety of cardiac diagnoses examined ventricular volumes at rest and during exercise in patients randomly programmed to either DDD or VVIR pacing. No significant difference was observed in cardiac output for a given level of work. Therefore, on the basis of these limited data, it appears that an increase in ventricular rate is more important than maintenance of A-V synchrony in order to maximize exercise performance in paced patients with complete A-V block.

Pacemaker syndrome

Another benefit of dual-chamber pacing is the prevention of pacemaker syndrome—the symptomatic intolerance of ventricular pacing. Pacemaker syndrome can cause a wide variety of symptoms such as palpitations, lethargy, dyspnea, presyncope, dizziness, and headache. A number of mechanisms have been proposed as the cause of these problems, including loss of A-V synchrony, valvular incompetence, abnormal ventricular activation sequence, inappropriate circulatory reflexes, and retrograde conduction into the atrium [46]. Between 7% and 20% of patients with ventricular pacemakers may have symptoms of pacemaker syndrome [47,48]. The diagnosis can be particularly difficult in elderly patients, since the symptoms are so nonspecific [48]. However, the onset and persistence of such symptoms after implantation of a ventricular pacemaker should prompt the consideration of pacemaker syndrome as a diagnosis, since revision of the system to dual-chamber pacing will result in resolution of symptoms [47].

Pacemaker-mediated tachycardia

A disadvantage of early dual-chamber pacemaker systems was the development of pacemaker-mediated tachycardias (PMTs). The most common PMT is the endless-loop tachycardia that occurs when a ventricular paced beat conducts retrogradely to the atrium with a ventriculoatrial (V-A) time longer than the pacemaker's atrial refractory period. The atrial depolarization is therefore detected by the atrial sensing channel of the pacemaker, triggering the programmed A-V delay and another ventricular paced beat. The tachycardia is most often initiated by a premature ventricular depolarization that conducts retrogradely to the atrium, and it will be maintained unless the pacemaker timing parameters are changed, retrograde V-A conduction fatigues, or the pacemaker software has the ability to detect and terminate an endless-loop tachycardia automatically. Elderly patients with complete A-V block are not spared susceptibility to PMT, since retrograde conduction may persist in patients with antegrade block [49].

Early dual-chamber pacemakers were particularly likely to cause PMT because of a short (155 msec), nonprogrammable atrial refractory period [50]. Subsequent pacemakers had longer atrial refractory periods (235 msec), but many patients remained susceptible. Current pacemakers have a number of features that, if used properly, dramatically reduce the frequency of endless-loop tachycardias. These include programmable atrial refractory periods, automatic prolongation of the atrial refractory period after a premature ventricular depolarization is sensed, and rate-adaptive A-V delay. Some dual-chamber pacemakers also have the ability to recognize and terminate PMT automatically.

Another issue to consider with dual-chamber pacing is the frequent need to abandon it and reprogram the pacemaker to a single-chamber pacing mode. Limited data are available describing the rationale and frequency with which dual-chamber pacing is abandoned [51,52]. Reasons for abandonment include development of atrial tachyarrhythmias, atrial lead dislodgement, and exit block or nonsensing from the atrial lead. In one preliminary study, 34% of DDD pacemakers had been reprogrammed to another mode 48 months after implantation [51]. However, recent improvements in design and programmability of dual-chamber pacemakers and leads have reduced the problems of atrial tachyarrhythmias and lead dislodgement. Pacemakers capable of DDI pacing allow dual-chamber pacing in patients with paroxysmal atrial tachyarrhythmias without rapid erratic ventricular pacing caused by tracking of pathologic atrial depolarizations [53]. In patients with coexisting sinus-node dysfunction, DDI pacing may also decrease the incidence of these arrhythmias [53]. It is unclear whether the same benefits will be seen in patients with complete A-V block. Atrial lead dislodgement is less common with the improvement in design of atrial leads and the use of active fixation systems.

Physicians now have the option of using pacing systems that increase pacing rate in response to various sensors (VVIR, DDDR, DDIR) [54]. These systems may be particularly useful in patients with complete A-V block and concomitant sinus-node disease, who are unable to appropriately increase their atrial rate in response to exercise. (The benefits of increased ventricular rate during exercise in patients with complete heart block were discussed earlier in this chapter.) A variety of sensors are under investigation for use in pacing systems, including vibration, respiratory rate, evoked Q-T interval, temperature, venous oxygen content, venous pH, and stroke volume [54]. At the time of this writing, two have been approved for clinical use in the United States: an actvity-based sensor (Actvitrax II, Synergist II, Medtronic Inc; Synchrony II, Pacesetter Systems Inc.) and a respiratory-rate sensor (Meta MV, Telectronics Inc.). Although the advantages and disadvantages of each system are beyond the scope of this discussion, the development of sensor-driven, rate-adaptive pacemakers is an important advance in pacing technology. Patients with complete A-V block (whether drug induced or due to conduction system disease) who may benefit from this mode of pacing include those with atrial fibrillation (VVIR pacing) and those with sinus-node dysfunction (DDDR, DDIR), in whom the ability to increase heart rate on demand is an important consideration.

One study has specifically examined the use of VVIR pacemakers in the elderly. VVIR pacing improved maximal exercise tolerance in elderly patients (mean age 75) with complete A-V block and atrial fibrillation compared to VVI pacing [55]. Rate-responsive pacing was also associated with decreased patient perception of difficulty when performing submaximal exercise [55].

Sinus-node dysfunction

As stated in the introduction to this chapter, sinus-node dysfunction (sick sinus syndrome or bradycardia–tachycardia syndrome) is a common indication for pacing in elderly patients [1]. Permanent pacing is indicated when symptomatic sinus bradycardia occurs as the primary manifestation of the syndrome or when symptomatic bradycardias follow abrupt termination (offset pause) of an episode of atrial tachycardia [24]. Permanent pacing may also be necessary when drug therapy to control symptomatic tachyarrhythmias produces significant sinus bradycardia or A-V block (table 9-5) [24].

Choosing a permanent pacing system for patients with sinus-node dysfunction may be as complicated as for patients with A-V block. Fortunately, there are more data with which to make recommendations. A recent literature review by Sutton and Kenny [53] addressed two important aspects of sinus-node dysfunction that impact on selecting a permanent pacing system: the development of atrial fibrillation and progression to A-V

Table 9-5. Indications for permanent pacing in sinus-node dysfunction

---

Class I

A. Sinus-node dysfunction with documented symptomatic bradycardia. In some patients, this will occur as a consequence of long-term essential drug therapy of a type and dose for which there is no acceptable alternative

Class II

A. Sinus-node dysfunction, occurring spontaneously or as a result of necessary drug therapy, with heart rates below 40 beats/min when a clear association between significant symptoms consistent with bradycardia and the actual presence of bradycardia has not been documented

Class III

A. Sinus-node dysfunction in asymptomatic patients, including those in whom substantial sinus bradycardia (heart rate <40 beats/min) is a consequence of long-term drug treatment.
B. Sinus-node dysfunction in patients in whom symptoms suggestive of bradycardia are clearly documented *not* to be associated with a slow heart rate.

Adapted and reprinted with permission of Elsevier Science Publishing Company, Inc. from Joint American College of Cardiology/American Heart Association Task Force on Assessment of Cardiovascular Procedures (1991). Guidelines for implantation of cardiac pacemakers and antiarrhythmic devices. J Am Coll Cardiol 18: 1–13.

block. Atrial fibrillation was initially identified in 8% of patients and developed in an additional 16% during a mean follow-up of 38 months [53]. Atrial demand pacing systems (AAI) dramatically reduced the incidence of atrial fibrillation [53,56]: 4% of patients with AAI pacers developed atrial fibrillation, compared with 22% of patients with VVI pacers in the series reported by Sutton and Kenny [53]. Not surprisingly, AAI pacing was associated with a much lower incidence of systemic embolization: 1% of AAI paced patients suffering embolic events versus 12% in patients paced in the VVI mode [53]. In this review by Sutton and Kenney [53], the incidence of clinically important A-V block at the time of diagnosis was 16%. During a mean follow-up of 34 months, an additional 8% of patients developed A-V block [53].

Thus, there is considerable evidence that the use of atrial demand pacing will diminish morbidity in patients with sinus-node dysfunction. Furthermore, a reasonable proportion (>20%) of patients with sinus-node dysfunction either have A-V block at the time of diagnosis or will have it develop within three years. Therefore, it may be reasonable to implant pacing systems capable of DDD pacing in patients with sinus-node dysfunction. Pacemakers capable of DDIR pacing (atrial demand, ventricular demand, rate responsive in both channels but with a ventricular channel not triggered by sensed atrial activity) may be particularly useful, since ventricular tracking of atrial tachyarrhythmias can be avoided.

Other considerations when making choices regarding single- versus dual-chamber pacing for either A-V block or sinus-node dysfunction include cost and longevity. Evaluation of the cost of dual-chamber pacing versus single-chamber pacing has become necessary as resources for medical care become more limited. Other than an obvious price differential at the time of implantation, little information is available regarding which system is more cost-effective in the treatment of patients. A 1986 comparison of estimated costs between the two types of systems found a $5100 higher cost over 12 years for dual-chamber systems, including the higher initial price of the generator and extra lead [57]. This study assumed similar morbidity and survival in patients with the two types of systems. As noted, however, there is reason to believe that patients with dual-chamber systems will have a much lower incidence of atrial fibrillation and systemic embolization. Hence, at least in patients with sinus-node dysfunction, dual-chamber pacing may actually be the most cost-effective form of pacing therapy.

REFERENCES

1. Levander-Lindgren M and Lantz B. 1988. Bradyarrhythmia profile and associated diseases in 1265 patients with cardiac pacing. PACE 11:2207–2215.
2. Harris A, Davies M, Redwood D, et al. 1969. Etiology of chronic heart block. A clinical-pathological correlation in 65 cases. Br Heart J 31:206–218.
3. Davies M and Harris A. 1969. Pathological basis of primary heart block. Br Heart J 31:219–226.
4. Chatterjee K, Harris A, Patrick J, et al. 1970. The electrocardiogram in chronic heart block. A histological correlation with ECG changes in 42 patients. Am Heart J 80:47–55.
5. Lenegre J. 1964. Etiology and pathology of bilateral bundle branch block in relation to complete heart block. Prog Cardiovasc Dis 6:409–444.
6. Lev M. 1964. The pathology of complete atrioventricular block. Prog Cardiovasc Dis 6:317–326.
7. Yater WM and Cornell WH. 1935. Heart block due to calcareous lesions of the bundle of His: review and report of a case with detailed histopathologic study. Ann Intern Med 8:777–785.
8. Lenegre J. 1962. Les blocs auriculoventriculaires complets chroniques. Etude des causes et des lesions a propos de 37 cas. Malattie Cardiovascolari 3:311–336.
9. Davies MJ. 1976. Pathology of the conduction system. In FI Caird, JLC Dall, RD Kennedy (eds), Cardiology in Old Age. New York: Plenum Press, pp 57–80.
10. Meltzer LE and Kitchell JB. 1966. The incidence of arrhythmias associated with acute myocardial infarction. Prog Cardiovasc Dis 9:50–63.
11. Stock RJ and Macken DL. 1968. Observations on heart block during continuous electrocardiographic monitoring in myocardial infarction. Circulation 38:993–1005.
12. Norris RM. 1962. Heart block in posterior and anterior myocardial infarction. Br Heart J 31:352–356.
13. Davies MJ, Anderson RH, and Becker AE. 1983. The Conduction System of the Heart. London: Butterworth.
14. Weed CL, Kulander BG, Mazzarella JA, et al. 1966. Heart block in ankylosing spondylitis. Arch Intern Med 117:800–806.
15. Liu SM and Alexander CS. 1969. Complete heart block and aortic insufficiency in rheumatoid spondylitis. Am J Cardiol 23:888–892.
16. Roberts WC and Waller BF. 1983. Cardiac amyloidosis causing cardiac dysfunction: analysis of 54 necropsy patients. Am J Cardiol 52:137–146.
17. Buja L, Khoi NB, and Roberts WC. 1970. Clinically significant cardiac amyloidosis. Am J Cardiol 26:394–405.
18. Steere AC, Batsford WP, Weinberg M, et al. 1980. Lyme carditis: cardiac abnormalities of lyme disease. Ann Intern Med 93:8–16.

19. Lee JK and Lewis JA. 1962. Myxedema with complete A-V block and Adams-Stokes disease abolished with thyroid medication. Br Heart J 24:253–256.
20. Singh JB, Searobin OE, Guerrant RL, et al. 1973. Reversible atrioventricular block in myxedema. Chest 63:582–585.
21. Amikam S, Lemur J, Roguin N, et al. 1976. Long-term survival of elderly patients after pacemaker implantation. Am Heart J 91:445–449.
22. Furman S, Hayes DL, and Holmes DR, Jr. 1989. A Practice of Cardiac Pacing. Mount Kisco. NY: Futura.
23. Barold SS and Mugica J. 1988. New Perspectives in Cardiac Pacing. Mount Kisco, NY: Futura.
24. Joint American College of Cardiology/American Heart Association Task Force on Assessment of Cardiovascular Procedures. 1991. Guidelines for implantation of cardiac pacemakers and antiarrhythmic devices. J Am Coll Cardiol 18:1–13.
25. Donmoyer TL, DeSanctis RW, and Austen WG. 1967. Experience with implantable pacemakers using myocardial electrodes in the management of heart block. Ann Thorac Surg 3:218–227.
26. Edhag O and Swahn A. 1976. Prognosis of patients with complete heart block or arrhythmic syncope who were not treated with artificial pacemakers: a long-term follow-up study of 101 patients. Acta Med Scand 200:457–463.
27. Dhingra RC, Denes P, Wu D, et al. 1974. The significance of second degree atrioventricular block and bundle branch block: observations regarding site and type of block. Circulation 49:638–646.
28. Donoso E, Adler LN, and Friedberg CK. 1964. Unusual forms of second-degree atrioventricular block, including Mobitz type II block, associated with the Morgagni–Adams–Stokes syndrome. Am Heart J 67:150–157.
29. Ranganathan N, Dhurandher R, Phillips JH, and Wigle Ed. 1972. His bundle electrogram in bundle-branch block. Circulation 45:282–294.
30. Akhtar M, Shenasa M, Denker S, et al. 1983. Role of cardiac electrophysiologic studies in patients with unexplained recurrent syncope. PACE 6:192–201.
31. Touboul P and Ibrahim M. 1972. Atrioventricular conduction defects in patients presenting with syncope and normal PR intervals. Br Heart J 34:1005–1011.
32. Dhingra RC, Wyndham C, Amat-Y-Leon F, et al. 1979. Incidence and site of atrioventricular block in patients with chronic bifascicular block. Circulation 59:238–246.
33. Altshuler H, Fisher JD, and Furman S. 1979. Significance of isolated H-V interval prolongation in symptomatic patients without documented heart block. Am Heart J 97:19–26.
34. Scheinman MM, Peters RW, Sauve MJ, et al. 1982. Value of H-Q interval in patients with bundle branch block and the role of permanent pacing. Am J Cardiol 50:1316–1322.
35. Strauss HD and Berman ND. 1978. Permanent pacing in the elderly. PACE 1:458–464.
36. Cobler JL, Akiyama T, and Murphy GW. 1989. Permanent pacemakers in centenarians. J Am Geriatr Soc 37:753–756.
37. Bernstein AD, Camm AJ, Fletcher RD, et al. 1987. The NASPE/BPEG generic pacemaker code for antibradyarrhythmia and adaptive-rate pacing and antitachyarrhythmia devices. PACE 10:794–799.
38. Miyatake K, Okamoto M, Kinoshita N, et al. 1984. Augmentation of atrial contribution to left ventricular inflow with aging as assessed by intracardiac doppler flowmetry. Am J Cardiol 53:586–589.
39. Miller TR, Grossman SJ, Schectman KB, et al. 1986. Left ventricular diastolic filling and its association with age. Am J Cardiol 58:531–535.
40. Kruse I, Arnman K, Conradson RB, et al. 1982. A comparison of the acute and long-term hemodynamic effects of ventricular inhibited and atrial synchronous ventricular inhibited pacing. Circulation 65:846–855.
41. Fananapazir L, Bennett DH, and Monks P. 1983. Atrial synchronized ventricular pacing: contribution of the chronotropic response to improved exercise performance. PACE 6:601–608.
42. Perrins EJ, Morley CA, Chan SL, et al. 1983. Randomized controlled trial of physiological and ventricular pacing. Br Heart J 50:112–117.

43. Kristensson B-E, Krister A, Smedgard P, et al. 1985. Physiological versus single-rate ventricular pacing: a double blind cross-over study. PACE 8:73–84.
44. Jordaens L, De Backer G, and Clement DL. 1988. Physiologic pacing in the elderly: effects of exercise capacity and exercise-induced arrhythmias. Jpn Heart J 29:35–44.
45. Ausubel K, Steingart RM, and Shimshi M. 1985. Maintenance of exercise stroke volume during ventricular versus atrial synchronous pacing: role of contractility. Circulation 72:1037–1043.
46. Ausubel K, Boal BH, and Furman S. 1985. Pacemaker syndrome: definition and management. Cardiol Clin 3:587–594.
47. Cohen SI and Frank HA. 1982. Preservation of active atrial transport: an important clinical consideration in cardiac pacing. Chest 81:51–54.
48. Escher DJW, Fisher JD, Furman S, et al. 1979. Dizziness in the paced patient: pacemaker malfunction or not? In C Meere (ed), Cardiac Pacing. Montreal: Pacesymp.
49. Furman S and Fisher JD. 1982. Endless loop tachycardia in an AV universal (DDD) pacemaker. PACE 5:486–489.
50. Klementowicz P, Ausubel K, and Furman S. 1986. The dynamic nature of ventriculoatrial conduction. PACE 9:1050–1054.
51. Klementowicz P, Oseroff O, Andrews C, and Furman S. 1987. An analysis of DDD pacing mode survival: the first 5 years (abstract). PACE 10:409.
52. Harthorne JW and Jansyn E. 1988. Pacemaker mediated tachycardia: unsolvable problem. In SS Barold and J Mugica (eds), New Perspectives In Cardiac Pacing. Mount Kisco, NY: Futura.
53. Sutton R and Kenny R. 1986. The natural history of sick sinus syndrome. PACE 9: 1110–1114.
54. Benditt DG, Milstein S, Buetikofer J, et al. 1987. Sensor-triggered, rate-variable cardiac pacing. Ann Intern Med 107:714–724.
55. Gammage M, Schofield S, Rankin I, et al. 1991. Benefit of single setting rate responsive ventricular pacing compared with fixed rate demand pacing in elderly patients. PACE 14:174–180.
56. Langenfeld H, Grimm W, Maisch B, and Kochsiek K. 1988. Atrial fibrillation and embolic complications in paced patients. PACE 11:1667–1672.
57. Eagle KA, Mulley AG, Singer DE, et al. 1986. Single-chamber and dual-chamber cardiac pacemakers: a formal cost comparison. Am Intern Med 105:264–271.

10. POSTURAL HYPOTENSION AND SYNCOPE

MICHAEL G. ZIEGLER
RICHARD R. BARAGER

The abrupt loss of consciousness is the second most common reason why people seek emergency medical care. The very old have a 6% yearly incidence of syncope, and those who do faint have a recurrence rate of 30% [1]. Vasovagal syncope, or the common faint, and psychogenic fainting are relatively less common in the elderly than in young persons. Serious treatable causes of syncope such as postural hypotension and cardiac arrhythmias are more frequent in the old (table 10-1).

The initial evaluation of the patient who has abruptly lost consciousness should distinguish *cerebral* from *circulatory* causes of loss of brain function. Cerebral causes of unconsciousness such as stroke and trauma leave persistent localizing neurologic signs, but patients usually fully recover from a seizure. The circulation may fail to provide adequate nutrients, oxygen, or blood flow. Inadequate blood flow to the brain results in syncope. Patients who have recovered from syncope or a seizure may state that they passed out but now feel better. However, several distinguishing characteristics allow the two to be differentiated by the history of their onset and by the behavior of the patient after regaining consciousness (table 10-2). A seizure can begin with the patient in any posture and may start with local tonic or clonic movements that spread. The patient will usually report a sudden blackout,

Franz H. Messerli (ed.), CARDIOVASCULAR DISEASE IN THE ELDERLY (Third Edition). Copyright © 1993 Kluwer Academic Publishers. ISBN 0-7923-1859-5. All rights reserved.

Table 10-1. Causes of fainting

Usual	Uncommon
Vasovagal	Glossopharyngeal neuralgia
Postural hypotension	Hypogylcemia
Cardiac arrhythmia	Hypoxia
Micturition	Anemia
Drugs	Basilar ischemia
Carotid sinus sensitivity	Acute hydrocephalus
	Psychogenic
	Pheochromocytoma
	Sleep apnea

Table 10-2. Differences between seizure and syncope

Characteristic	Seizure	Syncope
Onset	Rapid	Slow
Recovery	Slow with confusion	Rapid
Posture at onset	Any	Upright
Appearance at onset	Normal	Pale
Injury	Usual	Unusual
Tonic posturing	Usual	Unusual
Clonic movements	Usual	Unusual
Tongue biting	Usual	Unusual
Incontinence	Usual	Unusual

with no initial phase of dizziness or dimming of vision. The episode often occurs so rapidly that patients are injured by falling. Tongue biting, lacerations of the cheek, and a sore back from intense muscular contractions are characteristic of seizures. The postictal period brings about a slow return to consciousness, with confusion, headache, and weakness. Consciousness returns many minutes before full orientation, and this postical confusional state leaves the patient conscious but disoriented and impresses observers with the notion that "there is something wrong" with the patient. In the first hours after the seizure, the patient may have focal neurologic signs, such as dilated pupils, hemiparesis, reflex asymmetry, and evidence of trauma, tongue biting, and incontinence [2].

SYNCOPE

The patient who faints because of syncope is usually sitting or standing and is frequently exercising. A feeling of light-headedness and dimming of vision may precede the loss of consciousness. An observer will note that a fair-skinned person becomes pale. The patient often has time to slump to the floor and avoid trauma but may have some tonic posturing and a few clonic jerking movements if held upright. Tongue biting and incontinence are very rare in the syncopal patient, and there is no postical period. The postsyncopal patient recovers promptly and does not experience the period of confusion seen after seizure. Patients recovering from syncope sometimes feel exhausted and weak, but they do not have the excruciating headache, back pain, tongue lacerations, or other stigmata of a recent seizure. Syncope tends to occur gradually (over seconds), with a dimming of consciousness; it abates rapidly with full orientation shortly after consciousness is regained. Seizure, on the other hand, occurs rapidly but subsides with a confusional state.

SEIZURES

Etiology

If the history of a patient's loss of consciousness includes tonic–clonic movements, incontinence, postictal confusional state, or other indications of a seizure, then an evaluation of the brain is indicated [3]. Although most young patients with seizures have idiopathic epilepsy, the new onset of seizures in an elderly person is often due to a lesion that can be diagnosed and treated. Elderly patients may also be taking a variety of drugs; withdrawal of depressant medications, such as sleeping pills, alcohol, and benzodiazepines, may make the patient susceptible to seizures. If agitation from drug withdrawal is treated with a tricyclic antidepressant or a phenothiazine, seizures will frequently occur simply on the basis of combined drug effects. If there is no clear history of a precipitating cause for seizures, then the new onset of epilepsy in an adult is grounds for thorough investigation of treatable intracerebral lesions, such as tumor or infection. As people grow older, they become more susceptible to respiratory and renal failure and to seizures from hypoxia and uremia. Respiratory failure is usually obvious, but renal failure of sufficient degree to cause uremia, hypocalcemia, or hyponatremia may not be apparent without the pertinent laboratory investigations.

Evaluation

The sudden onset of seizures in the elderly patient is most often the result of an intracerebral infarct or tumor, drugs, or metabolic causes. Therefore, evaluation of the patient suspected of having a seizure should first include a careful history of all drugs taken and a physical exam for localizing signs of an intracerebral infarct or tumor. Bronchogenic carcinoma is such a common cause of intracerebral tumor that a chest x-ray is appropriate [3]. Common metabolic causes of a seizure can be determined on routine chemistry screening, but if these investigations do not reveal the cause of seizure, a computed tomography (CT) scan, electroencephalogram (EEG), and lumbar puncture are in order. The EEG will demonstrate an abnormality in 40% to 75% of the cases, usually a generalized paroxysmal three-per-second, spike-slow-wave complex. However, over 25% of patients with a seizure disorder will have a normal EEG, and about 25% of normal patients will have nonspecific abnormalities on their EEG. In contrast to the overwhelming

Table 10-3. Common causes of epilepsy in the elderly

Drugs and toxins	Intracranial causes	Metabolic	Miscellaneous

Intoxications
  Tricyclic
    antidepressants
  Phenothiazines
  Lidocaine
  Tocainide
  Aminophylline
  Lead
  Arsenic
Withdrawal
  Ethanol
  Barbiturates
  Sedatives
  Benzodiazepines
	Lesions
	  Head injury
	  Infarct
	  Tumor
	  Hemorrhage
	Infections
	  Viral encephalitis
	  Bacterial abcess
	  Fungi
	  Meningitis
	  Neurosyphilis
		Uremia
		Hypocalcemia
		Hypoglycemia
		Hypoxia
		Hyponatremia
			Hypertensive
			  encephalopathy
			Cerebral degenerative
			  disorders

appearance of idiopathic seizures that occur in younger individuals, seizures in elderly subjects are frequently due to a definable cause (table 10-3). Up to 30% of patients evaluated for unexplained syncope go on to have a documented seizure [4].

FAINTNESS IN THE ELDERLY

When blood supply to the brain diminishes, faintness and then syncope ensue. Over 90% of episodes of abrupt loss of consciousness are due to syncope, and syncope is an increasingly frequent problem with advancing age. Cardiac arrhythmias cause syncope, but failure of the neurogenic regulation of blood pressure is an even more common reason for fainting. In order to understand the causes of fainting in the elderly, it is necessary to first understand the normal regulation of blood pressure and how it is affected by aging.

Normal maintenance of blood supply to the brain

Blood supply to the brain remains constant over a wide range of blood pressures in normal individuals. During exercise, blood flow to the muscles increases greatly, renal blood flow decreases, and blood pressure increases, but blood flow to the brain remains constant. In the case of severe hypertension or hypotension, however, brain flow may change. Most elderly people have vascular disease of the carotid and basilar arteries. Atherosclerotic plaques can cause stenotic lesions that require higher pressure to maintain adequate blood flow to the brain. As a consequence, some elderly subjects become completely dependent on maintenance of a certain level of blood pressure to avoid postural dizziness. This vascular disease decreases autoregulatory capabilities of the cerebral arterial supply and makes older people subject to syncope from moderate changes in perfusion pressure.

The body possesses an elaborate system to maintain blood pressure and adequate perfusion of all organs. The system malfunctions at times in the majority of elderly subjects, however, as manifested by the frequency of hypertension and syncope. The whole system is driven by the heart, which must have an adequate filling pressure and blood supply in order to function properly. Blood supply to the heart may decrease during hypovolemia and from increased intrathoracic pressure caused by coughing or the Valsalva maneuver. Even if the heart fills properly, its output can be diminished by congestive heart failure or from aortic or subvalvular stenosis. Intermittent cardiac arrhythmias are a frequent cause of syncope in the elderly and can temporarily diminish or stop cardiac output [4].

Pressure sensors in the aortic arch and at the carotid bifurcation monitor blood pressure. When stretched, they decrease output from brainstem vasomotor centers to return blood pressure back to normal. These stretch receptors are usually stimulated by pressure inside the great vessels, but they may also be stimulated by the Valsalva maneuver, cough, adjacent tumors, or carotid massage. When they are stimulated, heart rate slows and peripheral vascular resistance decreases in response to increased vagal tone and diminished sympathetic tone. The carotid bodies and vasomotor centers are particularly important in maintenance of blood pressure when we stand. The brainstem vasomotor nuclei integrate signals from the carotid bodies and from the rest of the brain. In response to stress, hypotension, and upright posture, the sympathetic nerves are stimulated to release norepinephrine, which increases heart rate, myocardial contractility, vascular resistance, constriction of the large veins, and renin secretion. Several diseases of the elderly affect these vasomotor centers. Shy–Drager syndrome destroys medullary vasomotor centers and adjacent structures. Other degenerative diseases, such as Huntington's chorea and parkinsonism, are also associated with a decrease in blood pressure and postural hypotension. Vascular disease of the basilar artery is common in the elderly and when severe may affect the vasomotor centers, causing dizziness both from interruption of vestibular input and poor blood pressure control [5].

Effects of aging on autonomic function

The function of peripheral autonomic nerves that control heart rate and blood pressure changes with age [6]. There is an apparent decrease in parasympathetic vagal tone with aging, as evidenced by a decrease in the incidence of vasovagal fainting. Along with this decreased parasympathetic activity, there is an increase in sympathetic nervous activity, since both circulating levels of norepinephrine and sympathetic nerve electrical activity double in the period from youth to old age. Concomitantly, the number of beta-receptors decreases with aging, and to compensate, the elderly secrete increased amounts of norepinephrine. Alpha-receptor levels remain constant, however, so that the elderly develop increased alpha-receptor-stimulated vasoconstriction, and blood pressure increases with age. The arteries lose their compliance with aging, in response to both degenerative changes and atherosclerosis. This diminished compliance causes an increase in pulse pressure and the characteristic increase in systolic blood pressure seen in the elderly. When young people stand, their systolic and diastolic blood pressures remain fairly constant; however, by age 60, the average person decreases systolic blood pressure by 7 mmHg on standing [6].

The body has several defenses to try to maintain blood pressure in the face of upright posture, but when these defenses fail, syncope ensues. The autonomic nervous system causes an almost instantaneous increase in heart rate and blood vessel tone. Renin levels increase, and aldosterone production and sodium retention occur more slowly. The entire system of blood pressure maintenance can be disrupted by many diseases that cause degeneration of the autonomic nervous system. Uremia and diabetes lead to degeneration of the autonomic nerves over time, while toxins or idiopathic degeneration of the autonomic nerves can cause a more rapid onset of a syndrome of postural hypotension and syncope (see table 10-4).

Drugs

Drugs are one of the most common causes of postural dizziness and syncope in the elderly [7]. Agents such as chlorpromazine predispose to both syncope

Table 10-4. Causes of syncope and faintness

Reduced blood supply to the heart	Neurogenic with persistent postural hypotension
Hypovolemia	Autonomic neuropathies
Decreased plasma volume	Diabetic
Anemia	Uremic
Venous pooling	Toxic
Hemorrhage	Guillain–Barré
Valsalva maneuver	Amyloidosis
Cough	Idiopathic
Atrial myxoma	Central nervous system defects
Reduced cardiac output	Spinal (e.g., transsection, syringomyelia)
Left heart	Shy–Drager syndrome
Aortic stenosis	Degenerative disorders (e.g., parkinsonism,
Idiopathic hypertrophic subaortic	Huntington's chorea)
stenosis (IHSS)	Basilar artery disease
Right heart	Drugs
Pulmonary emboli	Antidepressants (tricyclics, MAO inhibitors)
Pulmonary stenosis	Diuretics
Pulmonary tamponade	Nitrates
Pericardial tamponade	Alpha-blockers (prazosin, phenothiazines)
Heart failure	Beta-blockers
Arrhythmias	Dopamine agonists (L-dopa, bromocriptine)
Neurogenic	Sedatives
Vasovagal	Altered composition of the blood
Carotid sinus syncope	Hypoxia
Micturition syncope	Anemia
Glossopharyngeal neuralgia	Hypoglycemia

and seizure, and any drug that interferes with cardiovascular function can cause syncope. The elderly are especially prone to the blood-pressure-lowering effects of certain drugs such as diuretics, and are relatively immune to hypotension from beta-blockers. When hypotension occurs in a patient with stenosis of the blood vessels supplying the brain, dizziness and syncope are likely outcomes.

Diuretics

Many elderly patients have diminished blood volume, and when they stand, their systolic blood pressure decreases, unlike the systolic pressure of younger individuals. These patients are susceptible to the hypotensive effects of a small dose of diuretic. Patients who receive a diuretic increase their sympathetic tone and renin activity in an attempt to maintain blood pressure [8]. Elderly patients with impaired function of the autonomic nervous system, or those with autonomic neuropathy or heart failure, are unable to fully activate these compensatory mechanisms, however, and are much more prone to syncope from diuretics. A young hypertensive may tolerate 50 mg of hydrochlorothiazide easily, while the same diuretic dose can cause hyponatremia, hypokalemia, postural hypotension, and syncope in the elderly.

Nitrates

Nitrate drugs, the first line of treatment in the therapy of angina pectoris, primarily dilate the veins. The patient with coronary artery disease may have syncope because of cardiac arrhythmia or congestive heart failure, but is also likely to have dizziness and syncope from overuse of nitrates. These drugs cause venous pooling, which decreases blood return to the heart and cardiac output. Since some of the agents are short acting and rapidly absorbed, they can transiently attain high blood levels, which can result in fainting. Nitrate levels are usually markedly diminished by the time the patient consults a physician for the episode of syncope.

Alpha-blockers

Alpha-blocking drugs are used in the treatment of hypertension. Among these, labetolol and prazosin are the most commonly prescribed agents and are particularly prone to cause syncope. A first or increased dosage of prazosin can dramatically decrease blood pressure and effect a marked postural drop in blood pressure. Many drugs that have as their primary action blockage of dopaminergic, serotonergic, histaminergic, or beta-receptors also have some alpha-receptor-blocking activity. Chloropromazine is a good example of such an agent (prescribed for its dopamine-receptor-blocking properties), which has clinically important alpha-receptor-blocking activity. Chloropromazine can thus cause postural hypotension, particularly in patients who are slightly volume depleted. Haloperidol possesses much less alpha-blocking activity, but is equally useful in treating the elderly. Other psychotherapeutic agents, such as tricyclic antidepressants and monoamine oxidase inhibitors, alter alpha-receptor sensitivity and can cause postural hypotension, dizziness, and syncope.

Beta-blockers

Beta-blockers usually do not lower blood pressure very much in the elderly, and when their use is associated with syncope, it is often due to heart block or congestive failure. When low doses of a beta-blocking drug are associated with dizziness or fainting, an electrocardiogram (ECG) or Holter monitoring should be obtained, since the drug may act by exacerbating an atrioventricular (A-V) conduction defect [9].

Other agents

Dopamine agonist drugs such as L-dopa and bromocriptine are very helpful in treating the motor disturbance of parkinsonian patients. However, patients with parkinsonism tend to have relatively low blood pressures, and these drugs inhibit the release of norepinephrine, causing postural hypotension, which is particularly prominent when the patient is volume depleted [10]. Any central nervous system disease that involves the basal ganglia and brainstem can impair brain control of blood pressure. A wide variety of sedative agents also act on these brain centers. Patients who "pass out" when receiving a sedative agent may have had an overdose of the drug, or may have tried to arise too quickly while under the drug's influence and had a temporary drop in blood pressure due to impaired activity of the brain vasomotor centers. Even ordinary therapeutic doses of antianxiety agents increase the frequency of episodes of dizziness and syncope in the elderly [11].

In addition to the already-mentioned agents that affect blood pressure control, other drugs alter cardiac electrical activity and may cause syncope through alterations in cardiac rate and rhythm. An enormous number of drugs are capable of causing syncope, and these usually act through the cardiovascular system or the autonomic nervous system. A quick review of the drugs a patient is receiving that can affect these systems can often determine the cause of syncope.

VASOVAGAL SYNCOPE

Vasovagal syncope occurs most commonly in individuals under 30 years of age, but is still a frequent cause of fainting in the elderly. Older people seem less prone to fainting from psychological stimuli, such as "the sight of blood," but are still quite susceptible to vasovagal episodes from physical stimuli, such as abdominal paracentesis or pleural biopsy. Vasovagal syncope always occurs with the individual upright, unless the heart responds to vagal stimulation with cardiac standstill of sufficient duration to cause unconsciousness.

Vasovagal episodes can usually be diagnosed from history alone. There is always an inciting stimulus, which may be physical stimulation of the pleura or peritoneum or which may be psychological in nature [12]. Psychological stimuli are usually those in which the individual would prefer to run from a perceived danger, but some social or physical constraint prevents escape. The stimulus may be simple venipuncture or a gruesome accident, but it leads to a very stereotyped reaction.

The attack begins with yawning, pallor, and diaphoresis, particularly around the forehead. At this time, bradycardia begins, and the subject starts to feel uncomfortable, may see spots before the eyes, and have dimming of vision. Intestinal peristalsis increases and is perceived as an uncomfortable abdominal sensation or nausea. Vision dims further, and the individual may lose consciousness at this point. If the person is held upright, a few motor movements may ensue until he or she is placed recumbent. Once recumbent, the individual quickly regains consciousness and full orientation but may feel exhausted and have a compensatory exaggeration in sympathetic nervous activity with tachycardia that can last for many minutes. These episodes are usually quite benign, but in the presence of cardiac or cerebrovascular disease, may be dangerous [12].

Atropine can prevent most manifestations of vasovagal attacks and is useful in situations likely to provoke one of these attacks. For example, if an abdominal paracentesis is to be carried out with the patient in the sitting posture, a small dose of atropine is a worthwhile precaution, particularly if the patient has any evidence of cardiac conduction defects.

POSTURAL HYPOTENSION

Recurrent faintness and syncope are common in the patient with postural hypotension. Every patient who reports an episode of syncope should have postural responses evaluated. With the patient recumbent, pulse rate and blood pressure should be measured, and the color and warmth of the hands should be noted. The examiner should next have the patient stand and note the change in heart rate in the first 20 seconds (which reflects withdrawal of vagal tone to the heart). A normal response at one minute is a decrease of less than 7 mmHg diastolic blood pressure, an increase of at least 8 beats/min heart rate, and mild vasoconstriction and cooling of the hands. The patient who is vasodilated due to drugs, fever, or heat will develop postural hypotension and tachycardia and maintain warm pink skin. Patients who are volume depleted develop hyperadrenergic postural hypotension with tachycardia and cool, vasoconstricted extremities. Patients with diseases of the autonomic nervous system develop hypoadrenergic postural hypotension with little change in heart rate and failure to vasoconstrict. The patient with a history of postural dizziness and no fall in blood pressure on standing should then be exercised and blood pressure and heart rate again measured. Exercise normally raises blood pressure but will decrease blood pressure in the various diseases that cause postural hypotension.

If a decrease in blood pressure on standing is found, the first step should be a careful inquiry as to what drugs the patient is taking. In the absence of serious heart disease, the heart rate response to standing can be used to classify the patient's postural hypotension as hyperadrenergic or hypoadrenergic [13].

Hyperadrenergic postural hypotension

Hyperadrenergic patients will have a marked increase in heart rate on standing if their blood pressure drops. It is distinctly abnormal for the heart rate to remain low or only slightly increased in the face of hypotension. Patients who develop tachycardia while their blood pressure drops usually do so because of poor cardiac output or a decrease in their effective blood volume. Blood volume may be low because of a decrease in either plasma or red cell fraction. Plasma volume can be decreased by diuretics, dehydration, and hypoalbuminemia [8]. The red blood cell volume is diminished in anemia and has also been found to be low in some diabetic patients who have a normal hematocrit but a contracted total blood volume. If the patient has a marked tachycardia on standing, and no serious heart disease, then decreased blood volume is the most likely cause, and plasma and red blood cell measurements may be appropriate. Some patients have a normal blood volume but increased pooling of blood in their extremities. This is most commonly seen in patients with venous varicosities, dependent edema, or obstruction of the inferior vena cava. In these patients, walking increases arterial blood flow to the legs, accelerates venous pooling there, and decreases the return of blood to the heart.

Patients with congestive heart failure, outflow obstruction, or pericardial tamponade may also have postural hypotension. Heart disease sufficiently severe to impair the ability to maintain normal blood pressure while standing is usually clinically apparent on the most cursory examination of the cardiovascular system. A clear differentiation between this cause of postural hypotension and volume depletion is imperative, however, since volume depletion is treated with fluid expansion and heart failure is treated with diuretics.

Hypoadrenergic postural hypotension

The sympathetic nervous system is essential to maintenance of blood pressure during upright posture. A variety of drugs and diseases can interfere with this system. Diseases that affect the autonomic nervous system are most common in the elderly [14]. If a patient stands and has a decrease in diastolic blood pressure and heart rate fails to increase by at least 10 beats/min, the response is abnormal. This failure to respond may be due to drugs, such as beta-blockers, or to heart disease or defective autonomic reflexes.

Patients with disease of the autonomic nervous system will report many other symptoms. The onset of autonomic dysfunction is usually gradual and in men begins with impotence and then incontinence, urinary retention, altered bowel habits, heat intolerance and the inability to sweat, and then a fixed heart rate with postural hypotension. Failure of the autonomic nervous system may be due to central nervous system disease, invariably accompanied by other symptoms of disease in the brainstem or spinal cord [14]. A variety of diseases of the elderly may cause degeneration of sympathetic nerve fibers. Diabetes is the most common of these, but various toxins, amyloidosis, uremia, and idiopathic causes may similarly cause deterioration of these nerves.

Patients with a peripheral autonomic neuropathy usually do not have serious disease of the central nervous system but have the same symptoms of autonomic dysfunction related above. These causes of postural hypotension can be distinguished by the plasma norepinephrine response to standing and exercise (see figure 10-1).

Management

Patients who experience syncope from hypoadrenergic postural hypotension can be treated with volume-expanding agents, such as fludrocortisone [15]. Low doses of this drug (0.1 to 0.2 mg per day) sensitize blood vessels to vasoconstriction. Higher doses cause fluid retention and hypertension. When the patient has an adequate blood volume, then Jobst stockings can be used to compress their lower extremities to prevent blood pooling in the legs while standing. Waist-high Jobst stockings are particularly helpful in patients with varicose veins, but loose-fitting elastic hose are useless in preventing postural hypotension.

Patients who have postural hypotension due to partial autonomic neuropathy can increase their blood pressure in response to indomethacin or other nonsteroidal anti-inflammatory drugs that suppress prostaglandin synthesis [16]. These drugs increase alpha-receptors and decrease beta-receptors, thereby enhancing the pressor response to norepinephrine. Patients who release only small amounts of norepinephrine due to a partial autonomic neuropathy can then improve their blood pressure control while receiving indomethacin. Patients who respond to indomethacin often have a favorable response to less toxic inhibitors of prostaglandin synthesis, such as ibuprofen or even aspirin. Metoclopramide has hemodynamic effects similar to those of indomethacin and is helpful for patients who have gastroparesis as well as postural hypotension from autonomic insufficiency [17]. Having 240 mg of caffeine, given as two cups of fresh-brewed coffee in the morning, helps maintain blood pressure and is also helpful in combatting the hypotension that sometimes accompanies meals or insulin in these patients [7].

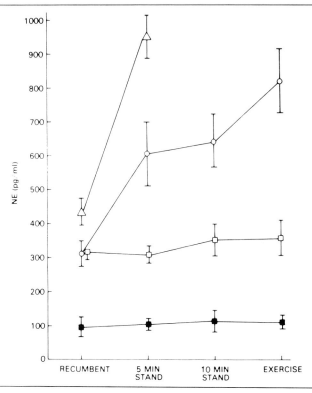

Figure 10-1. The response of plasma norepinephrine (NE) to standing and exercise. Normal subjects (○) double their NE levels after standing five minutes and have a further increase on exercise. Patients with volume depletion (△) have high NE levels and an exaggerated response to standing. Patients with neurologic disease of brain vasomotor centers (□) have normal NE levels at rest, but fail to increase NE appropriately in response to stress. Patients with autonomic neuropathy (■) have persistently low NE levels, since their sympathetic nerves cannot synthesize or release NE. (Reproduced with permission from the *Annual Review of Medicine*, Vol. 31. © 1980 by Annual Reviews, Inc.)

The beta-blocking drugs, dihydroergotamine, monoamine oxidase inhibitors, and pressor agents have all been reported helpful in treatment of autonomic insufficiency with postural hypotension and have all been associated with toxic side effects in these patients. Patients with autonomic insufficiency severe enough to cause postural hypotension are subject to unusual drug reactions. Over-the-counter decongestants can cause hypertensive reactions, and diuretics cause hypotension. Dysautonomic patients lack normal mechanisms for cardiovascular homeostasis, so drugs that alter blood pressure often have exaggerated and potentially dangerous side effects [7].

CAROTID SINUS SYNCOPE

The carotid sinus is a stretch receptor located at the bifurcation of the carotid arteries that responds to distention of these arteries by blood pressure. Although blood pressure is the physiologic stimulus to these structures, the carotid sinuses can be stimulated extrinsically by massage or a tight collar, and can be impinged upon by a growing tumor. Stimulation of the carotid sinuses activates cardioinhibitory centers of the medulla and leads to an increase in vagal discharge and a decrease in sympathetic nervous discharge. In most people, stimulation of the carotid sinus by carotid massage causes a bradycardia and lower blood pressure. However, in some subjects, vasodilation is a dominant effect of carotid sinus stimulation; in these subjects, heart rate may change little, but blood pressure still decreases [18].

Although syncope caused by the carotid sinus syndrome may be initiated by such ordinary stimuli as turning the head to one side or wearing a collar that is too tight, it most often occurs in the absence of definable stimuli. This syndrome is most frequently seen in the elderly and is more common in men than in women. Attacks occur when the patient is upright. Faintness lasts only a few minutes, and the usual syncopal attack is preceded by a prodrome of faintness that allows the individual to sink to the ground. There is some risk of trauma from falling. The attacks are unexpected and may occur in an otherwise healthy elderly person. There are several successful modes of treatment available for carotid sinus syncope, but diagnosis of the syndrome is sometimes difficult [18].

In most individuals, the hypotension that follows stimulation of the carotid sinus results from both slowing of the heart and vasodilation. Withdrawal of sympathetic tone causes systemic vasodilation, decreased heart rate, and inotropism, and parasympathetic stimulation causes cardiac slowing. All these effects lower blood pressure.

Testing for carotid sinus hypersensitivity

The carotid sinus can be stimulated by external massage at the area of greatest pulsation in the neck. This test can be hazardous in elderly patients with hypertension and extensive atherosclerosis of the carotid arteries and may cause transient or permanent paralysis. The test is safe in normotensive patients with no bruit and no history of cerebrovascular disease [19]. An explanation of the hazards of carotid massage to the patient may negate the value of the test. Anxiety about the procedure can raise heart rate and blood pressure and give a false-negative test.

When the carotid sinus is stimulated, it is normal for the heart rate to slow and for blood pressure to decrease. An abnormal response is one in which ventricular asystole lasts for three seconds or more, or a decrease in systolic and diastolic blood pressure greater than 50 mmHg occurs. Using these criteria, Walter et al. report that approximately one third of older men with coronary atherosclerotic and hypertensive heart disease have a hyperactive carotid sinus reflex [18]. Although these men had a high incidence of spontaneous syncope, most patients with a hyperactive carotid sinus reflex are asymptomatic. However, Davies et al. report that elderly men with normal electrocardiograms and no evidence of cardiac or neurologic disease have a very low incidence of hypersensitive carotid sinus responses [19]. Thus, in the patient who presents with fainting, carotid sinus stimulation cannot by itself produce a reliable diagnosis of carotid sinus syncope, but the maneuver can be a helpful guide to the diagnosis.

Carotid sinus syncope may be caused by *cardioinhibitory* or *vasodepressor* responses to carotid sinus stimulation [18]. If carotid sinus stimulation results in cardiac asystole for more than three seconds, then the patient should be given 1.2 mg atropine intravenously and the carotid sinus stimulation repeated within five minutes of drug administration while the patient is seated. Atropine will prevent cardiac slowing from carotid sinus stimulation, but some patients nonetheless will have a decrease in blood pressure as a result of vasodepressor activity of carotid sinus stimulation. A significant drop in blood pressure and dizziness during carotid sinus stimulation in the atropinized patient is indicative of vasodepressor carotid sinus syncope [20]. This occurs in about 20% of individuals with carotid sinus syncope, the remaining 80% having the more common cardioinhibitory type.

Management

If the patient has the cardioinhibitory type of carotid sinus syncope and is taking a drug that affects cardiac pacemaker activity or blood vessels, this drug should be withdrawn and the patient tested when the drug is no longer present. Methyldopa has been implicated as a cause of carotid sinus hypersensitivity [21]. Digitalis can increase carotid sinus neural discharge, and propranolol can aggravate cardiac slowing due to vagal stimulation. Diuretics and vasodilators, particularly the nitrates, may enhance the hypotensive response to carotid stimulation. If the cardioinhibitory form of carotid sinus hypersensitivity is present, even when the patient is not taking aggravating drugs, then cardiac pacemaker implantation is the preferred treatment for this type of syncope. Pacemaker treatment is highly successful and the results superior to those of any other form of therapy reported.

The vasodepressor form of carotid sinus syncope often cannot be adequately treated by cardiac pacing [22]. Several forms of treatment are available, but none is uniformly successful. Irradiation of the carotid sinus may decrease sensitivity to stimulation, but in some cases a total dose of over 2000 roentgens has been required. Irradiation results in complete to moderate relief in about 70% of subjects, usually without immediate serious complications. Surgery may be tried with carotid sinus denervation and periarterial stripping of the carotid sheaths above and below the carotid bifurcation. Sectioning of the carotid sinus nerve alone is technically difficult because this nerve is poorly defined. While surgery may be temporarily successful, a recurrence of symptoms after surgery is possible.

GLOSSOPHARYNGEAL NEURALGIA

Glossopharyngeal neuralgia is sometimes associated with bradycardia and syncope. The mechanism is similar to that involved in carotid sinus syncope, but is accompanied by pain mediated through the glossopharyngeal nerve. Pain usually occurs in the throat but may be present in the ear, neck, or face. Ninety percent of patients who experience syncope during glossopharyngeal neuralgia have an accompanying bradycardia. In about three fourths of cases, phenytoin or carbamazepine alleviate both the pain and syncope. Atropine can often prevent cardiovascular slowing, but it does not alleviate pain. When pharmacotherapy is ineffective, surgical interruption of the glossopharyngeal nerve is always effective. As with carotid sinus syncope, insertion of a cardiac-demand pacemaker can usually prevent syncope. It does not, however, alleviate the excrutiating pain these patients may undergo [23].

CARDIAC ARRHYTHMIAS

Cardiac arrhythmias in the elderly are discussed in detail in another chapter. Cardiac arrhythmias may cause syncope when they interfere with ventricular contraction, slow the heart rate to less than 40 beats/min, or increase it to greater than 185 beats/min. Changes in heart rate outside these limits may impair circulation sufficiently so that cerebral blood flow decreases and consciousness is impaired. Lesser alterations in heart rate may impair cerebral circulation in the presence of cerebrovascular disease, anemia, myocardial or valvular disease, and upright posture.

A Stokes–Adams attack is the association of complete heart block with syncope. Attacks may be intermittent, but the patient frequently has evidence of a secondary A-V block or bifascicular or trifascicular block. If this partial heart block becomes complete and no pacemaker below the block takes over, cardiac output ceases and syncope follows. These syncopal attacks may occur with the patient in any posture and with no more than a momentary feeling of weakness. When cardiac output is totally interrupted, the patient becomes gray and cyanotic, may have a few clonic jerks, and will develop confusion and neurologic signs due to cerebral ischemia if the attack is of sufficient duration. Occasionally, heart block is transitory, and an ECG taken later may not show any arrhythmia [4].

Heart slowing or cardiac standstill may be precipitated by increased vagal tone. Thus, a vasovagal episode, glossophrayngeal neuralgia, or carotid sinus supersensitivity may simulate a Stokes–Adams attack. If electrophysiologic testing is carried out on a patient who may have one of these syndromes, it is helpful to try to reproduce symptoms during testing by carotid massage or upright posture [24]. However, electrophysiologic testing may be of little overall benefit [25].

MICTURITION SYNCOPE

Distention of the urinary bladder causes a reflex increase in sympathetic nervous output and a subsequent elevation in blood pressure. In patients with section of the cervical cord, this reflex is not inhibited by brain influences, and urinary distention can lead to striking increases in circulating norepinephrine and blood pressure. Urination removes the stimulus for this reflex since sudden withdrawal of sympathetic tone causes a decrease in heart rate and blood pressure. About a third of the cases of micturition syncope occur in healthy young men, but the syndrome is more frequent in elderly men and women with multiple illnesses [26]. The majority of these elderly patients have postural hypotension, and therapy should be directed at the causes of the hypotension. Patients who complain of postmicturition syncope should be examined for urinary retention and instructed to urinate while sitting, especially at night.

UNUSUAL CAUSES OF SYNCOPE

Hyperventilation and hysterical syncope are among the more common causes of fainting in young people, but they become less common with advancing age. Paroxysms of coughing may lead to syncope, usually in obese patients with bronchitis. Coughing may increase intrathoracic pressure to 300 mmHg, which can almost entirely obstruct venous return to the heart and cause a marked decrease in cardiac output. Cerebrospinal fluid pressure increases at the same time; as a result, the brain is inadequately perfused. When coughing causes syncope, the association is usually obvious.

Swallowing may produce syncope in patients with esophageal diverticuli, peptic strictures, or glossopharyngeal neuralgia [27]. The condition is rare, and treatment is best directed at the anatomic cause.

Syncope may occur in pacemaker failure induced by electrical appliances, such as electric razors and microwave ovens. This problem has become less prevalent with the introduction of pacemakers that are adequately shielded from outside electrical interference.

CLINICAL APPROACH TO THE PATIENT WITH SYNCOPE

The abrupt loss of consciousness is usually due to seizure or syncope. A history of the episode often differentiates these causes, but when there is a question of a new onset of seizures in an elderly person, a thorough evaluation is indicated, since treatable causes such as infection or tumor may be involved [5]. A diagnosis of syncope should be made not simply by excluding seizure disorders, but by diagnosing the mechanism of the syncopal episode [28].

In an elderly person, the first line of inquiry should be toward drugs being used. The history should include a record of the patient's posture, level of exercise, emotional stress, premonitory symptoms, and rate of onset and recovery from syncope. In the physical exam, blood pressure and pulse rate should be measured with the patient recumbent, standing, and after moderate exercise. If upright posture brings about a drop in blood pressure with an increase in heart rate, then a clinical and laboratory evaluation of blood volume is indicated. If blood pressure falls but heart rate remains relatively fixed, then the patient should be asked about other symptoms of autonomic insufficiency, and the norepinephrine response to standing should be measured, if available. Auscultation of the carotid arteries and of the heart can help in evaluation of extracranial cerebrovascular disease and left ventricular outflow obstruction. If there is no contraindication for carotid massage, this can be performed with ECG monitoring to test for carotid sinus syncope. The ECG may indicate A-V block or a bilateral bundle branch block [28].

If these investigations fail to reveal the cause of syncope and the patient has experienced rapid loss of consciousness with only brief or no premonitory symptoms, then further investigations into a possible cardiac origin of syncope are indicated. Holter monitoring may reveal intermittent arrhythmias. Electrophysiologic studies are usually not diagnostic but are helpful in evaluating the probability of a patient developing cardiac arrhythmias.

Fifty to seventy percent of patients with syncope can have a diagnosis made on the basis of history, physical exam, ECG, and studies directly indicated by the history. Further evaluation has a low diagnostic yield and tends to be expensive, so it is only appropriate in patients at risk from their disease. Patients with vasovagal or psychogenic syncope and young patients with syncope of unknown cause have a benign prognosis [29]. At the other extreme, patients with a cardiovascular cause of syncope have a 24% incidence of sudden death and a 33% mortality at one year [30]. Most patients who faint can be placed into a very high risk or very low risk category and treated appropriately. However, elderly patients who experience syncope of undetermined origin are in a medium-risk category, and there is currently no firm consensus on how thorough their evaluation should be. It is not appropriate to carry out procedures such as invasive cardiovascular testing when there is an appreciable risk and a low diagnostic yield. On the other hand, 24-hour ECG monitoring is often indicated in an otherwise healthy elderly patient with syncope of undetermined origin. The presence of known heart disease is associated with a relatively high yield of syncopal patients who have cardiac arrhythmias detected on Holter or electrophysiologic testing [30].

Episodic loss of consciousness is one of the most common reasons for elderly people to seek medical care. Some of the causes, such as vasovagal episodes, are relatively benign, but potentially life-threatening disorders such as intracerebral masses or cardiac arrhythmias are more common in the elderly than in young people. Although simple studies usually reveal the

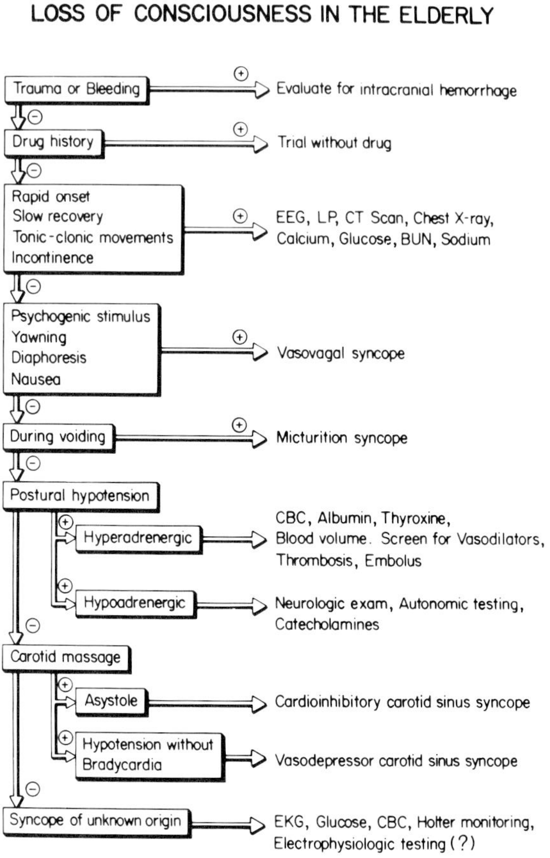

LOSS OF CONSCIOUSNESS IN THE ELDERLY

Figure 10-2. Loss of consciousness in the elderly.

probable cause of a syncopal episode, more detailed tests are appropriate when simple measures fail. (see figure 10-2).

GLOSSARY

Syncope	Loss of consciousness due to an interruption in the blood supply to the brain
Norepinephrine	The neurotransmitter of sympathetic nerves
Sick sinus syndrome	Sinoatrial dysfunction that can cause bradycardia, tachycardia or sinus arrest
Valsalva maneuver	Production of increased intrathoracic pressure by attempted expiration against a closed glottis

Vasovagal attack A response to an unpleasant stimulus consisting of decreased vascular resistance, yawning, sweating, and increased vagal activity

REFERENCES

1. Lipsitz LA, Wei JY and Rowe JW. 1985. Syncope in an elderly, institutionalized population: Prevalence, incidence, and associated risk. Q J Med 55(216):45–54.
2. Scherokman B and Massey EW. 1980. Evaluating loss of consciousness in the elderly. J Am Geriatr Soc 28(11):504–506.
3. Warlow CP. 1980. Blackouts. Practitioner 224:711–716.
4. Raviele A, Proclemer A, Gasparini G, et al. 1989. Long term follow-up of patients with unexplained syncope and negative electrophysiologic study. Eur Heart J 10:127–132.
5. Simon RP. 1981. Syncope and episodic loss of consciousness. Compr Ther 7:19–23.
6. Palmer GH, Ziegler MG and Lake CR. 1978. Response of norepinephrine and blood pressure increase with age. J Gerontol 33(4):482–487.
7. Ziegler MG. 1990. Therapy of postural hypotension. In FH Messerli (ed), Drugs for the Heart and Circulation. Philadelphia: pp 1608–1617.
8. Lake CR and Ziegler MG. 1978. Effects of acute volume alterations on norepinephrine and dopamine-beta-hydroxylase in normotensive and hypertensive subjects. Circulation 57: 774–778.
9. Amer MS. 1977. Mechanisms of action of beta blockers in hypertension. Biochem Pharmacol 26:171–175.
10. Ziegler MG, Lake CR, Williams AC, et al. 1978. Bromocriptine inhibits norepinephrine release. Clin Pharmacol Ther 25:215–224.
11. Hale WE, Stewart RB and Marks RG. 1985. Antianxiety drugs and central nervous system symptoms in an ambulatory elderly population. Drug Intell Clin Pharm 19(1):37–40.
12. Engel GL. 1978. Psychologic stress, vasodepressor (vasovagal) syncope and sudden death. Ann Intern Med 89:403–412.
13. Ziegler MG. 1980. Postural hypotension. Ann Rev Med 31:239–245.
14. Ziegler MG, Lake CR and Kopin IJ. 1977. The sympathetic nervous system defect in primary orthostatic hypotension. N Engl J Med 296:293–297.
15. Ziegler MG. 1981. Choosing therapy for postural hypotension. Drug Ther 11(10):97–115.
16. Ziegler MG and Lake CR. 1985. Noradrenergic responses in postural hypotension: implications for therapy. In CR Lake and MG Ziegler (eds), The Catecholamines in Psychiatric and Neurologic Disorders. Woburn, MA: Butterworth, pp 121–136.
17. Beretta-Piccoli C and Weidmann P. 1982. Metoclopramide alone or combined with flurbiprofen in the treatment of orthostatic hypotension associated with diabetes mellitus. Klin Wockenschr 60:863–865.
18. Walter PF, Crawley IS and Dorney ER. 1978. Carotid sinus hypersensitivity and syncope. Am J Cardiol 42:396–403.
19. Davies AB, Stevens MR and Davies AG. 1979. Carotid sinus hypersensitivity in patients presenting with syncope. Br Heart J 42:583–586.
20. Cohen FL, Fruehan CT and King RB. 1976. Carotid sinus syncope. J Neurosurg 45:78–84.
21. Morley CA, Perrins EJ and Sutton R. 1981. Alpha-methyldopa and carotid-sinus hypersensitivity. N Engl J Med 305:1418.
22. Almquist A, Gornick C, Benson W Jr, et al. 1985. Carotid sinus hypersensitivity: evaluation of the vasodepressor component. Circulation 71:927–936.
23. Jacobson RR and Russell RW. 1979. Glossopharyngeal neuralgia with cardiac arrhythmia: a rare but treatable cause of syncope. Br Med J 1:379–380.
24. Hammill SC, Holmes DR Jr, Wood DL, et al. 1985. Electrophysiologic testing in the upright position: improved evaluation of patients with rhythm disturbances using a tilt table. J Am Coll Cardiol 4(6):703–708.
25. Doherty JU, Pembrook-Rogers D, Grogen EW, et al. 1978. Electrophysiologic evaluation and follow-up characteristics of patients with recurrent unexplained syncope and presyncopes. Am J Cardiol 55(6):796–798.

26. Kapoor WN, Peterson JR and Karph M. 1985. Micturition syncope. A reappraisal. JAMA 253(6):796–798.
27. Brick JE, Lowther CM and Deglin SM. 1978. Cold water syncope. South Med J 71: 1579–1580.
28. Noble RJ. 1977. The patient with syncope. JAMA 237:1372–1376.
29. Eagle KA, Black HR, Cook EF and Goldman L. 1985. Evaluation of prognostic classifications for patients with syncope. Am J Med 79(4):455–460.
30. Kapoor WN, Karpf M, Wieand S, et al. 1983. A prospective evaluation and follow-up of patients with syncope. N Engl J Med 309:81–83.

11. VALVULAR HEART DISEASE IN THE ELDERLY

DAVID C. BOOTH
ANTHONY N. DEMARIA

Valvular heart disease in the elderly has commanded increasing attention in the past decade [1–5]. A prime reason has been the steady lowering of operative risk from open heart surgery [6–10]. Noninvasive diagnostic procedures such as echocardiography, radionuclide ventriculography, and Doppler echocardiography allow accurate confirmation of clinical diagnoses in most cases [11–17]. With regard to therapy, criteria based on noninvasive studies have been proposed for use in clinical decision making in selected disease states.

Many valvular lesions in the elderly are extensions of diseases begun earlier in life and may be acquired or even inherited [18]. Other pathologic processes may well be by-products of aging; for example, the usual fibrotic thickening of valvular tissue may become excessive, or the expected dilatation and calcification of a valve annulus may progress rapidly enough to produce hemodynamic abnormalities. We have chosen to organize this chapter according to the valve involved and, when appropriate, by specific pathogenetic process. Clinical presentation, key studies, and differential diagnoses are included.

Franz H. Messerli (ed.), CARDIOVASCULAR DISEASE IN THE ELDERLY (Third Edition). Copyright © 1993 Kluwer Academic Publishers. ISBN 0-7923-1859-5. All rights reserved.

AORTIC VALVULAR STENOSIS

Incidence and pathology

The incidence of calcific aortic stenosis in the aged population has been estimated at 1% [1]. In autopsy series, aortic stenosis represents approximately 8% of all heart disease [4]. It is to be distinguished from rheumatic aortic stenosis, which occurs as a result of commissural fusion [19], is less frequent than calcific aortic stenosis [20–22], and often is associated with significant aortic regurgitation and rheumatic mitral valvular disease [22,23]. In patients over age 65 with calcific aortic stenosis, the aortic valve is tricuspid in greater than 90% and congenitally malformed or bicuspid in less than 10% [3]. A recent necropsy study showed that minor inequalities in cusp size and height were the rule in hearts of patients who did not have aortic stenosis [24]. The presence of similar changes in stenotic valves suggests that aortic stenosis may represent an extreme in a spectrum of alterations that occur with aging. Valvular thickening and calcification, presumed to be due to years of mechanical stress on valve tissue, occur on the aortic aspect of the valve. Nodular deposits are distributed uniformly over the valve surface and anulus, rendering the valve rigid and stenotic. Because fusion of cusps and retraction of valve tissue do not occur unless they are preexistent in a biscuspid valve or of rheumatic etiology, significant aortic regurgitation in the absence of infective endocarditis is an uncommon finding [3,19].

Pathophysiology

Hemodynamically significant aortic stenosis produces angina pectoris, congestive heart failure, and syncope. Congestive heart failure may be precipitated by the onset of atrial fibrillation. The occurrence of congestive heart failure may be more ominous than syncope or angina pectoris, but from the onset of any of these symptoms, five-year survival is 50%, and the majority of untreated patients die within eight years [25]. Older patients are at risk for sudden death, as are patients with congenital aortic stenosis, but the exact incidence is unknown.

Clinical findings

On physical examination, the jugular venous pressure is normal unless congestive heart failure is present. The carotid contour to palpation is notched and slowly rising, though the abnormality may be indistinguishable from the normal carotid pulse of many older patients, in whom arterial wall compliance is reduced [26]. An aortic ejection sound is uncommon at auscultation; the absence of this finding has been attributed to lack of fusion of valve leaflets and to valve immobility. An atrial gallop sound is usually present as a result of left ventricular hypertrophy; however, this finding has little specificity, since atrial gallops are found in the majority of the elderly population due to an increase in myocardial stiffness that occurs with aging [2]. The murmur of aortic stenosis generally peaks in mid- to late systole, is harsh (the sound of one clearing one's throat), and is best heard at the right sternal edge in the second intercostal space. The murmur radiates widely over the precordium and to the carotid arteries. A thrill is usually felt in cases of hemodynamically significant aortic stenosis, when cardiac output is sufficient to generate a transaortic gradient of greater than 50 mmHg. The first heart sound is often soft. The second heart sound will split paradoxically if left ventricular decompensation is present, but it is usually single.

Differential diagnosis

Functional aortic outflow murmurs, such as occur in hypertension and which often radiate loudly to the carotid arteries, can mimic the murmur of aortic stenosis. In this regard, however, Wenger [1] has noted that diastolic blood pressure in excess of 100 mmHg essentially excludes aortic stenosis. The murmur of hypertrophic obstructive cardiomyopathy may also be confounded with aortic stenosis but usually does not radiate to the neck. Carotid palpation in this disease frequently reveals a bifid pulse with primary "spike" and secondary "dome" impulses characteristic of dynamic left ventricular outflow obstruction. Murmurs due to abnormalities of the posterior mitral leaflet apparatus may radiate in the distribution of an aortic valve murmur, but they are usually part of an acute clinical syndrome. Since the risk of sudden cardiac death exists in critical aortic stenosis, a history of chest pain compatible with angina pectoris in combination with an aortic outflow murmur considered to be significant constitutes a relative contraindication to exercise stress testing as a means of identifying coronary artery disease.

Evaluation

The chest x-ray commonly demonstrates post-stenotic dilatation of the aorta, and aortic valvular calcification may be seen. The heart size usually is normal. The electrocardiogram shows left ventricular hypertrophy and S-T and T-wave abnormalities. The occurrence of chest pain, syncope, or congestive heart failure is an indication for cardiac catheterization in aortic stenosis. However, strict adherence to this tenet has diminished as a result of the emergence of Doppler echocardiographic techniques. In our experience, both M-mode and two-dimensional echocardiography have proved useful in differentiating aortic stenosis from other causes of systolic murmurs, in estimating the aortic valve gradient, and in assessing left ventricular performance [23,27–29]. On M-mode, increased echoes and diminished leaflet excursion are present in the region of the aortic valve. Similar findings may be seen in many elderly patients with aortic sclerosis and systolic hypertension, but aortic-valve systolic excursion of 8 mm or more essentially excludes critical aortic stenosis. Two-dimensional echocardiography usually differentiates aortic stenosis from aortic sclerosis. Two-dimensional images show the calcified aortic valve to be highly echogenic, frequently giving the appearance of a dense mass of echoes, findings not observed in nonobstructive degenerative aortic disease.

Numerous studies have documented the accuracy of Doppler methods in the estimation of the transvalvular gradient of aortic stenosis [29–31]. Doppler techniques enable sampling of blood flow velocity at a given intracardiac location through processing of the frequency of the delivered and returning ultrasonic signal. In the case of the aortic valve, the frequency shift imparted to ultrasound by particulate components of moving blood in the region of the stenotic aortic valve orifice is transduced to a graphic depiction of flow velocity. Given the aortic flow velocity, the aortic valve gradient may be calculated from the modified Bernoulli equation [29]. More recently, several groups [32–35] have reported on noninvasive estimation of aortic valve area using the principle of continuity of flow. The refinement of echo and Doppler techniques has continued a trend toward valve-replacement surgery without preoperative catheterization, as has been advocated in selected centers [36,37]. Intuitively, this approach is more applicable in younger age groups less likely to have associated coronary artery disease [37]. On the other hand, general acceptance of noninvasive techniques may reduce the need for catheterization in elderly patients, i.e., valvular and ventricular function data will be obtained noninvasively, and invasive study limited to coronary arteriography. Catheterization data are still important for estimating aortic valve orifice size in patients in whom Doppler studies are technically unobtainable. Comparison of results obtained by invasive and noninvasive methods may be helpful in patients with left ventricular dysfunction, who may have critical aortic stenosis but not the high transaortic gradient usually seen in this disease.

Management

Like other open heart surgical procedures in the elderly, aortic valve replacement no longer carries a 15% to 25% mortality risk as it did before 1970. Surgical mortality in several current series is 5% to 10%—and less than 5% in selected patients with normal left ventricular function [6–10]. Aortic valve replacement for calcific aortic valve stenosis is accepted therapy for patients age 75 or younger and can be successfully performed in those over age 75. [10,38,39]. Although necropsy data indicate significant potential for degeneration of porcine heterografts [40], other investigators have demonstrated the durability of these valves through mean follow-up of 8 to 12 years [41–44]. This evidence, coupled with the fact that extended anticoagulation is unnecessary, makes the porcine valve the prosthesis of choice in the elderly [44]. Whether coexistent coronary artery disease should be submitted to myocardial revascularization has been questioned recently, but both procedures can be performed safely and successfully at the same operation [45–48]. The decision to replace the aortic valve in this age group, with or without concurrent coronary artery bypass, must be made on an individual basis and must account for factors other than cardiovascular status, such as associated diseases and the likelihood that surgery will significantly improve the elderly patient's functional status. A potential alternative in patients in whom aortic valve replacement is contraindicated is percutaneous balloon aortic valvotomy. A substantial experience with this palliative procedure [49] has now been reported, and its use as a bridge to aortic valve replacement in the critically ill patient may be its best indication [50]. Berland et al. [51] recently reported one-year clinical improvement in 20 of 55 patients (36%), mean age 77, with critical aortic stenosis and left ventricular ejection fraction of less than 40%; however, three in-hospital deaths occurred, as well as 21 aortic stenosis-related deaths over the one-year follow-up interval. Ferguson et al. [49] confirmed the high rate of restenosis following balloon aortic valvotomy and have documented poor outcomes for patients requiring a second balloon procedure. Isner et al. [52] reported a 6.3% incidence of catastrophic complications from the procedure, including ventricular rupture, ventricular fibrillation, and cardiogenic shock. The mortality rate for such complications was 77%. At this time, percutaneous aortic balloon valvotomy is a short-term palliative procedure with a substantial rate of clinical failure and complications. Its use should be reserved for the appropriate clinical presentation, namely, patients in whom aortic valve replacement is contraindicated.

AORTIC INSUFFICIENCY

Pathology

Frequently the underlying etiology of aortic regurgitation in the elderly is uncertain. Recent Doppler echo studies [53,54] have demonstrated the presence of aortic regurgitation in persons in whom auscultation fails to disclose a diastolic murmur, i.e., a phenomenon that has been termed *Doppler heart disease.* [55]. These investigations, in which patients with thickened leaflets, aortic root dilatation, and annular calcification were excluded, have shown an age-related increase in the prevalence of aortic regurgitation. Whether clinically significant aortic regurgitation can result from degenerative processes too subtle to be confirmed by two-dimensional echocardiography remains uncertain. Mild degrees of aortic insufficiency may accompany calcific aortic stenosis, and infective endocarditis accounts for a certain percentage of cases [3]. Rheumatic heart disease in most series accounts for one third of isolated aortic regurgitation in the general population [22,56,57], although Roberts [58] has seriously questioned this frequency. The aortic valve is the most commonly damaged valve in cases of closed-chest trauma, which presents as acute aortic regurgitation [59]. Rheumatic heart disease is a common cause of aortic regurgitation in the elderly, but it is usually seen in combination with some degree of mitral valve involvement [3,59]. Moreover, combined valvular disease of rheumatic origin generally presents in patients younger than age 60. Thus, isolated aortic regurgitation is relatively uncommon in the elderly. Other causes include bicuspid aortic valve, hypertension, rheumatoid processes such as ankylosing spondylitis, arteriosclerotic ascending aortic aneurysm, and syphilitic aortitis, which is rarely seen in the United States today but which nevertheless is more common in the elderly [3,60,61]. Aortic dissection or infective endocarditis may produce the syndrome of acute severe aortic regurgitation.

Pathophysiology

The left ventricle accommodates to aortic regurgitation by dilation and, as in aortic stenosis, by development of eccentric left ventricular hypertrophy. The chamber is thereby able to produce the large stroke volume made necessary by regurgitant filling from the aorta. The arterial system adjusts to a lowered vascular resistance to accept the larger stroke volume. This change has the beneficial effect of minimizing aortic regurgitation. Thus, patients may remain asymptomatic for many years. When the left ventricle can no longer manage its increased stroke work, significant symptoms begin. Dyspnea at rest or on exertion may occur, as well as angina pectoris.

Physical findings

On physical examination, the pulse pressure is increased, giving rise to low systemic diastolic pressures. The carotid pulse is brisk and may demonstrate a bisferiens or bifid peak with rapid runoff. In the elderly, noncompliant peripheral arteries in systolic hypertension may simulate the wide pulse pressure of aortic regurgitation. A variety of peripheral manifestations such as de Musset's sign (bobbing of the head with systole), Quincke's pulse (pulsating subungual capillary flow), Corrigan's pulse ("water hammer" pulse), and Durozier's sign (pistol-shot sound over a compressed peripheral artery) may be documented. Systolic and diastolic thrills may be present on the precordium. At auscultation the first heart sound is normal or soft. A loud systolic murmur due to increased aortic outflow is present. The second heart sound is physiologically split, but A_2 may be soft or not heard due to the high-frequency, early diastolic murmur of aortic regurgitation. The duration of the murmur is a more accurate reflector of the degree of regurgitation than is the murmur's intensity. Greater intensity to the right of the sternum suggests an aortic etiology such as aortic dilatation (whatever cause), while a murmur more intense on the left sternal edge suggests a valvular etiology. An atrial gallop is frequently present, as well as a third heart sound. An apical diastolic rumble, the so-called Austin Flint murmur, may be present. It is believed to be produced by antegrade flow across a mitral valve partially closed by early ventricular filling from the aorta [62]. It can be distinguished from the murmur of mitral stenosis by the absence of an opening snap, and it may be diminished or extinguished by administration of amyl nitrate. The syndrome of acute severe aortic regurgitation produces the constellation of tachycardia, significantly low diastolic blood pressure (in which the diastolic arterial pressure measured indirectly by cuff represents the left ventricular diastolic pressure, due to free aortic regurgitation), and a very soft or absent first heart sound. Because the left ventricle is unprepared to suddenly accept this degree of regurgitant volume, the diastolic murmur is decrescendo, harsh, and short, ending when the left ventricle is maximally filled [63].

Laboratory examination

In chronic aortic regurgitation, the chest x-ray usually demonstrates cardiomegaly with left ventricular enlargement. The electrocardiogram shows left ventricular hypertrophy and strain. The S-T segment and T-wave initially may be normal. Their conversion to a "strain" pattern should alert the clinician to the possible need for valve replacement, although all patients with aortic insufficiency must surely pass through this stage. Echocardiographic findings include fluttering of the anterior mitral leaflet in diastole and left ventricular enlargement. The echocardiogram also will show coexistence of mitral valve disease. Pulsed Doppler echo techniques [64,65], in which the extent of regurgitation may be assessed by intraventricular "mapping" of the penetration of the regurgitant aortic jet into the left ventricle, require significant operator experience and yield significant overlap between mild–moderate and moderate–severe degrees of aortic regurgitation. The technique can reliably distinguish mild and severe aortic regurgitation. Left ventricular end-diastolic pressure can be estimated using the diastolic cuff blood pressure and Doppler information [66]. Knowledge of the left ventricular end-diastolic pressure, in combination with echocardiographic data on left ventricular function such as the end-systolic dimension, may provide useful information on the timing of aortic valve replacement in aortic regurgitation. Color flow Doppler methods have allowed for rapid confirmation of the presence of aortic regurgitation [67], but whether the degree of aortic regurgitation may be accurately estimated by this technique remains controversial [68,69]. Regardless of method, the documentation of severe regurgitation continues to be one of the prerequisites for valve replacement in aortic insufficiency, underlining the potential utility of accurate noninvasive quantitation.

Management

Valve replacement in aortic insufficiency is indicated in symptomatic patients only, since an ideal aortic valve prosthesis, with excellent wear characteristics and no propensity for complications, does not yet exist. Patients in New York Heart Association functional class II may be managed with medical treatment. Pharmacologic afterload reduction, by decreasing the regurgitant fraction and facilitating left ventricular ejection, holds promise as therapy for these and selected class III patients, but it has not yet been shown to reverse left ventricular dysfunction once the process begins. The decision to operate must be individualized and is facilitated by knowledge of the patient's long-term course. Echocardiographic left ventricular dimensions offer an easily obtainable index of ventricular performance [70,71]. Enlarging dimensions in the presence of increased symptoms suggest the need for cardiac catheterization and aortic valve replacement [70]. An asymptomatic patient with normal left ventricular function, assessed by echocardiogram or radionuclide studies, should be followed conservatively. Preoperative resting left ventricular dysfunction identifies a patient with aortic regurgitation who is at risk of death or persistent left ventricular dysfunction after aortic valve replacement [72]. Early identification of left ventricular dysfunction from long-term follow-up studies may optimize the timing of surgery, resulting in improved survival and functional capacity. In most centers, the prognosis and outcome of valve replacement in aortic regurgitation approach the results for patients with aortic stenosis, with a surgical mortality between 5% and 15%. Valve replacement for aortic regurgitation in the elderly is a legitimate therapeutic alternative in carefully selected patients. In acute severe aortic regurgitation, valve replacement is the therapy of choice.

MITRAL REGURGITATION

Pathology

Roberts and Perloff [73] have noted that competence of the mitral valve is dependent on normal function of the mitral annulus, leaflets, chordae tendineae, papillary muscles, and left ventricular myocardium. Mitral regurgitation arises when one or more of these parts fails. Causes of mitral insufficiency in the general population may also produce this lesion in the elderly [3]. Myxomatous degeneration of the valve may lead to severe chronic mitral regurgitation [3,5]. Papillary muscle dysfunction due to coronary artery disease may produce any degree of mitral incompetence, from intermittent regurgitation during myocardial ischemia to acute severe mitral insufficiency occurring with papillary muscle rupture. Infective endocarditis can also cause varying degrees of mitral insufficiency, usually superimposed on another mitral abnormality. Spontaneous rupture of chordae tendineae is an infrequent cause of mitral regurgitation that can produce acutely disabling congestive heart failure. Calcification of the mitral annulus is a process peculiar to the elderly, except for its association with congenital diseases such as Hurler and Marfan syndromes [3,74–76], which can lead to significant mitral regurgitation. Rheumatic heart disease is among the more common causes of mitral regurgitation, but it usually produces mitral stenosis as well. As with aortic regurgitation, Doppler echocardiographic techniques identify instances of mitral regurgitation in which a murmur is not present on cardiac auscultation [53]. The long-term significance of these findings remains uncertain.

Papillary muscle dysfunction

Papillary muscle dysfunction is a frequent accompaniment of coronary artery disease. Acute necrosis, rupture, or chronic fibrosis leads to varying degrees of insufficiency. Left ventricular dilatation or scarring at the base of a papillary muscle may also contribute to this process [3,73]. Dysfunction may occur solely during angina pectoris, or a mild to moderate degree of regurgitation may exist as a result of chronic ischemic damage. Jeresaty [77] has described a click–murmur syndrome that may be produced by papillary muscle dysfunction. Chronic mitral incompetence due to papillary muscle dysfunction is easily distinguished from other causes of mitral regurgitation by its coexistence with coronary artery disease syndromes. Physical findings are variable due to their dependence on the degree of papillary muscle dysfunction. The most common manifestation is an early-midsystolic apical murmur, which can be mistaken for an aortic outflow murmur. Appropriate electrocardiographic findings should support the presence of coronary artery disease, and echocardiography usually reveals regional wall-motion abnormalities. In general, this degree of mitral regurgitation can be managed medically, and mitral valve replacement is not required when coronary artery bypass surgery is performed. In selected cases, mitral regurgitation may improve with relief of ischemia.

Infective endocarditis

Infective endocarditis can produce varying degrees of mitral regurgitation. The clinical presentation of subacute bacterial endocarditis in the elderly may be more subtle than that in younger populations [78], and a significant percentage of cases may not involve a murmur. While fever and murmur ultimately are present [79], the presenting sign of endocarditis may be progressive renal failure, acute neurologic abnormality, or severe pneumonia. Echocardiography has shown utility in imaging vegetations in a significant percentage of patients with endocarditis [79]. However, endocarditis is a microbiologic, not an echocardiographic, diagnosis. Antibiotic therapy should be based on blood cultures, and, although in many cases drugs must be initiated before identification of the organism, antibiotic dosage should be planned according to minimum bactericidal titers.

Acute mitral regurgitation

As in the general population, acute or fulminant bacterial endocarditis in the elderly is most frequently caused by *Staphylococcus aureus*. Acute endocarditis and clinically severe episodes of subacute bacterial endocarditis, papillary muscle rupture, and spontaneous rupture of chordae tendineae may produce the syndrome of acute severe mitral regurgitation. Acute hemodynamic abnormalities produced by acute mitral dysfunction dominate the clinical presentation, which involves tachycardia and pulmonary venous congestion. Palpation of the chest may disclose an apical systolic thrill. A late systolic impulse due to left atrial expansion may be felt at the left sternal border. At auscultation, S_1 is soft or absent and the pulmonary component of S_2 is loud, reflecting acute pulmonary hypertension due to pulmonary venous congestion. The murmur of acute mitral regurgitation depends on whether the acute event is superimposed upon chronic mitral insufficiency [80]. In patients with little or no preexisting mitral regurgitation, the murmur typically is a harsh, short, and early systolic murmur that ends when the relatively noncompliant left atrium can accept no further regurgitant blood. The murmur is more typically pansystolic when acute insufficiency is superimposed on chronic insufficiency. A ventricular diastolic sound is usually present, often with duration due to torrential antegrade mitral flow. An atrial gallop may be heard.

Laboratory examination in acute mitral regurgitation

The chest x-ray in acute mitral regurgitation demonstrates pulmonary venous congestion and pulmonary edema. In the absence of preexisting significant left ventricular dysfunction, the cardiac size is normal. The electrocardiogram may demonstrate increased QRS voltage and "volume overload" repolarization abnormality. Echocardiography consistently demonstrates a hyperkinetic left ventricle and, in instances of chordal or papillary muscle rupture, may demonstrate flail mitral leaflet. Transthoracic pulsed Doppler flow techniques confirm mitral regurgitation in the majority of cases [55]. Recent data [55] indicate that because of better temporal resolution (higher framing rates), transesophageal color flow Doppler is superior to transthoracic study in the imaging of acute mitral regurgitation. Swan–Ganz catheterization will disclose elevated pulmonary capillary wedge pressure with large regurgitant waves. Frequently, the regurgitant wave may be reflected to the pulmonary artery pressure, giving the appearance of dicrotic or bifid pressure.

Treatment of acute mitral regurgitation

When acute mitral regurgitation is due to papillary muscle rupture, the patient may be stabilized by pharmacologic therapy in combination with intra-aortic balloon counterpulsation [80]. Insertion of this device in this setting should be reserved for patients in whom emergency mitral valve surgery is planned. Cardiac catheterization should be performed after intra-aortic balloon insertion. Posterior papillary muscle rupture in the setting of inferior myocardial infarction is perhaps the most common cause of this presentation, and these patients may have excellent responses to mitral valve replacement combined with myocardial revascularization. Given appropriate coronary pathoanatomy, successful percutaneous transluminal coronary angioplasty will eliminate mitral regurgitation in acute ischemic papillary muscle insufficiency without rupture.

Chronic mitral regurgitation

Calcification of the mitral annulus

Calcification of the mitral annulus, myxomatous valve degeneration, and rheumatic mitral insufficiency are responsible for most cases of chronic mitral regurgitation in the elderly. Annular calcification results in mitral insufficiency by preventing normal annular systolic contraction, or perhaps by interfering with closure of the mitral leaflets [74,75]. This process appears to be accelerated by conditions that elevate left ventricular pressure, such as hypertension. Women are more frequently affected than men. Annular calcification has also been described in combination with hypercalcemia and in patients with renal failure on chronic hemodialysis [3]. Physical examination discloses a soft first heart sound and a holosystolic murmur that is loudest at the apex and radiates to the axilla and occasionally to the back. The electrocardiogram shows left ventricular hypertrophy. A ringlike or horseshoe-shaped opacification may be seen on chest x-ray, signifying annular calcification. Echocardiography demonstrates a dense structure below the posterior mitral leaflet, which is the reflected mass of the calcified annulus.

Mitral prolapse

Myxomatous degeneration of the mitral valve most frequently presents as mitral valve prolapse, with typical clinical and echocardiographic findings [77]. Management of mitral valve prolapse in the elderly is similar to that in the general population. Chest pain occasionally accompanies this syndrome in younger patients, but in the older population pain may be due to coexistent coronary artery disease. Atrial fibrillation is a frequent finding in mitral valve prolapse in the elderly, particularly when significant mitral regurgitation is present, but ventricular arrhythmias are an uncommon finding [14]. Antibiotic prophylaxis against infective endocarditis is recommended. Recent reports that mitral valve prolapse may be a causal factor in some types of transient cerebral ischemia are inconclusive [81,82]. One group has found that the incidence of mitral prolapse on echocardiography in a series of consecutive patients with transient ischemic attacks was low enough to preclude the need for routine echocardiography unless prolapse was specifically suspected [81]. As in other types of transient ischemic events, affected patients are most safely and effectively treated with aspirin.

A small percentage of patients with mitral valve prolapse may have progressive mitral dysfunction with severe mitral regurgitation [77,83]. Physical examination is similar to that in annular calcification. Electrocardiography and chest x-ray may not differentiate these two processes. In contrast, echocardiography shows prolapsing mitral valve motion in systole, as well as the left ventricular and left atrial enlargement seen in any form of chronic mitral regurgitation. Occasionally, flail mitral motion may be seen.

Doppler echocardiography in chronic mitral regurgitation

Doppler examination in chronic mitral regurgitation has proven to be sensitive in differentiating mitral regurgitation from other causes of systolic murmurs. Both pulsed Doppler mapping and color flow Doppler are sensitive and specific for the presence of mitral regurgitation when the duration of the regurgitant jet equals more than half of systole [55]. Results of studies assessing the accuracy of Doppler methods in the quantitation of mitral regurgitation, which admittedly have employed semiquantitative angiography as the standard for comparison, have been variable. Doppler techniques can distinguish between mild and severe mitral insufficiency, but estimates are less certain in cases with a moderate degree of insufficiency.

Management of chronic mitral regurgitation

Chronic mitral insufficiency may be managed for many years with medical therapy. Symptoms of heart failure generally respond to digitalization, diuresis, and left ventricular afterload reduction. The decision to replace the mitral valve is influenced primarily by the degree of symptoms but is a more complex problem than other types of valvular disease. At any given degree of contractility, the left ventricle is ejecting into a low-impedance conduit—the left atrium—such that following mitral replacement the left ventricular ejection fraction may fall in patients who were considered to have good left ventricular function preoperatively. The reduction in ejection fraction postoperatively has been attributed to the imposition of a higher afterload on the ventricle with a newly competent mitral valve; however, this theory has recently been questioned [84]. Echocardiographic criteria for mitral replacement have been proposed but are inconclusive [85,86]. Progressive left ventricular dilatation and increasing symptoms constitute a rationale for cardiac catheterization. While no generally accepted indices are available, the combination of severe mitral regurgitation and even slightly reduced ejection fraction defines the need for surgery, whether the disease process is calcific, myxomatous, or rheumatic. Surgical mortality of mitral valve replacement in the elderly is approximately 10% and rises steeply in individual cases as the left ventricular ejection fraction declines [6,7,87]. Reed and coworkers [88] recently noted that left atrial size is an important predictor of outcome in patients with chronic mitral regurgitation and that various catheterization parameters add little to the predictive power of noninvasive follow-up data. The decision to operate must be made in light of the patient's overall status.

Myxomatous degeneration and chordal rupture have the best options. In these syndromes, the mitral valve may be surgically reconstructed and buttressed with a ring [89]. The indications for mitral valvuloplasty, when the operation is technically feasible, are continuing to evolve. Since this operation has the distinct advantage of not necessitating permanent postoperative anticoagulation, it should be considered the procedure of choice. Actuarial studies in series of mitral regurgitation treated surgically indicate better survival in surgically treated subjects. However, the interpretation of data must be tempered by the patient's age and the performance of the left ventricle.

MITRAL STENOSIS

Presentation
Rheumatic heart disease more than rarely has its initial presentation after age 65 and is the predominant cause of mitral stenosis. Some degree of mitral insufficiency frequently coexists with mitral stenosis. The number of patients identified as having congestive symptoms in the fourth and fifth decade and responding to medical management into the sixth decade is perhaps larger than previously thought [12,90]. However, the presenting sign in the elderly may be stroke or other systemic embolization in combination with atrial fibrillation. Rarely, patients may present in the late stages of mitral stenosis with pulmonary hypertension and right ventricular failure, that have masqueraded for years as severe chronic obstructive pulmonary disease. The pathology of rheumatic stenosis is well described [90]. The rheumatic process gives rise to calcification and fibrosis of the mitral leaflets and chordal apparatus. Commissural fusion, not a part of other calcific cardiac processes in this age group, leads to valve retraction and stenosis.

On physical examination, the venous pressure may be elevated. The carotid pulse contour is brisk if rheumatic aortic regurgitation is also present. Precordial palpation may disclose a prominent right ventricular impulse. The presence of prominent right and left ventricular impulse with interposed retraction due to septal contraction suggests the presence of combined mitral disease with biventricular hypertrophy. The first heart sound is loud, even when coexistent mitral regurgitation is present, because mitral closing occurs at a higher, more rapidly rising left ventricular pressure. A protodiastolic snap of mitral opening is heard, followed by a diastolic rumble with presystolic accentuation that may be audible even when atrial fibrillation is present.

Laboratory examination
Electrocardiographic findings may vary from normal to overt right ventricular hypertrophy. The chest x-ray demonstrates findings consistent with left atrial enlargement. Echocardiography is diagnostic. Characteristic

M-mode findings include thickened mitral echoes, reduced diastolic motion, and parallel movement of the anterior and posterior leaflets in diastole. Left atrial myxoma can be differentiated easily from rheumatic disease, particularly on two-dimensional study. The two-dimensional echocardiogram also shows the characteristic "doming" diastolic mitral motion concave to the left atrium, the echocardiographic hallmark of rheumatic mitral stenosis. In contrast to assessment of the aortic valve, cross-sectional echocardiographic techniques have proven to be reliable for estimation of mitral valve area. Thus, when true chronic obstructive pulmonary disease and mitral stenosis exist simultaneously, a not infrequent finding in elderly patients, the severity of mitral valve disease may be determined noninvasively. The mitral valve may be imaged in this setting in 80% of patients. Doppler echocardiographic evaluation of the mitral valve has proven to be an accurate and useful means of assessing the severity of isolated mitral stenosis in patients with and without prior commissurotomy [91], and it promises to be equally accurate in patients with combined valvular disease. The specific method, the Doppler pressure half-time technique, provides a second noninvasive means of quantifying mitral valve area, allowing planimetry of the two-dimensional mitral echocardiogram and Doppler to be employed in a complementary fashion. Color flow Doppler, which is more confirmatory than diagnostic, demonstrates a characteristic diastolic "color flow mosaic" resulting from increased transmitral blood flow velocities. In patients with low cardiac output, hemodynamic formulas for the calculation of valve orifice size such as the Gorlin formula, which assumes a constant value for the hydraulic discharge coefficient, may be less accurate than Doppler indices derived from integrated flow velocity [92]. The decision to recommend mitral valve intervention is based on the presence of functional limitation and confirmation of critical mitral stenosis, a mitral valve area of $1.0\,cm^2$ or less. Pulmonary and right ventricular systolic pressure can also be estimated, when tricuspid regurgitation is present, by applying the modified Bernoulli equation to the tricuspid jet [93]. Thus, considerable hemodynamic information, previously the sole province of the catheterization laboratory, is now available from noninvasive studies.

Management

As in the general population, mitral stenosis in the elderly often responds to medical therapy. The ventricular response to atrial fibrillation may be controlled with digitalization. Verapamil may have a role in the treatment of atrial fibrillation due to rheumatic mitral disease [94]. With regard to anticoagulation, it has been strongly recommended that all patients with mitral stenosis and atrial fibrillation or a history of embolism be anticoagulated with warfarin sufficient to increase the prothrombin ratio (patient/control) to 1.5–2.0 [95,96]. Anticoagulation should also be considered for patients in sinus rhythm with left atrial enlargement [95].

Percutaneous balloon mitral valvotomy [97,98] provides a nonsurgical alternative in the management of symptomatic, critical mitral stenosis and is now the procedure of choice for elderly patients with mild to moderate mitral valve calcification and preserved pliability [98]. Complications from this procedure include mitral regurgitation in 8% to 20% and atrial septal defect in less than 5% (produced by dilation of the fossa ovalis after transseptal catheterization in order to facilitate passage of the mitral balloon). For patients in whom balloon valvotomy is considered inappropriate because of excessive calcification, open mitral commissurotomy may be performed. Surgical mortality in this age group is generally 5% or less, with excellent long-term survival [6]. Valve replacement may be necessary when the mitral valve is severely deformed. Ideally, porcine heterografts in the mitral position do not require permanent anticoagulation, and warfarin can be stopped after the 6 to 8 weeks required for endothelialization of the valve frame and sewing ring. In practice, only patients with sinus rhythm and normal left atrial size can be maintained without anticoagulation. This approach should also be used in valve replacement for mitral regurgitation. We maintain patients on warfarin treatment when left atrial size on M-mode echocardiography measures 4.5 cm or greater. Continued anticoagulation is strongly recommended for patients with persistent (chronic) atrial fibrillation. Mitral valve replacement carries a higher risk, particularly when significant mitral regurgitation is present and when aortic valve replacement is also performed. Prosthetic mitral valve function, as well as aortic replacement function, may be followed postoperatively by a combination of echocardiography and Doppler studies. Recently, Hammer et al. [76] described significant mitral valve gradients at catheterization in four patients with normal mitral leaflets but severe annular calcification and small, hypertrophied ventricles. Mitral "stenosis" was thought to have occurred due to reduced mitral function as a result of calcification and left ventricular stiffness. Such patients should be managed with medical therapy.

TRICUSPID VALVE DISEASE

Primary tricuspid valvular disease is rare in the elderly. Tricuspid stenosis due to rheumatic heart disease generally is associated with left-sided disease, and the combination produces severe functional limitation in the fourth or fifth decade of life. Tricuspid stenosis may be identified at the bedside by the presence of elevated venous pulsation with poor or absent Y-descent, and at auscultation by the presence of a diastolic rumble that augments with inspiration. The tricuspid valve more often is made insufficient in rheumatic disease by pulmonary hypertension and right ventricular failure due to long-standing mitral stenosis. Successful relief of mitral stenosis usually produces a fall in pulmonary pressure and relief of right ventricular overload, and tricuspid plication is seldom necessary. Acute tricuspid regurgitation with severe valvular damage from endocarditis is primarily a disease secondary to intravenous drug addiction. Ebstein's anomaly of the tricuspid valve rarely presents in the sixth decade. Tricuspid valve and right ventricular dysplasia in these patients is distinctly mild. Echocardiography is diagnostic, with two-dimensional study showing characteristic changes of the disease. Closed-chest trauma is a rare cause of new-onset tricuspid regurgitation [59], as is acute inferior myocardial infarction. Such patients usually respond to medical therapy. Carcinoid syndrome may produce severe tricuspid regurgitation, and in rare cases of pulmonary carcinoid, mitral involvement with regurgitation may occur [99]. Tricuspid valve replacement has been performed rarely, but cardiac disease tends to follow the course of the tumor.

PULMONARY VALVE DISEASE

Pulmonary valvular insufficiency in this age group is almost exclusively the result of high pulmonary artery pressure (secondary to intrinsic arterial disease, chronic obstructive pulmonary disease, or left heart disease) and requires no primary therapy. Pulmonary hypertension suspected on physical exam may be confirmed by the appearance of the pulmonic valve on M-mode echo and by Doppler methods. Congenital pulmonic stenosis has been identified in the fifth decade of life but to our knowledge has not been noted to be present in the elderly [100]. Dexter's group, however, found that patients with this disease could remain asymptomatic for long periods despite significant right ventricular hypertension relative to systemic arterial pressure [100]. Thus, presentation or follow-up of this disease into the seventh decade is possible, and decisions on therapy should be individualized in light of the patient's course. Two-dimensional echocardiography may be employed to confirm pulmonic stenosis; Doppler echocardiography may be used to assess its severity.

NONBACTERIAL THROMBOTIC ENDOCARDITIS

The combination of systemic embolization and extreme cachexia or known malignancy should alert the physician to this disease [101]. Its pathogenesis is poorly understood, but the association with chronic disease and inanition-producing states such as cancer is clear. The "hypercoagulability" of some patients with malignancy may have a role. Eighty percent of those affected are over age 60. These patients present classically with stroke and peripheral manifestations mimicking systemic bacterial endocarditis, without fever and frequently without leukocytosis. Microbiologic studies consistently show no bacterial growth. Postmortem study demonstrates the presence of valvular vegetations 1 to 20 mm in diameter from which organisms cannot be cultured. The diagnosis should be considered when endocarditis coexists with cancer. Two-dimensional echocardiography resolves objects 2 mm or greater in size and images the larger of these vegetations. Therapy is empiric and consists primarily of treatment of the underlying disease. Most such patients receive antibiotic therapy, although infective agents are not confirmed. Persistence of vegetations or embolic phenomena in these cases would support use of anticoagulation or antiplatelet therapy. Recently, *Streptococcus bovis* endocarditis had been described in association with carcinoma of the colon [102]. When this tumor is present and endocarditis is suspected, *S. bovis* must be excluded as a cause. This organism is highly sensitive to penicillin, and the course of valvular infection produced resembles that in systemic bacterial endocarditis due to *S. viridans*.

CARDIAC MYXOMAS

The majority of patients with cardiac myxomas are in the fourth, fifth, and sixth decades of life [103]. In one large series, 12% of patients with myxomas were over age 70 [103]. Debate continues on the pathogenesis of these lesions. Some authors have suggested that myxomas may be a form of organizing thrombus [103–105]. The majority of investigators, however, favor the view that myxomas are a true neoplastic process [104]. Clinical manifestations in the elderly are identical to those in younger age groups; signs and symptoms of mitral valve disease and embolic episodes are the most common presentations. Five percent of patients with cardiac myxomas die suddenly and unexpectedly. A useful clinical distinction is that congestive symptoms due to pulmonary venous hypertension in left atrial myxoma may worsen rather than improve when the patient assumes the upright position [103]. The most common clinical finding in right or left atrial myxoma is a diastolic murmur that mimics mitral stenosis. An opening snap is not present, but a "tumor plop" may be heard in cases of pedunculated myxoma, when the mass reaches its maximum excursion into the ventricle at mitral valve opening. Atrioventricular valve regurgitation may also occur as a result of interruption of valve closure or chronic impact on valve tissue by the myxomas. Both sessile and pedunculated myxomas can also occur in the ventricles [103]. Confirmation of cardiac myxoma is the province of two-dimensional echocardiography. A consensus exists that two-dimensional echocardiography will image nearly all such intracardiac masses [106]. In most cases, surgical removal may be undertaken without the need for cardiac catheterization and angiography [107]. Surgery is curative, though recurrence is possible [108]. Long-term follow-up is facilitated by echocardiography.

CONCLUSION

We have discussed diseases that produce valvular dysfunction in the elderly, some of which are unique but many of which are present in the general population. Diagnosis and follow-up have been enhanced significantly by noninvasive imaging techniques. Echocardiography is pivotal in differentiating many of the valvular diseases in the elderly. Methods of Doppler echocardiography have an equally valuable role in the assessment of severity of disease. Improvement in cardiopulmonary bypass and myocardial preservation techniques have decreased the risk of open-heart surgery in the older age group. When surgery is timed correctly, replacement valves can be expected to make the patient better and to have reasonable durability. Valve replacement need not be withheld purely on the basis of the patient's age. When indicated medically and warranted by the patient's general status, valve replacement is the preferred treatment.

REFERENCES

1. Wenger NK. 1979. Selected cardiac problems in the elderly patient. J Med Assoc Ga 68:1033–1041.
2. Burch GE. 1975. Interesting aspects of geriatric cardiology. Am Heart J 89:99–114.
3. Kotler MN, Mintz GS, Parry WR, et al. 1981. Bedside diagnosis of organic murmurs in the elderly. Geriatrics 36:107–125.
4. Sugiura M, Ohkawa S, Hiraoka K, et al. 1981. A clinicopathologic study on valvular heart diseases in 1000 consecutive autopsy of the aged. Jpn Heart J 22:1–13.
5. Collins P, Cotton RE and Duff RS. 1976. Symptomatic mitral myxomatous transformation in the elderly. Thorax 31:765–770.
6. Jamieson WRE, Dooner J, Munro AI, et al. 1981. Cardiac valve replacement in the elderly: a review of 320 consecutive cases. Circulation 64:II-177–II-183.
7. Fremes SE, Goldman BS, Ivanov J, et al. 1989. Valvular surgery in the elderly. Circulation 80:I-77-I-90.
8. Hochberg MS, Morrow AG, Michaelis LL, et al. 1977. Aortic valve replacement in the elderly. Encouraging postoperative clinical and hemodynamic results. Arch Surg 112:1475–1480.
9. Quinlan R, Cohn LH and Collins JJ. 1975. Determinants of survival following cardiac operations in elderly patients. Chest 68:498–500.
10. Murphy ES, Lawson RM, Starr A, et al. 1981. Severe aortic stenosis in patients 60 years of age or older: left ventricular function and 10-year survival after valve replacement. Circulation 64:II-184–II-191.
11. Feigenbaum H. 1975. The value of echocardiography in older patients. Geriatrics 30:106–111.
12. Tam PH. 1979. Mitral and aortic valvular disease in the elderly. NY State J Med 79:378–381.
13. Flohr KH, Weir EK and Chesler E. 1981. Diagnosis of aortic stenosis in older age groups using external carotid pulse recording and phonocardiography. Br Heart J 45:577–582.
14. Higgins CB, Reinke RT, Gosink BB, et al. 1976. The significance of mitral valve prolapse in middle-aged and elderly men. Am Heart J 91:292–296.
15. Schwartz A, Vignola PA, Walker HJ, et al. 1978. Echocardiographic estimation of aortic-valve prolapse in aortic stenosis. Ann Intern Med 89:329–335.
16. Borer JS, Bacharach SL, Green MV, et al. 1978. Exercise-induced left ventricular dysfunction in symptomatic and asymptomatic patients with aortic regurgitation: assessment with radionuclide cineangiography. Am J Cardiol 42:351–357.
17. Port S, Cobb FR, Coleman RE, et al. 1980. Effect of age on the response of the left ventricular ejection fraction to exercise. N Engl J Med 303:1133–1137.
18. Burch GE. 1969. Geriatric cardiology. Am Heart J 78:700–708.
19. Edwards JE. 1961. Calcific aortic stenosis: pathologic features. Mayo Clin Proc 36:444–451.
20. Roberts WC. 1970. The congentially bicuspid aortic valve: a study of 85 autopsy cases. Am J Cardiol 26:72–83.
21. Pomerance A. 1972. Pathogenesis of aortic stenosis and its relationship to age. Br Heart J 34:569–574.
22. Rotman M, Morris JJ, Behar VS, et al. 1971. Aortic valvular disease: comparison of types and their medical and surgical management. Am J Med 51:241–257.
23. Urrichio JF, Sinha KP, Bentivoglio L, et al. 1959. A study of combined mitral and aortic stenosis. Ann Intern Med 51:668–678.

24. Vollebergh FEMB and Becker AE. 1977. Minor variations of cusp size in tricuspid aortic valves. Possible link with isolated aortic stenosis. Br Heart J 30:1006–1011.
25. Rapaport E. 1975. Natural history of aortic and mitral valve disease. Am J Cardiol 35:221–227.
26. Spodick DH, Sugiura T, Doi Y, et al. 1982. Rate of rise of the carotid pulse. An investigation of observer error in a common clinical measurement. Am J Cardiol 49:159–162.
27. DeMaria AN, Bommer W, Joye J, et al. 1980. Value and limitations of cross-sectional echocardiography of the aortic valve in the diagnosis and quantification of valvular aortic stenosis. Circulation 62:304–312.
28. Williams DE, Sahn DJ and Friedman WF. 1976. Cross-sectional echocardiographic localization of sites of left ventricular outflow tract obstruction. Am J Cardiol 37:250–255.
29. Smith MD, Dawson PL, Elion JL, et al. 1985. Correlation of continuous wave Doppler velocities with cardiac catheterization gradients: an experimental model of aortic stenosis. J Am Coll Cardiol 6:1306–1314.
30. Hatle A, Angelsen BA and Transdal A. 1980. Noninvasive assessment of aortic stenosis by Doppler ultrasound. Br Heart J 43:284–291.
31. Stamm RB and Martin RP. 1983. Quantification of pressure gradients across stenotic valves by Doppler ultrasound. J Am Coll Cardiol 2:707–718.
32. Zaghbi WA, Farmer KL, Soto JG, et al. 1986. Accurate noninvasive quantification of stenotic aortic valve area by Doppler echocardiography. Circulation 73:452–459.
33. Ohlsson J and Wranne B. 1986. Noninvasive assessment of valve area in patients with aortic stenosis. J Am Coll Cardiol 7:501–508.
34. Otto CM, Pearlman AS, Comess KA, et al. 1986. Determination of the stenotic aortic valve area in adults using Doppler echocardiography. J Am Coll Cardiol 7:509–517.
35. Miller WE, Richards KL, Miller JF, et al. 1985. Aortic valve area and mean pressure gradient by combined imaging and Doppler echo (abstract). Circulation 72 (Suppl III):III-144.
36. St. John Sutton MG, St. John Sutton M, Oldershaw P, et al. 1981. Valve replacement without preoperative cardiac catheterization. N Engl J Med 305:1233–1238.
37. Brandenburg RO. 1981. No more routine catheterization for valvular heart disease? N Engl J Med 305:1277–1278.
38. Bessone LN, Pupello DF, Hiro SP, et al. 1988. Surgical management of aortic valve disease in the elderly: a longitudinal analysis. Ann Thorac Surg 46:264–269.
39. Fiore AC, Naunheim KS, Barner HB, et al. 1989. Valve replacement in the octagenarian. Ann Thorac Surg 48:104–108.
40. Ferrans VJ, Boyce SW, Billingham ME, et al. 1980. Calcific deposits in porcine bioprostheses: structure and pathogenesis. Am J Cardiol 46:721–734.
41. Bonchek LI. 1981. Current status of cardiac valve replacement: selection of a prosthesis and indications for operation. Am Heart J 101:96–106.
42. Cohn LH, Mudge GH, Pratter F, et al. 1981. Five- to eight-year follow-up of patients undergoing porcine heart-valve replacement. N Engl J Med 304:258–262.
43. Borkon AM, Soule LM, Baughman KL, et al. 1988. Aortic valve selection in the elderly patient. Ann Thorac Surg 46:270–277.
44. Jamieson WRE, Burr LH, Munro AI, et al. 1989. Cardiac valve replacement in the elderly: clinical performance of biologic prostheses. Ann Thorac Surg 48:173–184.
45. Kirklin JW. 1981. The replacement of cardiac valves. N Engl J Med 304:291–292.
46. Bonow RO, Kent KM, Rosing DR, et al. 1981. Aortic valve replacement without myocardial revascularization in patients with combined aortic valvular and coronary artery disease. Circulation 62:243–251.
47. Richardson JV, Kouchoukos NT, Wright JO III, et al. 1979. Combined aortic valve replacement and myocardial revascularization: results in 220 patients. Circulation 59:75–81.
48. Kirklin JW and Kouchoukos NT. 1981. Aortic valve replacement without myocardial revascularization. Circulation 63:252–253.
49. Ferguson JJ, Garza RA, et al. 1991. Efficacy of multiple balloon aortic valvuloplasty procedures. J Am Coll Cardiol 17:1430–1435.
50. Booth DC. 1988. Aortic stenosis and the potential role of balloon aortic valvuloplasty. Masters Cardiol 5:11–13.

51. Berland J, Cribier A, Savin T, et al. 1989. Percutaneous balloon valvuloplasty in patients with severe aortic stenosis and low ejection fraction. Immediate results and 1-year follow-up. Circulation 79:1189–1196.

52. Isner JM and the Mansfield Scientific Aortic Valvuloplasty Registry Investigators. 1991. Acute catastrophic complications of balloon aortic valvuloplasty. J Am Coll Cardiol 17:1436–1444.

53. Akasaka T, Yoshikawa J, Yoshida K, et al. 1987. Age-related valvular regurgitation: a study by pulsed Doppler echo. Circulation 76:262–265.

54. Kandath D and Nanda NC. 1990. Part I: Assessment of aortic regurgitation by noninvasive techniques. Curr Probl Cardiol 15:45–58.

55. Smith M. 1991. Evaluation of valvular regurgitation by Doppler echocardiography. Cardiol Clin 9:193–228.

56. Enghoff E. 1972. Aortic incompetence. Clinical hemodynamic and angiographic evaluation. Acta Med Scand 538(Suppl):3–17.

57. Stapleton JR and Harvey WP. 1969. Clinical analysis of aortic incompetence. Postgrad Med 46:156–165.

58. Roberts WC. 1970. Anatomically isolated valvular disease. The case against its being of rheumatic etiology. Am J Med 49:151–159.

59. MacKintosh AF and Fleming HA. 1981. Cardiac damage presenting late after road accidents. Thorax 36:811–813.

60. Walter BF, Zoltick JM, Rosen JH, et al. 1982. Severe aortic regurgitation from systemic hypertension (without aortic dissection) requiring aortic valve replacement. Am J Cardiol 49:473–477.

61. Prewitt TA. 1970. Syphilitic aortic insufficiency. Its increased incidence in the elderly. JAMA 211:637–639.

62. Fortuin NJ and Craige E. 1972. On the mechanism of the Austin Flint murmur. Circulation 45:558–570.

63. Morganroth J, Perloff JK, Zeldis SM, et al. 1977. Acute severe aortic regurgitation. Ann Intern Med 87:223–232.

64. Ciobanu M, Abbasi AS, Allen M, et al. 1982. Pulsed Doppler echocardiography in the diagnosis and estimation of severity of aortic insufficiency. Am J Cardiol 49:339–343.

65. Borras X, Carreras F, Auge JM, et al. 1988. Prospective validation of detection and quantitative assessment of chronic aortic regurgitation by combined echocardiographic and Doppler method. J Am Soc Echo 1:422–429.

66. Handshoe R, Handshoe S, Kwan OL, et al. 1984. Value and limitations of Doppler measurements in the estimation of left ventricular end diastolic pressure in patients with aortic regurgitation (abstract). Circulation 70 (Suppl II):II-117.

67. DeMaria AN, Smith MD, Branco M, et al. 1986. Normal and abnormal blood flow patterns by color Doppler flow imaging. Echocardiography 6:475–482.

68. Perry GJ, Helmcke F, Nanda NC, et al. 1987. Evaluation of aortic insufficiency by Doppler color flow mapping. J Am Coll Cardiol 9:952–959.

69. Smith MD, Grayburn PA, Spain MG, et al. 1988. Observer variability in the quantitation of Doppler color flow jet areas for mitral and aortic regurgitation. J Am Coll Cardiol 11:579–584.

70. Henry WL, Bonow RO, Boer JS, et al. 1980. Observations on the optimum time for operative intervention for aortic regurgitation. I. Evaluation of the results of aortic valve replacement in symptomatic patients. Circulation 61:471–483.

71. Henry WL, Bonow RO, Rosing DR, et al. 1980. Observations on the optimum time for operative intervention for aortic regurgitation. I. Serial echocardiographic evaluation of asymtomatic patients. Circulation 61:484–492.

72. Bonow RO, Picone AL, McIntosh CL, et al. 1985. Survival and functional results after aortic valve replacement for aortic regurgitation from 1976 to 1983: impact of preoperative left ventricular function. Circulation 72:1244–1256.

73. Roberts WC and Perloff JF. 1972. Mitral valvular disease. A clinicopathologic survey of the conditions causing the mitral valve to function abnormally. Ann Intern Med 77: 939–975.

74. Fulkerson PK, Beaver BM, Auseon JC, et al. 1979. Calcification of the mitral annulus. Etiology, clinical associations, complications and therapy. Am J Med 66:967–977.

75. D'Cruz I, Panetta, F, Cohen H, et al. 1979. Submitral calcification or sclerosis in elderly patients. M-mode and two-dimensional echocardiography in "mitral annulus calcification." Am J Cardiol 44:31–38.

76. Hammer WJ, Roberts WC and de Leon AC. 1978. "Mitral stenosis" secondary to combined "massive" mitral annular calcific deposits and small, hypertrophied left ventricles. Hemodynamic documentation in four patients. Am J Med 64:371–376.

77. Jeresaty RM. 1979. Mitral Valve Prolapse. New York: Raven Press.

78. Thell R, Martin FH and Edwards JE. 1975. Bacterial endocarditis in subjects 60 years of age or older. Circulation 51:174–182.

79. Robbins N, DeMaria AN and Miller MH. 1980. Infectious endocarditis in the elderly. South Med J 73:1335–1338.

80. Kusiak V, Brest AN. 1986. Acute mitral regurgitation. Pathophysiology and management. In WS Frankl, AN Brest (eds): Cardiovascular Clinics. Valvular Heart Disease: Comprehensive Evaluation and Management. Philadelphia: F. A. Davis, pp 257–280.

81. Barnett HJM, Boughner DR, Taylor DW, et al. 1980. Further evidence relating mitral valve prolapse to cerebral ischemic events. N Engl J Med 302:139–144.

82. Knopman D, Anderson DC, Greenland P, et al. 1980. Mitral valve prolapse and cerebral ischemic events in the elderly (letter). N Engl J Med 303:641.

83. Mills P, Rose R, Hollingsworth J, et al. 1977. Long-term prognosis of mitral valve prolapse. N Engl J Med 297:13–18.

84. Zile MR, Gaasch WH and Levine HJ. 1985. Left ventricular stress-dimension-shortening relations before and after correction of chronic aortic and mitral regurgitation. Am J Cardiol 56:99–105.

85. Schuler G, Peterson KL, Johnson A, et al. 1979. Temporal response of left ventricular performance to mitral valve surgery. Circulation 59:1218–1231.

86. Ross J. 1981. Left ventricular function and timing of surgical treatment in valvular heart disease. Ann Intern Med 94:498–504.

87. Hochberg MS, Derkae WM, Conkle DM, et al. 1979. Mitral valve replacement in elderly patients. Encouraging postoperative results. J Thorac Cardiovasc Surg 77:422–426.

88. Reed D, Abbott RD, Smucker ML, et al. 1991. Prediction of outcome after mitral valve replacement in patients with symptomatic chronic mitral regurgitation. Circulation 84:23–34.

89. Carpentier A, Chauvaud S and Fabiani JN. 1980. Reconstructive surgery of mitral valve incompetence. Ten-year appraisal. J Thorac Cardiovasc Surg 79:338–348.

90. Limas CJ. 1991. Mitral stenosis in the elderly. Geriatrics 26 (part 2):75–79.

91. Smith MD, Handshoe R, Handshoe S, et al. 1986. Comparative accuracy of two-dimensional echocardiography and Doppler pressure half-time methods in assessing severity of mitral stenosis in patients with and without prior commissurotomy. Circulation 73:100–107.

92. Segal J, Lerner DJ, Miller DC, et al. 1987. When should Doppler-determined valve area be better than the Gorlin formula?: variation in hydraulic constants in low flow states. J Am Coll Cardiol 9:1294–1305.

93. Hatle L, Brubakk A, Tromsdal A, et al. 1978. Noninvasive assessment of pressure drop in mitral stenosis by Doppler ultrasound. Br Heart J 40:131–140.

94. Lang R, Klein HO, Guerrero J, et al. 1981. Verapamil improves maximal exercise capacity in digitalized patients with chronic atrial fibrillation: a double-blind crossover study (abstract). Circulation 64 (Suppl IV):IV-296.

95. Chesebro JH, Adams PC and Fuster V. 1986. Antithrombotic therapy in patients with valvular heart disease and prosthetic heart valves. J Am Coll Cardiol 8:41B–56B.

96. American College of Chest Physicians and the National Heart, Lung, and Blood Institute. 1986. National Conference on Antithrombotic Therapy. Arch Intern Med 146:462–472.

97. Lock JE, Khalilullah M, Shrivastava S, et al. 1985. Percutaneous catheter commissurotomy in rheumatic mitral stenosis. N Engl J Med 313:1515–1518.

98. Abascal VM, Wilkins GT, O'Shea JP, et al. 1990. Prediction of successful outcome in 130 patients undergoing percutaneous balloon mitral valvotomy. Circulation 80:448–456.

99. Hendel N, Leckie B and Richards J. 1980. Carcinoid heart disease: eight-year survival following tricuspid replacement and pulmonary valvotomy. Ann Thorac Surg 30:391–395.

100. Johnson LW, Grossman W, Dalen JE, et al. 1972. Pulmonic stenosis in the adult: long-term follow-up results. N Engl J Med 287:1159–1163.
101. Chino F, Kodama A, Otake M, et al. 1975. Nonbacterial thrombotic endocarditis in a Japanese autopsy sample. A review of eighty cases. Am Heart J 90:190–198.
102. Klein RS, Rocco RA, Catalano MT, et al. 1977. Association of Streptococcus bovis with carcinoma of the colon. N Engl J Med 297:800–802.
103. McAllister HA. 1979. Primary tumors and cysts of the heart and pericardium. Curr Probl Cardiol 4:1–51.
104. Bashery RI and Nochumson S. 1979. Cardiac myxoma. Biochemical analyses and evidence for its neoplastic nature. NY State Med 79:29–32.
105. Salyer WR, Page DL and Hutchins GM. 1975. The development of cardiac myxomas and papillary endocardial lesions from mural thrombus. Am Heart J 89:4–17.
106. Lappe DL, Bulkley GH and Weiss JL. 1978. Two-dimensional echocardiography diagnosis of the left atrial myxoma. Chest 74: 55–58.
107. Donahoo JS, Weiss JI, Gardner TJ, et al. 1979. Current management of atrial myxoma with emphasis on a new diagnostic technique. Ann Surg 189:763–768.
108. Walton JA, Kahn DR and Willis PW. 1972. Recurrence of a left atrial myxoma. Am J Cardiol 29:872–876.

12. CORONARY ARTERY DISEASE

ANDREW P. REES
CARL J. LAVIE
CARL J. PEPINE

The elderly as a whole are a population at risk for coronary artery disease (CAD). The elderly, defined as those individuals over 65 years of age, also represent an increasing proportion of the United States population. It is estimated that 60% of all patients hospitalized for acute myocardial infarctions (MI) are older than 65 years, and this figure is expected to increase to 80% over the next 10 years [1]. In the last 35 years, this age group has doubled to a current estimate of 28 million people, accounting for 12% of the United States population. This is projected to grow to 17% over the next 35 years; by the year 2035, the elderly will constitute 20% to 25% of the United States population [2].

Mortality from CAD is high in the elderly. Patients older than 65 years account for 80% of deaths from myocardial infarction, with those older than 75 years accounting for 60% of such deaths [3]. The in-hospital infarct-related mortality of patients younger than 55 years is 5%, compared to 32% of patients older than 75 years. One-year survival is 94% and 77%, respectively [4]. One of the possible reasons for this is that elderly persons are more likely to have had prior MI or coexisting illnesses such as diabetes mellitus, hypertension, cerebrovascular disease, or valvular heart disease.

As health care attends to the elderly, health care expenditures will rise in a

Franz H. Messerli (ed.), CARDIOVASCULAR DISEASE IN THE ELDERLY (Third Edition). Copyright © 1993 Kluwer Academic Publishers. ISBN 0-7923-1859-5. All rights reserved.

proportionate if not exponential manner. In 1978, health care expenditures in the elderly were $50 billion, and these costs are projected to grow to $200 billion by the year 2000 [2]. The combined costs of cardiac catheterization, angioplasty, and pacemaker insertion equal about $4 billion annually, and coronary artery bypass surgery costs $5 billion annually; one third of these procedures are performed in the elderly [5]. Because of the population shift toward an elderly society, it is pertinent to address efficient and effective care of CAD in the elderly and to emphasize its prevention.

PATHOPHYSIOLOGIC CONSIDERATIONS

With aging come well-documented alterations in cardiovascular structure and function that impact upon therapeutic decisions. The endocardium thickens due to increased fat and collagen deposition, leading to a progressive de-crease in ventricular chamber distensibility. This results in an increase in the dependence of cardiac output upon venous return. Higher left ventricular filling pressures without proportionate increases in aortic diastolic pressure decrease coronary perfusion pressure. The coronary circulation itself develops atrophy of the vessel media and increasing fibrosis and calcification of atheroma. Collateral circulation may become extensive, particularly when significant long-standing CAD is present. The elderly myocardium displays reduced responsiveness to catecholamines.

Vascular changes include diminished distensibility of the vessel wall and subsequent systolic hypertension, which increases myocardial oxygen demand directly and perpetually by promoting left ventricular hypertrophy (LVH). LVH itself is associated with impaired coronary reserve. Baroreceptor responses become blunted, making accommodation to arterial hypotension more difficult. Additionally, extracellular volume, plasma volume, and volume of distribution of hydrophilic compounds all decrease in the elderly.

Coronary risk factors in the elderly

Age itself is one of the strongest risk factors for CAD [6]. As a whole, the male–female incidence of CAD is similar in the elderly [7,8]. Coronary disease predominates in men at an earlier age (30 to 60 years), with a progressive increase in risk through the sixth decade. After a decline in the seventh decade, coronary disease in men again rises during the eighth and ninth decades. Women show a slower and more progressive rise throughout their lifetime; a later onset may be due to the protective effect of estrogens, which lower low-density lipoprotein cholesterol (LDL-C) and increase cardioprotective high-density lipoprotein cholesterol (HDL-C). After menopause, CAD rates for women increase to those of males 5 to 10 years younger [6].

Hypertension persists as a risk factor for CAD in the elderly. In fact, with aging, the impact of blood pressure on CAD risk is greater [9]. Treatment of hypertension has been shown to reduce the incidence of cerebrovascular accidents [10]. It has long been believed that therapy for hypertension must certainly reduce morbidity and mortality from coronary events; however, data from some major trials have demonstrated that drug therapy has less impact on CAD than expected, and in individual trials the reductions in CAD events often are not statistically significant. However, the recent Systolic Hypertension in the Elderly Program (SHEP) Study [11] randomized 4736 hypertensive patients aged 60 years or older to receive either a placebo or stepped care therapy utilizing low-dose chlorthalidone, atenolol, and reserpine and followed patients for an average of 4.5 years. The goal systolic blood pressure was less than 160 mmHg for those starting at greater than 180 mmHg, with a reduction of at least 20 mmHg for those starting at 160 to 179 mmHg. In addition to a decrease in stroke rates, the incidence of all other cardiovascular events was consistently reduced with active therapy, including 25% fewer CAD events, both fatal and nonfatal, in the active treatment group. Benefit was observed in patients with and without baseline electrocardiographic abnormalities [11]. Therefore, the treatment of systolic hypertension in excess of 160 mmHg can be strongly recommended in elderly persons with a reasonable life expectancy, with the goal of reducing morbidity and mortality from CAD.

Obesity is an independent risk factor for CAD in the elderly. This has been confirmed in the elderly over eight years of follow-up in males and 14 years of follow-up in females [9]. The immobility and subsequent lack of exercise that may come with aging promote obesity. Achievement and maintenance of ideal body weight throughout life is a major goal of preventive cardiology.

In contrast to the strong correlation between tobacco use and cardiovascular morbidity in the middle-aged, no such relation has been documented in the aged. Over age 65, the data from the Framingham Study fail to show a positive relation between smoking history and CAD, although total mortality, particularly due to lung cancer, accelerates [9]. A possible explanation for this finding is that while tobacco use continues to contribute to CAD risk, elderly patients are dying of other tobacco-related illnesses such as malignancy and lung disease. Another possibility is that smoking contributes to the death of susceptible younger patients so that those at greatest risk are excluded (by premature death) from the elderly population under study. Smoking should be strongly discouraged in all persons, including the elderly.

Diabetes is an important risk factor for CAD in any person, regardless of age. In a recent evaluation of the Framingham cohort [9], elevated fasting blood sugar emerged as a risk factor for CAD in the elderly. In another study [12], the presence of diabetes in an elderly person doubled CAD risk. Multiple risk factors had an exponential effect on risk, with the combination of diabetes and hyperlipidemia producing a 15-fold elevation in CAD risk [12].

During the last two decades, great progress has been made in establishing the cholesterol–CAD hypothesis [13,14]. High total plasma cholesterol has been confirmed as a risk factor in numerous studies of patients older than age 60 [13]. As was previously documented in younger persons, new data from the Framingham Study [9] indicate that a 1% increase in total cholesterol produces a 2% increase in coronary disease risk in the 60- to 70-year-old age group. However, total cholesterol is less predictive of new-onset CAD in older persons than it is in young persons. The best explanation for this relationship is that with age, the rising prevalence of competing disease and other risk factors obscures the influence of total cholesterol [15]. Nevertheless, several elderly high-risk groups can be identified. Epidemiologic studies [16,17] have documented an inverse relationship between HDL-C and CAD risk in the elderly. A high HDL-C level has a protective effect even with coexisting elevations in total cholesterol and LDL-C. Additionally, a high ratio of total cholesterol to HDL-C is a significant risk factor in the elderly. The triglyceride level seems to be a better predictor of coronary heart disease development in women over age 50. Conversely, triglycerides alone are not predictive of coronary disease in men over age 50. The combination of high triglycerides ($>150\,mg/dl$) and low HDL-C ($<40\,mg/dl$) is a particularly strong risk factor in the elderly [9]. This group was identified by the Lipid Research Clinics Study [17,18] and could easily be missed in clinical practice.

In middle-aged patients, lipid interventions have been documented not only to reduce the incidence of CAD events but also to retard the rate of progression of angiographically assessed coronary atherosclerosis [19–23]. However, lipid intervention trials are lacking in the elderly, and no trials have utilized pharmacologic interventions in this age group. Nonetheless, there is some evidence to support the treatment of hyperlipidemia in elderly persons. Only one study, the Los Angeles Domiciliary Trial [24], has evaluated therapy for lipid disorders in the elderly. In this study, 846 men of mean age 67 years were randomized to a diet of high polyunsaturated, low satured fats versus a control diet. The intervention group displayed a significant 20% reduction in mean cholesterol level, from $233\,mg/dL$ to $187\,mg/dL$. Patients in the active treatment group whose initial total cholesterol was greater than $233\,mg/dl$ had a significant reduction in cardiovascular endpoints, including death from CAD, nonfatal MI, and cerebrovascular accident. This benefit was not evident for eight years, so successful intervention required a relatively long duration of therapy. Whether elderly patients as a group would be tolerant of or responsive to pharmacologic therapy for hyperlipidemia is unknown. The only data available on this topic are from the Lipid Research Clinics Primary Prevention Trial, which was not specifically designed to evaluated older persons [22]. Treatment in this study lasted 7 to 10 years, during which time patients reached ages 42 to 69. Patients were treated with weight loss, dietary therapy, and cholestyramine. Study participants had a sustained reduction in LDL-C; in fact, older men had greater reductions in total cholesterol and LDL-C than younger patients. A reasonable recommendation would be that in patients over age 50 who are candidates for lipid intervention and whose total cholesterol is greater than 200 mg/dl, full lipid profiles should be evaluated. Dietary therapy should be started in any individual as a first step. The decision to begin drug therapy will be inversely related to patient age, since between 5 and 10 years of treatment may be necessary to achieve benefits. The elderly, however, should not be categorically denied the potential benefits of aggressive lipid treatment.

A final risk factor to be included is LVH, which when present by electrocardiographic criteria markedly increases coronary disease risk in elderly men and women. Nonspecific S-T- and T-wave abnormalities alone are significant risk factors in elderly women only (ages 65 to 94). Intraventricular conduction defects are not significant as a risk factor [9]. Echocardiographic evaluation of LVH is more sensitive than electrocardiographic evaluation and has recently been proven to be a strong risk factor for CAD in the elderly. In this study [25], left ventricular mass was indexed by height in a group of 1141 patients ranging in age from 60 to 90 years. Over four years, coronary heart disease risk increased progressively with greater left ventricular mass independent of smoking, systolic blood pressure, and cholesterol. In fact, in elderly men, left ventricular mass corrected for height was the strongest independent predictor of CAD events.

Clinical findings

Symptoms referrable to CAD may be difficult to elicit in the elderly due to hearing loss, expressive communication deficits, and memory impairment. A careful history, preferably with corroboration from a family member, can be invaluable. Although typical angina pectoris occurs less frequently than in younger patients, roughly one third of elderly patients will have a typical ischemic presentation. The elderly are more functionally limited, and angina may not occur due to simple lack of exertion. Frequently, slow ambulation may be tolerated, and more stressful arm activity may provoke angina [26]. A long duration of symptoms increases the likelihood of left main or three-vessel disease. In one angiographic study [27], patients with a history of angina dating 20 years or more had a 90% incidence of three-vessel coronary disease and a 28% incidence of left main disease. The elderly are certainly more predisposed to other symptoms, which must be discriminated from angina. Neck, shoulder, and arm pain, as well as pain originating in the gastrointestinal tract, may all mimic angina.

Approximately one third of elderly patients have symptoms other than angina. Dyspnea on exertion may be an anginal equivalent for the patient; however, coexisting lung disease often is a contributing cause. More ominous is dyspnea at rest, which may represent pulmonary edema [28].

This signals that mechanical dysfunction has occurred as a consequence of ischemia and that a critical amount of myocardium is in jeopardy. Other potential causes are ischemic mitral regurgitation or ventricular septal defect due to necrosis of infarcted septal myocardium. While current estimates of the incidence of these complications with MI are difficult to quantify, estimates are 1% and 2% to 4%, respectively [29]. Sudden cardiac death may occur, most frequently due to ventricular fibrillation. However, other mechanisms include asystole, profoundly diminished flow due to pump failure, and cardiac rupture. The latter is more commonly seen in elderly women with their first MI.

Finally, many elderly patients present with asymptomatic CAD that is discovered incidentally on electrocardiogram. In the Framingham study, this occurred in 35% of the hypertensive male population [30].

Physical examination frequently reveals an S_4 gallop in the aged, indicative of diminished ventricular compliance. Murmurs of aortic stenosis and mitral regurgitation are commonly present due to calcific valvular disease. Careful evaluation for carotid bruits is necessary, since evidence of cerebrovascular disease is a risk factor for concomitant CAD. In fact, patients with asymptomatic cervical bruits have a higher incidence of a cardiac ischemic event than of a cerebrovascular accident over only a three-year period [31]. Findings that are not cardiovascular frequently impact on therapeutic decisions. Examples are prostatic disease, other atherosclerotic vascular disease, and obstructive lung disease. The patient's functional status and general health should be assessed.

Diagnostic testing

Electrocardiography is indispensable in evaluation for prior and acute ischemic cardiac events. However, age-related morphologic changes occur that may make interpretation more difficult. With time, the P axis shifts rightward and the QRS axis shifts leftward. After age 75, prolongation of the P-R interval occurs. The amplitude of the T-wave diminishes with age, and nonspecific T-wave abnormalities become more common [32,33].

Chest radiography is useful for identifying pulmonary vascular congestion. While cardiomegaly increases with aging, it should be noted that elderly persons have a reduced thoracic diameter and may not inspire deeply, causing an increased cardiothoracic ratio regardless of cardiac chamber enlargement.

Exercise stress testing serves as an excellent screening tool to identify those young and middle-aged patients at risk for CAD events. Sensitivity and specificity for angiographically confirmed coronary disease are well documented in the 60% to 65% range and the 80% to 85% range, respectively. However, the sensitivity of the test is impaired in elderly patients because they have a diminished ability to increase myocardial oxygen consumption by increasing the heart rate. Specificity is impaired by resting S-T- and T-wave abnormalities, which are common in the elderly. In one preliminary report comparing exercise testing in patients younger than age 65 with those older than age 65 [34], S-T-segment depression of 1 mm or more was a much less specific parameter in older (29%) than in younger (67%) patients. The addition of radionuclide testing to stress electrocardiographic changes increases both the sensitivity and specificity of the test. Elderly patients, especially those older than 75 years, have progressive limitation of ambulation and mobility such that performing treadmill exercise may be difficult or impossible. In these persons, pharmacologic stress testing, discussed elsewhere, has emerged as a very useful test for assessing the presence and extent of CAD [35] (see the chapter on diagnostic tests). The overall sensitivity and specificity of these tests make them comparable to exercise thallium testing [36].

Echocardiography is useful to evaluate left ventricular wall motion abnormalities, wall thickness, and concomitant valvular heart disease. Chest deformities and lung disease will detract from the quality of the images obtained. Stress and dobutamine echocardiography are currently under investigation, and the latter may become applicable in elderly patients with limited exertional capacity.

The most definitive test for CAD is coronary arteriography. The indications for arteriography in the elderly are no different from those in younger persons, given that the patient's quality of life is of a level worth preserving with percutaneous transluminal angioplasty or coronary artery bypass surgery. Clear indications for coronary arteriography in eligible persons include angina unacceptably controlled by medical therapy, unstable angina, stress testing results suggestive of poor outcome, and mechanical complications of acute MI.

PHARMACOLOGIC THERAPY

Anti-ischemic medications

When considering pharmacologic anti-ischemic therapy in the aged, several principles should be emphasized. Extracellular volume, and therefore plasma volume, diminishes with age. Hydrophilic substances will therefore have a decreased volume of distribution. Additionally, hydrophilic substances are cleared primarily by the kidney, and as creatinine clearance falls with aging, drug elimination slows. In contrast, lipophilic substances are generally fat-stored and hepatically metabolized. Because the elderly have reduced extracellular volume, adipose tissue accounts for proportionately more body mass, increasing the volume of distribution of lipophilic drugs. Hepatic metabolism diminishes with aging, delaying the elimination of lipophilic substances.

Beta-adrenergic blocking agents

One of the more effective classes of anti-ischemic medications known is the beta-adrenergic blocking agents. These drugs are certainly of benefit in patients with symptomatic CAD and in the post-MI patient, and they may be of benefit in patients at risk for CAD, such as elderly hypertensives. The medications in this class relieve symptoms of ischemia such as angina through their negative inotropic and chronotropic actions on myocardial tissues. Because heart rate is directly related to myocardial oxygen consumption, the negative chronotropic action is both potent and effective in improving exercise tolerance and reducing the severity of ischemia-related symptoms. Myocardial oxygen consumption is also reduced directly by reduction of blood pressure as systolic wall stress declines. In addition to symptomatic benefits, patients derive the benefit of reduced morbidity and mortality from beta-adrenergic blockers. Currently, this is the only entire class of medications with such established benefits. It has been well established through three large, multicenter trials [37–39] that, in the postinfarction period, propranolol, timolol, and metoprolol effect reductions in mortality ranging from 26% to 45% over follow-up of 3 to 30 months. It is not clear whether this occurs through a reduction of the incidence of ischemic or arrhythmic death, but it is probably a combined effect. It is important to note that, in these studies, reinfarction was also consistently reduced. In two of these trials [37,38], patients aged 65 to 75 were evaluated separately, and the same *or greater* mortality benefits were observed. Therefore, these data may be especially applicable to the elderly post-MI patient. It must be stressed that beta-blockers are most useful in patients with larger infarcts, such as those with mechanical complications and congestive heart failure during the acute event [40].

While the coronary event rate has not been reduced in several antihypertensive trials in asymptomatic individuals, these studies have used beta-blockers infrequently and inconsistently [41]. More recent primary prevention data are encouraging, although they do not specifically refer to an elderly population. The Metroprolol Atherosclerosis Prevention in Hypertensives (MAPHY) trial [42] randomized asymptomatic men ages 40 to 64 years with CAD risk factors and diastolic hypertension to treatment with metoprolol or a thiazide diuretic in order to investigate potential reductions in coronary event rate with beta-blocker therapy. Diastolic hypertension was defined as a diastolic pressure of 100 to 130 mmHg. The population had several risk factors for coronary disease: males, mean age 53 years, systolic hypertension, elevated total cholesterol, and smoking (approximately one third). The risk for symptomatic or asymptomatic coronary events (sudden death, fatal and nonfatal MI) was 24% lower in the group receiving metoprolol. Smokers and nonsmokers benefited from beta-blocker therapy. Total cardiovascular mortality was also significantly lower in the metoprolol group [43]. Over the 12-year follow-up, the mean age increased to 65 years, with the elder persons in the cohort reaching an age of 76 years. While these findings are not strictly applicable to the elderly, even asymptomatic hypertensive males may derive tangible benefits from beta-blocker therapy.

Table 12-1. Beta-adrenergic blocker pharmacology

Medication	Lipid Solubility	Cardioselectivity	ISA	Metabolism	Half-life (hrs)
Atenolol	+	+	−	renal	6–7
Nadolol	+	−	−	renal	20–24
Acebutolol	+	+	+	60% hepatic	3–4
Betaxalol	++	+	−	80% hepatic	14–22
Metoprolol	++	+	−	hepatic	3–7
Labetalol	++	−	+	hepatic	6–8
Pindolol	++	−	+++	60% hepatic	8
Timolol	++	−	−	80% hepatic	4
Propranolol	+++	−	−	hepatic	3–6

ISA = intrinsic sympathomimetic activity

The pharmacologic properties of these drugs vary widely and must be considered to avoid toxicity and side effects (table 12-1). In general, the blood levels of patients taking hydrophilic beta-blockers tend to fluctuate less than for patients taking lipophilic beta-blockers, but peak levels may be increased because of diminished renal function. The effects of lipophilic drugs will be more persistent due to their increased volume of distribution and delayed hepatic clearance. Also, these drugs more commonly interact with other drugs. For example, the plasma concentration of propranolol increases in combination with cimetidine, furosemide, hydralazine, and verapamil [44–47]. Choosing a cardioselective (β-1 antagonist) agent may reduce the untoward effects seen with nonselective (β-1, β-2 antagonists) agents such as bronchospasm, the masking of hypoglycemic reactions, and worsening symptoms of peripheral vascular disease. Agents with intrinsic sympathomimetic activity (ISA) produce less reduction of resting heart rate and cardiac output and are less likely to exacerbate bradycardia or peripheral vascular disease. The influence of ISA is reduced during exercise, so that exertional hemodynamic responses approximate those seen in patients using beta-blockers without ISA [48]. However, beta-blocking agents with ISA have not been consistent in their ability to reduce CAD events among infarction survivors. (For example, alprenolol, practolol, and acebutolol have shown positive results, while pindolol and oxprenolol have not shown benefit.) Central nervous system side effects due to beta-blockers are particularly troublesome in the elderly, who may already have cognitive impairment. Fatigue, memory deficits, anorexia, and depression may occur with all beta-blockers and are more common in the elderly [49]. These side effects tend to be less severe with the more hydrophilic drugs [50]. Cardiovascular side effects such as bradyarrhythmia or congestive heart failure occur with all beta-blockers and are more common in the elderly [51]. Because hydrophilic beta-blockers are well tolerated, they appear to be a good choice in elderly patients with documented CAD and possibly in elderly hypertensive patients at risk for coronary events.

Calcium-channel blocking agents

A second class of anti-ischemic medications which have grown in popularity for use in the elderly because of their efficacy and desirable side effect profile are the calcium-channel antagonists. These drugs seem to be particularly effective antihypertensive agents in elderly patients, who have low plasma renin activity. Calcium antagonists generally are less likely to produce orthostatic hypotension than other antihypertensive agents. They are clearly effective antianginal agents [52]. All preparations to date are hepatically metabolized. As with other hepatically metabolized compounds, half-lives of calcium-channel antagonists may be prolonged in the elderly by as much as 50% [53,54]. Calcium-channel antagonists have differing effects on the cardiovascular system and may be separated into at least two groups based on these properties. It is important to be well acquainted with these in order to individualize therapy (table 12-2). The first commercially available dihydropyridine calcium-channel blocker was nifedipine. Soon to follow were nicardipine, felodipine, and isradipine. All of these drugs increase stroke volume and cardiac output after the first dose due to their predominantly vasodilatory action. Their negligible negative inotropic effects are offset by a favorable reduction in afterload. Increases in cardiac output return to baseline with chronic therapy. Dihydropyridines have essentially no cardiodepressant effects on the conduction system and, in fact, may cause a reflexive increase in heart rate. Generally, no net effect on heart rate is observed with chronic use, and therefore combination of these agents with beta-blockers is well tolerated. In survivors of MI, neither recurrent infarction nor mortality is reduced with administration of nifedipine [55]. It is disturbing that there is a trend toward an increased incidence of cardiac events in patients with unstable angina who are treated with nifedipine in the absence of concurrent beta-blocker use [56,57]. However, dihydropyridines remain very effective antihypertensive and antianginal preparations, particularly when combined with beta-blockers. They should be used with

Table 12-2. Calcium-channel antagonists

Medication	AV Conduction	SA Automaticity	Coronary Vasodilatation	Peripheral Vasodilatation	Hypotension
Dihydropyridines Nifedipine Nicardipine Felodipine Isradipine Amlodipine	N	↑↓	↑↑↑	↑↑↑	↑↑↑
Diltiazem	↓	↓↓	↑↑↑	↑	↑
Verapamil	↓↓	↓	↑↑	↑↑	↑↑

AV = atrioventricular
SA = sinoatrial

caution in combination with nitrate preparations to avoid orthostatic hypotension. Although negative inotropic effects usually do not occur in vivo, a recent trial of patients with congestive heart failure [58] demonstrated worsening in functional class and an increase in frequency of hospitalizations in nifedipine-treated patients. Therefore, these agents are all relatively contraindicated in patients with important left ventricular dysfunction. If a patient with congestive heart failure requires a calcium-channel blocker, either nicardipine, amlodipine, or isradipine, which possesses little detectable direct negative inotropic effect, is probably the best choice.

Two calcium-channel blockers should be separated from the dihydro-pyridine compounds because they possess more significant negative inotropic and chronotropic properties. While both verapamil and diltiazem have significant negative inotropic effect, verapamil causes the greatest reduction in systolic performance. These drugs are generally not tolerated in patients with impaired left ventricular function. In fact, each of these agents has been proven to be of no benefit or even detrimental in patients following MI when clinical indicators of left ventricular dysfunction (i.e., rales, S_3 gallop, or pulmonary congestion on chest radiography) are present [59,60]. It is important to realize, however, that each of these medications may be applicable in some specific post-MI patient subsets. Diltiazem has been shown to prevent early enzymatic evidence for reinfarction and angina after non–Q-wave MI [61]. The elderly composed a majority of this particular study group; therefore, these findings are specifically applicable to this discussion. In the trial, 57% of the patients were age 60 or older, and roughly 7% were older than age 75. In another study [62] of patients post-MI (Q-wave or non-Q-wave), in which roughly one third of the patients were age 65 or older, long-term treatment with verapamil significantly decreased the recurrence of cardiac events. Subgroup analysis confirmed this benefit in patients both older than and younger than age 65. The verapamil treatment group as a whole had a nearly 20% reduction in all major cardiac events post-MI, with nearly a 35% reduction in patients without clinical evidence of congestive heart failure. Pooled data from two large studies of verapamil versus placebo [60,62], which included approximately 4000 patients post-MI, suggested statistically significant reductions in all-cause mortality, reinfarction, and major cardiac events by 22%, 27%, and 23%, respectively. In contrast to trials of beta-adrenergic blocking drugs, no reduction in cardiac mortality has been observed with any individual calcium-channel antagonist after MI. Therefore, the calcium-channel blockers diltiazem and verapamil appear most beneficial in patients with smaller non-Q-wave MIs and infarcts without congestive heart failure, in contrast to beta-adrenergic blockers, which appear to be most beneficial in a subset of patients at higher risk after large MIs. Both verapamil and diltiazem depress sinus-node impulse formation and conduction through cardiac tissues and thus must be used cautiously in combination with beta-blockers. The combination of verapamil and beta-blockers should probably be avoided in elderly patients in order to avoid bradyarrhythmic complications or excessive depression of left ventricular function.

In summary, calcium-channel antagonists serve as excellent first-line antianginal medications in the elderly. These agents are known to reduce arterial pressure (particularly in patients with low-renin hypertension, such as the elderly), have a favorable lipid profile, and impede atherosclerosis both in vitro and in vivo. Additionally, these agents may reduce the prevalence and complexity of ventricular arrhythmias in hypertensive patients with LVH and permit regression of LVH [63–65]. Specific preparations have been shown to reduce nonfatal recurrent coronary artery disease events following MI; however, calcium-channel antagnoists have not reduced cardiac mortality in individual secondary prevention trials (although pooled data with verapamil suggest there is a benefit). No evaluation in primary prevention trials has been done. Calcium-channel blockers can be combined with beta-blockers or nitrates, with the understanding that medications with similar side effect profiles should be used cautiously, particularly in the elderly.

Nitrates

The third class of antianginal medications useful in the elderly is nitrates. Nitrate preparations have a pronounced effect on venous capacitance and are effective preload-reducing agents. The vascular and particularly the venous smooth muscle action of nitroglycerin is maintained and, in fact, increased in the elderly. There are at least two reasons for this: 1) the slower hepatic glutathione reductase metabolism seen in the elderly delays metabolism; and 2) nitrates are highly lipophilic compounds, and increased adipose stores in the elderly may allow accumulation of the drug [66]. Because nitrates have such an effect on preload, they have proven quite useful in elderly patients with CAD and reduced left ventricular function. They are the anti-ischemic medication of choice in this setting and can be easily combined with angiotensin-converting enzyme (ACE) inhibitors, diuretics, and digitalis in these patients. Because nitrates have no direct inotropic or chronotropic effects, they are easily combined with other classes of anti-anginal agents. Sublingual nitroglycerin remains effective for relief of anginal episodes in the elderly. Because elderly persons may have decreased saliva production and may be mouth breathers, dissolution of sublingual tablets may be delayed. One small study [67] found that sublingual isosorbide dinitrate spray relieved angina more rapidly than tablets in older patients. Also, because elderly persons are predisposed to impairments of visual and motor skills, nitroglycerin spray may allow for easier self-administration.

Because of the cardiovascular changes that occur with aging, the elderly are more susceptible to orthostatic hypotension with nitrate therapy. Decreased vascular distensibility and decreased extracellular fluid volume hinder the patient's ability to accommodate to postural changes. Additionally, decreased myocardial compliance with aging causes increased sensitivity to the preload state (and nitrates are potent preload-reducing agents). Severe hypotension is certainly more common in the elderly in the setting of acute MI and can be aggravated by nitrates [56,68,69].

Antiplatelet and anticoagulant agents

Although the role of thrombus in acute ischemic events was first suggested by Herrick in 1912 [70], extensive data during the past decade [71–75] have confirmed that a thrombus occurring on an atherosclerotic plaque is involved in the pathogenesis of most acute ischemic syndromes, including unstable angina, acute MI, and sudden cardiac ischemic death. Not surprisingly, much emphasis in cardiology during the past decade has focused on the prevention and treatment of coronary thrombosis. More recent evidence from the Physicians' Health Study [76], in which 22,071 physicians in the United States were randomized to receive either placebo or aspirin (325 mg every other day), supports the benefit of aspirin for both primary and secondary prevention of coronary events. The treatment group displayed a 44% lower risk of fatal and nonfatal MI than the placebo group. Risk reduction was apparent *only* in those age 50 or older, with beneficial effects persisting through age 79. While there was a trend of increased hemorrhagic strokes in the group receiving aspirin, the actual numbers were quite small, and total strokes were statistically similar in both groups. A British physicians' study [77] showed no such benefits with aspirin therapy; however, this study differed considerably from the American study, which may have affected the results. First, the British study was single-blinded, and compliance was significantly poorer in the group receiving aspirin than in the group receiving a placebo (70% versus 98%, respectively). Additionally, 500 mg of aspirin daily was used, which represents a threefold higher total dose than that used in the American study. Finally, the British study was only one fourth the sample size of the American study. Low doses of aspirin are recommended in elderly patients with cardiac risk factors as primary prevention for ischemic coronary events. Care should be taken in patients with severe hypertension to avoid provocation of hemorrhagic cerebrovascular events. In fact, prophylactic aspirin therapy may not be indicated in the rare patient with only hypertension as a risk factor for CAD, and arterial pressure should be reasonably well controlled in all patients before initiation of prophylactic aspirin therapy.

Therapy with aspirin is clearly beneficial as prophylaxis for recurrent coronary ischemic events. Multiple studies in post-MI populations show roughly an 8% reduction in mortality and a 23% reduction in recurrent infarction [75]. Based on multiple studies [75], aspirin is recommended after coronary artery bypass surgery to maintain graft patency, with treatment instituted within two days postoperatively and continued for life. Enteric coated aspirin preparations are less likely to cause gastric irritation and are safer in the elderly. Side effects are dose related. Current evidence suggests that as preventive therapy for coronary ischemic events, low doses (80 to 325 mg/day) are as effective as high doses. Therefore, we recomend 325 mg of enteric coated aspirin at least every other day for primary and secondary prevention of coronary ischemic events.

Other antiplatelet and anticoagulant medications have been extensively evaluated for primary and secondary prevention of coronary and cerebral ischemic events. Dipyridimole has had inconsistent effects and appears to offer no clear benefit over aspirin alone [75,78]. In addition, side effects from dipyridimole are common in the elderly. One second-generation platelet-active agent, ticlopidine, has been shown to prevent nonfatal stroke or death in patients with cerebrovascular disease [79]. Although warfarin therapy is not considered standard therapy for patients with stable ischemic heart disease, long-term anticoagulant therapy has been shown to reduce reinfarction in some elderly patients after MI [80]. However, due to the significantly increased risk of hemorrhagic complications with anticoagulants such as warfarin, these agents currently have a minor role in preventive therapy, except in patients at risk for thromboembolic events (i.e., atrial fibrillation, mitral valvular disease, or cardiomyopathy).

Lipid-lowering medications

While lipid interventions cannot be recommended with the same degree of enthusiasm in elderly persons as in young or middle-aged adults, many carefully selected elderly patients may benefit from such therapy. Other modifiable risk factors such as tobacco use, obesity, and hypertension should be addressed initially. Current data from large-scale trials [81–83] in middle-aged adults show that a minimum of 5 to 10 years of lipid intervention is required to significantly alter the morbidity and mortality associated with CAD. Therefore, an elderly candidate for lipid intervention should have a projected lifespan of at least that length of time, if not more. It may be that very aggressive lipid intervention aimed at both LDL-C and HDL-C can reduce cardiac events more rapidly, as has been shown in younger patients, but this awaits confirmation in the elderly. An additional consideration is maintenance of quality of life. An active, robust person has more to gain from such therapy than someone who is sedentary. Because the correlation between total cholesterol and CAD diminishes with aging, lipid interventions should be tailored to the patient's lipid profile, including HDL-C, LDL-C, and triglycerides, which, as described elsewhere, are closely correlated with CAD in the elderly.

While the National Cholesterol Education Program [84] has provided clear guidelines for the treatment of high blood cholesterol in young and middle-aged adults, there are no such guidelines for elderly persons (over age 60 years) due to the lack of clinical data. Dietary therapy is most easily tolerated, and therefore initial intervention in elderly patients at risk for or with documented CAD should be a vigorous nonpharmacologic approach, including implementation of a step-one diet as detailed by the American Heart Association [85]. A step-two diet is more restrictive of saturated fatty acid and cholesterol intake and can be adopted if three or more months of a step-one diet fail to produce the desired results. Increasing dietary intake of soluble fiber (e.g., oat bran and psyllium) can reduce total cholesterol and LDL-C, and should be considered an extension of other dietary measures. Additional benefits of increased fiber intake in the elderly are reduced risk of colon cancer and maintenance of bowel regularity in a population predisposed to constipation. While detailed analysis is beyond the scope of this chapter, it should be emphasized that the elderly need a nutritionally balanced diet, and care should be taken to provide this within the bounds of these measures. At least six months of dietary therapy should be adhered to before more aggressive lipid-modifying therapy is recommended [15]. Although the prescription of vigorous nonpharmacologic therapy is unusual in the elderly, we have recently demonstrated that such therapy is equally beneficial in elderly and young persons for improving coronary risk factors and functional capacity [86,87].

Pharmacologic lipid intervention in the elderly must be weighed carefully because the risk-to-benefit ratio may be less than it is in younger persons over the long term. These measures are applied with the knowledge that there is no documentation of benefit in the elderly but with the reasoning that the dramatic benefits observed in middle-aged adults may be extrapolated to certain carefully chosen older individuals. Since the prevalence of CAD is much higher in the elderly than in younger groups, even greater benefits may be produced when vigorous lipid intervention is applied to this age group. Good therapeutic choices for reduction of LDL-C in the elderly include low doses of bile acid sequestrants or hydroxymethylglutaryl-coenzyme A (HmG CoA) reductase inhibitors (table 12-3). Lower doses initially will help to avoid drug toxicity, and progressively increased doses of each agent can follow as necessary [16]. Because HDL-C cholesterol has such a major influence on CAD in the elderly, it is possible that elevation of HDL-C may retard the progression of disease, as suggested in several trials [81,83,88]. Agents known to impact favorably on HDL-C include nicotinic acid, gemfibrozil, and HmG CoA reductase inhibitors which may be associated with hepatotoxicity as well and with other side effects (table 12-3). [13]. Gemfibrozil and niacin have also been shown to substantially lower serum triglycerides, which are particularly of concern in older women.

REVASCULARIZATION THERAPY
Detailed discussion of revascularization strategies and their application in the elderly is provided elsewhere in this text. Indications for coronary artery

Table 12-3. Drug therapy for lipid disorders*

Drug	Daily Dose (g)	Frequency	Effect on				Adverse Effects
			Cholesterol	Triglycerides	LDL-C	HDL-C	
Cholestyramine	12–24	BID	↓	N↑	↓	N↑	Taste, bloating, nausea, gout, constipation, diarrhea
Colestipol	15–30	BID	↓	N↑	↓	N↑	As above
Nicotinic acid	1.5–6	TID	↓	↓	↓	↑↑	Pruritis, flushing, GI upset, glucose intolerence, gout, rash, dizziness, liver dysfunction, atrial arrhythmias
Gemfibrozil	600–1200	BID	↓	↓	↓	↑	Myositis, cholelithiasis, GI upset
Probucol	0.5–1	BID	↓↑	N→	N↓	↓→	Diarrhea, prolonged QT, GI upset
Eicosapentaenoic acid (fish oil)	1–8	BID	↑↓	↓	↓	N↑	Weight gain, immune dysfunction
Lovastatin	20–80 mg	QD, BID	↓	N↓	↓	N↑	Liver dysfunction, myositis
Pravastatin	20–80 mg	QD	↓	N↓	↓	N↑	As above
Simvastatin	5–40 mg	QD	↓	N↓	↓	↑	As above

*adapted with permission from Lavie et al, Mayo Clin Proc 1988;63:613.

bypass surgery become more stringent in the elderly because prolongation of life is not an indication for the procedure in many patients. Instead, reducing the severity of symptoms and maintaining quality of life are the major issues. The risks of coronary artery bypass surgery are certainly greater in the elderly. Operative mortality in patients younger than age 60 is roughly 1% to 2%, compared to an operative mortality of roughly 9% in patients older than age 70. Because of the increasing surgical mortality associated with coronary artery bypass surgery in patients older than age 70, angioplasty, when possible, should be considered the revascularization procedure of choice in such patients [89].

SUMMARY

The elderly are a population at proportionately increased risk for CAD. Aging itself imposes an impressive risk for CAD development. In addition, most of the risk factors for CAD initially discovered in younger persons have recently been confirmed as risk factors in the elderly. Not only are a significant number of these modifiable, but also risk-factor modification produces clear reductions in morbidity and mortality. While elderly patients continue to pose a diagnostic challenge, the therapeutic armamentarium available to treat CAD in the elderly continues to grow. Enthusiasm for treatment must be tempered with practical considerations such as life expectancy and the preservation of quality of life.

REFERENCES

1. National Center for Health Statistics. 1987. 1986 Summary: National Hospital Discharge Survey. Advance Data from Vital and Health Statistics. No. 145. Hyattsville, MD: Public Health Service, p 6 (DHHS Publication No. PHS 87–1250).
2. Pifer A and Bronte L. 1986. Squaring the pyramid. In A Pifer and L Bronte (eds), Our Aging Society. New York: W. W. Norton, pp 3–13.
3. Kapantais G and Powell-Griner E. 1989. Characteristics of Persons Dying of Diseases of the Heart: Preliminary Data from the 1986 National Mortality Follow-up Survey. Hyattsville, MD: National Center for Health Statistics; Advance Data, p 172.
4. Goldberg RJ, Gore JM, Gurwitz JH, et al. 1989. The impact of age on the incidence and prognosis of initial acute myocardial infarction: the Worcester Heart Attack Study. Am Heart J 117:543–549.
5. Statson WB, Sanders CA and Smith HC. 1987. Cardiovascular care of the elderly: economic considerations. J Am Coll Cardiol 10:18A–21A.
6. Doyle TR. 1980. Incidence of coronary heart disease, stroke, and peripheral vascular disease. In TR Dawber (ed), The Framingham Study: The Epidemiology of Atherosclerotic Disease. Cambridge, MA: Harvard University Press, pp 59–76.
7. Gordon T, Castelli WP, Hjortland MC, et al. 1977. Predicting coronary heart disease in the middle-aged and older persons. The Framingham Study. JAMA 238:497–499.
8. Kennedy RD, Andrews GR and Caird FI. 1977. Ischaemic heart disease in the elderly. Br Heart J 39:1121–1127.
9. Castelli WP, Wilson PW, Levy D, et al. 1989. Cardiovascular risk factors in the elderly. Am J Cardiol 63:12H–19H.
10. Amery A, Birkenhager W, Brixko P, et al. 1985. Mortality and morbidity results from the European Working Party on High Blood Pressure in the Elderly trial. Lancet 1:1349–1354.
11. SHEP Cooperative Research Group. 1991. Prevention of stroke by antihypertensive drug treatment in older persons with isolated systolic hypertension. JAMA 265:3255–3264.

12. Assmann G and Schulte H. 1989. Diabetes mellitus and hypertension in the elderly: concomitant hyperlipidemia and coronary heart disease risk. Am J Cardiol 63:33H–37H.
13. Lavie CJ, Gau GT, Squires RW, et al. 1988. Management of lipids in primary and secondary prevention of cardiovascular diseases. Mayo Clin Proc 63:605–621.
14. Lavie CJ, O'Keefe JH, Blonde L, et al. 1990. High-density lipoprotein cholesterol. Recommendations for routine testing and treatment. Postgrad Med 87:36–44,47,51.
15. Denke MA and Grundy SM. 1990. Hypercholesterolemia in elderly persons: resolving the treatment dilemma. Ann Intern Med 112:780–792.
16. Gordon T, Castelli WP, Hjortland MC, et al. 1977. High density lipoprotein as a protective factor against coronary heart disease. The Framingham Study. Am J Med 62:707–714.
17. Lavie CJ and Milani RV. 1991. National Cholesterol Education Program's recommendations, and implications of "missing" high-density lipoprotein cholesterol in cardiac rehabilitation programs. Am J Cardiol 68:1087–1088.
18. Criqui M, Heiss G, Cohn R, et al. 1987. Triglycerides and coronary heart disease mortality. The Lipid Research Clinics Follow-up Study (abstract). CVD Epidemiol News 41:13.
19. Rubin SM, Sidney S, Black DM, et al. 1990. High blood cholesterol in elderly men and the excess risk for coronary heart disease. Ann Intern Med 113:916–920.
20. Blankenhorn DH, Nessim SA, Johnson RL, et al. 1987. Beneficial effects of combined colestipol-niacin therapy on coronary atherosclerosis and coronary venous bypass grafts. Circulation 69:3233–3240.
21. Levy RI, Brensike JF, Epstein SE, et al. 1984. The influence of changes in lipid values induced by cholestyramine and diet on progression of coronary heart disease: results of the NHLBI Type II Coronary Intervention Study. Circulation 69:325–337.
22. Lipid Research Clinics Program. 1984. The lipid research clinics coronary primary prevention trial results: I. Reduction in the incidence of coronary heart disease. JAMA 251:351–364.
23. Lipid Research Clinics Program. 1984. The lipid research clinics coronary primary prevention trial results: II. Reduction in the incidence of coronary heart disease. JAMA 251:365–374.
24. Dayton S, Pearce ML, Hashimoto S, et al. 1969. A controlled clinical trial of a diet high in unsaturated fat: in preventing the complication of atherosclerosis. Circulation (Suppl II): II-1–II-63.
25. Levy D, Garrison RJ, Savage DD, et al. 1989. Left ventricular mass and incidence of coronary heart disease in an elderly cohort. The Framingham Heart Study. Ann Intern Med 110:101–107.
26. Rothbaum DA. 1981. Coronary artery disease. Cardiovasc Clin 12:105–118.
27. Hamby RI, Hamby B and Hoffman I. 1986. Symptomatic coronary disease for 20 or more years: clinical aspects, angiographic findings, and therapeutic implications. Am Heart J 112:65–70.
28. Pathy MS. 1967. Clinical presentation of myocardial infarction in the elderly. Br Heart J 29:190–199.
29. Labovitz A et al. 1984. Mechanical complications of acute myocardial infarction. Cardiovasc Rev Rep 5:948.
30. Kannel WB, Dannenberg AL and Abbot RD. 1985. Unrecognized myocardial infarction and hypertension: The Framingham Study. Am Heart J 109:581–585.
31. Chambers BR, Norris JW. 1986. Outcome in patients with asymptomatic neck bruits. N Engl J Med 315:860–865.
32. Olbrich O and Woodford-Williams E. 1953. Normal precordial electrocardiogram in aged. J Gerontol 8:40–55.
33. Campbell A, Caird FI and Jackson TFM. 1974. Prevalence of abnormalities of electrocardiogram in old people. Br Heart J 36:1005–1011.
34. Vasilomanolakis E, Damian A, Mahan G, et al. 1984. Treadmill stress testing in geriatric patients (abstract). J Am Coll Cardiol 3:520.
35. Lavie CJ, Ventura HO and Murgo JP. 1991. Assessment of stable ischemic heart disease. Which tests for which patients? Postgrad Med 89:44–50,57–60,63.
36. Coyne E, Belveder D, Streek P, et al. 1991. Thallium-201 scintigraphy after intravenous infusion of adenosine compared with thallium testing in the diagnosis of coronary artery disease. J Am Coll Cardiol 17:1289–1294.

37. The Norwegian Multicenter Study Group. 1981. Timolol-induced reduction in mortality and reinfarction in patients surviving acute myocardial infarction. N Engl J Med 304:801–807.
38. Hjalmarson Å, Herlitz J, Málek I, et al. 1981. Effect on mortality of metoprolol in acute myocardial infarction: a double-blind randomized trial. Lancet 2:823–827.
39. ß-blocker Heart Attack Study Group. 1981. The ß-blocker Heart Attack Trial. JAMA 246:2073–2074.
40. Lichstein E, Hager WD, Gregory JJ, et al. 1990. Relation between beta-adrenergic blocker use, various correlates of left ventricular function and the chance of developing congestive heart failure. The Multicenter Dilitazem Post-Infarction Research Group. J Am Coll Cardiol 16:1327–1332.
41. Staessen J, Fagard R, Van Hoof R, et al. 1988. Mortality in various intervention trials in elderly hypertensive patients: a review. Eur Heart J 9:215–222.
42. Wikstrand J, Warnold I, Tuomilehto J, et al. 1991. Metoprolol versus thiazide duretics in hypertension. Morbidity results from the MAPHY Study. Hypertension 17:579–588.
43. Olsson G, Tuomilehto J, Berglund G, et al. 1991. Primary prevention of sudden cardiovascular death in hypertensive patients. Mortality results from the MAPHY Study. Am J Hypertens 4(2, Part 1):151–158.
44. Feely J, Wilkinson GR and Wood AJJ. 1981. Reduction of liver flow and propranolol metabolism by cimetidine. N Engl J Med 304:692–695.
45. Chiariello M, Volpe M, Rengo F, et al. 1979. Effect of furosemide on plasma concentration and ß-blockade by propranolol. Clin Pharmacol Ther 26:433–436.
46. McLean AJ, Skews H, Bobik A, et al. 1980. Interaction between oral propranolol and hydralazine. Clin Pharmacol Ther 27:726–732.
47. Pieper JA. 1984. Serum protein binding interactions between propranolol and calcium channel blockers (abstract). Drug Intell Clin Pharm 18:492.
48. Choong CY, Roubin GS, Harris PJ, et al. 1986. A comparison of the effects of beta-blockers with and without intrinsic sympathomimetic activity on hemodynamics and left ventricular function at rest and during exercise in patients with coronary artery disease. J Cardiovasc Pharmacol 8:441–448.
49. Griffin SJ and Freidman MJ. 1986. Depressive symptoms in propranolol users. J Clin Psychiatr 47:453–457.
50. Westerlund A. 1985. Central nervous system side-effects with hydrophilic and lipophilic beta blockers. Eur J Clin Pharmacol 28 (Suppl):73–76.
51. Greenblatt DJ and Koch-Weser J. 1973. Adverse reactions to propranolol in hospitalized medical patients: a report from the Boston Collaborative Drug Surveillance Program. Am Heart J 86:478–484.
52. Frishman WH, Charlap S, Kimmel B, et al. 1986. Calcium-channel blockers for combined angina pectoris and systemic hypertension. Am J Cardiol 57:22D–29D.
53. Abernethy DR, Schwartz JB, Todd EL, et al. 1986. Verapamil pharmacodynamics and disposition in young and elderly hypertensive patients. Altered electrocardiographic and hypotensive responses. Ann Intern Med 105:329–336.
54. Morselli P, Rovel V, Mitchard M, et al. 1979. Pharmacokinetics and metabolism of diltiazem on man (observations on healthy volunteers and angina pectoris patients). In RJ Bing (ed), New Drug Therapy With a Calcium Antagonist: Diltiazem. Hakone Symposium 1978. Amsterdam: Excerpta Medica, pp 152–167.
55. The Israeli SPRINT Study Group. 1988. Secondary Prevention Reinfarction Israeli Nifedipine Trial (SPRINT). A randomized intervention trial of nifedipine in patients with acute myocardial infarction. Eur Heart J 9:354–364.
56. Lavie CJ and Gersh BJ. 1990. Acute myocardial infarction: initial manifestations, management, and prognosis. Mayo Clin Proc 65:531–548.
57. Lavie CJ, Murphy JG and Gersh BJ. 1988. The role of beta-receptor and calcium-entry-blocking agents in acute myocardial infarction in the thrombolytic era: can the results of thrombolytic reperfusion be enhanced? (Editorial.) Cardiovasc Drugs Ther 2:601–607.
58. Elkayam U, Amin J, Mehra A, et al. 1990. A prospective, randomized, double-blind, crossover study to compare the efficacy and safety of chronic nifedipine therapy with that of isosorbide dinitrate and their combination in the treatment of chronic congestive heart failure. Circulation 82:1954–1961.

59. The Multicenter Diltiazem Postinfarction Trial Research Group. 1988. The effect of diltiazem on mortality and reinfarction after myocardial infarction. N Engl J Med 319: 385–392.
60. Danish Study Group on Verapamil in Myocardial Infarction. 1990. Secondary prevention with verapamil after myocardial infarction. Am J Cardiol 66:331–401.
61. Gibson RS, Boden WE, Theroux P, et al. 1986. Diltiazem and reinfarction in patients with non-Q-wave myocardial infarction. Results of a double-blind, randomized trial. N Engl J Med 315:423–429.
62. The Danish Study Group on Verapamil in Myocardial Infarction. 1990. Effect of verapamil on mortality and major events after acute myocardial infarction. (The Danish Verapamil Infarction Trial II—DAVIT II.) Am J Cardiol 66:779–785.
63. Lavie CJ, Ventura HO and Messerli FH. 1991. Regression of increased left ventricular mass by antihypertensives. Drugs 42:945–961.
64. Lavie CJ, Milani RV and Messerli FH. 1991. How antihypertensives affect lipid levels. Intern Med 12:36–46.
65. Messerli FH, Nunez BD, Nunez MM, et al. 1989. Hypertension and sudden death. Disparate effects of calcium entry blocker and diuretic therapy on cardiac dysrhythmias. Arch Intern Med 149:1263–1267.
66. Marchionni N, Schneeweiss A, Di Bari M, et al. 1988. Age-related hemodynamic effects of intravenous nitroglycerin for acute myocardial infarction and left ventricular failure. Am J Cardiol 61:81E–83E.
67. Reisen LH, Landau E, Darawshi A. 1988. More rapid relief of pain with isosorbide dinitrate oral spray than with sublingual tablets in elderly patients with angina pectoris. Am J Cardiol 61:2E–3E.
68. Come PC and Pitt B. 1976. Nitroglycerin-induced severe hypotension and bradycardia in patients with acute myocardial infarction. Circulation 54:624–628.
69. Lavie CJ and Gersh BJ. 1990. Mechanical and electrical complications of acute myocardial infarction. Mayo Clin Proc 65:709–730.
70. Herrick JB. 1912. Certain clinical features of sudden obstruction of the coronary arteries. Trans Assoc Am Phys 27:100.
71. Sherman CT, Litvack F, Grunfest W, et al. 1986. Coronary angioscopy in patients with unstable angina pectoris. N Engl J Med 315:913–919.
72. DeWood MA, Spores J, Notske R, et al. 1980. Prevalence of total coronary occlusion during the early hours of transmural myocardial infarction. N Engl J Med 303:897–902.
73. Davies MJ and Thomas A. 1984. Thrombosis and acute coronary-artery lesions in sudden cardiac ischemic death. N Engl J Med 310:1137–1140.
74. White C, Ramee S, Mesa J, et al. 1990. Percutaneous coronary angioscopy in stable and unstable angina. Circulation 82 (Suppl III):III-677.
75. Lavie CJ and Genton E. 1991. Hemostasis, thrombosis, and antiplatelet therapy: implications for prevention of cardiovascular diseases. Cardiovasc Rev Rep 12:24–44.
76. Steering Committee of the Physicians' Health Study Research Group. 1989. Final report on the aspirin component of the ongoing physicians health study. N Engl J Med 321:129–135.
77. Peto R, Gray R, Collins R, et al. 1988. Randomised trial of prophylactic daily aspirin in British male doctors. Br Med J 296:313–316.
78. Klimt CR, Knatterud GL, Stamler J, et al. 1986. Persantine-aspirin Reinfarction Study. Part II. Secondary coronary prevention with persantine and aspirin. J Am Coll Cardiol 7: 251–269.
79. McTavish D, Faulds D and Goa KL. 1990. Ticlodipine. An updated review of its pharmacology and therapeutic use in platelet-dependent disorders. Drugs 40:238–259.
80. A double-blind trial to assess long-term oral anticoagulant therapy in elderly patients after myocardial infarction. Report of the sixty plus Reinfarction Study Research Group. 1980. Lancet 1:989–993.
81. Brown G, Albers JJ, Fisher LD, et al. 1990. Regression of coronary artery disease as a result of intensive lipid-lowering therapy in men with high levels of apolipoprotein B. N Engl J Med 323:1289–1298.
82. Cashin-Hemphill L, Mack WJ, Pogoda JM, et al. 1990. Beneficial effects of colestipol-niacin on coronary atherosclerosis. A 4-year follow-up. JAMA 264:3013–3017.

83. Buchwald H, Varco RL, Matts JP, et al. 1990. Effect of partial ileal bypass surgery on mortality and morbidity from coronary heart disease in patients with hypercholesterolemia. Report of the Program on the Surgical Control of the Hyperlipidemias (POSCH). N Engl J Med 323:946–955.

84. The Expert Panel. 1988. Report of the National Cholesterol Education Program on Detection, Evaluation, and Treatment of High Blood Cholesterol in Adults. Arch Intern Med 148:36–69.

85. O'Keefe J, Lavie CJ and O'Keefe J. 1989. Dietary prevention of coronary artery disease. Postgrad Med 85:243–261.

86. Milani R and Lavie C. 1991. Benefits of secondary coronary prevention in the elderly (abstract). Circulation 84 (Suppl II):II-221.

87. Lavie CJ and Milani RV. 1991. Benefits of cardiac rehabilitation and exercise training in the elderly (abstract). J Am Coll Cardiol 19:377A.

88. Frick MH, Elo O, Haapa K, et al. 1987. Helsinki Heart Study: primary-prevention trial with gemfibrozil in middle-aged men with dyslipidemia: safety of treatment, changes in risk factors, and incidence of coronary heart disease. N Engl J Med 317:1237–1245.

89. DeBakey ME. 1989. Surgical treatment of atherosclerotic heart disease. Am J Cardiol 63:9H–11H.

13. ACUTE MYOCARDIAL INFARCTION

NOBLE O. FOWLER

Who are the elderly? They are generally considered to be those beyond middle age—which is currently often defined as being between 40 and 60 years. Most medical writings on coronary artery disease consider the elderly to be those either beyond 65 years or beyond 70 years. Thus, for this writing, we shall use these same criteria in order to provide suitable literature citations. Two recent papers [1,2] have pointed out that in convalescent patients with cardiac infarction over age 75, death is often due to an ischemic event. These papers urge that these older patients also receive consideration for coronary revascularization procedures when indicated by symptoms and noninvasive studies.

In the United States, approximately 1.3 million people per year suffer from acute myocardial infarction [3]. Although many die outside hospitals, and some recover without treatment, a large number reach hospitals for diagnosis and treatment. In 1987, approximately 750,000 patients with acute myocardial infarction were admitted to hospitals in the United States [4]. Of these, what proportion of patients may be defined as elderly? In a one-year study at Baptist Memorial Hospital in Memphis [5], 50 patients with acute infarction were under 65 years of age and 55 were over 65 years of age. In another hospital study, among survivors of acute infarction who did not have

Franz H. Messerli (ed.), CARDIOVASCULAR DISEASE IN THE ELDERLY (Third Edition). Copyright © 1993 Kluwer Academic Publishers. ISBN 0-7923-1859-5. All rights reserved.

a revascularization procedure, 111 were older than 65 years, and 133 were between 55 and 65 years [6]. In a study at University Hospitals of Cleveland, 225 patients had definite evidence of acute infarction in 1970; of these, 83 were over age 70, 81 were between ages 31 and 60, and 61 were between ages 61 and 70 years [7]. Thus, elderly patients comprise 50% or more of patients hospitalized for acute myocardial infarction.

This chapter will examine a number of aspects of the diagnosis and treatment of acute cardiac infarction in elderly patients. The presenting symptoms in elderly patients should be carefully evaluated, since they may be atypical. The acute care of myocardial infarction in elderly patients may need modification, since prognostic outlook and tolerance of medications are different; the usual indications for acute interventions may need reconsideration. Indications for in-hospital exercise testing, predischarge ECG monitoring, coronary arteriography, and myocardial revascularization procedures may be different in elderly patients. Long-term management of the postinfarction patient needs evaluation as well, since the elderly patient might have different tolerance for beta-adrenergic blocking drugs, which are now generally recommended for postinfarction patients. Certain secondary preventive measures, such as dietary modifications or cessation of smoking, may be less cogent in the elderly. The risks and benefits of myocardial revascularization procedures for postinfarction angina in elderly patients need consideration. The usefulness of rehabilitation programs for elderly patients must be evaluated.

PATHOGENESIS

The great majority of patients with acute cardiac infarction have fixed obstructive coronary arterial lesions. Although as many as 17% to 45% of patients younger than age 36 with acute infarction lack fixed lesions on follow-up coronary arteriographic study [8], this percentage decreases with advancing age. The absence of fixed lesions in elderly patients is exceptional. Current studies of all patients during the first few hours of acute infarction show that 80% to 90% also have acute thrombotic lesions superimposed upon fixed lesions [9].

PRESENTING FEATURES

A previous history of angina pectoris (50% vs. 44%) or congestive heart failure (23% vs. 14%) was more common in patients over age 75 than in those aged 65 to 75 [1]. A history of previous infarction was present in 33% of both groups [1]. It is generally believed that the presenting features of acute cardiac infarction in the elderly are more likely to be atypical than in younger patients. The Framingham Study reported that in an active general population, 10% of acute infarctions were painless and another 10% were associated with atypical symptoms [10]. One study of 387 patients over age 65 found typical symptoms in only 75 patients; 77 had instead sudden dyspnea or exacerbation of heart failure [11]. In a study of 52 patients over age 60 with myocardial infarction, Rodstein [12] found silent infarctions in 16 aged 71 to 90 years and atypical symptoms in 21 aged 71 to 90 years. A recent hospital study [5] reported atypical pain or no pain in 38% of patients over 65, compared to only 4% of patients under 65. MacDonald [13] found that 90% of elderly patients with acute infarction had as presenting features either chest pain, breathlessness, or syncope. Chest pain was present in 55% to 64%% of patients in review of four series, and was less likely with increasing age. Tinker [14], in a study of 87 patients older than 65 years with acute infarction, found that 51 had either classical chest pain or tightness. Nineteen presented with dyspnea or exacerbation of heart failure. Six presented with stroke, four with syncope, three with giddiness, two with weakness, and one with confusion. One of the 87 had a "silent" infarction.

DIAGNOSIS

The diagnosis of acute myocardial infarction in the elderly is based upon the same three criteria used in other age groups. These are the history, the electrocardiogram, and changes in myocardial serum enzymes. At least two of these three criteria should be present. Q-wave infarctions are diagnosed from the electrocardiogram when there is an evolving pattern of pathologic Q-waves associated with typical S-T segment and T-wave changes of myocardial injury and ischemia. Non-Q-wave infarctions are diagnosed when there are S-T- and/or T-changes of myocardial injury or ischemia plus typical changes in serum enzymes. Additional aid may be obtained from nuclear scintigraphy, which may show increased myocardial uptake of technetium-99m pyrophosphate during the period 2 to 5 days after the infarction. In addition, thallium[201] scanning usually shows decreased myocardial uptake of the radioisotope in the ischemic area, especially when made 12 to 24 hours after the onset of symptoms. Certain aspects of the diagnostic criteria may be modified in elderly patients with acute cardiac infarction. The historical features were commented upon in the preceding paragraph. Serum enzyme changes in the elderly following acute infarction follow the same pattern as in younger patients: serum CPK and SGOT values rise within 6 to 8 hours of onset, with values exceeding the control by 100% or more within 24 to 48 hours (see figure 13-1). CPK-MB isoenzyme values should exceed 4% of the total rise in CPK; a rise in total CPK without a significant rise in CPK-MB may be owing to skeletal muscle damage, including intramuscular injection of medications. Of note, the typical electrocardiogram (ECG) changes of infarction are less frequent in elderly patients (5). Applegate et al. [5] found typical QRS changes in only 47% of patients over age 65, but in 72% of those under age 65. This is owing, at least in part, to the fact that as many as 50% of patients over age 65 have abnormal baseline ECGs. Furthermore, a larger number of elderly patients have had a prior infarction, the ECG changes of which may tend to obscure the Q-waves and S-T- and T-changes of a fresh infarction.

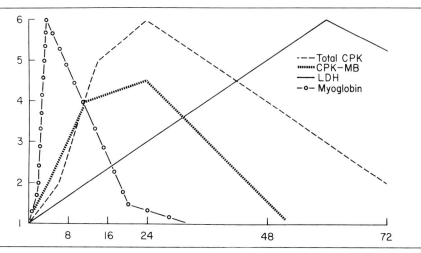

Figure 13-1. Changes in serum enzymes and serum myoglobin following acute cardiac infarction. Horizontal axis = time elapsed from onset of pain; vertical axis = multiples of normal value. (Courtesy Dr. Evan A. Stein, Assistant Professor of Medicine and Pathology, University of Cincinnati Medical Center.)

PROGNOSIS

The in-hospital mortality rate for acute infarction in elderly patients is higher than in younger patients. Two studies reported in the 1970s [15,16] described mortality rates of 27% to 40% for patients over age 70 with acute infarction. This was twice the mortality rate for younger patients. Kincaid and Botti [7] found a mortality rate of 27% in patients over age 80, compared to an overall mortality rate of 15% in patients with acute infarction. Applegate et al. [5] reported a hospital mortality rate of 16% in patients over age 65 and of only 4% in patients under age 65. Peterson et al. [17] found an in-hospital mortality rate of 12% for patients under age 60 and of greater than 50% for acute infarction patients over 80 years of age.

In part, the greater mortality in older patients is due to more frequent and more severe complications (see table 13-1). Applegate et al.]5] found congestive heart failure in 44% of patients with acute infarction who were over age 65 and in 16% of those under age 65. In a long-term evaluation, Kitchin and Milne [18] found a five-year mortality rate of 67% for those ages 70 to 79 years old and 74% for those over age 80. In a more recent analysis, Smith et al. [1] reported an in-hospital death rate of 19.9% in patients over age 75, compared with a death rate of 12.2% for patients between ages 65 and 75 ($p < 0.01$). In the present era of thrombolytic therapy, reported mortality rates are generally lower, but the age-related differential in mortality rate probably still exists.

Prognosis may be more precise when certain observations are made during

Table 13-1. Effects of age on complications of acute myocardial infarction (%)[a]

Complication	Age < 70	Age > 70
Pulmonary edema	52	74
Cardiogenic shock	15	25
Congestive cardiac failure	8	22
Pericarditis	11	9
Heart block and conduction disturbances	21	35
Atrial flutter or fibrillation	8	14
Ventricular fibrillation	6	4
Hospital stay	26	31
Hospital mortality	17	39

[a] Adapted from Williams BO, Begg TB, Semple T, et al. 1976. The elderly in a coronary unit. Br Med J 2:451–453. Used with permission.

hospitalization. For example, Green et al. [19] studied 36 patients over age 70 with acute cardiac infarction. A left ventricular ejection fraction (MUGA scan) below 30% was predictive of an increased mortality rate. Long-term prognosis may be evaluated more accurately by the ability to perform an exercise test before hospital discharge. Deckers et al. [20] studied 159 patients over 65 years of age. Those ineligible for a stress test had a one-year mortality rate of 37%, whereas those able to perform an exercise test had a one-year mortality rate of only 4%. The latter figure was comparable to a 6% one-year mortality rate in patients age 55 to 64 who were able to perform a stress test. Patients were ineligible for a stress test for various reasons: congestive heart failure, angina pectoris, peripheral vascular disease, cerebrovascular disease, or poor general condition.

TREATMENT

The goals of treatment of acute myocardial infarction are several. These include relief of symptoms, observation in a coronary care monitoring unit for prompt recognition and treatment of complications, reduction in mortality rate, reduction of infarct size and preservation of myocardial function, maintenance of an acceptable quality of life, and prevention of recurrences.

The treatment of acute myocardial infarction in the 65- to 75-year age group is similar to that in younger patients. In patients over age 75, some modifications may be required, especially with regard to use of thrombolytic agents, lower tolerance for certain drugs, and the presence of associated diseases. The American College of Cardiology and the American Heart Association (ACC/AHA) jointly have recently published guidelines for the early management of acute myocardial infarction [4].

EARLY PHASE: THE FIRST SIX HOURS

During the first six hours of acute infarction, there are a number of important considerations. The patient should be hospitalized without delay in a coronary care unit with ECG monitoring. A tertiary care facility is especially to be recommended when there has been cardiac arrest, symptomatic bradycardia, ventricular tachyarrhythmia, or hypotension prior to hospitalization. In such a facility, cardiologists, cardiac surgeons, and high-technology procedures will be available. Kincaid and Botti [7] pointed out that cardiac monitoring continues to be valuable in detecting ventricular tachycardia in patients over age 70, many of whom can be resuscitated successfully.

Oxygen

Oxygen by nasal prongs, 2–4 L/min, is generally recommended for patients with acute ischemic pain, at least for the first few hours. This is continued if there is continued pain, congestive heart failure, or hypotension.

Intravenous line

An intravenous infusion of 5% dextrose in 1/2 normal saline is begun at a rate of 10 ml/h so as to be available for prompt administration of medications.

Pain relief

Nitroglycerin and morphine are the mainstays of pain relief. Sublingual nitroglycerin in doses of 0.2 to 0.4 mg is recommended for the treatment of acute ischemic pain. This dosage may be repeated if there is no relief within five minutes. Nitroglycerin should be avoided when systolic blood pressure is below 90 to 100 mmHg, when there is significant bradycardia or tachycardia, or when there is cerebrovascular disease. It may be hazardous in patients with right ventricular infarction. Elderly patients are more susceptible to the hypotensive effects of nitroglycerin. After the diagnosis of infarction is established, or with pain that does not respond to nitroglycerin, morphine is employed for pain relief in intravenous doses of 2 mg. Three doses at five-minute intervals may be used if needed. However, in elderly patients, morphine tolerance may be reduced. When pain is continuing and difficult to control, one may employ intravenous nitroglycerin, beginning at 10 μg/min and increasing by 5 μg/min every five minutes to a maximum of 200 μg/min. Systolic blood pressure should not fall below 90 mmHg, and pulse rate should not rise above 110 beats per minute. Long-acting oral nitrates are not recommended [4]. Usually intramuscular injections of medications are not used in order to avoid an effect upon serum CPK enzymes (vide supra).

Thrombolytic therapy

Eighty to ninety percent of patients with acute infarction who are studied by coronary arteriography within a few hours of onset are found to have an occlusive thrombus. Studies by Rentrop et al. [21] and Ganz et al. [22] in

1981 demonstrated that intracoronary infusion of streptokinase could lyse intracoronary clots and improve myocardial perfusion in the majority of patients treated within the first 4 to 6 hours of infarction. Both the Gruppo Italiano por lo Studio della Streptochinasi nell' Infarcto Miocardico (GISSI) trial [23] and the Second International Study of Infarct Survival (ISIS-2) trial [24] showed that thrombolysis produced significant improvement in early mortality rate (evaluated at 21 days for GISSI and five weeks for ISIS-2). Intravenous infusion of 1.5 million units of streptokinase was given within the first six hours of infarction in the GISSI trial and within the first 24 hours in ISIS-2. The improvement was still present at 12 months in the GISSI trial. At present the ACC/AHA guidelines recommend the use of thrombolytic therapy (either streptokinase or tissue plasminogen activator) in patients under 70 who present with chest pain consistent with acute infarction who have at least 1 mm S-T-segment elevation in at least two contiguous precordial ECG leads and in whom therapy can be started within six hours of pain onset. Patients up to 75 years of age are considered for thrombolytic therapy at our institution, and age greater than 75 is not a definite contraindication. Although with increasing age the risk of bleeding complications may be greater, the benefits appear to be maintained in patients over age 70. Contraindications to thrombolytic therapy include active internal bleeding, a hemorrhagic disorder, suspected aortic dissection, prolonged or traumatic cardiopulmonary resuscitation, recent head trauma, diabetic hemorrhagic retinopathy, pregnancy, previous allergic reaction to the thrombolytic agent, blood pressure >200/120 mmHg, or history of a hemorrhagic cerebrovascular accident. The merit of thrombolytic therapy in patients with non-Q-wave infarction is currently under investigation.

Anticoagulants

If there are no contraindications, patients are given oral aspirin 160–325 mg immediately and daily thereafter. Following the initiation of thrombolytic therapy, heparin is given intravenously; a bolus of 5000 units is followed by 600 to 800 units/per hour for 24 hours, maintaining the active partial thromboplastin time at 1.5 to 2 times control values. Intravenous heparin is continued until hospital discharge in patients with large Q-wave anterior infarcts. Intravenous heparin is also recommended for patients with non-Q-wave infarction. In patients not receiving intravenous heparin, subcutaneous heparin (5000 units every 12 hours) is recommended for patients over 70, or those with prior infarction, obesity, continued immobilization, or who have heart failure or shock. This is continued until the patient is fully ambulatory.

Beta-adrenergic blockade

The TIMI-II trial demonstrated a significant improvement in recurrent infarction or ischemia in patients with acute infarction given intravenous beta-blockers within a few hours of the onset of symptoms, as compared to a group in whom oral beta-blocker therapy was deferred until day 6 [25]. Patients received three 5-mg doses of atenolol intravenously at two-minute intervals and then 100 mg orally daily thereafter. Early intravenous beta-blocker therapy was recommended for patients with acute infarction and reflex tachycardia or systolic hypertension, those with tachyarrhythmias, and those with postinfarction angina while awaiting further study [4]. Contraindications to beta-blocker therapy include a heart rate below 55 to 60 beats per minute, systolic blood pressure below 100 mmHg, moderate to severe left ventricular failure (pulmonary rales extending over more than the lower third of the lungs), peripheral hypoperfusion, atrioventricular (A-V) conduction abnormalities (P-R interval >0.22 seconds, second- or third-degree A-V block), or severe chronic obstructive pulmonary disease. A history of bronchial asthma is a relative contraindication.

Lidocaine

In many institutions lidocaine is given intravenously to prevent ventricular arrhythmias in all patients with acute infarction who are not allergic to this drug. The dose used at our institution is 100 mg as an intravenous bolus, followed by 2 mg/min for the first few days. The ACC/AHA guidelines [4] recommend lidocaine in acute infarction only when there are definite indications, e.g. ventricular premature beats that exceed six per minute or are closely coupled, are multiform, or occur in bursts of three or more. The drug is also used in patients who have had ventricular tachycardia or fibrillation. The guidelines advise against using this agent in patients over age 70 without these indications. Elderly patients are more prone to respiratory center depression and central nervous system effects of lidocaine.

Coronary angioplasty

Coronary angioplasty is not considered to be a routine therapy for patients with acute infarction. It can be considered, when adequate facilities are available, in patients seen within six hours of onset of acute infarction in whom thrombolytic therapy is contraindicated, or in patients who present in cardiogenic shock. The procedure also may be considered in patients who are otherwise suitable and who have postinfarction angina. Angioplasty is not recommended as a routine treatment for patients who have undergone thrombolytic therapy and may actually increase patient risk. The TIMI-II trial showed no advantage in mortality rate or recurrent infarction within 42 days when angioplasty was performed routinely after thrombolysis in patients up to 75 years of age [25].

TREATMENT DURING THE FIRST SEVEN DAYS

In the first seven days of hospitalization of a patient with acute cardiac infarction, the emphasis is upon continuation of necessary medications begun during the first six hours and upon the prompt recognition and treatment of complications.

Coronary care unit ECG monitoring is carried out for the first 48 to 72 hours, and is prolonged beyond that time for such complications as continued ischemic pain, arrhythmia, or hemodynamic instability. Step-down unit monitoring may be continued for an additional 48 hours.

Anticoagulants

Therapy with intravenous or subcutaneous heparin is continued when indicated, as described previously. Oral aspirin, 160 to 325 mg per day, is used in all patients who tolerate it. Coumadin therapy maintaining the prothrombin time between 1.3 and 1.5 times control is recommended for patients with large Q-wave anterior infarcts, and for those with areas of dyskinesia or with mural thrombus demonstrated on echocardiography.

Beta-adrenergic blocking agents

In a review of seven randomized clinical trials of beta-blocking drugs in postinfarction patients, Frommer and Furberg [26] noted a 28% decrease in all-cause mortality over an average period of 12 to 25 months. Beta-adrenergic blocking agents have several effects that may tend to reduce the incidence of sudden death or recurrent myocardial infarction. Among these are reduction in cardiac work as the result of decreasing blood pressure and heart rate, intrinsic antiarrhythmic activity, and effects on platelet aggregation. Thus, oral therapy with beta-blocking agents, e.g. propranolol 180–240 mg daily or atenolol 50–100 mg daily, is begun 12 hours after onset of acute infarction in patients with no contraindications to beta–adrenergic blockade (vide supra). A possible exception to this recommendation is a low-risk patient who has had no complications, good residual left ventricular function, no angina or arrhythmia, and no evidence of ischemia on ECG stress testing. Hutchison and Campbell [27] reviewed the use of beta-blocking drugs in the elderly and concluded that the beneficial effect of beta-blockade after cardiac infarction is not altered in patients over age 65. The Timolol study [28] showed no greater incidence of side effects in the age group 65 to 75 than in younger patients. The value of beta–adrenergic blocking agents in non-Q-wave infarction is uncertain at this time.

Calcium-channel blocking agents (nifedipine, verapamil, and diltiazem)

Until recently there has been no evidence to support the routine use of calcium-channel blocking agents in the treatment of Q-wave infarctions. There is evidence to support their use after non-Q-wave infarction, beginning within 48 hours and continued for the first year postinfarction [4]. In selected patients under 76 years of age without heart failure or A-V block, and not receiving beta-blockers, administration of verapamil was found to reduce both death and reinfarction rates. Verapamil was started during the second week after infarction and continued up to 18 months [28a]. Calcium-channel blocking agents may be used in postinfarction angina patients awaiting coronary arteriography. Diltiazem, when used routinely in post-Q-wave infarction patients with an ejection fraction below 40%, may be associated with an increased incidence of late-onset heart failure [29].

Diet
Because of the risk of nausea and vomiting, a liquid diet is used for the first 24 to 36 hours. Afterward, a 1500-calorie diet without added salt is recommended.

Physical activity
After the first 24 hours, patients free of shock, hypotension, or continued ischemia should begin to sit in a chair at the bedside while ECG monitoring is continued. A bedside commode is preferable to a bedpan. For patients free of major complications, an instructional and rehabilitation program is begun after the first 24 to 48 hours. Patients free of major complications generally walk to their bathroom by the fourth day and begin to walk in the halls by the seventh day. Blood pressure and heart rate should be monitored to be certain that these activities are well tolerated.

MANAGEMENT OF COMPLICATIONS
Complications of acute cardiac infarction in the elderly are managed as in younger patients, with due consideration for the effect of age upon tolerance of various medications, e.g. morphine, lidocaine, and digitalis. Details of the management of all complications of acute myocardial infarction are beyond the scope of this presentation.

Swan–Ganz catheter placement
Balloon flotation right heart catheter placement and hemodynamic monitoring are recommended in patients with severe or progressive heart failure, hypotension not related to blood volume depletion, cardiogenic shock, or such mechanical complications as ventricular septal defect or papillary muscle rupture [4].

Temporary pacemakers
Temporary pacemakers are recommended for the following complications of acute myocardial infarction: asystole, complete A-V block, right bundle branch block with left anterior or left posterior hemiblock developing in acute myocardial infarction, left bundle branch block developing in acute myocardial infarction, Mobitz type II second-degree A-V block, and symptomatic bradycardia unresponsive to atropine [4].

Ventricular tachycardia

Sustained ventricular tachycardia is treated with an intravenous bolus of lidocaine, 1 mg/kg body weight, followed by an infusion of lidocaine in a dosage of 2 to 4 mg/min and a second bolus of 0.5 mg/kg body weight 10 to 20 minutes after the first. Patients who fail to respond are candidates for D.C. cardioversion. Elderly patients may have respiratory depression and cerebral effects of lidocaine, especially in doses above 2 mg/min. It may be desirable to measure blood levels after 12 hours of infusion.

Shock

Patients with shock who fail to respond to fluid challenge are given dobutamine or dopamine, 3–10 µg/kg/min intravenously, and may require intra-aortic balloon counterpulsation.

Congestive heart failure

Congestive heart failure is treated with sodium restriction and diuretics, e.g. furosemide 20 to 160 mg orally per day. Patients who fail to respond may require vasodilators, e.g. captopril 6.5 mg to 50 mg b.i.d. or t.i.d. Refractory heart failure may be an indication for Swan–Ganz catheter placement and the use of intravenous dopamine or dobutamine, 3–10 µg/kg body weight/min. Diastolic aortic balloon pumping may be necessary.

Atrial flutter and fibrillation

Atrial flutter or fibrillation is an indication for digitalization to control ventricular rate, e.g. with digoxin 0.75 to 1 mg as a loading dose in divided doses. Maintenance doses of digoxin may range from 0.125 mg to 0.5 mg daily, and serum levels should be evaluated. Digoxin should be employed with particular caution in the elderly, owing to the increased sensitivity of the ischemic myocardium to ventricular arrhythmias and to the reduced creatinine clearance usually found in the aged.

Major mechanical complications

Major mechanical complications, such as papillary muscle dysfunction or rupture with severe mitral incompetence, or ventricular septal rupture, should be considered for early operative repair, especially when complicated by shock, refractory heart failure, or pulmonary edema. Aortic balloon pumping may be useful temporarily and was employed preoperatively in the series reported by Weintraub et al. [30]. They described early operative repair of postinfarction ventricular septal defect in 12 patients aged 66 to 82 years. Seven were hospital survivors. The survivors were observed for 10 months to 7.5 years. One died suddenly after 7.5 years. Five were in NYHA class I and one was in class II. The authors concluded that the operation is worthwhile, since the two-month mortality rate with medical treatment was estimated to be 86%.

Coronary arteriography and cardiac surgical procedures

The principal indication for early coronary arteriography in the postinfarction elderly patient is persistent postinfarction angina. Coronary artery bypass grafting may be recommended for patients in whom coronary angioplasty cannot be done. Patients with non-Q-wave infarction (nontransmural infarction) should also be considered for angiography, especially those with ischemic changes in the distribution of the left anterior descending coronary artery, since they are likely to have a large area of healthy myocardium at risk. In these patients, elective operation is recommended if there is either left main or three-vessel disease. Operation is also recommended for two-vessel disease with significant proximal left anterior descending coronary disease or an ejection fraction below 40% [4]. In general, the risk of coronary artery bypass grafting in elderly patients is acceptable. Knapp et al. [31] reviewed their results in elderly patients who had disabling angina as an indication for coronary bypass. Forty-eight percent of their patients had had a prior infarction, 28% had abnormal Q-waves on electrocardiogram, 23% had cardiomegaly, and 83% had unstable angina pectoris. Of 121 patients over age 70, the in-hospital mortality rate for the procedure was 1.6%, as compared to 1.1% in 2850 patients under 70 years of age. The 36-month survival rate was 95% in both age groups. The authors concluded that patients over 70 need not be denied coronary bypass grafts because of their age, but extensive calcification of the ascending aorta was considered a relative contraindication for the procedure.

Although emergency coronary revascularization operations for acute evolving myocardial infarction have been carried out successfully during the first six hours, simultaneous randomized control studies were not done [32,33]. This procedure has not been shown superior to thrombolysis or angioplasty and cannot be recommended as a routine at present [4].

THE PREHOSPITAL DISCHARGE PERIOD (7–10 DAYS AFTER ONSET)

Most patients with uncomplicated infarction are considered for hospital discharge after 7 to 10 days. At this time the emphasis is upon evaluation of prognosis and whether or not early coronary arteriography is indicated. Long-term medications, such as anticoagulants and beta-blocking drugs, will be continued. At this time a 24-hour Holter ECG, a rate-limited ECG stress test, a radioisotope ventriculogram (MUGA scanning), and an echocardiogram should be considered.

MUGA scanning may be employed to identify patients with impaired left ventricular ejection fraction who have a poorer outlook. This study is recommended in postinfarction patients unless determination of ventricular function has been made by other means [4]. The increased risk of complications in postinfarction patients with an ejection fraction less than 40% suggests that coronary arteriography be considered in this group [36].

Heart-rate-limited ECG exercise tests also may be used just prior to hospital discharge (6 to 10 days postinfarction), using 100 to 120 beats per minute as the target heart rate. Exercise thallium[201] scintigraphy should be used when baseline ECG abnormalities compromise its interpretation. Those with angina or positive tests at a low level of exercise fall into a group with poor prognosis [34–36]. Failure to increase left ventricular ejection fraction by at least five units indicates an increased probability of complications after infarction [34]. As already described, patients unable to exercise at all fall into a group with very poor prognosis. Dipyridamole–thallium[201] scintigraphy may be considered in this group. Coronary arteriography may be recommended when these tests show evidence of ischemia, especially in the 65- to 75-year age group.

The 24-hour Holter ECG may be used to evaluated prognosis. This study should be done just prior to hospital discharge and not in the first 48 hours of infarction. Although ventricular ectopic activity is strongly associated with left ventricular dysfunction, it must be considered as an independent risk factor. Postinfarction patients with less than one premature beat per hour have a two-year mortality rate of less than 5% [4].

Patients with multiple premature ventricular contractions exceeding 10 per hour, those with ventricular couplets, and those with runs of ventricular tachycardia constitute a group with poor prognosis following infarction. Those with ≥10 ventricular premature beats per hour have a two-year mortality rate exceeding 20%. Although the value of intervention is not proved, this group may be considered for antiarrhythmic drugs or coronary arteriography. There is a risk of proarrhythmic effects with drug therapy, however, and treatment of asymptomatic or mildly symptomatic ventricular ectopic beats with encainide or flecainide may increase the death rate [37]. Since the Cardiac Arrhythmia Suppression Trial study, antiarrhythmic drugs are being used less frequently in this group. One may wish to consider an electrophysiologic study in patients with reduced left ventricular ejection fraction and bouts of ventricular tachycardia. Routine electrophysiologic testing is not recommended in myocardial infarction patients at this time.

Two-dimensional echocardiography

This study is principally recommended for detection or confirmation of suspected complications of infarction: myocardial rupture, aneurysm or pseudoaneurysm formation, infarct extension or expansion, mural thrombus, and right ventricular infarction. It may also be used to evaluate left ventricular function in predicting a low-risk subgroup for early ambulation [4].

CONVALESCENT PERIOD: SECOND THROUGH EIGHTH WEEKS POSTINFARCTION
During this period, the emphasis is upon evaluation of risk for future events, development of a satisfactory life-style, and prevention of recurrent infarction. Aspirin is continued indefinitely; beta-adrenergic blocking drugs are continued for at least two years unless they are contraindicated; coumadin is continued for three months or more when indicated (vide supra).

Long-term anticoagulant therapy
In the Netherlands, the effect of long-term oral anticoagulants (coumarin derivatives) was evaluated in a double-blind study of 578 postinfarction patients over 60 years of age [38]. The two-year mortality rate was 13.4% in the placebo group and 7.6% in the group receiving anticoagulants ($p <$ 0.017). Recurrent infarction took place in 58 patients in the placebo group and in 20 in the anticoagulant group ($p = 0.001$). Despite this encouraging study, the routine use of anticoagulants after cardiac infarction is not firmly established in the United States. Patients with a history of systemic or pulmonary embolism, congestive failure, atrial fibrillation, ventricular aneurysm, ventricular mural thrombi, or limited physical activity should be considered for such therapy. The risks must be weighed as well; as age increases, there is an increased danger of complications, especially intracranial bleeding.

Stress ECG
A late stress ECG (6 to 8 weeks postinfarction) is recommended to evaluate prognosis and to evaluate functional capacity. Exercise thallium[201] scintigraphy is recommended for those whose baseline ECG would render the interpretation of the stress ECG difficult. A dipyridamole–thallium[201] scintigram may be considered for those unable to exercise. When there is evidence of ischemia from one of these tests, coronary arteriography is recommended.

Kannel and McGee [39] discussed risk-factor modification in post-infarction patients. These modifications include control of hypertension, cessation of cigarette smoking, lowering of serum cholesterol levels through diet, exercise, and correction of obesity. Some of these measures are more applicable to elderly patients than others. Cessation of cigarette smoking and control of hypertension are usually readily achievable and have some likelihood of benefit in the shortened remaining life span of the elderly patient. On the other hand, extensive dietary modification is of less certain short-term benefit and may be unacceptable psychologically. Patients, especially those under age 70, with LDL cholesterol values of 160 mg or above, may be considered for lovastatin therapy if unresponsive to diet [40].

Physical exercise is to be encouraged in the postinfarction elderly patient as in other age groups. Williams et al. [41] recommend that cardiac rehabilitation programs be considered in elderly patients, since these programs improve physiologic capacity. Akman [42] also recommended an active rehabilitation program for elderly postinfarction patients. However, such a program should not be recommended routinely, and there is no convincing evidence that these programs improve survival. For those who do not wish to be participants in such programs, this author finds that a walking program beginning 6 to 8 weeks postinfarction is very satisfactory. Winter walking may be done in gymnasia or enclosed malls. Walking is begun with one block only at four weeks postinfarction and increased every few days, aiming for a goal of 2 to 4 miles daily as a rate of one mile in 20 minutes if tolerated. Exertional dyspnea, angina with minimum effort, gross cardiac enlargement, S_3 gallop rhythm, or congestive failure indicate patients who are not candidates for such active exercise programs.

Sexual activity

Both partners are often fearful of resuming sexual activity post-infarction. According to Marron [43], the general rule is to resume sexual activity three months after cardiac infarction. Earlier sexual activity could be considered in those without evidence of ischemia on exercise tests 6 to 8 weeks postinfarction. Approximately one third of elderly patients return to their previous level of sexual activity; the majority have a permanent reduction in sexual activity, and 10% abstain.

REFERENCES

1. Smith SC Jr, Gilpin E, Ahnve S, et al. 1990. Outlook after acute myocardial infarction in the very elderly compared with that in patients aged 65 to 75 years. J Am Coll Cardiol 16:784–792.
2. Adolph RJ. 1990. The elderly, the very elderly and traditional practice patterns (editorial comment). J Am Coll Cardiol 16:793–794.
3. Hillis LD and Braunwald E. 1977. Medical progress. Myocardial ischemia. N Engl J Med 296:971–980.
4. ACC/AHA Guidelines for the early management of patients with acute myocardial infarction. 1990. A report of the American College of Cardiology/American Heart Association Task Force on assessment of diagnostic and therapeutic cardiovascular procedures. Circulation 82:664–707.
5. Applegate WB, Graves S, Collins T, et al. 1984. Acute myocardial infarction in elderly patients. South Med J 77:1127–1129.
6. Fioretti P, Deckers JW, Brower RW, et al. 1984. Predischarge stress test after myocardial infarction in the old age: results and prognostic value. Eur Heart J 5 (Suppl E):101–104.
7. Kincaid DT Botti RE. 1973. Acute myocardial infarction in the elderly. Chest 64:170–172.
8. Glover MU, Kuber MT, Warren SE, et al. 1982. Myocardial infarction before age 36: risk factor and arteriographic analysis. Am J Cardiol 49:1600–1603.
9. Rentrop KP. 1985. Thrombolytic therapy in patients with acute myocardial infarction. Circulation 71:627–631.
10. Stokes J III and Dawber TR. 1959. The "silent coronary": the frequency and clinical characteristics of unrecognized myocardial infarction in the Framingham study. Ann Intern Med 50:1359–1369.

11. Pathy MS. 1967. Clinical presentation of myocardial infarction in the elderly. Br Heart J 29:190–199.
12. Rodstein M. 1956. The characteristics of nonfatal myocardial infarction in the aged. Arch Intern Med 98:84–90.
13. MacDonald JB. 1984. Presentation of acute myocardial infarction in the elderly—a review. Age Ageing 13:196–200.
14. Tinker GM. 1981. Clinical presentation of myocardial infarction in the elderly. Age Ageing 10:237–240.
15. Chaturvedi NC, Shivalingappa G, Shanks B, et al. 1972. Myocardial infarction in the elderly. Lancet 1:280–281.
16. Williams BO, Begg TB, Semple T, et al. 1976. The elderly in a coronary unit. Br Med J 2:451–453.
17. Peterson DR, Thompson DJ and Chinn N. 1972. Ischemic heart disease prognosis. A community-wide assessment (1966–1969). JAMA 219:1423–1427.
18. Kitchin AH and Milne JS. 1977. Longitudinal survey of ischaemic heart disease in randomly selected sample of older population. Br Heart J 39:889–893.
19. Green SJ, Ong LY, Reiser P, et al. 1985. The role of early radionuclide ejection fraction in predicting early mortality after acute myocardial infarction in the elderly. Mt Sinai J Med 52:618–622.
20. Deckers JW, Fioretti P, Brower RW, et al. 1984. Ineligibility for predischarge exercise testing after myocardial infarction in the elderly: implications for prognosis. Eur Heart J 5 (Suppl E):97–100.
21. Rentrop P, Blanke H, Karsch KR, et al. 1981. Selective intracoronary thrombolysis in acute myocardial infarction and unstable angina pectoris. Circulation 63:307–317.
22. Ganz W, Buchbinder N, Marcus H, et al. 1981. Intracoronary thrombolysis in evolving myocardial infarction. Am Heart J 101:4–13.
23. Gruppo Italiano por lo Studio della Streptochinasi nell'Infarcto Miocardico (GISSI). 1987. Long-term effects of intravenous thrombolysis in acute myocardial infarction: final report of the GISSI study. Lancet 2:871–874.
24. ISIS-2 (Second International Study of Infarct Survival) Collaborative Group. 1988. Randomised trial of intravenous streptokinase, oral aspirin, both, or neither among 17,187 cases of suspected acute myocardial infarction: ISIS-2. Lancet 2:349–360.
25. The TIMI Study Group. 1989. Comparison of invasive and conservative strategies after treatment with intravenous tissue plasminogen activator in acute myocardial infarction. Results of the Thrombolysis in Myocardial Infarction (TIMI) Phase II trial. N Engl J Med 320:618–627.
26. Frommer PL and Furberg C. 1985. Beta-blocking drugs in the prevention of sudden cardiac death. In J Morganroth and LN Horowitz (eds), Sudden Cardiac Death. Orlando, FL: Grune & Stratton, pp 249–256.
27. Hutchison S and Campbell LM. 1983. Review. Beta-blockers and the elderly. J Clin Hosp Pharm 8:191–199.
28. Gundersen T, Abrahamsen AM, Kjekshus J, et al. 1982. Timolol-related reduction in mortality and reinfarction in patients ages 65–75 years surviving acute myocardial infarction. Circulation 66:1179–1184.
28a. The Danish Study Group on Verapamil in Myocardial Infarction. 1990. Effect of verapamil on mortality and major events after myocardial infarction. The Danish verapamil infarction trial II (DAVIT II). Am J Cardiol 66:779–785.
29. Goldstein RE, Boccuzzi SJ, Cruess D, et al. 1991. Diltiazem increases late-onset congestive heart failure in postinfarction patients with early reduction in ejection fraction. Circulation 83:52–60.
30. Weintraub RM, Thurer RL, Wei J, et al. 1983. Repair of postinfarction ventricular septal defect in the elderly. Early and long-term results. J Thorac Cardiovasc Surg 85:191–196.
31. Knapp WS, Douglas JS Jr, Craver JM, et al. 1981. Efficacy of coronary artery bypass grafting in elderly patients with coronary artery disease. Am J Cardiol 47:923–930.
32. Phillips SJ, Kongtahworn C, Zeff RH, et al. 1979. Emergency coronary artery revascularization: a possible therapy for acute myocardial infarction. Circulation 60:241–246.

33. Flameng W, Sergeant P, Vanhaecke J, et al. 1987. Emergency coronary bypass grafting for evolving myocardial infarction. Effects on infarct size and left ventricular function. J Thorac Cardiovasc Surg 94:124–131.
34. Corbett JR, Dehmer GJ, Lewis SE, et al. 1981. The prognostic value of submaximal exercise testing with radionuclide ventriculography before hospital discharge in patients with recent myocardial infarction. Circulation 64:535–544.
35. Mukharji J, Rude R, Gustafson N, et al. 1983. Late sudden death following myocardial infarction: inter-dependence of risk factors (abstract). J Am Coll Cardiol 1:585.
36. Moss AJ, Bigger JT Jr, Case RB, et al. 1983. Risk stratification and prognostication after myocardial infarction (abstract). J Am Coll Cardiol 1:716.
37. The Cardiac Arrhythmia Suppression Trial (CAST) Investigators. 1989. Preliminary report: effect of encainide and flecainide on mortality in a randomized trial of arrhythmia suppression after myocardial infarction. N Engl J Med 321:406–412.
38. Report of the Sixty Plus Reinfarction Study Research Group. 1980. A double-blind trial to assess long-term oral anticoagulant therapy in elderly patients after myocardial infarction. Lancet 2:989–994.
39. Kannel WB and McGee DL. 1985. Modifiable risk factors for sudden coronary death. In J Morganroth and LN Horowitz (eds), Sudden Cardiac Death. Orlando, FL: Grune & Stratton, pp 267–284.
40. The Expert Panel. 1988. Report of the National Cholesterol Education Program Expert Panel on detection, evaluation, and treatment of high blood cholesterol in adults. Arch Intern Med 148:36–69.
41. Williams MA, Maresh CM, Aronow WS, et al. 1984. The value of early out-patient cardiac exercise programmes for the elderly in comparison with other selected age groups. Eur Heart J 5 (Suppl E):113–115.
42. Akman D. 1983. Treatment of acute myocardial infarction in the elderly. Geriatrics 38: 46–52.
43. Marron KR. 1982. Sexuality with aging. Geriatrics 37(9):135–136, 138.

14. DISEASES OF THE MYOCARDIUM, PERICARDIUM, AND ENDOCARDIUM

CELIA M. OAKLEY

DISEASES OF THE MYOCARDIUM

Overview of terms

Cardiomyopathies are disorders of the myocardium of unknown cause (figure 14-1).

Specific heart muscle diseases have causes or associations by which they are known, such as amyloid, sarcoid, or alcoholic heart disease. Heart failure caused by structural abnormalities or systemic or pulmonary hypertension is so designated. Although the terms *alcoholic cardiomyopathy* and *ischemic cardiomyopathy* are in common usage with clear meaning, they transgress World Health Organization (WHO) agreed terminology. *Dilated cardiomyopathy* is the approved term for what used to be known as congestive cardiomyopathy or idiopathic cardiomegaly in Africa. *Hypertrophic cardiomyopathy* is the approved term for what was known as idiopathic hypertrophic subaortic stenosis, muscular subaortic stenosis, or asymmetric hypertrophy.

Cardiomyopathies are divided into three types—*dilated, hypertrophic,* and *restrictive*—by which they can be recognized both clinically and pathologically [1].

Specific heart muscle diseases may assume any of the three functional forms, their pathogenesis being determined after clinical investigation that includes cardiac biopsy [1] (table 14-1).

Franz H. Messerli (ed.), CARDIOVASCULAR DISEASE IN THE ELDERLY (Third Edition). Copyright © 1993 Kluwer Academic Publishers. ISBN 0-7923-1859-5. All rights reserved.

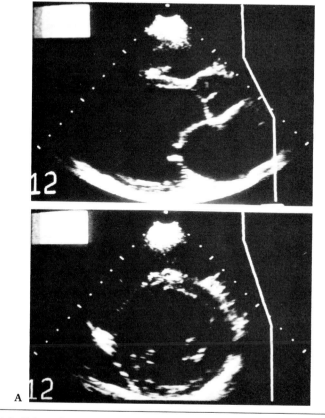

Figure 14-1. Echocardiograms in dilated (**A**: long- and short-axis views) and hypertrophic

Assessment of age-related changes in the elderly heart in relation to possible myocardial disease

Heart failure is common in the elderly, and most diseases of the myocardium can cause heart failure. Changes in the heart that occur with increasing age greatly modify the clinical appearance of heart muscle disease and blur the distinctions between the three functional types of cardiomyopathy, which are usually clear in younger people.

The older heart has increased collagen content and consequent changes in filling characteristics, with increased stiffness and an enhanced atrial contribu-

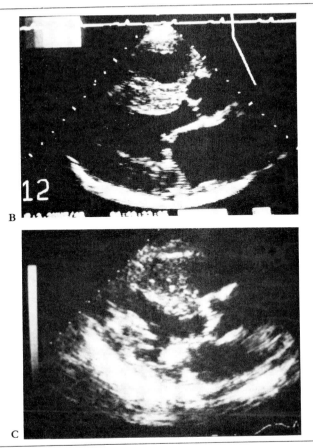

Figure 14-1. (*continued*) (**B**: long-axis view) cardiomyopathy shows the three main functional and pathologic types. The fault is mainly systolic in dilated cardiomyopathy and wholly or mainly diastolic in the hypertrophic and restrictive types. Since the heart tends to develop increasing restriction to filling with aging as well as a tendency to wall hypertrophy related to hypertension, the distinction between the three types of cardiomyopathy tends to be blurred in the elderly patient. (**C**: long-axis view) shows the heart of a patient with senile pseudo-hypertrophic cardiomyopathy showing a small cavity, wall thickening, and dense mitral annular calcification.

tion. Hypertension, particularly systolic hypertension, is common in the elderly and is responsible for the development of left ventricular hypertrophy (LVH) with an increase in wall thickness recognizable on echocardiography. This contributes further to diastolic abnormality. Although systolic function is usually well maintained in healthy old age, degenerative changes in the

Table 14-1. Specific heart muscle diseases seen in the elderly

Dilated	Hypertrophic[a]	Restrictive
Alcoholic Hemochromatosis	Amyloid	Advanced amyloid Adriamycin toxicity Postirradiation Carcinoid Sarcoid Hypereosinophilic syndrome

[a] Echocardiography does not distinguish hypertrophy from wall thickening due to infiltration.

Table 14-2. Differential diagnosis of cardiomyopathy and specific heart muscle disease in the elderly

Dilated	Hypertrophic	Restrictive
Hypertensive heart disease Coronary Aortic stenosis	Hypertensive heart disease Aortic stenosis Mitral valve prolapse	Constrictive pericarditis

myocardium, particularly infiltration by senile amyloid, is now recognized to be of functional importance. Senile amyloid has a slow evolution but can contribute further to diastolic restriction.

The older heart shows configural differences recognized on echocardiography, particularly a sigmoid ventricular septum projecting into and sometimes narrowing the left ventricular outflow tract. Mitral annular calcification is common, particularly in women, and is often associated with some mitral regurgitation due to splinting of the annulus. The functional importance of degenerative changes in the aortic and mitral valves may be underestimated or may complicate the interpretation of possible myocardial disease. Aortic stenosis due to degenerative changes with calcification in an anatomically normal tricuspid valve is extremely common and very likely to be missed or dismissed as aortic "sclerosis." *Sclerosis* means *stenosis*. These changes make it more likely for an older patient to develop heart failure postoperatively or with the advent of atrial fibrillation, anemia, thyrotoxicosis, or myocardial infarction. A "cardiomyopathy" or specific heart muscle disease may be overdiagnosed, just as heart failure itself is often mistakenly diagnosed in this age group, but it may also be missed (table 14-2).

DILATED CARDIOMYOPATHY

Dilated cardiomyopathy results from contractile failure of the left ventricle or both ventricles, with consequent dilatation. Rarely, only the right ventricle is affected. In older patients the clinical syndrome of heart failure is often seen when left ventricular systolic function is only mildly impaired. This is because the filling pressure rises when there is only a modest increase in ventricular residual volume. In other words, there is an earlier restrictive component to systolic failure in older patients. Failure to dilate while maintaining low filling pressures, as is usual in the young, means a lower stroke volume with a higher filling pressure and clinical heart failure while left ventricular systolic function is only moderately impaired, with the ejection fraction still between 40% and 50%. Younger patients with dilated cardiomyopathy are rarely in clinical failure when the ejection fraction is above 40% and may even be asymptomatic.

Etiology

Dilated cardiomyopathy is probably heterogenous in origin. It is important to exclude alcohol abuse because improvement in myocardial function may follow abstinence (figure 14-2) [2]. Patients with systolic hypertension should be treated vigorously. When systolic hyperteasion is present it should be regarded as the cause of heart failure. Failure of the heart may have resulted in a fall in blood pressure down to normal levels, but a history of high blood pressure and increased left ventricular wall thickness on echocardiography will suggest a diagnosis of hypertensive heart failure rather than of cardiomyopathy. Viral infection may contribute to heart failure but is usually difficult to prove. Much recent interest has been directed toward recognition of viral residue in cardiac biopsy samples using modern in vitro hybridization techniques, but the contribution of recent viral infection to heart failure in dilated cardiomyopathy remains uncertain. Equally uncertain is whether a replicating virus may contribute to the progression of heart failure after myocarditis or whether heart failure after myocarditis is due to an immune response to a previous virus. This has importance when one is considering the use of immunosuppression in patients with serologic [3] or biopsy [4] evidence of recent viral infection, and the question has not been answered. The etiology of dilated cardiomyopathy remains unknown.

Pathogenesis

Heart failure is the usual mode of presentation. Heart failure in the elderly is often labeled as coronary in origin, but this is rarely the case in the absence of previous angina, infarction, or focal abnormality on the ECG. There is often no clinical reason for diagnosing coronary disease in older patients with heart failure, and no evidence of major coronary artery obstruction may be found if coronary angiography or subsequent autopsy is undertaken, although coronary disease may, of course, coexist with cardiomyopathy. Elderly patients who develop heart failure in the absence of uncontrolled atrial fibrillation, thyroid dysfunction, anemia, heart murmur, or positive evidence of coronary disease may have a cardiomyopathy. Distinction of cardiomyopathy from other heart muscle diseases involves recognition that

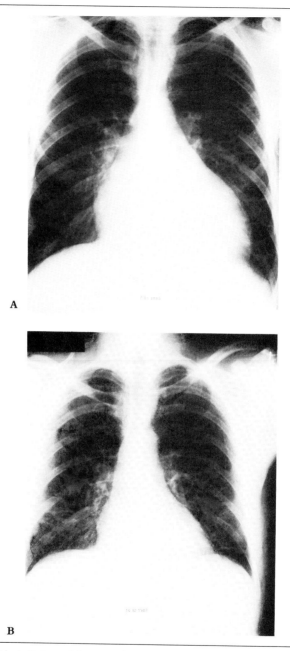

Figure 14-2. Alcoholic heart failure may be wholly or entirely reversible following abstinence. **A**: The grossly dilated heart of an alcoholic patient whose ventricular function returned virtually to normal after he had stopped drinking and measured so (**B** & **C**).

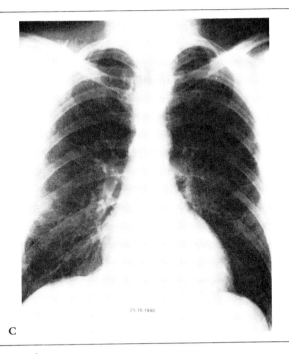

C

Figure 14-2. (*continued*)

the left ventricle is dilated and poorly contracting. This may readily be determined by echocardiography. Coronary heart failure is, of course, the major differential diagnosis. Both hypertrophic cardiomyopathy and amyloid heart disease are usually associated with an undilated and thick-walled left ventricle. In dilated cardiomyopathy, the left ventricular cavity is increased in size, but the wall thickness is normal or subnormal with reduced systolic thickening and reduced excursion. There is usually some functional mitral regurgitation.

Clinical findings

There may be a short history with sudden onset of breathlessness mistakenly attributed to respiratory infection. The heart may be in regular rhythm or in atrial fibrillation. If it is in sinus rhythm there may be pulsus alternans. The venous pressure is usually raised unless diuretics have been given. Left ventricular displacement may be palpable and a third heart sound or mitral regurgitant murmur heard. The chest x-ray usually shows considerable left ventricular enlargement and pulmonary venous congestion. The ECG may show left atrial P-waves and typically rather low voltage in the standard leads but increased voltage in the chest leads with an intraventricular conduction defect and T-wave inversion.

Treatment

The first administration of a diuretic usually results in complete disappearance of the signs of failure both clinically and radiologically, but these signs tend to recur with continued treatment. The smallest dose of diuretic that controls pulmonary venous congestion should be used, and the venous pressure in the neck should be permitted to remain raised. Overuse of diuretics is common. Digoxin is always indicated for patients in atrial fibrillation. In sinus rhythm the use of digoxin has been controversial, but a small positive benefit is likely. Assessment of dosage is difficult for patients in sinus rhythm. Inotropic benefit is related linearly to the dose; however, toxicity is easily produced, and the risks of toxicity are high in the elderly. An angiotensin-converting enzyme (ACE) inhibitor should be introduced early, even in patients who respond well to diuretics. The potassium-retaining effect of ACE inhibitors may make it unnecessary or even dangerous, particularly in the elderly, to prescribe a potassium-sparing agent such as amiloride in addition to the diuretic. Potassium supplements also should be avoided. Serum potassium should be followed serially, since hyperkalemia may develop gradually in patients receiving these agents. The advantage of ACE inhibitors over other dilators is now established. The main disadvantage is hypotension, particularly a marked first-dose effect. This can be avoided by introducing an ACE inhibitor even before starting a diuretic or by stopping the diuretic for 24 hours before giving the first dose of ACE inhibitor, which should be taken after retiring. ACE inhibitors are especially useful when blood pressure is well maintained or raised, but they may be combined with other dilators. Chronic heart failure necessitates individualized drug combinations [5]. Anticoagulants should be considered because of a risk of both systemic and pulmonary embolism in these patients, even when the rhythm is regular. The advantages of anticoagulants have to be weighed against the risks in this age group. Patients should be warned against the use of alcohol because it is a potent myocardial depressant.

Prognosis

For patients with only slight left ventricular dilatation, the situation may remain stable over many years. However, in patients with advanced class III or IV heart failure, very large hearts, hypotension, hyponatremia, or reduced renal function, the outlook tends to be poor. Ventricular arrhythmias, usually asymptomatic and shown on Holter ECG taping associated with late potentials on signal-averaged ECGs, have a poor prognosis. The mode of death is often sudden in these patients, about half of whom die unexpectedly rather than after a period of increasing heart failure [6].

HYPERTROPHIC CARDIOMYOPATHY

Hypertrophic cardiomyopathy (HOCM) is defined as idiopathic hypertrophy and characterized by hypertrophy of the left and often also the right ventricle, usually with a raised diastolic pressure. HOCM is often asymmetrical, with the septum more hypertrophied than the free wall. Outflow tract gradients are common, and about one half of patients have a family history with an autosomal dominant mode of inheritance.

Although HOCM was originally considered to be a disease mainly affecting adolescents and young adults, it has been increasingly diagnosed in older patients, with an increased proportion of older patients in recently reported series [7,8]. The escalation of the diagnosis among older people reflects an increasing intensity of diagnostic endeavor among this age group, particularly with the use of echocardiography. Important differences between HOCM in the elderly and in the young emphasize the heterogeneity of the disease and indicate that HOCM in the elderly is probably the result of disease processes different from the "classic" disorder. Thus, a high proportion of older patients with a diagnosis of HOCM are hypertensive, giving rise to the term *hypertensive hypertrophic cardiomyopathy* [9]. Such patients tend to have concentric hypertrophy that is regarded as excessive for the degree of hypertension. Other older patients have murmurs and outflow tract gradients, as in the classical disease in the young, but the cardiac morphology is different [10]. These patients show an exaggeration of the elderly sigmoid septum and protrusion of a hump into the left ventricular outflow tract, causing it to be narrowed. In distinction to the classical disease, such patients have less hypertrophy of the septum, and it is seen to contract actively. This is unlike the thick immobile septum seen in young patients with HOCM; moreover, in the elderly, the posterior wall does not move excessively as it does in younger patients. There may also be calcification of the mitral annulus or mitral leaflet prolapse and mild or even moderate mitral regurgitation, which, in the absence of left ventricular cavity dilatation, reduces the stroke volume and contributes to a raised filling pressure (figure 14-c).

The natural history of HOCM first diagnosed in old age differs from the disease in the young. The prognosis is relatively benign [7]. Sudden death is less common, and a positive family history of the disorder is rare. HOCM may be found unexpectedly at autopsy of elderly patients who have died from noncardiac causes [11]. Some may show coronary artery disease that may have contributed to their demise. The usual history is one of good health throughout life until a complaint of dyspnea and anginal type chest pain or syncope—the same symptoms as in younger patients. There may be a history of raised blood pressure, but it may be normal. Examination may reveal a forceful left ventricular impulse with atrial beat and late systolic murmur, or there may be no abnormal physical signs.

The ECG tends to show marked changes of LVH with absent Q-waves and T-wave inversion in the left ventricular leads, also often an intraventricular conduction delay. The chest x-ray may be unimpressive or may show some cardiac enlargement and pulmonary venous congestion.

The natural history is unknown because of the lack of previous documentation of patients who are first seen late in life. The fact that they have been regarded as healthy without a heart disorder until this time makes it unlikely that the hypertrophy has been present since adolescence, as in the classical disease, although it could be speculated that a benign form of the disorder had developed early but failed to progress or that the patient survived because excellent hemodynamic performance and electrical stability were maintained. Past hypertension as well as systolic hypertension occurring on effort should be excluded before making a diagnosis of HOCM.

The echocardiographic criteria for the diagnosis of HOCM include 1) left ventricular septal thickness equal to or more than 15 mm; 2) a nondilated left ventricle with normal or hyperkinetic systolic function, with or without systolic anterior motion of the mitral valve; ±3) a left ventricular outflow tract gradient detected by Doppler echocardiography either at rest or after provocation with a sympathetic stimulus.

Differential diagnosis

The clinical differential diagnosis is primarily from nonrheumatic mitral regurgitation due to leaflet prolapse, but it may also be from aortic stenosis. The character of the arterial pulse may not help, since it frequently is not slow rising in elderly patients with aortic stenosis (table 14-2).

The other major differential diagnosis is from amyloid heart disease (table 14-1). This diagnosis can be very difficult, since the echocardiographic features of both diseases may be almost identical. Amyloid heart disease tends to cause a concentric increase in left ventricular wall thickness with thickening of the right ventricular wall, as in HOCM, but with thickening of all four cardiac valves and of the atrial septum as well. Increased echocardiographic reflectivity is typical of amyloid but also is seen to some extent in hypertrophic cardiomyopathy.

Complications

Patients with outflow tract gradients may develop a fixed deformity of the mitral valve due to degenerative changes in it caused by turbulence at the site. These patients may develop increasing mitral regurgitation and benefit from mitral valve replacement with a low-profile valve. This automatically removes outflow tract turbulence and gradients and corrects mitral regurgitation. Infective endocarditis is a risk for patients with HOCM who have mitral regurgitation and outflow tract gradients, and these patients also may develop severe mitral regurgitation requiring surgery.

Treatment

Patients with anginal chest pain benefit from beta-adrenergic blockers. These patients may have associated coronary artery disease that may be severe enough to require coronary bypass surgery, which should be undertaken for the same indications as in patients without HOCM. Calcium antagonists, particularly verapamil, may through their depressant effect on myocardial contraction give rise to pulmonary edema, or the vasodilatation may cause marked hypotension. Digoxin is not contraindicated in patients with atrial fibrillation, but amiodarone is the only drug effective in restoring and maintaining sinus rhythm, and it may also be used for suppressing ventricular ectopic activity if this causes symptoms. Diuretics may be needed for congestive features persisting after the correction of heart rate and rhythm.

THE RELATION BETWEEN HYPERTENSION AND HYPERTROPHIC CARDIOMYOPATHY

HOCM is a diagnosis of exclusion. The term *hypertensive hypertrophic cardiomyopathy* is an admission that one is hedging one's bets. Many older patients with normal or barely raised resting blood pressures show an excessive increase in systolic blood pressure on exercise, which explains the LVH. In the past, although discussion about the treatment of hypertension has illogically been based on the lowest values obtained at rest, ambulatory blood pressure monitoring has shown that the blood pressure may be at a much higher level during the normal exertions of the day. In recent reports of HOCM in the elderly, the proportion of patients over the age of 60 or 65 years has been high. In an echocardiographic study carried out in an old peoples' home, the majority of residents showed increased left ventricular wall thickness [12]. A rise of systolic blood pressure at rest and excessively on exercise is common in old age and is related to inelasticity of the conducting arteries, which fail to dilate in order to damp the pressure wave (absence of Windkessel function). Myocyte fallout and hypertrophy are components of aging that, together with increase in interstitial tissue, account for a tendency toward increasing wall thickness as the years go by. The benign nature of so-called HOCM in the elderly is not unexpected if we consider most of them to simply have hypertension.

RESTRICTIVE CARDIOMYOPATHY

Restrictive cardiomyopathy is characterized by diastolic impairment and an increased increment in diastolic pressure for each increment in volume. This results in raised left and right ventricular filling pressures. Preservation of normal or near normal systolic function is characteristic of "pure" restrictive physiology. This is seen infrequently in patients with fine interstitial fibrosis, normal left ventricular wall thickness, and preserved left ventricular function. This fine fibrosis is quite different from the coarser patchy fibrosis seen in dilated cardiomyopathy. Other patients may show myocyte hypertrophy with fibrosis and disarray.

The features may closely resemble constrictive pericarditis both clinically and on echocardiographic examination, but patients with restrictive

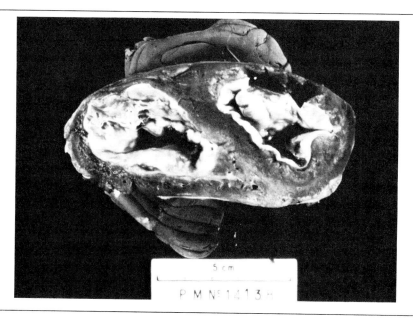

Figure 14-3. The heart in endomyocardial fibrosis. Restriction to filling is caused by fibrous scarring of the endocardium of the inflow tracts of one or both ventricles. This cross–section across the left and right ventricle shows bilateral involvement. The patient was a British woman who had never been to the tropics.

cardiomyopathy are distinguished by the frequent development of tricuspid regurgitation and marked right atrial dilatation, both of which are rare in constrictive pericarditis. Left ventricular and left atrial diastolic pressures usually exceed right ventricular and right atrial diastolic pressures, but with the development of tricuspid regurgitation these pressures may become roughly equal, increasing the superficial resemblance of restrictive cardiomyopathy to pericardial constriction. Marked tricuspid regurgitation is rare in constrictive pericarditis, but if the diagnosis is uncertain, pericardial thickening can be identified by computerized tomography or magnetic resonance imaging. Indeed, it is usually possible to see the potential pericardial space and thence the thickness of the parietal pericardium by echocardiography in good echocardiographic subjects. It is, of course, extremely important not to miss constrictive pericarditis, which is a relatively rare condition but no respecter of age.

HOCM, like dilated cardiomyopathy in older patients, also overlaps into restrictive physiology in the elderly. Patients with classical HOCM who survive into their later years very often develop restrictive features associated with progressive wall thinning together with some loss of systolic function but little or no left ventricular cavity dilatation. This results in a state of low output failure with atrial fibrillation and often no clues to the pathogenetic origin of hypertrophic cardiomyopathy. In fact, HCOM may not be recognized unless the patient was seen earlier, when its features were more typical.

Eosinophilic heart disease and endomyocardial fibrosis (figure 14-3), previously regarded as the classical examples of restrictive cardiomyopathy, really belong with the specific heart muscle diseases and are uncommon in the elderly. In temperate climates, eosinophilic heart disease develops in association with a hypereosinophilic syndrome. This disease is characterized by an eosinophil count equal to or in excess of 15^9/dl. Rarely, it is associated with carcinoma, leukemia, asthma, allergy, or parasitic infection. Much more often it exists as a disease seemingly on its own without cytologic features of malignancy but with a malignant clinical course. The eosinophilia is characterized by hypermature eosinophils, and patients who develop cardiac disease show morphologic abnormalities in the eosinophils with vacuolation and degranulation. Cardiac damage has been attributed to extrusion of the cationic protein from the eosinophil. The cardiac changes may go through a sequence of endocardial necrosis followed by thrombosis and eventual fibrosis. Nests of eosinophils are found perivascularly in the myocardium. This condition should be differentiated from the Churg–Strauss variant of polyarteritis nodosa, which is characterized by a vasculitis, usually absent in the hypereosinophilic syndrome, and by the occasional development of pericardial constriction.

AMYLOID HEART DISEASE

Amyloid heart disease is the specific heart muscle disease usually cited as exemplifying restrictive physiology. In cardiac amyloidosis, amyloid is progressively laid down in the interstitium between the myocardial cells as well as in the walls of small coronary arteries. It is a progressive disorder with increasing deposition causing the left and right ventricular walls to gradually thicken and the functional diastolic disorder to change from an early delay in relaxation with slow filling to a restrictive disorder in which filling is completed early (figure 14-4). Left ventricular systolic function is normal early but gradually deteriorates, often with little or no dilatation, so that these patients have a very low forward cardiac output and very high left and right ventricular filling pressures. When the amyloid deposition is mainly in the walls of small coronary arteries, angina may be prominent, and systolic failure with dilatation may be seen [13].

Amyloid is an abnormal eosinophilic fibrillar protein laid down intercellularly. It may be formed from a number of different precursor proteins, but in all cases it is bound to a nonfibrillar glycoprotein that is a normal plasma constituent. The particular precursor protein determines the appearance of the amyloid fibrils, which can be identified by distinctive appearances on electron microscopy.

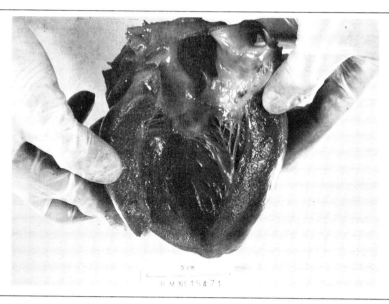

Figure 14-4. Gross anatomy of the amyloid heart, which is thickened and stiff. It does not collapse on the postmortem table. Staining reactions may be atypical.

Most clinically recognized cases of amyloid heart disease result from the deposition of amyloid AL fibrils derived from monoclonal immunoglobulin light chains and associated with myeloma, macroglobulinemia, or malignant B-cell lymphomas. In some cases in which this type of amyloid is deposited, no immunocyte dyscrasia can be identified. The amyloid may be limited to certain organs or generalized. The heart or the heart and tongue (with or without skeletal muscle) and autonomic and peripheral nerves are commonly involved. In other cases, massive infiltration of the spleen, gastrointestinal tract, and kidney may occur and influence the clinical picture. Deposition of amyloid in small blood vessels in the mucosa and in skin may give rise to skin purpura, which is often periorbital and sometimes associated with swelling of the lips, gums, and tongue.

Senile amyloid used to be thought to be a clinically unimportant component of increasing age; however, it is now apparent that amyloid infiltration not only contributes to the functional abnormality of the senile heart but also can be the cause of heart failure and death [14,15]. In senile amyloid, the amyloid fibrils are derived from a variant of plasma prealbumin (now renamed transthyretin), and no monoclonal protein is found in plasma or urine. It is often clinically unrecognized in the very old, but some younger patients who develop senile amyloid show a milder and more slowly advancing disease than is usual in AL amyloid. In reactive amyloidosis associated with chronic inflammation or suppuration as in rheumatoid arthritis or bronchiectasis, the heart is usually not clinically involved. However, there are exceptions. In reactive amyloidosis the AA fibrils are derived from serum amyloid A protein.

Natural history

Early in the course of disease, the patient with cardiac amyloidosis is asymptomatic. However, left ventricular Doppler ultrasound inflow recordings may show abnormal relaxation with a reduced peak early velocity, a prolonged deceleration time, and an increased peak late velocity. These may be recognized before an increase in ventricular wall thickness is detectable. As the amyloid deposition increases, isovolumic relaxation and passive filling are prolonged, the left ventricular wall thickens, and the heart becomes ever stiffer. Late filling is then diminished or abolished. Eventually the amyloid heart becomes so stiff that filling is completed early by diastolic suction during the period of shape change following the isovolumic relaxation period and while left ventricular diastolic pressure is still falling after early opening of the mitral valve because of the high left atrial pressure. Cardiac output becomes very low, and cardiac failure is further worsened with the beginning of deterioration of systolic function. Serial echocardiography has been the means through which this gradual process has been appreciated (figure 14-5) [16].

Electrocardiography shows low voltage and sometimes sinoatrial or atrioventricular conduction defects with a fascicular block. Occasionally the ECG is almost normal. An unexpectedly low-voltage ECG may bring the diagnosis to mind.

The chest x-ray characteristically shows a small heart with pulmonary venous congestion, but pericardial effusions are not uncommon, and this may increase the size of the heart shadow.

Patients with amyloidosis tend to look pale and sick. They may have lost weight, perhaps from malabsorption. They may have muscle wasting or, less often, amyloid deposition may give the skeletal muscles increased bulk. Mononeuritis or carpal tunnel syndrome may bring the amyloidosis to attention before cardiac abnormality has become overt.

A low output state with cool extremities, peripheral cyanosis, and hypotension that may be orthostatic due to involvement of autonomic nerves is typical. Jugular venous pressure is usually high but may rarely be normal. The heart is usually quiet, without added sounds or murmurs.

In patients who undergo invasive investigation, left ventricular angiography may show a deceptively normal appearance, but sometimes exaggeration of the internal architecture caused by subendocardial amyloid infiltration coarsens trabeculation and increases the size of papillary muscles.

The differential diagnosis in amyloid heart disease is from HOCM, and the differentiation may be surprisingly difficult [13]. Both the clinical and the echocardiographic features may be similar, but in HOCM with true

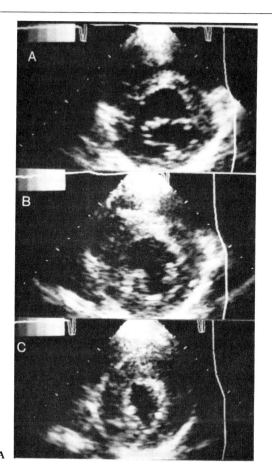

A

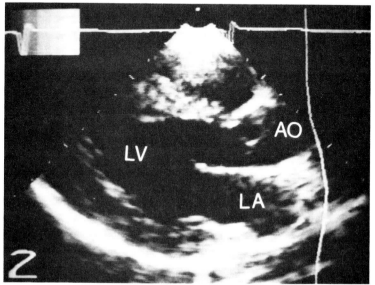

B

hypertrophy the ECG voltage is usually high, whereas in amyloid—an infiltrative disease—the ECG voltage is low. One feature of advanced cardiac amyloidosis is thickening of the valves and atrial septum due to amyloid infiltration, which is not seen in HOCM.

Endomyocardial biopsy reveals the diagnosis but staining reactions may be atypical in AL amyloid. If staining is negative, the amyloid may be missed except on electron microscopy when the fibrillar masses are readily recognized.

In the past, congo red used to be injected as a diagnostic test for amyloid, the pigment being removed from the plasma in proportion to the amount of amyloid deposited. However, false negatives were common because the test was insensitive and the amyloid did not always have the usual physical affinity for the pigment. Allergic reactions also occurred, and the test was abandoned. A newly developed technique involves radioiodine labeling of the purified serum amyloid protein P component with I^{123} [17]. Patients with amyloidosis show uptake of the label by amyloid deposits, and high-resolution scintigraphy can then reveal even small deposits. Unfortunately, this technique is insensitive for the detection of cardiac amyloid because of the large blood pool containing the label.

Treatment

No medical treatment yet exists that prevents progression of amyloidosis or causes it to be removed. Cardiac transplantation in younger patients with amyloidosis can offer quite long-term palliation even when there is amyloid infiltration of other organs and even though amyloid may be detected on cardiac biopsies of the transplanted heart within months after the transplant. The progression of deposition appears to be very slow, permitting normal activity for many years.

OTHER RESTRICTIVE HEART MUSCLE DISORDERS

Sarcoidosis and hemochromatosis may also cause a restrictive picture. Sarcoidosis tends to cause massive focal replacement of myocardium by granuloma and finally by fibrous scar tissue with a predilection for the inflow portion of the left ventricle and the ventricular septum. Symptoms may be absent. Angina is not uncommon, yet other patients may have supraventricular arrhythmias, repetitive ventricular tachycardia, or atrio-ventricular block even in the absence of detectable focal granulomatous masses [18,19]. Cardiac sarcoidosis is not always accompanied by evidence of

Figure 14-5. Echocardiography in amyloid heart disease is often diagnostic, although, as with the gross specimen, it can be difficult to distinguish amyloid from hypertrophic cardiomyopathy of the type with symmetrical hypertrophy but without outflow tract gradient. Thickening of valves and atrial septum is common in amyloid heart disease and helps to distinguish between the two. The short-axis view of the left ventricle at different levels (**A**) shows concentric wall thickening, prominent papillary muscles, and a thickened mitral valve, also seen on the long-axis view (**B**). LV = left ventricle; LA = left atrium; AO = aorta.

Table 14-3. Pericardial syndromes

- Acute pericarditis
- Subacute constrictive–effusive pericarditis
- Chronic relapsing pericarditis
- Pericardial tamponade
- Chronic lax pericardial effusion
- Constrictive pericarditis

---

sarcoid elsewhere or by a history of pulmonary or cutaneous sarcoidosis and is therefore readily missed. Hypercalcemia may be absent and serum angiotensin-converting enzyme (ACE) is not raised unless the granulomatous masses are extensive. Treatment is unsatisfactory in cardiac sarcoidosis partly because of difficulty in monitoring response and partly because only immunosuppressive treatment is available.

Hemochromatosis tends to produce a restrictive picture when it presents in middle-aged men with a short history of breathlessness and congestive failure. In such patients, who may still have relatively normal-sized ventricles, repeated venesection may be followed by reduction of myocardial iron deposition as revealed by serial cardiac biopsy and restoration of function. However, in the typical elderly bronzed diabetic, the cardiac picture is more one of dilated cardiomyopathy, and treatment brings little improvement in cardiac function.

PERICARDIAL DISEASES

Tuberculosis is now rare in the indigenous population of the West, and antibiotics have reduced the incidence of acute purulent pericarditis. Consequently, patients with pericardial disease now compose only a small proportion of the patients seen by cardiologists. Many are referred from other specialties, particularly rheumatology and oncology, because the pericardium is often involved in systemic diseases [20].

The various pericardial syndromes are shown in table 14-3. Acute *idiopathic pericarditis* of presumed (but rarely proven) viral origin can occur at any age and may progress rapidly to constriction, of which it now appears to be the commonest cause. The post-myocardial infarction syndrome of Dressler and the postcardiotomy syndrome may pursue a relapsing course. *Relapsing pericarditis* may also occur after acute idiopathic pericarditis. *Subacute constrictive effusive pericarditis* may be tuberculous, but it is also seen in rheumatoid arthritis and in malignancy. A *chronic lax pericardial effusion* is sometimes found accidentally following radiography of the chest or because of rather nonspecific complaints. The cause of such effusion usually remains occult after exclusion of hypothyroidism, tuberculosis, and malignancy. *Chronic constrictive pericarditis* is now rarely tuberculous in origin and rarely calcified. It is thought usually to follow acute idiopathic pericarditis of viral origin, but there is often no history of this; the patient may be first seen with no past history of cardiac illness or disability.

Acute pericarditis

The cardinal features of acute pericarditis are precordial pain, a pericardial friction rub, and concordant S-T-segment elevation on the electrocardiogram. Infective, immunologic, and neoplastic causes should be thought of as well as postirradiation, traumatic, and uremic pericarditis.

Acute pericarditis thought to be of viral origin is rarely associated with evidence of myocarditis and only uncommonly gives rise to cardiac tamponade. Pericardiocentesis is therefore carried out for diagnostic purposes.

Pericarditis may occur in rheumatoid arthritis and Reiter's disease, in systemic lupus erythematosus, and in the Churg–Strauss variant of polyarteritis nodosa. It may also occur in Whipple's disease, and inflammatory bowel disease; therefore, all of these conditions should be sought when a patient has unexplained pericarditis or pericardial effusion.

A major differential diagnosis of acute pericarditis in the elderly is acute anterior myocardial infarction. The chest pain and ECG changes may be superficially similar, but infarction is associated with focal S-T-segment elevation, usually most marked in leads V_2 to V_6, and with reciprocal S-T-segment depression in leads III and AVF. It is important to make the distinction early because there is a risk of causing hemorrhage into the pericardium if thrombolytic treatment is given to a patient with acute pericarditis. There is a similar risk in an elderly patient with a benign condition that does not need treatment.

Relapsing pericarditis

Whatever the cause of the original pericarditis, a relapsing picture of recurrent chest pain with friction rub, ECG changes, and small effusions may develop. The patient may be made quite miserable. The physician who is asked by the patient to prevent these painful recurrences may be tempted to use steroids. While acute steroid treatment quickly suppresses the symptoms of the acute attack, chronic maintenance treatment fails to prevent recurrences. The tendency therefore is for the physician or the patient to gradually increase the dose, though still without preventing recurrence. Maintenance steroids should be avoided. Acute attacks may respond to aspirin. Indomethacin suppositories can be useful. Acute attacks may be treated very effectively with colchicine given as for acute gout, in a dose of 1 mg followed by 500 ug two or three hourly until the pain goes or vomiting occurs. A severe attack may be treated with prednisolone in a dose of 60 mg daily for two days, decreasing to nothing over the next 10 days. No maintenance therapy is given, but a further attack may be treated in a similar fashion. However, it is better to avoid steroids altogether; particularly in patients who have been treated unsuccessfully with maintenance steroids, it is important to treat acute flares with colchicine while continuing to diminish the steroid dose.

Pericardiectomy has been carried out but is unsuccessful in preventing recurring pain. This is perhaps because relapsing pericarditis is due to an autoimmune process resulting from misrecognition of damaged native myocardial protein as foreign. If so, removal of the parietal and even of the visceral pericardium is unlikely to be curative. In the long term, resolution invariably occurs and constriction is not a risk, probably because the recurrent effusion prevents adherence and also stretches the fibrous pericardium.

Constrictive pericarditis

Constrictive pericarditis limits cardiac filling and thus the forward output. Because the tight pericardium constricts the heart as a whole, right-sided features are prominent with high venous pressure, hepatomegaly, and sometimes ascites. However, pulmonary venous congestion is rare. The blood pressure is usually low. Pulsus paradoxus is seen in about half of patients but is not as florid as in cardiac tamponade. The venous pressure is raised with an M-shape due to exaggerated X- and Y-descents in patients with sinus rhythm. The venous pressure rises on inspiration (Kussmaul's sign), but this sign is difficult to elicit and is nonspecific. The enlarged liver is often said to be nonpulsatile, but although the pulsations are not as great as in tricuspid regurgitation it is certainly pulsatile. The cardiac impulse is quiet, but occasionally a diastolic impulse is felt that terminates in a third heart sound. Typically this is early and of high frequency, but it may be absent, particularly in severe constriction. The second heart sound is rather widely split.

The chest x-ray may show "step-ladder" P-waves indicative of biatrial hypertrophy, but many cases are in atrial fibrillation. The QRS complex is normal, but S-waves tend to be seen as far as V_6, and there may be repolarization abnormalities.

The chest x-ray usually shows a normal-sized heart, now rarely with any calcification, and the lungs are usually free from evidence of interstitial congestion.

Computed tomography shows thickening of the pericardium as well as a sinusoidal shape of the ventricular septum caused by equalization of the left- and right-sided diastolic pressures (figure 14-6).

Echocardiography shows normal chamber sizes and wall thickness with well-maintained systolic function and rapid outward excursion in diastole with rapid cessation. Doppler inflow recording shows an enhanced E and reduced or absent A due to increased early filling, sometimes with differential changes in mitral and tricuspid inflow with respiration. Thus inspiration may be associated with increased tricuspid and diminished mitral inflow, showing

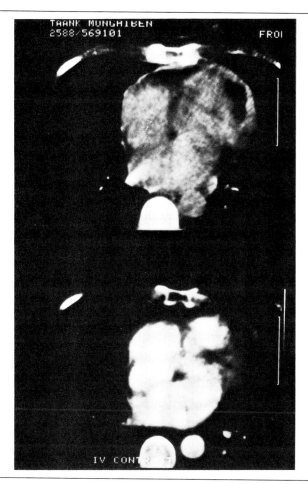

Figure 14-6. Computerized tomography of the thorax from a patient with constrictive effusive pericarditis. The thickened pericardium is clearly seen separated from the myocardium by the epicardial fat layer and a small amount of fluid.

the interdependence of the two ventricles in the presence of pericardial constriction [21].

Cardiac catheterization is unnecessary in typical cases of constrictive pericarditis, but when carried out it shows equalization of the diastolic pressure in all four cardiac chambers to within a few millimeters. Typically the raised right ventricular diastolic pressure is equal to at least one half of systolic pressure. Pulmonary hypertension is rare and, if found, militates against the diagnosis.

In restrictive cardiomyopathy, endomyocardial fibrosis, and amyloid heart

Table 14-4. Important points in the differential diagnosis
of pericardial constriction from restrictive heart muscle disease

	Constriction	Restrictive syndromes
Arterial pulse	Paradox in 50%	No paradox
Venous pulse	High, small excursion	Often regurgitant V-wave
Murmurs	Usually absent	Often mitral or tricuspid regurgitation
Chest x-ray	Small heart, ± calcification No pulmonary congestion	Often large atria Often pulmonary congestion
ECG	± atrial fibrillation "normal" QRS	± atrial fibrillation Often fascicular blocks (low voltage in amyloid)
Echo	Differential tricuspid and mitral Doppler inflow velocities with respiration	No differential Doppler inflow with respiration
CT or MRI	Thickened pericardium	Thick ventricular walls in amyloid and valves
Catheterization	Diastolic pressures equal in all four cardiac chambers	Left ventricular and left atrial diastolic pressures > 5 mm above right-sided pressures (except when severe tricuspid reflux)
	No pulmonary hypertension	Pulmonary hypertension common

Note: ECG = Electrocardiogram; CT = computed tomography; MRI = magnetic resonance imaging; Echo = echocardiography.

disease, the left diastolic pressures are usually much higher than those on the right side and pulmonary hypertension is not uncommon (table 14-4).

Pericardiectomy carries a low risk and has excellent results both in idiopathic constrictive pericarditis and in constriction associated with rheumatoid arthritis (figure 14-7). The venous pressure may remain elevated in the early weeks after the operation.

Constriction may occur after cardiac surgery, usually coronary artery bypass grafting. This is a rare complication, and its cause is still debated. Some have associated it with perioperative infarction, but it seems more likely that it follows a combination of a postoperative pericardiac collection (seen on ultrasound in about one quarter of early postoperative cases) and low-grade infection. Constriction usually develops fairly rapidly but is often not recognized for weeks or months after the operation. Pericardiectomy may be needed but is technically difficult because of the need to preserve the bypass grafts [22].

Cardiac tamponade

Cardiac tamponade is usually recognized quickly when it develops in a hospital patient with a condition known to carry this risk, but when it occurs outside the hospital in a previously fit individual it is frequently fatal.

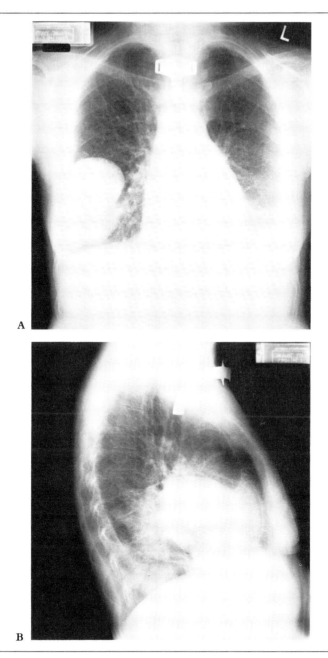

Figure 14-7. Chest radiograph (**A**: PA; **B**: lateral) from a patient with rheumatoid pericardial constriction showing a normal-sized heart and loculated pleural effusions. This patient had a permanent tracheostomy as the result of rheumatoid involvement of the arytenoid cartilages.

Tamponade may occur in pericarditis due to any cause, although it is uncommon in idiopathic pericarditis, post-myocardial infarction pericarditis, and pericarditis associated with connective tissue disorders and uremia. It is common in acute bacterial, tuberculous and malignant pericarditis. Acute hemopericardium may cause tamponade, as in acute or subacute cardiac rupture following myocardial infarction or in dissection of the ascending thoracic aorta when this ruptures into the pericardium, the usual fatal model of termination of this surgically treatable disorder. Tamponade is a relatively common early complication of cardiac surgery. Pericardial tumors, lymphoma, and mesothelioma may first be seen on account of tamponade, and the same is true for the much more common metastatic carcinoma. Chronic tamponade may occur in tuberculosis or uremia, and following irradiation for carcinoma of the breast or for Hodgkin's or non-Hodgkin's lymphoma.

Patients complain of shortness of breath, sweating, weakness, or fainting. Tachycardia and pulsus paradoxus with disappearance of the pulse on inspiration are usual. The blood pressure is low and the venous pressure high, with prominent X- but absent Y-descent. The liver is enlarged and the heart sounds quiet, but a pleuro-pericardial friction rub may be heard.

In tamponade there is an inspiratory increase of blood flow into the right ventricle, but this is accommodated at the expense of inflow into the left ventricle because the total diastolic volume of the heart cannot increase. The ventricular septum can be seen on echocardiography to move sharply towards the left ventricle on inspiration, thereby reducing left ventricular inflow and stroke volume.

The Y-descent of the venous pulse is lost because right atrial filling can only occur in systole, when the cardiac volume is diminishing through ejection into the aorta and pulmonary artery. Blood accepted into the right atrium in systole flows into the right ventricle early in diastole until the pericardial pressure rises above the intracardiac pressure, thereby causing further inflow to cease. At this time diastolic collapse of the walls of the right atrium and of the right ventricular outflow tract may be seen on echocardiography.

The ECG shows tachycardia and low-voltage and sometimes electrical alternans caused by the heart swinging in the pericardial sac. The chest radiograph is unhelpful, except perhaps in revealing an underlying bronchial carcinoma.

The need for paracentesis is urgent, and if it is performed under echocardiographic control, this increases the safety. Use of the Seldinger technique permits placement of a soft catheter with multiple side holes in the pericardial space, which allows continuous drainage of fluid.

Chronic lax pericardial effusions without compression may occur in myxedema or amyloid heart disease and following irradiation. They may also be idiopathic [23].

DISEASES OF THE ENDOCARDIUM

Subacute bacterial endocarditis (SBE)

Incidence in the elderly

The incidence of SBE is not completely known in the United Kingdom, where it is not a disease that has to be reported. Recent evidence suggests that the incidence is increasing, with 13,000 cases a year in the United States and more than 3000 in the United Kingdom. The increase is in old people, people with surgically palliated congenital heart disease, and drug abusers [23].

The proportion of cases occurring in people over age 65 has steadily increased. More people are living long enough to develop degenerative valve disease, and they are living more often with their own teeth and with prosthetic heart valves. Other more important factors are 1) more elderly people are being referred for a precise diagnosis and are having more diagnostic procedures that may cause bacteremia and 2) the diagnosis of infective endocarditis is now more frequently made correctly in the elderly. Nonetheless, more cases are likely to be missed in the elderly than in younger people. Many obvious factors contribute to this problem, including underrating of the significance of murmurs, greater difficulties in accurate auscultation, occasional modification of constitutional response, and the presence of other pathology, which is very common in the elderly.

The recognition of SBE depends greatly on the interest and awareness of the physician. Infective endocarditis is a well-known and classic disease, but one that is comparatively rare in the experience of most physicians. This fact combined with the multiplicity of possible presenting features that lead the patient to almost any medical or surgical specialist no doubt accounts for the many delays in diagnosis and treatment. Such delays account for the continuing mortality in what should be a totally curable disease.

Organisms and their possible sources

About 75% of cases of *medical* SBE are caused by streptococci of the *Viridans* group. In the elderly, the proportion of other organisms is higher because of sources of infection in the gastrointestinal and genitourinary tracts and a higher incidence of skin staphylococci. But streptococci still account for nearly 50% of cases of *geriatric* SBE. Edentulous patients are not immune from such infections, possibly because of retained tooth roots or ill-fitting dentures or because these organisms are not confined to the mouth. *Streptococcus bovis*, a group D streptococcus, is a gastrointestinal organism that when identified indicates a search for hidden carcinoma or polyp, an association that can be accounted for more often than by chance. Gram-negative organisms are uncommon causes of SBE, perhaps because blood bactericidal activity is more efficient toward gram-negative organisms or because they produce no dextrans. The higher incidence of enteric streptococci and other gastrointestinal organisms in the elderly points to sources of bacteremia from these areas. This is especially likely when the organism is unusual, as in the case of an elderly man with SBE who was found to harbor *Salmonella typhi suis* in his gallbladder.

Cases of SBE due to enteric organisms have shown such a close temporal relationship to intestinal biopsy, prostatic biopsy, or cystoscopy that the origin could not be doubted. *Staphylococcus epidermidis* is a not infrequent primary infecting organism in the elderly, even when there has been no preceding surgical procedure. Staphylococcal infection due to a coagulase-positive organism can more often be linked to skin sepsis, which is sometimes also associated with diabetes.

Predisposing heart disease

Less than half of our patients with SBE have had preexisting heart disease [23]. How many had entirely normal hearts is quite unknown, although autopsy specimens from patients dying from SBE may show no evidence of previous rheumatic, congenital, or even degenerative abnormality. This question is fascinating in relation to prophylaxis but of little relevance to diagnosis, since nearly all patients with SBE have a murmur when they are first seen. The greater frequency of both aortic and mitral systolic murmurs in the healthy elderly adds to difficulties of diagnosis. Rheumatic and even congenital heart lesions in the elderly patient become infected, but the most common site of SBE in the elderly remains the aortic valve. The valve may show a minor congenital fault, some variant of the bicuspid aortic valve such as two or three cusps of unequal size with varying amounts of degenerative change, atheroma, and calcification. The increased wear-and-tear changes can be related to the abnormal hemodynamics with turbulent flow and endothelial damage.

The greater frequency of these abnormalities in males accounts in part for the male predominance of SBE. With advancing age, even normally constructed aortic valves may undergo degenerative changes, even to the extent of developing severe aortic stenosis. The older the patient with aortic valve stenosis, the less the congenital abnormality and the greater the degenerative changes contributing to obstruction. Aortic systolic murmurs should not be underestimated in the elderly, because they indicate some degree of stenosis and some risk from infection.

The second most common predisposing condition is mitral regurgitation, again of degenerative cause but usually in a valve that originally was anatomically normal. The anterior leaflet of the mitral valve is the most common and earliest site of atheroma in the normal aging heart, and this leads to stiffening of the leaflet. Mitral regurgitation may be contributed to by calcification in the fibrous skeleton of the heart and mitral annulus. This prevents contraction of the ring and leads to mild mitral regurgitation. Prolapse of part of the mitral leaflet (usually posterior) may result from elongation of supporting chordae even without rupture. All of these or a

Table 14-5. Changes in infective endocarditis

1. The patients are older
2. Males predominate
3. Underlying heart disease is usually degenerative and previously unknown to patient and doctor
4. Increase in immunologic phenomena: Renal failure and vasculitis
5. Prosthetic valve endocarditis accounts for up to one third of cases

combination may give rise to a mitral systolic murmur and regurgitation, which may be of no importance clinically unless infection occurs.

Prosthetic valve endocarditis (PVE) now accounts for up to one third of cases in most series. Early PVE is caused by organisms that gain access during or soon after surgery through wound infections. These are staphylococci, fungi, or opportunistic organisms such as *Diphtheroids* and *Klebsiella*. The mortality is still very high, and reoperation is usually required. Late cases are caused by the same organisms that infect natural valves.

Underlying general disease

Bacteremias are a daily occurrence in the healthy. The big question is this: What determines the development of SBE? People with immune paresis from any cause are more vulnerable, particularly to pyogenic infections, which are now otherwise uncommon. SBE is sometimes recurrent in patients with myeloma and in patients with indwelling venous lines for cancer chemotherapy or parenteral feeding. Patients with systemic lupus erythematosus may develop infection of previously sterile thrombotic vegetations (Libmann–Sacks endocarditis). In patients with sterile thrombotic endocarditis (marantic endocarditis) usually associated with adenocarcinoma in the pancreas, stomach, or prostate, secondary infection may occur.

Diagnosis

The clinical spectrum of SBE as commonly seen has changed since the classic descriptions (table 14-5). Recognition of early cases depends on a high index of suspicion in any patient with fever and a murmur without a good explanation for the fever [24]. The responsibility rests initially on the patient to report sick without delay and on prompt action by the general practitioner or internist. Any additional symptoms or signs reside in longer-established disease and therefore mean a neglected diagnosis, but patients may be first seen because of embolism to any site with a history of few or no symptoms. Patients with embolism should be regarded as having SBE until it is disproved whether they are in sinus rhythm or in atrial fibrillation.

The old adage that SBE is uncommon in patients with atrial fibrillation is unfounded. The classic triad of signs of infection, embolism, and a heart disorder indicates established untreated disease as it was described in the

Table 14-6. Infective endocarditis—the classic triad

Signs of infection	Signs of "embolism"	Signs of a cardiac disorder
Fever	Petechiae	Cardiac murmur
Sweating	Vasculitic rash	New murmur
	Embolic stroke	
	Coronary or limb embolism	
Anemia	Hematuria	Acute or progressive heart failure
Clubbing	Proteinuria	
Weight loss	Osler's nodes	
Splenomegaly	Mycotic aneurysm	
Pigmentation		

Note: Below the line are signs of established and therefore neglected disease. Most patients seen now have only fever and a murmur ± embolic features.

Table 14-7. Immunologic phenomena in infective endocarditis

Skin	Purpura
	Vasculitis
	Osler's nodes
Retina	Roth's spots
Joints	Arthralgia
	Arthritis
Pericardium	Sterile effusion
Kidney	Proliferative glomerulonephritis, usually focal
Plasma	Polyclonal gammopathy
	Rheumatoid factor
	Hypocomplementemia

days before antibiotics (table 14-6). Fever and night sweats may be prominent with a virulent organism and inapparent with a less vigorous one. Weight loss, anemia, clubbing, and splenomegaly all take weeks to develop. Most of the classic skin lesions originally attributed to embolism may be immunologic, including vasculitic lesions on the skin, hematuria, Roth's spots on the retina, or renal failure. Any patient with unexplained renal failure and a heart murmur should also be regarded as having SBE until it is disproved. Elderly patients with SBE may be afebrile with an illness marked by vasculitis and renal failure (figure 14-8), perhaps with a seemingly unimportant heart murmur (table 14-7). Positive blood cultures and vegetations seen on two-dimensional echocardiography (figure 14-9) leave no room for doubt, particularly when administration of appropriate antibiotics leads to a steady recovery, but negative blood cultures are common with some fastidious streptococci or when previous antibiotics have been given. Echocardiography can never exclude the diagnosis because vegetations may not be visualized if they are laminar or on a calcified thickened valve. The

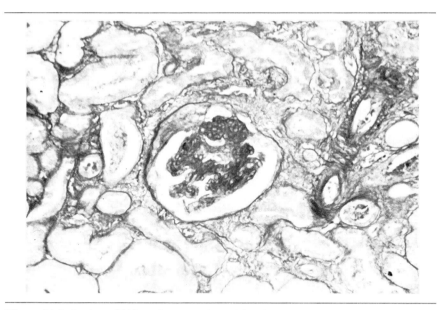

Figure 14-8. Section of kidney from a patient with infective endocarditis showing crescentic glomerulonephritis. Immunofluorescent staining showed clumps of IgG on the basement membrane.

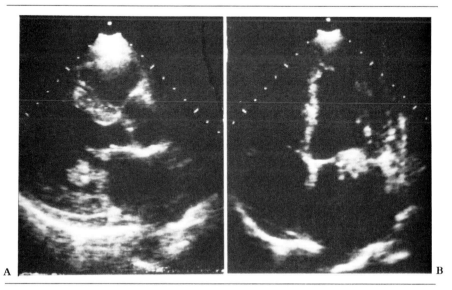

A   B

Figure 14-9. Echocardiogram (transthoracic window) showing a large vegetation on the mitral valve. (**A**: Long-axis view; **B**: apical four-chamber view.)

transesophageal approach greatly increases the quality of the images and facilitates recognition of vegetations or abscess formation in a much higher proportion of cases [25].

Coxiella endocarditis

These infections are often very indolent, and patients are unable to say when they first became unwell. Specific features are often slow to develop, so diagnosis is late and the presentation is more likely to point to extracardiac disease. Patients with *Coxiella* infections often have prominent malaise, weight loss, and sometimes evidence of an autoimmune illness with jaundice or renal failure. Clubbing is usual. Splenomegaly may be minor or massive. Although the organism is common in rural areas, not all patients with *Coxiella* infection come from the country or can relate their infection to a country holiday or visit. Neither can they usually remember any respiratory illness. When they can do so, the interval between these possible causes and presentation is usually 2 or 3 months but may be very much longer, even years.

The drug of choice for *Coxiella* endocarditis is a tetracycline, because long-term treatment is necessary. Doxycycline, which is partly metabolized in the liver, may be preferred if there is renal dysfunction or if chronic hepatic infection with the organism is present. It used to be thought that tetracycline treatment never cured *Coxiella* endocarditis because the organisms are intracellular and the antibiotics are not cidal against *Coxiella* in vitro. Nonetheless, it seems that a cure can sometimes be obtained. The decision to cease therapy is always a difficult one because relapse may occur. It is often simpler to continue tetracycline in a low dose as suppressant therapy. Treatment should begin with 2 to 3 g of tetracycline daily. Clinical response is usually rapid. The dose should not be reduced until complement fixation titers have fallen. Then a decision should be made about continuing suppressant treatment in a low dose with doxycycline, 100 mg daily, or stopping treatment altogether after 3 to 6 months. Excision of a valve infected by this organism should be based only on hemodynamic deterioration, because if the valve is functioning adequately long-term tetracycline appears to be very effective. Rifampicin is an alternative choice, but there can be problems associated with resistance or anticoagulant control in patients on warfarin because the drug causes liver enzyme induction.

Prosthetic valve endocarditis (PVE)

The organisms encountered in late prosthetic valve endocarditis (PVE) are no different from those met with in SBE on native valves except for the late-appearing fungal infections and continuing higher incidence of staphylococcal infection in the first year. Infection by fungi, most commonly *Candida*, may produce anything from a severe constitutional illness to almost no host reaction at all. Indeed, some fungi apparently live in symbiotic harmony with their host until this symbiosis breaks down and the fungus starts to propagate. This can make the diagnosis of fungal infection exceedingly difficult, and any odd syndrome in a prosthetic valve wearer should be taken seriously. Unfortunately, the first hard evidence of something wrong may be massive embolic obstruction of a limb artery or a stroke. Vegetations are usually large and easily visualized on echocardiography.

There seem to be no differences in susceptibility to infection between mechanical and tissue valves nor between the various styles of prosthesis.

The diagnosis of PVE is based on the same criteria that apply to SBE of native valves. Diagnosis should be rapid because both patient and doctor are forewarned, but the mistaken belief that infection will cause some change in prosthetic valve sounds often delays diagnosis. This is a late event because vegetations have to be large before they interfere with moving parts or cause a paraprosthetic leak. Indeed, prosthetic valve sounds may remain unchanged in the presence of paravalvular abscess and massive infection outside the immediate vicinity of the valve. Echocardiography may not reveal vegetations on mechanical prostheses, but they are much easier to visualize on bioprostheses. Transesophageal passage of the transducer greatly improves the quality of the images and the sensitivity to detection of vegetations on prosthetic valves as well as thrombus formation and paravalvular abscess.

Treatment

The principles of treatment of endocarditis are the same in the elderly as in the young; however, older people are much more likely to be damaged by gentamicin, and poorer renal function may result in higher-than-expected blood levels of antibiotics excreted by the kidney. Caution should be exercised when giving any part of the treatment by mouth unless the swallowing of tablets is witnessed.

In view of the 30% chance that endocarditis in the elderly is caused by an enteric streptococcus, treatment must begin with penicillin plus an aminoglycoside. Penicillin plus gentamicin is a more efficient synergistic combination against some enteric streptococci, which can show ribosomal resistance to streptomycin, but streptomycin is safer in the elderly. If the laboratory results indicate that gentamicin is preferable to streptomycin, it should be given with care to avoid peaks above 5 mg/L or troughs above 1 mg/L. Ampicillin may be preferable to penicillin once the organism is known. Netilmicin is a semisynthetic antibiotic with properties similar to gentamicin but allegedly reduced toxicity [26].

We prefer a subclavian venous line in the elderly (as in younger subjects), because once in place it is painless, and because old people tend to get hematomata from peripheral and intramuscular injections. The subclavian venous line is put in under maximal sterile precautions, and the puncture site is covered with a transparent occlusive dressing. Penicillin, gentamicin, or streptomycin is given by bolus injection through a two-way tap, which is then closed off after the line is filled with heparin. The subclavian line should be left untouched unless there is some cause to remove it, and it should not be used for any other purpose, such as taking blood for laboratory tests.

Even with proper care and accurate laboratory aid, some elderly people still develop irreversible vestibular damage. Since vestibular damage is a great disadvantage to an elderly person, gentamicin should not usually be continued for more than two weeks.

The principle of treatment with intravenous bolus dosage is the achievement of high peak levels of antibiotics. The organisms situated within vegetations and relatively far removed from the bloodstream receive a lower concentration of antibiotic than is measurable in the blood. Neither intramuscular injection nor oral dosage provides high peak levels, even with well-absorbed drugs such as amoxycillin. Probenecid is no longer advised because its use in blocking renal excretion results only in boosting the trough values, with a higher chance of toxic side effects; however, probenecid may be used with oral amoxycillin for the second two weeks of treatment after intravenous therapy.

The duration of treatment is an individual decision dependent upon four considerations: 1) the organism; 2) the duration of symptoms before diagnosis; 3) the rapidity of clinical response; and 4) the presence of prosthetic material.

The shortest course for a fully sensitive *Viridans* infection would be two weeks of intravenous penicillin plus streptomycin, followed by two weeks of oral amoxycillin 1 g four times daily. PVE caused by *Viridans* organisms can usually be cured with 4 to 6 weeks of intravenous therapy. The aim in the treatment of SBE should be to have a patient who is clinically well and afebrile for the last two weeks of treatment. Infection by enteric streptococci usually requires six weeks of intravenous treatment.

Staphylococcal endocarditis

Resistance may develop during the course of treatment unless staphylococcal endocarditis is treated with two drugs to which the organism is sensitive. The choice is usually from a combination of flucloxacillin, gentamicin, sodium fusidate, and rifampicin. Only about 10% of nosocomal staphylococci are now sensitive to penicillin G. Most *Staphylococcus aureus* infections should be treated with flucloxacillin in a dose of at least 12 g in 24 hours plus either gentamicin or fusidic acid for the first two weeks [26,27]. The flucloxacillin–fusidic acid combination may be antagonistic in vitro and sometimes in vivo. Some recent reports have recommended flucloxacillin alone for *S. aureus*. Combinations are needed for *S. epidermidis*, which more often exhibits multiple resistance. A diagnosis is usually made quickly when the infection is caused by coagulase-positive staphylococci because the patient usually becomes ill very fast and because the organisms are quickly grown

Table 14-8. Indications for surgery in infective endocarditis

1. Acute hemodynamic deterioration	Usually due to aortic or mitral regurgitation
2. Failure to respond despite sensitive organism	Usually due to paravalvular abscess
3. Failure to respond due to resistant organism	
4. Leaking infected prosthetic valve	Paraprosthetic leak due to paravalvular abscess Destroyed bioprosthesis
5. Obstructed infected prosthesis	Thrombus or vegetation
6. Embolism with persisting large vegetations on echocardiography	

and recognized. Infection by *S. epidermidis* is usually more indolent and the organisms more difficult to eradicate. A longer period of treatment is therefore generally required for skin staphylococci than for the more virulent coagulase-positive staphylococci. It should be remembered that embolic abscesses in distant parts are a feature of infection by coagulase-positive staphylococci. If a patient who has had SBE due to these organisms reports focal symptoms, this possibility should be borne in mind.

The choice of antibiotic treatment always depends on bacteriologic evidence. Tests for bactericidal efficiency of the patient's plasma are made against the organism. If possible, the patient's serum should show at least eight times the minimal bactericidal concentration (mbc) at the peak. This is arbitrary. It may be insufficient to eradicate sensitive organisms if they are far removed from the bloodstream, and it may be impossible to attain even this concentration when using more toxic antibiotics against organisms that are not fully sensitive to them. When treating a patient whose infection is slow to respond despite seeming sensitivity of the organism and in whom dosage cannot be raised further with safety, the possibility of abscess formation is high.

Because penicillin itself is more effective than any other antibiotic against sensitive organisms, it should be chosen in preference to the newer synthetic penicillin whenever possible.

When blood cultures are repeatedly negative and the clinical diagnosis is firmly based, with exclusion of other causes of fever, the cause of infection is usually either a streptococcus sensitive to penicillin plus aminoglycoside or a cell-dependent organism such as *Coxiella* or *Chlamydia*.

Indications for surgery

Indications for surgery in the elderly are in general the same as for younger people, though based on common sense (table 14-8) [24,28]. The development of serious acute aortic or mitral regurgitation in a previously fit elderly person must be treated by urgent surgery. The timing is dependent on the hemodynamic urgency rather than on the duration of antibiotic treatment. Persisting bacteremia is often an indicator of paravalvular abscess, particularly when it is associated with calcific aortic stenosis where actual valve disruption by infection is not very common because organisms tend to spread outward in the paravalvular tissues. The development of conduction fault on ECG may give a clue to this complication.

Infection by a relatively resistant organism such as *Coxiella* or *Chlamydia* does not necessarily represent an indication for excision of an infected valve in the elderly. The clinical response is usually gratifying and the patient is well, so a conservative attitude with long-continued antibiotics is preferred when possible. Decisions have to be individual, with, again, a tendency toward a more conservative policy in elderly patients. It should be remembered that vegetations are to be expected in SBE, and their demonstration by echocardiography does not amount to an automatic indication for valve excision in order to prevent embolization. Nevertheless, embolism is more common in patients with large mobile vegetations seen on echocardiography.

Previously fit old people with an acute cardiac problem tolerate cardiac valve replacement remarkably well. This is particularly true for aortic valve replacement. Age itself is no contraindication to surgery.

Prophylaxis

The question of antibiotic prophylaxis for SBE remains under scrutiny. Many conventional ideas on the subject are founded on logic and circumstantial evidence rather than on scientific facts. The continuing prevalence of streptococcal endocarditis itself testifies to the failure of prophylaxis. The fact that more than half of patients with SBE had not been known to have heart disease until their illness means that selective prophylaxis misses at least half of patients who will later contract SBE. Even if prophylaxis were completely effective and invariably given to all patients with heart disease before predictable bacteremia, and even if unpredictable bacteremias were never responsible for SBE, the number of cases could only be reduced by less than one half [23].

Only a small proportion of cases of streptococcal endocarditis have anything to do with previous dental work. In cases in which dental treatment appeared to have been relevant, the interval between treatment and the onset of symptoms was measured in days up to almost 2 to 3 weeks, rather than the period of up to three months that has often been suggested. It is known that patients with heart disease may be so afraid of infection that they prefer to remain away from the dentist. This has led to a level of oral hygiene in patients with heart disease that is inferior to that of the general population. Since most infections follow spontaneous rather than dentally induced bacteremias, the basis for effective prophylaxis must be optimal oral hygiene.

Even though it has been shown that dental treatment is responsible for only a minority of infections caused by oral organisms, dental extraction produces a short-lived bacteremia of predominantly penicillin-sensitive organisms, and it is necessary to try to protect susceptible individuals. A single oral dose of 3 g of amoxycillin is followed by a high and sustained bactericidal concentration in the blood for as long as 10 hours. We have shown that all primary blood cultures were sterile in patients who had received 3 g of amoxycillin for dental prophylaxis.

Patients having dental extractions carried out under general anesthesia should receive a single intramuscular dose of ampicillin or amoxycillin 1.5 g. Patients allergic to penicillin should reveive clindamycin 600 mg orally as a single dose. If they are undergoing extractions under general anesthesia in the hospital, they should receive intravenous vancomycin through an intravenous infusion cannula over 100 minutes.

Most clinical procedures to evaluate the intestinal and urinary tracts are carried out in the hospital and should be covered by intramuscular amoxycillin, 1.0 g, plus gentamicin, 80 mg one hour before plus a further oral dose of amoxycillin, 0.5 g, six hours later. Procedures that should be covered include cystoscopy as well as prostatic or intestinal biopsy, and there is logic to giving prophylaxis to unselected patients over age 65 because of the high incidence of unknown degenerative valve changes as well as the high linkage found between such procedures and the subsequent development of endocarditis.

Patients with prosthetic valves have higher susceptibility as well as a generally higher mortality and morbidity from SBE. We therefore extend the indications for antibiotics to procedures with a lower incidence of predictable bacteremia and therefore a lower risk of infection. These include investigations such as barium enema, which is followed by about a 20% incidence of low-grade bacteremia.

Sterile thrombotic endocarditis

The development of fibrin platelet vegetations on the heart valves unassociated with bacterial infection may occur to a small extent in any severely debilitated subject, but it is seen especially with adenocarcinoma (particularly of the pancreas) and in patients with systemic lupus erythematosus (Libmann–Sacks endocarditis). The presence of these vegetations may only become known because of embolism. However, the most common presentation is because of the development of a murmur due to mitral regurgitation or, less often, to aortic valvar regurgitation. It is likely but unproven that secondary bacterial infection of such vegetations may account for SBE developing in a minority of these patients. This converts nonerosive endocarditis into a destructive form. Patients with systemic lupus erythematosus are usually on both steroids and immunosuppressive drugs, and the constitutional reaction may be minimal. If blood cultures are negative because of recent antibiotic treatment or because the organism is a fragile streptococcus, the diagnosis may have to be made on the basis of other evidence.

REFERENCES

1. Oakley CM. 1987. Cardiomyopathies/Specific heart muscle disorders. In DJ Weatherall, JGG Ledingham, and DA Warrell (eds), Oxford Textbook of Medicine, 2nd ed. Oxford: Oxford University Press.
2. Regan TJ, Harder B, Ahmed S, et al. 1977. Whiskey and the heart. Cardiovasc Med 2:165.
3. Muir P, Nicholson F, Tilzey AJ, et al. 1989. Chronic relapsing pericarditis and dilated cardiomyopathy: serological evidence of persistent enterovirus infection. Lancet 1:804–807.
4. Tracy S, Wiegand V, McManus B, et al. 1990. Molecular approaches to enteroviral diagnosis in idiopathic cardiomyopathy and myocarditis. J Am Coll Cardiol 15:1688–1694.
5. Packer M. 1989. Therapeutic options in the management of chronic heart failure. Is there a drug of first choice? Circulation 79:198–204.
6. Luu M, Stevenson WG, Stevenson LW, et al. 1989. Diverse mechanisms of unexpected cardiac arrest in advanced heart failure. Circulation 80:1675–1680.
7. Fay WP, Taliercio CP, Ilstrup DM, et al. 1990. Natural history of hypertrophic cardiomyopathy in the elderly. J Am Coll Cardiol 16:821–826.
8. Shenoy MM, Khanna A, Nejat M, et al. 1986. Hypertrophic cardiomyopathy in the elderly: a frequently misdiagnosed disease. Arch Intern Med 146:658–661.
9. Topol EJ, Traill TA and Fortuin NJ. 1985. Hypertensive hypertrophic cardiomyopathy of the elderly. N Engl J Med 312:277–283.
10. Lever HM, Karam RF, Currie PJ, et al. 1989. Hypertrophic cardiomyopathy in the elderly: distinctions from the young based on cardiac shape. Circulation 79:580–589.
11. Pomerance A and Davies MJ. 1975. Pathological features of hypertrophic obstructive cardiomyopathy (HOCM) in the elderly. Br Heart J 37:305–312.
12. Perin TJ and Tavel ME. 1979. Idiopathic hypertrophic subaortic stenosis as observed in a large community hospital: relation to age and history of hypertension. J Am Geriatr Soc 27:43–46.
13. Oakley CM. 1985. Amyloid heart disease. In JF Goodwin (ed), Heart Muscle Disease. England: MTP Press, pp 141–153.
14. Hodkinson HM and Pomerance A. 1977. The clinical significance of senile cardiac amyloidosis: a prospective clinico-pathological study. Q J Med 46:381–387.
15. Gertz MA, Kyle RA and Edwards WD. 1989. Recognition of congestive heart failure due to senile cardiac amyloidosis. Biomed Pharmacother 43:101–106.
16. Klein AL, Hatle LK, Taliercio CP, et al. 1990. Serial Doppler echocardiographic follow-up of left ventricular diastolic function in cardiac amyloidosis. J Am Coll Cardiol 16:1135–1141.
17. Hawkins PN, Myers MJ, Lavender JP, et al. 1988. Diagnostic radionuclide imaging of amyloid: biological targeting by circulating human serum amyloid P component. Lancet 1:1413–1418.
18. Wait JL and Movahed A. 1989. Anginal chest pain in sarcoidosis. Thorax 44:391–395.
19. Oakley CM. 1989. Cardiac sarcoidosis (editorial). Thorax 44:371–372.
20. Oakley CM. 1989. Pericardial diseases. In Diseases of the Heart. London: Bailliere-Tindall, pp 974–1000.
21. Ribeiro P, Sapsford R, Evans T, et al. 1984. Constrictive pericarditis as a complication of coronary artery bypass surgery. Br Heart J 51:205–210.
22. Hatle LK, Appleton CP and Popp RL. 1989. Differentiation of constrictive pericarditis and restrictive cardiomyopathy by Doppler echocardiography. Circulation 79:357–370.
23. Brown AK. 1966. Chronic idiopathic pericardial effusion. Br Heart J 28:609–614.
23. Bayliss R, Clarke C, Oakley CM, et al. 1986. Incidence, mortality and prevention of infective endocarditis. J R Coll Phys 20:15–20.
24. Nihoyannopoulos P, Oakley CM, Exadactylos N, et al. 1985. Duration of symptoms and the effects of a more aggressive surgical policy. 2. Factors affecting prognosis of infective endocarditis. Eur Heart J 6:380–390.

25. Ellis SG, Goldstein J and Popp RC. 1985. Detection of endocarditis associated perivalvular abscesses by two-dimensional echocardiography. J Am Coll Cardiol 5:647–653.
26. British Society for Antimicrobial Chemotherapy. 1985. Antibiotic treatment of streptococcal and staphylococcal endocarditis. Report of a working party. Lancet 2:815–817.
27. Karcher AW. 1985. Staphylococcal endocarditis. Laboratory and clinical basis for antibiotic therapy. Am J Med 78:116–127.
28. Alsop SG, Blackstone EH, Kirklin JW, et al. 1985. Indications for cardiac surgery in patients with active infective endocarditis. Am J Med 78:138–147.

15. DISEASES OF THE AORTA AND ARTERIAL TREE

DONALD J. BRESLIN
NICHOLAS P. TSAPATSARIS

Diseases of the aorta and arterial tree in the elderly are common and most often are complications of atherosclerosis. These conditions frequently are potent markers of severe coronary artery disease and should prompt careful cardiac evaluation. Although a single pathologic disease is present, clinical manifestations are diverse and depend on the particular expression of atherosclerosis (aneurysm formation, stenosis, and occlusion or embolism) and on its specific anatomic location (thoracic aorta and its cervical and intracranial branches, or abdominal aorta and its visceral and extremity branches).

Temporal arteritis and aortic dissection also occur with sufficient frequency in the elderly to merit discussion. In the past, luetic aortitis was a major cause of thoracic aortic disease, but modern antibiotic therapy has rendered this a disease infrequently seen by the clinician.

ARTERIAL PATHOPHYSIOLOGY

Aging changes in the normal aorta

In recent years, the normal aging process affecting the aorta has been well described by Schlatmann and Becker [1]. They studied 100 aortas of patients of various ages and described the changes they thought represented the

Franz H. Messerli (ed.), CARDIOVASCULAR DISEASE IN THE ELDERLY (Third Edition). Copyright © 1993 Kluwer Academic Publishers. ISBN 0-7923-1859-5. All rights reserved.

normal aging process: cystic medial necrosis, defined as pooling of mucoid material; elastin fragmentation, characterized by disruption of elastin lamellae; fibrosis, defined as an increase in collagen at the expense of smooth muscle cells; and medionecrosis, defined as areas with apparent loss of nuclei. These changes correlated well with age and were considered phenomena of injury and repair caused by hemodynamic events. Such changes result in widening and uncoiling of the aorta.

Pathophysiology

The pathophysiologic mechanisms leading to the atherosclerotic process and the histologic features of progression of fatty streaks to complicated atherosclerotic plaques have been well described and will not be reviewed here.

Calcification of the aorta and its vessels is usually a complication of atherosclerosis. Nonatheromatous calcification of the media described by Mönckeberg is found mainly in the arteries of limbs of middle-aged and elderly persons [2]. While these arteries are stiff and brittle, they are not stenotic.

Giant-cell arteritis affects large-sized and medium-sized arteries. The media is infiltrated by mononuclear cells, predominantly lymphocytes. The internal elastic membrane is fragmented, and closely associated with these fragments are the giant cells characteristic of the disease. However, the presence of giant cells is not mandatory for diagnosis. Arterial involvement is typically patchy. This inflammatory process leads to obliteration of the arterial lumen and ischemia or infarction of the organs distal to the obstruction [3,4]. Lie et al. [5] published an illustrated histopathologic classification and criteria for the vasculitis syndrome, including giant-cell arteritis. This review constitutes the best summary of the clinical and pathologic distinctions of the various vasculitides.

Atherosclerotic aneurysms

In modern clinical practice, most arterial aneurysms are atherosclerotic in origin, particularly in the elderly population [6,7]. Increasing life span and the refinement of treatment for syphilis have largely been responsible for this occurrence [7].

The pathogenesis of atherosclerotic dilation of arteries is less clearly understood than the process of progressive atherosclerotic stenosis. The media of the wall of a small atherosclerotic aneurysm contains less elastin, collagen, and muscle than that of a nonaneurysmal atherosclerotic artery [8]. It is uncertain how many of these alterations in the media are primary rather than secondary to the anatomic changes that occur as the vessel dilates [9,10].

Aneurysms tend to occur in anatomically unfixed areas of arteries, whereas the greatest involvement of atherosclerosis tends to be in portions of the artery that are relatively fixed. Constitutional weakness in the wall, systemic hypertension, and possibly the stress of vibration in a relatively mobile vessel and decreased flow through the vasa vasorum play a role in the formation of aneurysms [10]. Severe thickening of the intima reduces diffusion of blood into the arterial wall from the lumen and causes injury and weakening of the media [7]. Physical laws support the concepts of increased lateral pressure on the arterial wall in the poststenotic vessel (Bernoulli effect). Once dilation has commenced, increased tension on the wall should be directly proportional to the radius of the viscus (LaPlace's law). Wall stress should be inversely proportional to wall thickness [10].

Abdominal aortic aneurysms

Natural history

Abdominal aortic aneurysms occur most frequently with an estimated incidence of 2% at autopsy [7]. Approximately 95% are infrarenal [11]. They occur at least six times more often in men than in women [7], and the incidence rises with increasing age. More than one fifth of these aneurysms are found in individuals aged 70 years or more [12]. Between 40% and 60% of such patients have systemic hypertension [13–15].

Although most abdominal aortic aneurysms contain intraluminal clot, thrombotic occlusion of the artery or clinically significant emboli from the aneurysm are much less common complications than arterial rupture. The larger the aneurysm, the more likely it is to rupture. However, even small aneurysms are vulnerable. In an autopsy study [16], as many as 10% of aneurysms less than 4 cm in diameter had ruptured. Clinically, however, the incidence of rupture of such small aneurysms seems much less common [6], although some will rupture unpredictably. The risk that an aneurysm initially measuring 4 cm in diameter will rupture in five years is estimated to be less than 15% in contrast to more than 75% for an aneurysm 8 cm in width [17]. Szilagyi and coworkers [18] reported on 156 patients rejected for surgical correction of abdominal aortic aneurysm because they were considered poor risks. Overall survival at 1 to 2 years was 72% for patients with aneurysms less than 6 cm in diameter and 39% for those greater than 6 cm in diameter. Of those who died, the cause of death was aortic rupture in 31% of those with smaller aneurysms and 42.5% of those with aneurysms more than 6 cm wide. This implies a risk of death by rupture in 1 to 2 years of 8.7% for patients with aneurysms less than 6 cm in diameter and 26% for patients with larger aneurysms.

Nevitt et al. [19] have suggested that the risk of rupture of small aneurysms may actually be lower. They argue that referral-based and autopsy studies are subject to considerable selection bias. In the population-based cohort study, they reported that the diameter of the abdominal aortic aneurysm increased by a median of 0.21 cm per year and that 24% of aneurysms were associated with a rate of expansion of 0.4 cm or more per year. These authors [19] found a cumulative incidence of rupture of 6% after five years and 8% after ten years. The risk of rupture during a five-year period was 0% for patients with an aneurysm less than 5 cm in diameter and 25% for patients with an aneurysm 5.0 cm or greater [19]. Crawford and Hess [20] faulted this study for the elimination from the study of five patients who had leakage or rupture of an abdominal aortic aneurysm within 48 hours after the first ultrasound examination. In addition, 31% of patients had aneurysms less than 3.5 cm in diameter. The size range was not given, and the ratio of diameters of uninvolved to involved aorta was not measured. Therefore, some of the patients may not have had aneurysms by the definition of Crawford and Hess [20].

The risk of rupture increases in aneurysms observed to be enlarging rapidly. Of aneurysms less than 6 cm in diameter, expansion occurs at an average rate of 0.4 cm per year, but individual rates of growth are unpredictable [21].

In addition to increasing size of the aneurysm, some symptoms indicate an urgent need for surgical repair. With improving technology and increased awareness, many more aneurysms are being discovered when they are small and asymptomatic. For example, in a group of 144 patients treated surgically between 1968 and 1976, 82% were free of symptoms [14] when they were first seen. Symptoms may be related to sudden enlargement, pressure on adjacent structures, or rupture [10].

Clinical aspects

Abdominal, flank, or back pain sometimes associated with aortic tenderness may occur as the aneurysm enlarges. Back or abdominal pain or both and cardiovascular collapse were present in most patients with ruptured abdominal aortic aneurysms, with one tenth also complaining of flank or groin pain or diarrhea [21]. Rarely, aching in the flank or back, which may be associated with ureteral obstruction, can occur in the presence of retroperitoneal fibrosis induced by an inflammatory response to an abdominal aortic aneurysm [22]. In this rare instance, pain does not necessarily indicate impending rupture.

Upper gastrointestinal tract bleeding from duodenal mucosal hemorrhage can reflect the presence of an enlarging aneurysm. Aortoduodenal or aortoesophageal rupture may occur with or without external bleeding [23].

On physical examination, abdominal aortic aneurysms can be felt in the middle and upper part of the abdomen above the bifurcation of the aorta, which lies at the level of the umbilicus. They may be palpable when they attain a size of 4.5 cm in diameter [15], but in moderately obese individuals, a palpable aneurysm is usually more than 6 cm in diameter. Its expansile character distinguishes it from other masses transmitting pulses. Deep palpation will often reveal a border extending to the right of the midline, which is a feature not usually found in the tortuous but undilated abdominal aorta [17]. Tenderness usually indicates imminent or actual rupture, which may result in abdominal rigidity. The rare occurrence of aortocaval rupture can be associated with an abdominal bruit, widened pulse pressure, venous hypertension, and congestive heart failure [24].

Laboratory examination

Ultrasound will detect virtually all abdominal aortic aneurysms and is superior to radiography in determining their size [25]. It can also detect associated retroperitoneal fibrosis [22], although computed tomography is sometimes more effective for detecting that rare condition. If intestinal gas and obesity interfere with an adequate ultrasound evaluation, computed tomography enhanced by administration of intravenous contrast material is equally helpful, although more expensive, and it may be superior in demonstrating extravasated blood. Aortography is inadequate to detect abdominal aortic aneurysms, since intraluminal clot may create a misleadingly narrowed central channel and not reveal the surrounding arterial dilation. However, aortography is used to demonstrate renal artery stenosis or anomalies of renal circulation, extension of the aneurysm above the level of the renal arteries, and the status of the mesenteric circulation and of the outflow arteries distally. Surgeons vary in the extent of their use of aortography in this context. Some will obtain aortography in all such patients preoperatively, accepting the small risk of the procedure. Many will limit this investigation to patients with hypertension, azotemia, or abdominal or flank bruit. In addition, arteriography will help to define the proximal limit of the aneurysm and its relation to the renal arteries more accurately than ultrasound or computed tomography. It will also help clarify the status of the mesenteric and peripheral arterial circulation.

Ligation of the inferior mesenteric artery is common during aortic surgery. It results in marked colon ischemia in approximately 1% of patients [26], the remainder being protected by the collateral circulation. Arteriography can alert the surgeon to the status of the protective mesenteric collateral circulation preoperatively.

The presence of renal anomalies, such as a horseshoe kidney, and the rare occurrence of anomalous renal arterial circulation, retroperitoneal fibrosis with ureteral obstruction, and impaired arterial perfusion of a kidney are important in planning aortic surgery. If aortography is not performed, intravenous pyelography or computed tomography with contrast is necessary to detect such problems preoperatively.

Surgical therapy

The decision to excise an abdominal aortic aneurysm involves balancing operative risk against the risk of dying of aortic rupture. Such decisions can only be made on an individual basis. In general, the patient with overt cardiovascular disease is more likely to die of myocardial infarction than aortic rupture [6]. In the absence of clinically apparent heart disease, the cause of death is likely to be rupture [6]. The larger the aneurysm, the more likely it is that death will result from rupture.

Of the total group of patients undergoing resection for abdominal aortic aneurysm at the Cleveland Clinic [25] between 1969 and 1973, most (69%) had features of coronary heart disease by history or electrocardiography. Myocardial infarction accounted for 37% of postoperative deaths after resection of the aneurysm in that series, with a total postoperative death rate of 9.6% associated with elective repair, 26.5% with symptomatic aneurysms, and 46.5% with ruptured aneurysms.

In another group [14], 21% had a myocardial infarction intraoperatively or postoperatively, and half of the patients died as a result. Although no randomized series has been reported, in selected patients, myocardial revascularization seems indicated before such aortic surgery to decrease the mortality from myocardial infarction. The mortality from aortocoronary bypass in a group of patients who required peripheral vascular surgery (5.3% at Cleveland Clinic) is outweighed by the potential benefit for the patient requiring resection for abdominal aortic aneurysm who also has severe coronary disease [27].

The mortality rate associated with elective resection of abdominal aortic aneurysm has improved with time. Thus, the postoperative mortality rate in one series [14] for the years 1958 through 1968 was 15.6% compared with 6.3% for 1968 through 1976. Such improvement has not occurred in the mortality rate associated with surgery for ruptured aneurysm, which remains more than 50% [14].

Thoracic aortic aneurysms

Surgery for thoracic aortic aneurysm is associated with a higher postoperative mortality than surgery for abdominal aneurysms. When the surgical team is experienced, the mortality rate associated with surgery of the ascending aorta [28] and for the thoracoabdominal aorta [29] is approximately 10%. For relatively rare aneurysms of the transverse aorta, it is higher at about 25% [30].

Serious complications of surgery for aneurysms involving the descending thoracic aorta are ischemia and paraplegia of the spinal cord, which occurred in 4.8% of a large series [30].

In a series [31] from the Mayo Clinic, published at a time when the residua of syphilis were still encountered in considerable numbers, arteriosclerotic thoracic aortic aneurysms were found in 73%; 19% were thought to have a syphilitic origin, the remainder being from traumatic or congenital sources. Of the total group, 68% of patients survived three years, and 50% survived five years; one third of the patients died of rupture, and approximately one half died of cardiovascular disease. A large aneurysm or the presence of symptoms related to it, with accompanying systemic hypertension, increased the risk of rupture.

As in the abdomen, symptomatic aneurysms have a higher risk of rupture. In a series [32,33] of 90 thoracic arteriosclerotic aneurysms, of which 80 were in the descending aorta and 42% were associated with chest or back pain, 44% of the deaths were caused by rupture.

Pain from enlarging thoracic aortic aneurysm is most commonly substernal but may extend to the dorsum, neck, and shoulders. Pain increasing in severity suggests rapid dilation and possible rupture [34]. Compression of surrounding structures can cause respiratory distress, hoarseness, or dysphagia. Aneurysm of the ascending aorta with annular dilation may result in aortic insufficiency.

Most aneurysms of the thoracic aorta are first noted on chest radiography. A lateral film is sometimes sufficient to differentiate tortuosity from dilation. Fluoroscopy may be inadequate to differentiate other chest masses from aneurysm.

Computed tomography [35] with contrast enhancement is extremely helpful in distinguishing thoracic aortic aneurysm from other conditions that may resemble it radiographically. Aortography is usually required to delineate the extent of the aneurysm and its relation to vessels originating from the aorta.

Popliteal aneurysms

Aneurysms of the popliteal artery [36,37] comprise 70% of all peripheral aneurysms. With few exceptions, they occur in men [38]. The major risks they impose are thrombosis and distal embolization, often requiring amputation. Rupture is much less common.

In the series reported by Gifford and coworkers [39], of 80 popliteal aneurysms managed nonsurgically, 23% required amputation. In another series [36] of 111 such aneurysms, 65 were thrombosed, 30 had associated venous occlusion, 6 ruptured, and 23 were the source of peripheral emboli.

An important feature of these aneurysms is the association with aneurysms at other sites. In one series [36], 45% had this finding, particularly in the abdominal aorta, and to a lesser degree in the femoral or common iliac arteries. In another series [40], abdominal aortic aneurysms were found in 48% of patients with bilateral popliteal aneurysms and in 22% of patients in whom only one popliteal artery was involved. Discovery of a popliteal aneurysm makes a search for other aneurysms obligatory.

Most of these aneurysms are readily palpable. Ultrasonography is helpful in evaluating the size of the aneurysm and the presence of a contained thrombus. It may detect an aneurysm not readily palpable but that is suspected as a source of peripheral emboli [41]. Arteriography is useful to determine the status of vessels proximal and distal to the dilated vessel and to demonstrate whether any residual patency is present or whether the vessel is totally thrombosed. If the aneurysm is totally occluded, the need for surgery is determined by the presence of ischemia of the distal limb, since the threat of emboli is no longer present.

Because of the poor prognosis associated with these aneurysms, surgical repair of patent popliteal aneurysms is the treatment of choice when they are discovered. The operation consists of bypass grafting and ligation of the aneurysm or occasionally excision with an interposition graft [42]. Many of these patients have coronary artery disease and require careful cardiac evaluation before operation.

Aortic dissection

Aortic dissection is the most catastrophic illness affecting the aorta. If the disease is unrecognized and untreated, more than 90% of affected patients will die within one month. Even now, this disease can go unrecognized on initial presentation, often being confused with acute myocardial infarction. A high index of suspicion is necessary, and the clinician should be aware of the manifestations and treatment of aortic dissection, since more than 70% of patients with aortic dissection survive the initial episode if treated aggressively [43]. The diagnosis of aortic dissection should be considered in any patient with acute severe chest, back, or epigastric pain or in the patient with stroke, acute aortic insufficiency, or pulseless extremities.

Classification

DeBakey et al. [44] have classified aortic dissections as follows: type I, initimal tear in the ascending aorta and dissection extending into the descending aorta; type II, dissection confined to the aortic arch; and type III, dissection confined to the descending aorta. Wheat and others [45] have favored a simplified staging system: type A, proximal dissections (DeBakey types I and II) and type B, distal dissection (DeBakey type III), since the treatment of types I and II are similar.

Pathogenesis

The pathogenesis of aortic dissection remains obscure in many patients. In the past, cystic medial necrosis of Erdheim was thought to be a specific lesion of aortic dissection. In recent years, however, Schlatmann and Becker [46] have cast considerable doubt on this assumption. They believe that cystic medial necrosis is present in normal aortas and represents a normal aging process in the aorta. Atherosclerosis probably does not contribute appreciably to the pathogenesis of types I and II aortic dissection. Rupture of an atherosclerotic intimal plaque may be a contributory factor in type III dissections, although it is uncertain whether atherosclerosis is an incidental finding in this group [47]. Aortic dissection has been described in histologically normal aortas.

In 70% of aortic dissections, an intimal tear in the ascending aorta is the initiating event. In the remainder, the intimal tear is located distal to the left subclavian artery or, rarely, in the aortic arch [48].

Aortic dissection is not a disease confined only to the elderly. In fact, Larson and Edwards [47] reported the mean age of patients with aortic dissection and tricuspid, bicuspid, and unicommissural aortic valves to be 63, 55, and 40 years, respectively. They thought the major risk factors for aortic dissection were hypertension (52% for types I and II and 75% for type III), the Marfan syndrome, and for types I and II dissections, congenitally bicuspid or unicommissural valves. Aortic dissection has also been associated with the third trimester of pregnancy, coarctation of the aorta, and giant-cell arteritis. Uncommonly, aortic dissection may result from angiographic procedures.

Clinical aspects

The clinical manifestations of aortic dissection are diverse. Pain is the most common initial symptom (90%); it is described as sudden onset of an intense tearing or ripping sensation but is often nonspecific in character [48]. Often, the location of pain corresponds to the site of initial dissection—that is, anterior chest pain (proximal dissection) and back pain (distal dissection). The pain can radiate to the neck, back, and extremities as the dissection propagates along the aorta.

Hypertension is commonly present. Hypotension may result from aortic rupture into the pericardium, pleural space, or peritoneal cavity. In 50% of proximal dissections, blood pressure and pulse may be absent or decreased in one or both arms, a useful physical finding to differentiate acute myocardial infarction from aortic dissection and one which should be sought specifically in all patients with severe chest pain. Other frequent and ominous physical findings include aortic insufficiency, disturbances of consciousness, cerebrovascular accidents, and ischemic paraparesis.

Laboratory examination

Radiographic confirmation of a suspected aortic dissection should be sought. In 80% of patients, radiography of the chest shows a widened mediastinum, pleural effusion, or separation of intimal calcification from the outer border of the aorta [49]. Aortography is still mandatory to plan surgical approach. Computed tomography using high-volume contrast material and closely spaced tomographic planes is also accurate in identifying aortic dissections [50,51]. However, it will not demonstrate aortic insufficiency or accurately identify occlusion of major branch arteries—information that would be of great value to the surgeon. The major usefulness of computed tomography may be in excluding aortic dissection in patients whose condition is stable with a low or medium probability of having the disease. It is also valuable in confirming the diagnosis in patients who, for various reasons, are thought to be candidates for medical therapy only.

Two-dimensional echocardiography supplemented with Doppler color flow echocardiography is an accurate diagnostic technique when aortic dissection is suspected and when transesophageal echocardiography is used [52,53]. Magnetic resonance imaging holds promise in the diagnosis of aortic dissection and has the advantage of avoidance of contrast material. Gated magnetic resonance imaging is only suitable in hemodynamically stable patients who do not have pacemakers or metallic prosthetic valves [53].

Therapy

Initial treatment of all aortic dissections is medical and is aimed at relieving pain, lowering blood pressure in the hypertensive patient, and at treating hypotension by administration of parenteral fluids before angiography. The degree of hypertension and the rate of elevation of arterial pressure (DP/ DT) are the most important factors in the propagation of the dissection [54]. Infusion of nitroprusside to lower blood pressure, combined with intravenously administered propranolol (Inderal) to decrease heart rate and left ventricular contractility, is most frequently used. If the use of beta-blockers is contraindicated, alpha-methyldopa can be substituted. Clonidine is also useful but cannot be given intravenously. Intravenously administered trimethaphan (Arfonad) alone is an alternative to nitroprusside and propranolol.

Operation is the recommended treatment for proximal dissections. Distal dissections may initially be treated medically, since the operative mortality associated with emergency surgery is higher than the mortality with medical therapy. However, the presence of persistent pain, uncontrollable hypertension, or obstruction of a major branch vessel is an indication for immediate surgery [43].

Surgical mortality rates for acute proximal dissection may be as high as 40%; 50% of all patients treated aggressively may be alive at ten years [55]. Recurrent dissection and aneurysmal dilation are late complications. Chronic aggressive treatment of hypertension is mandatory and should include beta-blocking agents. Close follow-up, including carefully taken physical examination, serial films of the chest, and ultrasound or computed tomography of the aorta, may be helpful in the early detection of recurrent dissection.

OCCLUSIVE DISEASE OF ABDOMINAL VISCERAL VESSELS

Chronic intestinal ischemia

Although mesenteric arterial stenosis is common, chronic symptoms of the disorder are rare [56]. In an autopsy study of patients aged 28 to 86 years, atherosclerotic narrowing of the superior mesenteric artery was noted in 37% and of the celiac axis in 44% [57]. Atherosclerosis is the commonest cause of mesenteric artery disease, usually at the origins of vessels. As this process progresses gradually, the abundant collateral blood flow supplied by the adjacent mesenteric circulation and by the systemic circulation usually permits adequate support of intestinal circulation and prevents symptoms of ischemia. When disease of the mesenteric vessels is widespread or when major sources of collateral flow have been destroyed by previous operations, symptoms of intestinal ischemia will appear. The more rapid the progression of impaired blood flow, the more likely it is to produce symptoms.

Clinical aspects

Of the three major sources of mesenteric blood flow—namely, the celiac axis and the superior and inferior mesenteric arteries—reduction of flow in two of these major channels is usually necessary to produce symptoms [58]. In most such symptomatic patients, the superior mesenteric artery is involved. Rarely, symptoms have occurred with occlusion of only one mesenteric vessel with associated poor collateral circulation [59].

The diagnosis of chronic intestinal ischemia depends on the pattern of symptoms, since stenosis of the mesenteric vessels is a common finding in asymptomatic persons. Usually, no clinical findings are present other than the history, which will establish presence of the syndrome if arterial stenoses are demonstrated.

Postprandial abdominal pain [60], associated with a history of weight loss [56,61] of weeks' to months' duration, is the usual presentation of the disorder. The pain typically is epigastric or periumbilical, occasionally radiating to the back, is dull or cramping, and occurs usually from a few minutes to an hour after eating. The larger the amount of food ingested and the more severe the diminution in intestinal blood flow, the more frequently will pain be induced, and the more persistent it becomes. As the disease progresses, the amount of food that can be tolerated decreases, and the pain becomes more persistent and atypical in pattern. From a study at the Mayo Clinic [56,60], an atypical pain pattern was noted in 21 of 43 patients thought to have this syndrome. Under these circumstances, the diagnosis becomes extremely difficult to ascertain and depends on alert consideration of the possibility after all other potential causes of abdominal pain and weight loss have been excluded.

Although malabsorption may play a role [61,62], weight loss is primarily caused by decreased intake of food in an effort to avoid pain. The onset of this pattern may be insidious, and specific questioning is often required of the patient to elicit its presence. Abnormal bowel function may be present, manifested by constipation [63], bloating, or occasional diarrhea [56].

Physical examination yields no diagnostic findings. Evidence of under-nutrition, the occasional finding of an abdominal bruit, and the presence of arteriosclerosis elsewhere in the body, while consistent with the diagnosis, are nonspecific in their implications.

Laboratory examination

Evidence of malabsorption, including abnormal responses to d-xylose testing [64], and infrequently found abnormalities on barium study of the small intestine, such as segmentation, mucosal edema, and hypomotility [65], are also consistent with but not diagnostic of the disease.

Duplex ultrasound mesenteric arterial scanning is being evaluated as a screening technique for chronic visceral arterial occlusive disease. It has proved to be a helpful study that is sometimes supplemented by provocative ingestion of a high-calorie liquid meal [66]. However, duplex ultrasound scanning lacks the accuracy of biplane angiography, which remains the standard diagnostic study [67]. The need for screening techniques to detect mesenteric ischemia continues. Noninvasive methods to assess mucosal perfusion are being studied [66].

Arteriography is necessary [68] to demonstrate occlusion or flow-reducing stenosis diminishing the arterial orifice by at least 50% in diameter in at least two mesenteric vessels, usually including the superior mesenteric artery. Lateral views are important in addition to anteroposterior projections. Aortography demonstrates arteriosclerotic involvement at orifices of vessels better than selective angiography [65]. Both techniques are of value depending on individual anatomy.

Occlusive disease often resembles intra-abdominal cancer. The diagnosis of chronic intestinal ischemia is difficult to establish because it shares symptoms with a variety of other gastrointestinal disorders, including both malignant and benign diseases. Some of these are often difficult to exclude, as in carcinoma of the pancreas. Stenosis of the mesenteric artery may appear coincidentally with these diseases. Only by careful exclusion of those other entities with attention to the history of the initial appearance of the disorder and constant awareness of its potential existence will the diagnosis be made.

Therapy

Surgical treatment includes endarterectomy [69], arterial reimplantation, and more commonly, bypass grafting using synthetic grafts or autologous vein [65,70]. An operative mortality rate has been reported in the range of 9% [59,71], although no operative mortality was reported in one series [69]. More than 90% of patients are relieved of symptoms, with recurrence rates varying from 3% to 26.5% in 2 to 4 years [59,69,71]. Percutaneous balloon angioplasty of the superior mesenteric artery may have rare applicability as a therapeutic test to determine whether atypical symptoms are relieved by dilation of a stenosed vessel, but it has limited, if any, use as definitive therapy [66].

Acute intestinal ischemia

Acute intestinal ischemia has four major causes. The most common is a result of emboli to the superior mesenteric artery, which account for more than half of such cases [72]. Most mesenteric emboli originate from the left side of the heart, usually in association with atrial fibrillation [73]. Poor intestinal perfusion without vascular occlusion, owing to impaired cardiac output and splanchnic vasoconstriction, is a second major cause of acute ischemia [74]. It is estimated to be responsible for ischemia in 35% to 40% of patients [75,76]. The remainder are attributable either to acute mesenteric artery thrombosis, usually in vessels that are arteriosclerotic, or to mesenteric vein thrombosis [72,77]. Rarely, sacrifice of the inferior mesenteric artery in the course of aortic surgery will result in infarction of the colon if the mesenteric collateral circulation is poor [26].

In only 10% of patients with acute intestinal ischemia can the cause be related directly to stenosing disease of the mesenteric arteries [72]. Of that group with underlying arterial disease, half have a history of chronic intestinal ischemia [78] with prior symptoms of pain after eating, weight loss, and change in bowel habits preceding the acute event [77].

In mesenteric artery thrombosis, onset of symptoms of acute ischemia may be gradual. In contrast, emboli usually cause an abrupt onset of severe abdominal pain. In the latter condition, prior emboli will often have been found elsewhere in the body [79]. Underlying cardiac disease or arrhythmia will frequently suggest a potential embolic source [80].

Mesenteric ischemia without associated vascular occlusion is the result of low cardiac output and associated splanchnic vasoconstriction [77]. It may occur in such conditions as shock, sepsis, or head injury [81]. Mesenteric vasoconstriction causes ischemia of the bowel and damaged intestinal mucosa, which becomes infected. Associated sepsis and hypovolemia with reduction of cardiac output further stimulate the sympathetic nervous system and increase vasoconstriction, which further aggravates the process [77].

The presentation of acute intestinal ischemia can be typified by that resulting from emboli to the superior mesenteric artery. This consists of a triad, including abdominal pain, "gut emptying," and leukocytosis [77,82]. The pain may be periumbilical, generalized, or in the right upper quadrant of the abdomen. It is described as being out of proportion to physical findings, which initially may consist of no more than mild tenderness in a soft abdomen.

Peristaltic sounds can be heard until late in the course of the ischemic process when hemorrhagic infarction has developed. Vomiting and diarrhea are usually present. A white blood cell count of more than 15,000 per mm^3 is common.

Adequate diagnosis and management require angiography whenever acute intestinal ischemia is suspected. Treatment [77,83] includes volume replacement, correction of acidosis, and administration of antibiotics and intra-arterial vasodilators, such as papaverine, by catheter in the mesenteric artery. Embolectomy [83] or aortomesenteric graft in the case of arterial thrombi [77] is undertaken as early as possible. Such treatment may prevent the tragically high mortality rate of more than 80%, which can result from intestinal resection for mesenteric infarction [77]. Heparin must be administered for embolic disease to prevent recurrence, although optimal timing is uncertain. To avoid hemorrhage into ischemic intestine, this therapy is sometimes deferred for 48 hours. The usefulness of anticoagulants in the treatment of nonembolic intestinal ischemia is unknown and carries a considerable risk of bleeding.

Mesenteric vein thrombosis is an uncommon cause of intestinal infarction. Computed tomography may detect resulting changes in the intestinal wall, and when enhanced with contrast material, it can detect thrombus in the mesenteric vein [84]. Treatment consists of resection of involved intestine and postoperative anticoagulation [85] as well as a search for an underlying cause.

Renal artery stenosis

Renal artery stenosis is important both as a rare reversible cause of systemic hypertension and because it can produce life-threatening renal failure when it affects both kidneys. In the elderly, as surgical risks increase, emphasis on renal preservation as a basis for surgical intervention increases. Hypertension must be severe and medically uncontrollable to justify the risks of such surgery in the elderly patient. The alternative approach of renal artery dilation—percutaneous balloon angioplasty—is associated with a lower risk than the various types of vascular reconstruction. However, this procedure is less effective in the treatment of atherosclerotic renal artery disease than it is for stenosing fibromuscular dysplasia of the arteries of younger persons [86].

Pathogenesis

Renal artery stenosis as a cause of systemic hypertension was suggested in 1934 by the experiments of Goldblatt et al. [87]. They produced hypertension in the dog by experimental constriction of a renal artery. This led to surgical efforts to cure hypertension directed at the kidney. In subsequent years, such attempts initially met with a high failure rate [88] because the patho-physiology of renal ischemia was not understood. It was not recognized that renal artery stenosis is common in normotensive individuals [89,90]. The presence of occlusive disease of a renal artery in a hypertensive individual does not necessarily imply that it is responsible for raising blood pressure in that person.

Subsequently, differential renal function tests analyzing urine obtained by ureteral catheter were used to establish the functional importance of renal ischemia [91,92]. Such studies were later supplanted by ratios of plasma renin obtained from both renal veins [93,94]. Understanding the role of the renin-angiotensin system improved identification of renal artery stenosis as a functionally significant cause of systemic hypertension.

Renin, a proteolytic enzyme, is released by the ischemic kidney. It acts on a glycoprotein made by the liver to produce angiotensin I, a decapeptide, subsequently transformed by converting enzyme to an octapeptide, angiotension II. Angiotensin II is 50 times more potent than norepinephrine in raising blood pressure [95].

Improved screening tests for renal artery stenosis causing hypertension continue to be sought. Response of peripheral plasma renin activity to a challenge of the angiotensin-converting enzyme inhibitor, captopril, has been reported [96–98] with varying sensitivity and specificity, ranging from poor to excellent. Further study and standardization of this test will be required before its general clinical applicability can be decided.

Comparison of renin levels in the venous blood of both kidneys provides a ratio that is a guideline to detection of hypertension-producing renal artery stenosis. Marks and coworkers [93] reviewed several series that defined renin ratios varying between 1.4 and 2.5 as abnormal values. Cure or improvement of hypertension with surgery occurred in 93% of patients with these renin ratios.

However, renal vein renin ratios may fail to predict improvement of hypertension with renovascular reconstruction on occasion. In a series from the Lahey Clinic [99], this was true in 20% of patients with unilateral renal artery disease and in 35% of patients with bilateral renal artery stenosis.

Prevalence

Renovascular hypertension is not common. Among 2552 hypertensive patients carefully studied in a referral center [100], renal artery stenosis was found in 9.5% of patients, but only 4.2% were believed to have renovascular hypertension. Arteriographic study [101] of renal artery stenosis in hypertensive patients revealed atherosclerosis in 63%, fibromuscular dysplasia in 32.4%, and other diseases in 4.6%. Dysplastic disease occurs predominantly in young women, and atherosclerotic disease is found in an older age group, with the greatest prevalence in men over age 65 [102–104]. In the elderly population, atherosclerosis is by far the major cause of renal artery stenosis. Bilateral involvement was noted [101] in 31.3% of patients with atherosclerotic disease. It usually involves the aortic orifice or proximal one third of the renal artery [102].

Clinical aspects

New onset or increased severity of hypertension in an individual more than 50 years of age should raise the question of underlying renal artery stenosis. Unexplained increasing azotemia should also suggest this possibility, particularly in the presence of atherosclerosis in extrarenal arteries [105] or risk factors for atherosclerosis.

Detection of an abdominal bruit increases the likelihood of underlying renal artery disease. Such bruits are typically high pitched, prolonged, and blowing. When originating from the renal artery, they are best heard in the upper part of the abdomen and may radiate to the flank [106].

Laboratory examination

For many years, rapid sequence intravenous pyelography has been the most commonly utilized screening technique for detection of an ischemic kidney. Disparity in size between the two kidneys, delayed appearance time of intrarenal dye, and late hyperconcentration are the major criteria for renal ischemia. A review [107] of the literature revealed a false-negative rate of 25.5% and a false-positive rate of 13.9% when this approach was used compared with arteriographic findings.

Since 1980, intravenous renal digital subtraction arteriography has gained increased popularity as a screening technique [108]. This study enables visualization of arteries after intravenous injection of contrast material using computed subtraction of venous images. Spatial resolution is inferior to standard arteriography; hence, distal and intrarenal vessels are less well visualized. Most surgeons require standard angiography if surgery is planned. Reviewing the literature, Havey and coworkers [107] reported that 7.4% of intravenous renal digital subtraction angiograms could not be interpreted because of motion artifacts of overlying vessels. Of the remainder, 12.4% false-negative and 10.5% false-positive results were obtained. This technique requires more contrast agent and is more expensive than intravenous pyelography. Nevertheless, it gives specific information about the renal arteries and is therefore a superior screening procedure.

Contrast-induced renal impairment is possible in patients who already have renal dysfunction, particularly in the elderly hypertensive population. Care that the amount of contrast agent is kept low and attention to adequate hydration before it is given help to decrease occurrence of this complication.

Radioisotope renography has the advantage of not using a contrast agent. The advent of the angiotensin-converting enzyme inhibitor, captopril, to enhance isotope renal scanning has improved the accuracy of radionuclide studies for renovascular disease. Studies [109–111] using technetium-99m-labeled diethylene triamine pentaacetic acid (^{99m}Tc-labeled DTPA) and iodohippurate sodium I 131 (^{131}I-labeled hippuram) have shown improved diagnostic accuracy after a provocative challenge with captopril. This approach shows promise of improved noninvasive screening for stenosis of the renal artery and for reversible renovascular hypertension. Its role in bilateral renal artery stenosis appears limited. Its final clinical place compared with other techniques requires further investigation. Meier et al. [111] described use of captopril renal scintigraphy and DTPA scanning in patients suspected of having renovascular hypertension. Of seven patients with normal results, one patient was improved after operation or angioplasty. Of eight patients with positive results, one patient was cured, five patients were improved, and two patients with bilateral renal artery stenosis failed to improve or worsened in terms of response of hypertension.

If renal artery stenosis is strongly suspected, it would be reasonable to go directly to standard arteriography rather than to resort to screening tests. Standard arteriography is usually required if surgery is being planned because of the limitations of intravenous digital angiography. Oblique and selective angiography is necessary to avoid missing some proximal stenosed arteries and those hidden by overlying vessels and to detect segmental artery stenoses [112]. Computed digital subtraction enhancement can be used with arterial injection to see greater detail with relatively small amounts of contrast agent.

Therapy

In the elderly population, hypertension caused by renal artery stenosis should be treated medically when possible. Approximately two thirds of patients with renovascular hypertension respond satisfactorily to standard anti-hypertensive drugs [113]. Although converting enzyme inhibitors are logical choices for treatment, they must be used with caution because of aggravation of azotemia in the presence of renal artery stenosis, particularly when stenosis is bilateral [114]. In medically treated patients, underlying renal artery disease and renal ischemia may progress [115,116], requiring periodic monitoring of renal function, including renal perfusion scans or digital subtraction renal angiography.

In recent years, progressive impairment of renal function caused by renal artery stenosis has been halted or improved by measures reversing the impairment of renal artery perfusion [117,118]. Preservation of renal function has become an important indication for renovascular reconstruction. The treatment of renal artery stenosis includes percutaneous transluminal angioplasty, thromboendarterectomy, renal artery bypass, and renal artery reimplantation. Aortorenal bypass is the most frequently used of these approaches.

Percutaneous transluminal renal artery dilatation using a balloon-tipped catheter is a low-risk, effective procedure of value when anticipated operative mortality is high. The recurrence rate of renal artery stenosis in patients with atherosclerotic disease with evidence of restenosis is high, occurring in 11 of 16 patients in one series [86] with a follow-up period of 3 to 24 months. When used for renal failure or hypertension associated with atherosclerotic renal artery stenosis or both, one study [119] of 55 patients showed initial cure or improvement in 53% but in only 34% at a follow-up time of 4 to 42 months (mean, 22 months). In another similar series [120] of 55 patients with atherosclerotic renal artery stenosis, a successful clinical outcome was described in 26.1%. Repeated dilations are possible, but further long-term study of this approach is needed. Patients with fibromuscular disease fare much better. However, atherosclerosis rather than fibromuscular disease is the cause of renal artery stenosis in the elderly.

Thromboendarterectomy is often suitable for atherosclerotic lesions limited to the orifice of the renal artery [121]. Renal artery bypass in various forms is the most widely used surgical technique. In a cooperative study [122] from several institutions, bypass was associated with a mortality rate of 5.4% and a complication rate of 13%. A remarkably low operative mortality rate of 0% to 1% associated with focal renal artery atherosclerosis [101,123] in highly specialized centers contrasts with a mortality rate of 8.5% in the same expert hands when diffuse atherosclerosis is present [123]. A high operative mortality is associated with aneurysmal or stenosing atherosclerosis of the abdominal aorta. In this situation, hepatorenal or splenorenal bypass sometimes presents an alternative that avoids mobilization of the abdominal aorta [124]. However, if an aneurysm is large, many surgeons prefer to replace the abdominal aorta at the time of renal revascularization. Diffuse atherosclerosis is commonly found in the elderly population with atherosclerotic disease of the renal arteries. Surgery for renal reperfusion should only be undertaken in this high-risk group when other therapeutic alternatives have failed and the situation is potentially life-threatening.

CEREBROVASCULAR DISEASE

Prevalence

Cerebrovascular diseases are the third most common cause of death in the United States. Between 1974 and 1978, the mortality associated with stroke was 0.83 per 1000 annually [125], or more than 180,000 deaths per year. Even more devastating is the associated crippling morbidity. Various studies have reported 3 to 9 strokes occurring for every stroke-related death [126,127]. Age is a decided risk factor for stroke. For patients more than 55 years of age, the incidence of stroke more than doubles for each successive decade [128]. Men are approximately 30% more susceptible to stroke than women, although this sex difference decreases slightly over 65 years of age [128].

Pathogenesis

Three fourths of patients who have had a stroke have hypertension [129]. Elevated blood pressure as a risk factor for stroke applies to both sexes, and all ages correlate with diastolic and even more closely with systolic blood pressure [130]. Correlation with systolic blood pressure increases with age and is independent of arterial rigidity [131].

An accelerating downward trend in the incidence of stroke has occurred in recent years [132]. The incidence of fatal strokes decreased in the United States by 45% in the past decade [133]. Although antihypertensive therapy has had a major effect on this declining rate [133], other unknown factors are present because stroke rates have been diminishing since 1914, long before antihypertensive therapy was available [132].

The effectiveness of antihypertensive therapy in the prevention of stroke is evident both in mild [134] and severe hypertension [135] and includes older age groups. Among hypertensive patients aged 60 to 69 years, a 45% reduction in the frequency of stroke was reported [125] in patients who had standardized aggressive treatment of hypertension in a clinic setting compared with patients with variable treatment by practitioners in the community.

Computed tomography has greatly increased the accuracy of distinguishing between cerebral hemorrhage and infarction and has helped to clarify the effects of preventive treatment. When this technique was used, intracerebral hemorrhage was detected relatively frequently [136]. However, a study at the Mayo Clinic [137] showed that from 1945 through 1954, intracerebral hemorrhage accounted for 17% of strokes in autopsied patients. Antihypertensive therapy is said to have a greater impact on decreasing the incidence of cerebral hemorrhage compared with the incidence of infarction [136]. However, in the Framingham study [130], increasing severity of hypertension was not associated with greater risk for cerebral hemorrhage compared with the risk of cerebral infarction.

The role of the heart as a source of cerebral emboli has been clarified with the increased use of echocardiography and radionuclide angiography and long-term ambulatory cardiac monitoring. Cardiogenic emboli account for approximately 15% of ischemic strokes [136], and depending on associated cardiac lesions, the risk may be increased much more. Atrial fibrillation increases the risk of stroke fivefold [138]. Almost half of cerebral emboli from the heart are the result of ischemic heart disease, rheumatic mitral stenosis, or prosthetic cardiac valves. Approximately 3% of patients who have an acute myocardial infarction have an ischemic stroke within four weeks with a strong correlation with mural thrombi. This is particularly true of anterior transmural myocardial infarctions, which account for 90% of the ischemic strokes associated with myocardial infarction [138].

Less common causes of cerebral emboli from the heart include mitral valve prolapse, calcification of the mitral annulus, nonbacterial thrombotic endocarditis, calcific aortic stenosis, cardiac myxomas, paradoxical embolism and congenital heart disease, nonischemic dilated cardiomyopathy, and infective endocarditis [138]. Good randomized trials comparing the efficacy of decreasing cardiogenic embolism by anticoagulants against the risk of bleeding from such therapy now exist for atrial fibrillation [139]. In such instances as mitral stenosis with atrial fibrillation requiring prosthetic valve replacement, the risk of embolization is high, exceeding the risk of anticoagulation. For such conditions as atrial fibrillation without valvular disease, guidelines for treatment are now available [139].

The relative importance of some findings, such as segmental hypokinesis of the left ventricle in the absence of a recent myocardial infarction, or the discovery of a mural thrombus years after a large myocardial infarction has occurred, remains unknown. Such findings are becoming increasingly frequent with the widespread use of echocardiography. In the absence of evidence of cardiac abnormality by history, physical examination, and electrocardiography to suggest a possible embolic source, the likelihood of finding a cardiac cause of cerebral embolism by echocardiography is low [139].

The incidence of ischemic heart disease in patients with symptoms of cerebral ischemia is high. Myocardial infarction is the most common cause of death in patients presenting with transient cerebral ischemia [140]. This has an important bearing on decisions for management of patients with cerebral ischemia and emphasizes the need for careful cardiac evaluation and treatment in this group of patients with underlying coronary disease.

Carotid artery disease

Recognition of the role of extracranial disease in the internal carotid arteries as a source of cerebral ischemia and infarction has stimulated aggressive efforts to detect and treat such disease. In an important necropsy study in 1965, Fisher and associates [141] noted that symptomatic atherosclerotic disease in the internal carotid arteries tended to be extracranial and that symptomatic disease in the vertebral basilar system was usually intracranial. At a clinical level, atherothrombotic disease involving major extracranial cerebral arteries is associated with one third of strokes, and such disease in a surgically accessible area comprises less than 15% of strokes [128]. Extracranial atherosclerotic occlusive disease in the internal carotid arteries without signs or symptoms of cerebral ischemia is common both at autopsy [141,142] and clinically [143].

The natural history of asymptomatic extracranial cerebrovascular disease is not well defined. Relatively little information is based on arteriographic studies. Other series are based on noninvasive study of cervical vessels, and some identify disease by the presence of an audible bruit in the neck, which is a relatively nonspecific finding. It is difficult, therefore, to assess the desirability of prophylactic measures to prevent stroke in such asymptomatic disease. The problem is further compounded by an absence of any randomized studies comparing treated with control groups.

The progression of asymptomatic carotid disease has been studied by Javid and coworkers [144] by arteriography in patients with atherosclerotic stenosis involving the internal carotid artery at the level of the carotid bifurcation. Initially, all had less than 60% stenosis of the carotid artery. Rapidly progressive stenosis with more than 25% change per year was found in 22% of the total group, but in 40% progression of stenosis was not appreciable during a period of 1 to 9 years of follow-up. In another group of patients studied noninvasively [145], progression of stenosis of the carotid artery occurred less often in persons over age 65 years. Diabetes mellitus and cigarette smoking increased the tendency to progression in one series [145], and systemic hypertension indicated a trend to progressing stenosis in another group [144]. As noted previously, an occluded internal carotid artery may produce no symptoms or findings of cerebral ischemia [141–143] if collateral flow is adequate. Most asymptomatic persons in whom carotid occlusion or symptoms of cerebral ischemia developed over a mean follow-up period of three years had preceding stenosis of the carotid artery of more than 80% demonstrable by ultrasound scanning [145]. In one series [146], asymptomatic carotid artery stenosis in the range of 80% to 99% determined by noninvasive studies was associated with a stroke rate of 47% over a mean of 36 months. Based on available community studies [147], the stroke rate in asymptomatic carotid disease is in the range of 1% to 2% per year. Stroke may be preceded by one or more transient ischemic attacks (TIAs), but it may also occur without warning in this asymptomatic group [147,148].

Transient cerebral ischemia
Transient cerebral ischemia has been defined as a temporary focal episode of transient neurologic dysfunction of presumed vascular origin, typically lasting 2 to 15 minutes but occasionally as long as 24 hours, clearing without residua [149]. Migraine is excluded when it can be identified as such. Certain symptoms, such as vertigo, dysarthria, and diplopia, are excluded from the definition of TIAs if they are isolated in occurrence [150]. However, transient blindness in one eye (amaurosis fugax) is considered a TIA. Nonspecific symptoms, such as confusion, lightheadedness, or syncope, are also not considered in themselves to represent a TIA [150]. Symptoms referable to the carotid artery include contralateral weakness or numbness, transient blindness in the ipsilateral eye, and if the dominant hemisphere is involved, dysphasia or apraxia. In the vertebrobasilar system, visual field loss, diplopia, unilateral or bilateral numbness or weakness, vertigo, dysarthria, dysphagia, and weakness or paralysis in both legs or in all extremities (drop attacks) without loss of consciousness may occur.

What are the implications of TIAs? In two articles, Millikan [151,152] described the characteristics of these attacks and their implications as precursors of cerebral infarction. Many of them are believed to be the result of emboli of platelet fibrin or atheroma from a proximal atherosclerotic artery [152]. Some are believed to be caused by small cardiac emboli [153]. In the presence of stenosed cerebral arteries, transient local shifts in cerebral blood flow must be responsible for some of these attacks, but this remains poorly understood. Transient hypotension [154] and cardiac dysrhythmia [155] superimposed on cerebrovascular disease in reality are probably rare precipitating causes of TIAs. Rarely, anemia, polycythemia, or thrombocytosis may be responsible for transient focal cerebral ischemia. Similar symptoms are sometimes produced by lacunar infarctions [156].

These tiny areas of cerebral ischemic necrosis, often found in the brainstem, are caused by local endarteriolar wall thickening and stenosis frequently caused by systemic hypertension. They are often productive of purely motor or purely sensory symptoms. By computed tomography, it may not be possible to distinguish a small infarction due to an embolus from a lacunar infarction due to arteriolar disease. In an angiographic analysis [156] of TIAs in the carotid territory distribution, half of the patients had tight stenosis or occlusion of the internal carotid artery extracranially. Transient monocular blindness and transient hemispheric symptoms occurring separately in the same individual had a strong correlation with the occurrence of tight stenosis in the extracranial internal carotid artery. Prolonged symptoms of cerebral ischemia lasting an hour or more tended to occur in patients with little or no extracranial carotid stenosis. This raises the question of whether some of the latter group were caused by cardiac emboli [156] since they were associated with a relatively open proximal carotid system.

Only about 10% of all strokes are preceded by TIAs [128,157], but this figure is much higher for patients with known carotid disease [158]. Of patients who have a TIA, approximately one third will have a stroke within five years [150]. Of patients who have a stroke preceded by TIA, cerebral infarction will occur within the first month after TIA in 20% and within one year in half the group [159]. After the first year following onset of a TIA, the stroke rate in subsequent years averages 5% to 6% per year [160,161]. Patients who come to attention as potential stroke risks are either those who have suggestive symptoms as described or those who have physical or laboratory findings raising the possibility of underlying cerebrovascular disease. A blowing bruit heard high in the lateral neck may indicate carotid disease. A prolonged bruit, extending through systole into diastole, indicates severe stenosis and suggests disease in the internal rather than the external carotid system. The internal carotid artery supplies a low-resistance system, which is not true of the external carotid artery; hence, a bruit heard into diastole is associated with the internal carotid system.

Even the most expert observer will misinterpret cervical bruits. Severe arterial stenosis often produces no bruit. At the Cleveland Clinic [162], 13% of patients without bruits had severe internal carotid stenosis, and 14% with a "carotid" bruit had no internal or external carotid disease at angiography. In addition, 7% without a bruit had a totally occluded carotid artery.

In the Framingham group [163], the presence of a carotid bruit increased in incidence with age to 7% of patients 65 to 79 years old. The stroke rate was doubled for individuals matched for age and sex with patients with a bruit, and the mortality rate was also increased 1.7 to 1.9 times in men and women, respectively. However, the location of the bruit did not tend to indicate the territory of a subsequent stroke. In that sense, it was simply a nonspecific sign of underlying atherosclerosis [163].

Rarely, examination of the retina will reveal bright yellowish-orange plaques at the bifurcations of retinal arterioles. Hollenhorst [164] noted them in 27 of 235 patients with carotid stenosing disease. They are small emboli of cholesterol emanating from the proximal atheromatous artery. They may persist for months but may disappear within two weeks after they are first seen [165]. These emboli are associated with an appreciable increase in the risk of stroke and a decrease in the expectancy of survival [166,167]. Of patients with this finding, 54% were dead within seven years, the majority of coronary artery disease [166]. The annual stroke mortality was 4 to 5 times greater than expected [167].

In addition to the cholesterol emboli described, small pale retinal intra-arteriolar aggregates, consisting of platelets and fibrin also thought to be of carotid origin [165], are rarely seen. They are difficult to visualize and tend to be evanescent.

In one series [168] of patients whose presenting complaint was amaurosis fugax, 110 patients were treated with antiplatelet agents and antihypertensive therapy when indicated. Patients were instructed to stop smoking. In this retrospective study of more than six years, 43% of patients remained asymptomatic, monocular blindness developed in 6%, and cerebral infarction occurred in 13%. The mortality rate was 38%, primarily of cardiac cause.

Laboratory examinations

Many laboratory techniques have been devised and are available for the study of the brain and cerebrovascular system. Some of these tests are still primarily research tools, but many have wide clinical application. Only the most frequently used will be mentioned here [169,170]. High-frequency sound waves (ultrasound) are utilized to visualize extracranial cerebrovascular vessels and to analyze flow characteristics through the cervical vessels. Detailed anatomy of the cervical arteries can be visualized in a two-dimensional manner by standard ultrasound. Detailed information of the characteristics of an endothelial plaque can be obtained in this way. Results of such tests have an important bearing on prognosis, and one study [171] supports the concept that a noncalcified, nonfibrosed plaque of low density has a greater tendency toward subintimal hemorrhage, ulceration, or embolization than a more organized plaque. Imaging with ultrasound has the disadvantage of inability to penetrate a calcified arterial wall. Doppler ultrasound utilizes the concept of a shift in frequency of sound waves proportional to the velocity of red blood cells from which it is reflected [169]. Although pulsed Doppler ultrasound can also be used for imaging vessels [172], Doppler studies are most frequently used to determine flow velocity and direction of flow, and to detect evidence of turbulence. Since stenosis increases velocity of flow, and a poststenotic scattering of wave frequencies (turbulence) occurs, the degree of stenosis can be measured. This technique is not always reliable in distinguishing severe stenosis from occlusion of a vessel. Also, any disorder that will increase flow velocity, such as compensatory flow because of a contralateral occluded vessel, anemia, or hyperthyroidism, may give a false impression of the degree of stenosis. Vertebral artery assessment is less accurate than that of the cervical carotid artery, but with use of the directional Doppler, retrograde flow through the vertebral artery from subclavian artery stenosis (subclavian steal) can be detected. Since asymptomatic patients who have severe carotid stenosis are said to be at highest risk for strokes [145], screening of the asymptomatic group with Doppler ultrasound is useful. To detect evidence of stenosis by Doppler flow measurement, more than 50% diameter narrowing of the vessel must have occurred. Ultrasound imaging and Doppler flow analysis are complementary techniques. When they are used in conjunction, accuracy in detecting carotid stenosis is improved. In one series [173], 91% correct responses were obtained compared with arteriography.

The addition of other techniques further enhances accuracy and specificity. Oculoplethysmography indirectly estimates decreased flow in the internal carotid system by assessing flow to each eye either by pressure measurement (Gee oculoplethysmography) [174] or by measuring pulse-volume changes in the eye (Kartchner oculoplethysmography) [175]. In conjunction with phonoangiography (visualization of audible cervical bruit), the latter technique is said to have a high correlation with detection of flow-reducing lesions in the internal carotid system, with an overall accuracy of 90% compared with arteriography [175]. Since results depend on comparison of blood flow in one eye to blood flow in the other, assessment of severity of carotid stenosis using the Kartchner method is inaccurate when bilateral lesions are present.

Noninvasive techniques do not replace arteriography but supplement it because they supply physiologic information reflecting collateral flow to add to the anatomic data of arteriography. In the presence of symptomatic disease (TIAs), these tests do not supply adequately detailed information, and standard arteriography is indicated.

Intravenous digital subtraction angiography, referred to elsewhere in this chapter, has also been used in assessing the cerebrovascular system [176]. It does not depict intracranial vessels, and the degree of resolution is inferior to that obtained with standard angiography. We have not found that information obtained by this technique adds to that derived by the noninvasive studies mentioned.

The advent of cerebral computed tomography marks a giant stride forward in the evaluation of patients suspected of having symptoms of cerebral ischemia. It has made possible prompt differentiation of intracerebral hematoma, hemorrhagic and non-hemorrhagic infarction, and subdural hematoma [176]. It detects intracranial tumors that may be associated with symptoms mimicking a TIA [176] and can aid in the diagnosis of cerebrovascular emboli and lacunar infarctions, some of which may be "silent" with regard to symptoms. The advent of magnetic resonance imaging adds still a further modality in such evaluation, with further experience needed to assess its role in this area. Positron emission tomography also has a potential for studying such patients in the future.

Prevention and therapy

The availability of noninvasive techniques has permitted increased awareness of a large number of individuals with extracranial cerebrovascular disease, much of it asymptomatic. Since treatment of completed cerebral infarction is relatively ineffective, much effort has been directed toward prevention of stroke in individuals at risk. This includes those with asymptomatic as well as symptomatic disease. Unfortunately, no satisfactory randomized trials have determined the desirability of different treatment modalities in many subgroups [150,177–180]. Controversy surrounds the major forms of treatment, including anticoagulation, use of antiplatelet agents, and surgery, including carotid endarterectomy. However, there is now good evidence to support endarterectomy in symptomatic severely stenosed internal carotid arteries [184].

Any decision considering operation must take into account the perioperative morbidity and mortality in the surgeon's experience. Based on studies of natural history, an operative stroke complication rate of more than 2.9% is unacceptable for carotid endarterectomy [147]. Yet, reported perioperative complication rates of stroke and death vary between 1.5% and 21.1% [147].

In asymptomatic disease, Thompson and colleagues [181] reported a fourfold incidence of stroke in nonoperated patients compared with those who had carotid endarterectomy. Yet, the overall incidence of stroke in asymptomatic disease is low (1% to 2% annually) [147] in community studies, making it difficult to justify the risk of carotid surgery [182]. Most of the asymptomatic group may well be currently unacceptable for carotid endarterectomy [147]. Reported perioperative complication rates of stroke and death vary between 1.5% and 21.1% [147].

Life expectancy must be considered carefully before a decision is made for carotid endarterectomy. Overt coronary disease, age over 65 years, and systemic hypertension are indications of shortened survival [183]. Surgical treatment for asymptomatic carotid artery disease for uncertain benefits should not be undertaken if life expectancy is brief. All patients must be instructed carefully in the symptoms of TIA that would place them in a much higher risk category for stroke and justify prompt treatment. Evidence [184] now exists that carotid endarterectomy is of definite benefit to patients with recent hemispheric transient ischemic attacks or nondisabling strokes and high-grade stenosis (70% to 99%) of the appropriate internal carotid artery. Study continues concerning the possible benefits of carotid endarterectomy to patients with symptomatic moderate internal carotid stenosis (30% to 60%) and for asymptomatic patients. The trial on which this conclusion was based includes 50 centers in the United States and Canada, involving 595 patients randomized to medical or surgical therapy with a mean follow-up time of 18 months. Including perioperative events, more than 24% of medical patients but only 7% of surgical patients died of fatal or nonfatal ipsilateral stroke by 18 months.

The use of anticoagulants for carotid or vertebrobasilar TIAs of noncardiac origin is controversial because the largest studies [150,177] favoring their use were not randomized. No unequivocal data support their use in cerebral ischemia that is not the result of cardiogenic emboli [177]. Suggestive evidence in nonrandomized trials has supported their use, but no statistically significant data for the prevention of stroke have been reported for patients with TIAs in the carotid distribution [150]. *Progressing stroke*, defined as a stroke with increasing signs of neurologic deficit in recent minutes, is said to benefit from anticoagulants commencing with heparin [178]. This, too, remains uncertain, however. In patients aged 55 to 74 years with TIAs, the risk of intracranial hemorrhage was increased eight times by anticoagulants, even when prothrombin times were in a therapeutic range [150]. This was true particularly for patients who had received anticoagulants for a year or more. However, when the prothrombin time was kept in the range of 1.2 to 1.5 times the baseline value, major bleeding did not exceed that of control subjects in one group [185] with a mean follow-up time of 2.2 years, although the incidence of minor bleeding was increased in the treated group by 55%.

Antiplatelet agents include aspirin, sulfinpyrazone, and dipyridamole. No evidence exists that sulfinpyrazone used alone prevents stroke in patients with transient cerebral ischemia [186] or that the addition of dipyridamole to the use of aspirin increases protection from stroke in patients who have sustained a prior cerebral ischemic event [187].

The effectiveness of aspirin in decreasing the rate of stroke and death in men who had a prior TIA has been supported [186]. In one study [187], aspirin, 1 g daily, given to individuals with a prior cerebral ischemic event decreased the rate of stroke in both sexes. Benefits of newer antiplatelet agents such as ticlopidine are being studied.

Patients with carotid TIA with a surgically remediable significant carotid lesion and a low expected complication rate should undergo carotid endarterectomy. The value of this approach in those patients with only moderate but hemodynamically significant internal carotid artery stenosis or in patients with milder stenoses by large heterogeneous atherosclerotic-complicated plaques requires further study. Its benefit is proved in patients with symptomatic internal carotid artery stenosis of 80% to 99%. If patients have nonoperable carotid disease and in most instances of vertebrobasilar TIA, anticoagulant—that is, sodium warfarin (Coumadin)—therapy is recommended for 1 [179] to 3 [150] months if no contraindications exist, followed by aspirin, 1 g daily, after administration of Coumadin has been stopped. Each patient must be evaluated individually to determine whether the benefits to be derived outweigh the potential complications of treatment.

GIANT-CELL TEMPORAL ARTERITIS

Giant-cell arteritis is an arteritis of unknown cause involving large-sized and medium-sized arteries. The clinical presentation and pathologic features are sufficiently distinct to separate it from other arteritides. The annual incidence of giant-cell arteritis has been estimated to be 16.3 to 17.4 per 100,000 in the population aged 50 years or more [188–190]. The mean age of patients at presentation is 71 years.

Clinical manifestations are diverse. In a large series reported by Malmvall et al. [191], 71% had polymyalgia rheumatica characterized by pain or stiffness or both in at least two muscle groups. Polymyalgia rheumatica most often involved shoulders or hip girdle but also muscles of the neck and lumbar region. Of these patients, 39% had symptoms classically related to temporal arteritis—local or diffuse headache, neck pain, facial pain, temporal artery or other cranial artery tenderness, and claudication of the jaw. The majority of patients in these two groups also had systemic symptoms; 8% complained of general symptoms only—fever, fatigue, anorexia, and weight loss. This latter group of patients can pose diagnostic difficulties, since initially they are suspected of harboring other diseases—namely, occult infection or malignant disease.

Blindness, either unilateral or bilateral, a dreaded complication of giant-cell arteritis, is seen in 7% to 20% of patients before therapy is instituted [189]. This rate has fallen from earlier reports that were as high as 30% to 60% and most likely reflects earlier diagnosis and prompt treatment. Occasionally, blindness is the first manifestation of giant-cell arteritis; fortunately, other symptoms usually are apparent before loss of vision occurs.

The actuarial survival for patients with temporal arteritis was not believed to be different from the survival for the general population of the same age [189,192,193]. A recent review [194] suggested an increased mortality from temporal arteritis in the initial phase of the disease only. However, severe complications and death occur but remain rare in well-treated patients. These complications include myocardial infarction, aortic dissection, and stroke, and are related to specific involvement of the coronary arteries, aorta, and internal carotid or vertebral arteries, respectively, by giant-cell arteritis [195].

Prompt diagnosis and treatment are essential to prevent complications. Diagnosis is firmly established by temporal or other cranial artery biopsy. However, because of patchy involvement of arteries, the biopsy is positive in only up to 60% of patients. If the biopsy is negative, diagnosis can be supported on clinical grounds—the presence of typical head symptoms or polymyalgia rheumatica associated with a Westergren erythrocyte sedimentation rate greater than 40 mm per hour or both and age over 50 years. An anemia of chronic disease is frequently present. Prompt response to corticosteroid treatment, with rapid and lasting relief of symptoms, fall in erythrocyte sedimentation rate, and resolution of anemia, is supportive of the diagnosis.

Attempts to increase the yield of temporal artery biopsy by localization of stenoses by temporal artery angiography or Doppler ultrasound [196] have been reported, but experience is limited, and results are equivocal using these techniques. Temporal artery biopsy should be directed at a clinically affected area identified by symptoms, tenderness, or palpable abnormality. When the artery is not clearly abnormal, as is true in the majority of patients, an ample biopsy sample of up to 4 cm should be obtained. The artery should be examined segmentally by frozen section, and when results are negative, biopsy of the opposite artery should be performed at the same time. This strategy has proved to be the best method for diagnosing temporal arteritis in as high a percentage of patients as possible in the experience of the Mayo Clinic [197].

When results of temporal artery biopsy are negative, treatment can be considered for patients who fulfill certain clinical criteria. Based on the experience of Fernandez-Herlihy [198] at the Lahey Clinic, prolonged steroid treatment can be started when the patient has an erythrocyte sedimentation rate of 50 mm per hour or more and has tenderness of the scalp, claudication of the jaw, recent visual symptoms, and polymyalgia rheumatica and has shown a good response to 48 hours of treatment with corticosteroids. Althernative criteria would be one or more of the following clusters of symptoms: claudication of the jaw plus recent headaches and tenderness of the scalp and an erythrocyte sedimentation rate of 50 mm per hour or more or visual symptoms with an erythrocyte sedimentation rate of 50 mm per hour or more. Hunder et al. [199] reviewed various criteria for the classification of giant-cell arteritis. From a traditional format classification, they selected five criteria: age 50 years or more at the onset of disease, new onset of localized headache, tenderness or decreased pulse of the temporal artery, erythrocyte sedimentation rate of 50 mm per hour or more, and a biopsy sample that included an artery showing necrotizing arteritis characterized by a predominance of mononuclear-cell infiltrates or a granulomatous process with multinucleated giant cells. The presence of three or more of these five criteria was associated with a sensitivity of 93.5% and a specificity of 91.2%. Hunder et al. [199] also analyzed this classification tree using six criteria. The criteria were the same as for the traditional format except that the elevated erythrocyte sedimentation rate was excluded and two other variables, tenderness of the scalp and claudication of the jaw or tongue on deglutition, were included. This classification tree was associated with a sensitivity of 95.3%. and a specificity of 90.7%.

The mainstay of therapy is corticosteroids. Prednisolone, in doses of 30 to 60 mg, can be administered initially [192,200]. Prompt initiation of treatment is recommended to prevent ischemic optic infarction, and therapy should be started before biopsy in patients with convincing clinical symptoms. Treatment should not affect the diagnostic efficacy of biopsy if performed within a week of the onset of therapy. Doses of prednisolone are subsequently gradually reduced if symptoms and signs are absent. In most patients, arteritis remains well controlled with maintenance doses of prednisolone of 5 to 10 mg daily. Alternate-day therapy is limited and is reported to be of variable efficacy by different authors [201,202], but it is not usually recommended. Therapy is believed to be suppressive and must be continued until the underlying inflammatory process resolves spontaneously, usually over a period of six months to several years [203].

ATHEROSCLEROSIS OF THE SKELETAL ARTERIES

Chronic limb ischemia

Occlusive peripheral vascular disease is a common and easily recognized problem in the elderly. With few exceptions, it is a complication of the atherosclerotic process. Diabetes mellitus, hypertension, hyperlipidemia, and cigarette smoking are recognized risk factors. Its presence, even in asymptomatic individuals, should be sought because it is commonly associated with severe coronary artery disease.

The most common areas affected by atherosclerosis are major arterial bifurcations in areas of posterior fixation and acute angulation. The most commonly involved lower-extremity site is the distal superficial femoral artery lying in Hunter's canal. Atheromas involving the common femoral artery extend into the superficial femoral artery with almost similar frequency. The distal abdominal aorta and aortic bifurcation are also commonly involved [204–206].

The presence of diabetes changes the distribution and increases the frequency of lower-limb atherosclerosis. The popliteal, tibial, and profunda femoris arteries are more severely involved, while the aorta and iliac arteries may remain largely spared.

Clinical aspects

The commonest symptom of chronic limb ischemia is intermittent claudication characterized by pain, ache, or fatigue in a functional muscle group. It is precipitated by a consistent amount of exercise and is promptly relieved by rest. Intermittent claudication is caused by an inability to increase blood flow to the exercising muscles to meet their metabolic demands.

The location of the pain often corresponds to the anatomic level of involvement. Claudication of the calf indicates superficial femoral artery stenosis. Claudication of hip and buttock most often indicates aortoiliac stenosis, and when associated with impotence in the male is termed *Leriche syndrome* and is caused by occlusion of the aortoiliac and internal pudendal arteries [207,208].

Some patients with claudication will ultimately have ischemic rest pain. Pain at rest is caused by a reduction of blood flow in the extremity to a level below that required for resting tissue metabolism. This pain is located in the foot as opposed to calf or thigh; it is experienced as painful paresthesias or aching when the leg is elevated and is relieved by dangling the leg or standing. Patients with ischemic rest pain are limited by their pain and are at increased risk for ulceration, infection, and subsequent limb loss.

The physician, aided by a carefully taken physical examination, should have little difficulty in making the diagnosis of peripheral vascular disease when the patient has classic symptoms. The patient with aortoiliac disease will have diminished femoral pulses, and bruits can be heart over the femoral arteries. The patient with superficial femoral artery stenosis will have normal femoral pulsations, but more distal pulses will be reduced. Grading of elevation pallor and venous filling time can help estimate the severity of the disease [209]. Dependent rubor, atrophy of the skin, and absent hair on toes are signs of advanced disease. Because patients with claudication usually have diffuse atherosclerotic disease, the physical examination should be extended to include auscultation of the carotid arteries to identify bruits in the neck and palpation of the arteries in the arm to identify subclavian stenosis.

In recent years, the noninvasive vascular laboratory has been a great help in assessing the severity, progression, and improvement after therapy of peripheral vascular disease. Pressures can be measured easily at various levels in the arm or leg using a Doppler flow detector and an appropriately sized blood pressure cuff. An index of systolic ankle blood pressure divided by systolic brachial blood pressure has been used to determine the severity of peripheral vascular disease. This index is usually 1 or greater in the normal individual. Patients with claudication but no rest pain usually have indexes greater than 0.5 [210]. Systolic pressures may be useful to predict healing in patients with ischemic ulceration. When the systolic ankle pressure index is less than 0.55 in the nondiabetic patient and less than 0.8 in the diabetic patient, healing of the ulcers is unlikely [211].

Occasionally, segmental blood pressures can be misleading in patients with calcified arteries, a condition most frequently associated with diabetes. Since these calcified arteries are not compressible by the blood pressure cuff, a falsely high blood pressure reading can be obtained. This gives the impression of mild reduction of blood flow when in fact severe reduction is present. Some centers have found analysis of arterial waveform to be helpful in such situations [210,212].

Occasionally, in some patients with a history suggesting intermittent claudication, results of physical examination and noninvasive data may be normal. In such patients, palpation of the arteries or noninvasive arterial testing after exercise will commonly reveal a loss of pulse or drop in systolic blood pressure.

Spinal stenosis of the cauda equina caused by hypertrophic ridging or protruded lumbar discs, called *pseudoclaudication*, can mimic the pain of claudication in elderly patients. In pseudoclaudication, the discomfort is often brought on by standing and movements involving the back. The discomfort is described as numbness, aching, or sometimes weakness. The pain is relieved by sitting, stooping forward, or lying down. In contrast to claudication, the pain of pseudoclaudication does not resolve promptly with rest, and the level of activity that induces it is more variable than with claudication. Usually, a carefully taken history and physical examination are sufficient to differentiate claudication from pseudoclaudication. Occasionally, neurologic evaluation, including lumbar computed tomography and myelography, is necessary [213].

Therapy

In making recommendations regarding treatment, the physician should consider the natural history of peripheral vascular disease. In the nondiabetic patient, the risk of ultimate loss of a limb is low. Symptoms remain stable over five years in 75% of patients with intermittent claudication. Less than 10% will require amputation of the extremity [214]. Patients with peripheral vascular disease should be advised of the relatively good prognosis regarding amputation, since many of them harbor this fear and do not express it to their physician.

Thus, for the majority of patients with peripheral vascular disease, treatment is conservative. Since many amputations may arise from avoidable trauma, patients should be instructed in care of the feet. This can be accomplished quickly and effectively by use of patient instruction sheets.

Modification of risk factors may play a role in stabilizing or improving the symptoms of claudication. Patients who continue to smoke may face a higher risk of losing a limb than those who stop smoking [215]. Cessation of smoking and a regular walking program may increase walking distance in one half to two thirds of patients, perhaps the most effective treatment for claudication that exists [216,217].

Drug therapy

Oral vasodilator drugs have not been proven to be helpful in the treatment of patients with peripheral vascular disease. Pentoxifylline (Trental), a hemorrheologic agent, is available for the treatment of patients with intermittent claudication. It may increase walking distance in some patients, but its effectiveness remains uncertain [217].

Vasoconstrictive drugs, such as ergot, should not be given. Beta-blockers may aggravate symptoms of peripheral vascular disease and should be avoided if no major indication for their use exists.

Treatment of hyperlipidemia in the elderly remains controversial. Studies [218] in the general population have shown decreased risks of myocardial infarction and death by lowering the low-density lipoprotein using a low fat, low cholesterol diet and instituting drug therapy. Correction of hyperlipidemia may retard angiographic progression of symptomatic femoral atherosclerosis [219]. It has been shown [220] to cause regression of coronary atherosclerosis in some patients. However, whether the rigors of strict diet and the adherence to costly drug therapy will result in substantial benefit to the older patient with peripheral vascular disease is uncertain. At this time, no conclusive recommendations can be made, and treatment must be individualized, taking into account the impact such treatment may have on the quality of life of the patient with limited life expectancy.

Likewise, whether strict control of diabetes in the patient with established peripheral vascular disease will affect progression of the disease is unknown. Hopefully, treatment of diabetes will decrease the incidence of peripheral neuropathy, which can complicate the management of patients with peripheral vascular disease and make the treatment of patients with infected ulcers easier. Strict control of diabetes in the elderly must be weighed against the risks of hypoglycemia in that age group.

The concept of small-vessel disease and its contribution to ischemia of the limb have been questioned. Ulcerations of the foot in the diabetic patient have been attributed to small-vessel disease when frequently they are related to severe large-vessel disease or to peripheral neuropathy. The concept of small-vessel disease may lead to inappropriate therapy and the withholding of arteriography and reconstructive vascular surgery in some patients [221].

Angioplasty and vascular surgery
Currently, angioplasty and vascular surgery are reserved for the patient with disabling claudication or threatened loss of a limb. Some active elderly patients with moderately limiting claudication may find their symptoms intolerable and will press their physician for surgery. Surgical enthusiasm should be tempered, however, by the small but definite risks of death and loss of limb from surgical procedures. In the elderly, functional exercise capacity may not be restored satisfactorily after successful surgical vascular bypass unless an extensive exercise rehabilitation program is provided.

Angiography, an integral part of the assessment of this group of patients, should include views of the abdominal aorta, anteroposterior and oblique projections of the iliac vessels, and views of the femoral arteries and popliteal and tibial arterial system to the foot. If the lesion is of uncertain hemodynamic importance, gradients can be measured manometrically following flow augmentation by contrast agents or injection of papaverine [222]. Intravenous digital angiography provides poor resolution of distal vessels and should not be used to assess peripheral vascular disease.

In recent years, considerable experience has been gained in the use of balloon catheter angioplasty of atherosclerotic lesions. The low morbidity associated with this procedure makes it an attractive alternative to operation in high-risk patients. It has been useful when applied to short segments (less than 10 cm) in the iliac arteries [223]. As measured by noninvasive testing, a patency rate of 83% at five years has been reported [224]. Angioplasty of femoropopliteal disease has had less success and durability [225,226]. A three-year patency rate of 70% for stenoses and more than 55% for complete occlusions has been described [227]. After careful evaluation, only a minority of patients requiring revascularization will be candidates for angioplasty. However, angioplasty may be the treatment of choice in patients with isolated iliac artery stenosis. Iliac angioplasty has also been used preoperatively and intraoperatively to improve arterial inflow before distal vascular reconstructive surgery.

Cardiac study with thallium has proved useful in assessing risk before major vascular surgery, particularly in patients whose clinical presentation places them in an intermediate cardiac risk group [228]. The physician should be mindful that as high as 60% of patients with peripheral vascular disease will have severe coronary artery disease [229]. Patients, particularly those considered for operation, should undergo careful cardiac examination. Since many patients are sedentary and are limited by claudication, they may have no cardiac symptoms and will be unable to perform adequate stress testing. Limited stress electrocardiography, however, may detect coronary artery disease in a considerable number of patients [230]. Arm ergometer stress testing can be substituted for the usual treadmill test. Intravenous dipyridamole (Persantine) thallium scanning performed at rest has been shown to be helpful in detecting patients who are high surgical risks [231]. A few centers [27] have performed cardiac catheterization in all patients before vascular surgery and have recommended coronary artery bypass grafting in patients with severe coronary artery disease before peripheral vascular surgery. However, in present practice only selected patients require cardiac catheterization. This strategy may decrease postoperative cardiac mortality but may be unsuitable for the elderly, frail patient who may not be able to rebound from multiple surgical procedures. In such patients, a reasonable alternative is to choose a procedure, such as extra-anatomic bypass (femoral to femoral or axillo bifemoral), which carries less surgical morbidity and mortality.

Sympathectomy

The role of sympathectomy in the treatment of peripheral vascular disease is limited and remains controversial. Usually, sympathectomy should be reserved for patients with peripherally distributed stenoses, mild pain at rest, and superficial ulcerations who are not candidates for vascular reconstruction [232]. It may help heal skin lesions but will not improve claudication. Diabetic patients with peripheral neuropathy may have autosympathectomy and usually will not benefit from sympathectomy.

The goal of treatment of the elderly patient with peripheral vascular disease is restoration of normal locomotion to maintain an independent life-style. In patients who unfortunately require amputation of the limb, current surgical procedures often permit preservation of the knee joint and accommodation to limb prostheses, which can provide full locomotion. If possible, above-knee amputation should be avoided because of the associated poor rates of rehabilitation and higher surgical mortality.

Acute limb ischemia

Acute limb ischemia should be recognized and treated promptly to avoid loss of limb. It is characterized by the sudden onset of the five P's: pain, pulselessness, pallor, paresthesia, and paralysis. If untreated, ischemia can advance to severe gangrene over a short time. Acute arterial occlusion can occur as a result of thrombosis of a previously stenotic diseased artery or as the result of embolism to a previously healthy artery.

Standard treatment requires arteriography and prompt surgical embolectomy. Thrombolytic therapy with streptokinase or urokinase by intravenous or local intra-arterial routes has been employed with some success and may obviate the need for surgery [233,234]. Local perfusion of thrombus by intra-arterial administration of high-dose urokinase has been reported [235] to be successful and to be associated with a low risk of hemorrhagic complications compared with systemic thrombolytic therapy.

Treatment after restoration of blood flow includes a search for an embolic source, anticoagulation for cardiac embolization, and revascularization or angioplasty of stenotic vessels.

SYNDROMES OF MULTIPLE MICROATHEROEMBOLI

A syndrome that has been well described but occasionally not recognized is that of multiple microatheroemboli. This syndrome can occur in three settings: spontaeous embolization frequently associated with abdominal aortic aneurysm or atherosclerotic aorta [236,237]; aortic manipulation by surgery, angiography, or cardiac catheterization [238,239] or, rarely, external trauma; and as a complication of anticoagulant therapy with Coumadin (blue toes syndrome) [237,240]. These atheromatous emboli are small and primarily consist of cholesterol in large and small arteries (50 to 90 µm diameter).

Clinical presentation can be diverse, depending on the distribution and number of emboli. Multiple small emboli involving the leg can cause livedo reticularis, skin infarction, painful digital ischemia with gangrene, and muscle pain in the presence of normal pedal pulses. When they are present in visceral vessels, renal failure [241,242], bowel ischemia, and pancreatitis can result. Occasionally, multiple emboli can cause systemic symptoms and a high erythrocyte sedimentation rate, eosinophilia, proteinuria, or an elevated level of creatine phosphokinase leading to an erroneous diagnosis of vasculitis, polyarteritis nodosa, subacute bacterial endocarditis, or polymyositis.

In the appropriate clinical setting, diagnosis is usually not difficult to make given a high index of suspicion and characteristic skin changes. Occasionally, a skin or renal biopsy, which can demonstrate multiple cholesterol emboli, is necessary.

Treatment for the sequelae of embolization is largely supportive. Anticoagulation has not been helpful, and in the case of Coumadin, may be a precipitant of cholesterol emboli. The role of antiplatelet agents in prevention is uncertain. A careful search for an embolic source, such as an abdominal aortic aneurysm, severely atheromatous ulcerated abdominal aorta, or more distal vessel, is recommended. If microatheroemboli are found, surgical removal of the affected aortic segment should be carried out.

REFERENCES

1. Schlatmann TJ and Becker AE. 1977. Histologic changes in the normal aging aorta: implications for dissecting aortic aneurysm. Am J Cardiol 39:13–20.
2. Silbert S, Lippmann HI and Gordon E. 1953. Mönckeberg's arteriosclerosis. JAMA 151:1176–1179.
3. Heptinstall RH, Porter KA and Barkley H. 1954. Giant-cell (temporal) arteritis. J Pathol Bact 67:507–519.
4. Parker F, Healey LA, Wilske KR and Odland GF. 1975. Light and electron microscopic studies on human temporal arteries with special reference to alterations related to senescence, atherosclerosis and giant cell arteritis. Am J Pathol 79:57–80.
5. Lie JT. 1990. Illustrated histopathologic classification criteria for selective vasculitis syndromes. American College of Rheumatology Subcommittee on Classification of Vasculitis. Arthritis Rheum 33:1074–1087.
6. Schatz IJ, Fairbairn JF II and Juergens JL, 1962. Abdominal aortic aneurysms: a reappraisal. Circulation 26:200–205.
7. Gore I and Hirst AE Jr. 1973. Arteriosclerotic aneurysms of the abdominal aorta: a review. Prog Cardiovasc Dis 16:113–150.
8. Sumner DS, Hokanson DE and Strandness DE Jr. 1970. Stress-strain characteristics and collagen-elastin content of abdominal aortic aneurysms. Surg Gynecol Obstet 130:459–466.
9. Sumner DS. 1984. Hemodynamics and pathophysiology of arterial disease. In RB Rutherford (ed), Vascular Surgery, 2nd ed. Philadelphia: W.B. Saunders, pp 19–44.
10. Rutherford RB. 1984. Arterial aneurysms: overview. In RB Rutherford (ed), Vascular Surgery, 2nd ed. Philadelphia: W.B. Saunders, pp 745–754.
11. Brewster DC, Retana A, Waltman AC and Darling RC. 1975. Angiography in the management of aneurysms of the abdominal aorta: its value and safety. N Engl J Med 292:822–825.
12. DeBakey ME, Crawford ES, Cooley DA, et al. 1964. Aneurysm of abdominal aorta: analysis of results of graft replacement therapy one to eleven years after operation. Ann Surg 160:622–639.
13. Bernstein EF, Fisher JC and Varco RL. 1967. Is excision the optimum treatment for all abdominal aortic aneurysms? Surgery 61:83–93.
14. Young AE, Sandberg GW and Couch NP. 1977. The reduction of mortality of abdominal aortic aneurysm resection. Am J Surg 134:585–590.
15. Sommerville RL, Allen EV and Edwards JE. 1959. Bland and infected arteriosclerotic abdominal aortic aneurysms: a clinicopathologic study. Medicine 38:207–221.
16. Darling RC, Messina CR, Morrison G and Brewster DC. 1976. Autopsy study of unoperated abdominal aortic aneurysms (AAA): the case for early resection (abstract). Circulation 54:II-11.
17. Rutherford RB. 1984. Infrarenal aortic aneurysms. In RB Rutherford (ed), Vascular Surgery, 2nd ed. Philadelphia: W.B. Saunders, pp 755–771.
18. Szilagyi DE, Elliott JP and Smith RF. 1972. Clinical fate of the patient with asymptomatic abdominal aortic aneurysm and unfit for surgical treatment. Arch Surg 104:600–606.
19. Nevitt MP, Ballard DJ and Hallett JW Jr. 1989. Prognosis of abdominal aortic aneurysms: a population-based study. N Engl J Med 321:1009–1014.
20. Crawford ES and Hess KR. 1989. Abdominal aortic aneurysm (editorial). N Engl J Med 321:1040–1042.
21. Bernstein EF, Dilley RB, Goldberger LE, et al. 1976. Growth rates of small abdominal aortic aneurysms. Surgery 80:765–773.

22. Henry LG, Doust B, Korns ME and Bernhard VM. 1978. Abdominal aortic aneurysm and retroperitoneal fibrosis: ultrasonographic diagnosis and treatment. Arch Surg 113:1456–1460.
23. Ferguson MJ and Arden MJ. 1966. Gastrointestinal hemorrhage secondary to rupture of aorta. Arch Intern Med 117:133–140.
24. Baker WH, Sharzer LA and Ehrenhaft JL. 1972. Aortocaval fistula as a complication of abdominal aortic aneurysms. Surgery 72:933–938.
25. Hertzer NR. 1980. Fatal myocardial infarction following abdominal aortic aneurysm resection: three hundred forty-three patients followed 6–11 years postoperatively. Ann Surg 192:667–673.
26. Young JR, Humphries AW, deWolfe VG and LeFevre FA. 1963. Complications of abdominal aortic surgery. Part II. Intestinal ischemia. Arch Surg 86:65–73.
27. Hertzer NR, Beven EG, Young JR, et al. 1984. Coronary artery disease in peripheral vascular patients: classification of 1,000 coronary angiograms and results of surgical management. Ann Surg 199:223–233.
28. Kidd JN, Reul GJ Jr, Cooley DA, et al. 1976. Surgical treatment of aneurysms of the ascending aorta. Circulation 54:III-118–III-122.
29. Crawford ES. 1974. Thoraco-abdominal and abdominal aortic aneurysms involving renal, superior mesenteric, and celiac arteries. Ann Surg 179:763–772.
30. Crawford ES and Rubio PA. 1973. Reappraisal of adjuncts to avoid ischemia in the treatment of aneurysms of descending thoracic aorta. J Thorac Cardiovasc Surg 66:693–704.
31. Joyce JW, Fairbairn JF III, Kincaid OW and Juergens JL. 1964. Aneurysms of the thoracic aorta: a clinical study with special reference to prognosis. Circulation 29:176–181.
32. Pressler V and McNamara JJ. 1980. Thoracic aortic aneurysm: natural history and treatment. J Thorac Cardiovasc Surg 79:489–498.
33. McNamara JJ and Pressler VM. 1978. Natural history of arteriosclerotic thoracic aortic aneurysms. Ann Thorac Surg 26:468–473.
34. DeBakey ME and Noon GP. 1975. Aneurysms of the thoracic aorta. Mod Conc Cardiovasc Dis 44:53–58.
35. Pond GD and Hillman B. 1981. Evaluation of aneurysms by computed tomography. Surgery 89:216–223.
36. Wychulis AR, Spittell JA Jr and Wallace RB. 1970. Popliteal aneurysms. Surgery 68:942–952.
37. Evans WE and Vermilion BD. 1982. Popliteal aneurysms. In JJ Bergan and JST Yao (eds), Aneurysms: Diagnosis and Treatment. New York: Grune & Stratton, pp 487–492.
38. Cole CW, Thijssen AM, Barber GG, et al. 1989. Popliteal aneurysms: an index of generalized vascular disease. Can J Surg 32:65–68.
39. Gifford RW Jr, Hines EA Jr and Janas JM. 1953. An analysis and follow-up study of one hundred popliteal aneurysms. Surgery 33:284–293.
40. Vermilion BD, Kimmins SA, Pace WG and Evans WE. 1981. A review of one hundred forty-seven popliteal aneurysms with long-term follow-up. Surgery 90:1009–1014.
41. Pathria MN, Zlatkin M, Sartoris DJ, et al. 1988. Ultrasonography of the popliteal fossa and lower extremities. Radiol Clin North Am 26:77–85.
42. Reilly MK, Abbott WM and Darling RC. 1983. Aggressive surgical management of popliteal artery aneurysms. Am J Surg 145:498–502.
43. Wheat MW Jr. 1980. Acute dissecting aneurysms of the aorta: diagnosis and treatment—1979. Am Heart J 99:373–387.
44. DeBakey ME, Cooley DA and Creech O Jr. 1955. Surgical considerations of dissecting aneurysm of the aorta. Ann Surg 142:586–612.
45. Wheat MW Jr, Palmer RF, Bartley TD and Seelman RC. 1965. Treatment of dissecting aneurysms of the aorta without surgery. J Thorac Cardiovasc Surg 50:364–373.
46. Schlatmann TJM and Becker AE. 1977. Pathogenesis of dissecting aneurysm of aorta. Am J Cardiol 39:21–26.
47. Larson EW and Edwards WD. 1984. Risk factors for aortic dissection: a necropsy study of 161 cases. Am J Cardiol 53:849–855.
48. Hirst AE Jr, Johns VJ Jr and Kime SW. 1958. Dissecting aneurysm of the aorta: a review of 505 cases. Medicine 37:217–279.

49. Earnest FIV, Muhm JR and Sheedy PF II. 1979. Roentgenographic findings in thoracic aortic dissection. Mayo Clin Proc 54:43–50.
50. Oudkerk M, Overbosch E and Dee P. 1983. CT recognition of acute aortic dissection. AJR 141:671–676.
51. Thorsen MK, San Dretto MA, Lawson TL, et al. 1983. Dissecting aortic aneurysms: accuracy of computed tomographic diagnosis. Radiology 148:773–777.
52. Erbel R, Mohr-Kahaly S, Rennollet H, et al. 1987. Diagnosis of aortic dissection: the value of transesophageal echocardiography. Thorac Cardiovasc Surg 35:126–133.
53. Kotler MN. 1989. Is transesophageal echocardiography the new standard for diagnosing aortic aneurysms? J Am Coll Cardiol 14:1263–1265.
54. Prokop EK, Palmer RF and Wheat MW Jr. 1970. Hydrodynamic forces in dissecting aneurysms. Circ Res 27:121–127.
55. Doroghazi RM, Slater EE, DeSanctis RW, et al. 1984. Long-term survival of patients with treated aortic dissection. J Am Coll Cardiol 3:1026–1034.
56. Osmundson PJ and Bernatz PE. 1980. Occlusive disease of abdominal visceral arteries. In JL Juergens, JA Spittell and JF Fairbairn II (eds), Peripheral Vascular Diseases, 5th ed. Philadelphia: W.B. Saunders, pp 295–325.
57. Derrick JR, Pollard HS and Moore RM. 1959. The pattern of arteriosclerotic narrowing of the celiac and superior mesenteric arteries. Ann Surg 149:684–689.
58. Reiner L. 1964. Mesenteric arterial insufficiency and abdominal angina. Arch Intern Med 114:765–772.
59. Hollier LH, Bernatz PE, Pairolero PC, et al. 1981. Surgical management of chronic intestinal ischemia: a reappraisal. Surgery 90:940–946.
60. Shaw RS and Maynard EP III. 1958. Acute and chronic thrombosis of the mesenteric arteries associated with malabsorption: a report of two cases successfully treated by thromboendarterectomy. N Engl J Med 258:874–878.
61. Bercher J, Bartholomew LG, Cain JC and Adson MA. 1966. Syndrome of intestinal arterial insufficiency ("abdominal angina"). Arch Intern Med 117:632–638.
62. Watt JK, Watson WC and Haase S. 1967. Chronic intestinal ischaemia. Br Med J 3:199–202.
63. Palmer WL. 1966. Clinical features of mesenteric artery insufficiency. J Tenn Med Assoc 59:152–160.
64. Fry WJ and Kraft RO. 1963. Visceral angina. Surg Gynecol Obstet 117:417–424.
65. Bergan JJ and Yao JST. 1984. Chronic intestinal ischemia. In RB Rutherford (ed), Vascular Surgery, 2nd ed. Philadelphia: W.B. Saunders, pp 964–971.
66. Hallett JW Jr, James ME, Ahlquist DA, et al. 1990. Recent trends in the diagnosis and management of chronic intestinal ischemia. Ann Vasc Surg 4:126–132.
67. Jäger K, Bollinger A, Valli C, et al. 1986. Measurement of mesenteric blood flow by Duplex scanning. J Vasc Surg 3:462–469.
68. Siegelman SS, Sprayregen S and Boley SJ. 1974. Angiographic diagnosis of mesenteric arterial vasoconstriction. Radiology 112:533–542.
69. Stoney RJ and Wylie EJ. 1966. Recognition and surgical management of visceral ischemic syndromes. Ann Surg 164:714–722.
70. Zelenock GB, Graham LM, Whitehouse WM Jr, et al. 1980. Splanchnic arteriosclerotic disease and intestinal angina. Arch Surg 115:497–501.
71. Baur GM, Millay DJ, Taylor LM Jr and Porter JM. 1984. Treatment of chronic visceral ischemia. Am J Surg 148:138–144.
72. Pierce GE and Brockenbrough EC. 1970. The spectrum of mesenteric infarction. Am J Surg 119:233–239.
73. Batellier J, Kieny R. 1990. Superior mesenteric artery embolism: eighty-two cases. Ann Vasc Surg 4:112–116.
74. Ende N. 1958. Infarction of the bowel in cardiac failure. N Engl J Med 258:879–881.
75. Butt LG and Cheek RC. 1969. Nonocclusive mesenteric vascular disease: clinical and experimental observations. Ann Surg 169:704–711.
76. Ottinger LW and Austen WG. 1967. A study of 136 patients with mesenteric infarction. Surg Gynecol Obstet 124:251–261.
77. Bergan JJ and Yao JST. 1984. Acute intestinal ischemia. In RB Rutherford (ed), Vascular Surgery, 2nd ed. Philadelphia: W.B. Saunders, pp 948–963.

78. Bynum TE and Jacobson ED. 1971. Blood flow and gastrointestinal diseases. Digestion 4:109–116.
79. Bergan JJ, Dean RH, Conn J Jr and Yao JST. 1975. Revascularization in treatment of mesenteric infarction. Ann Surg 182:430–438.
80. Laufman H, Nora PF and Mittelpunkt AI. 1964. Mesenteric blood vessels: advances in surgery and physiology. Arch Surg 88:1021–1044.
81. Price WE, Rohrer GV and Jacobson ED. 1969. Mesenteric vascular diseases (editorial). Gastroenterology 57:599–604.
82. Bergan JJ. 1969. Recognition and treatment of superior mesenteric artery embolization. Geriatrics 24:118–125.
83. Boley SJ, Feinstein FR, Sammartano R, et al. 1981. New concepts in the management of emboli of the superior mesenteric artery. Surg Gynecol Obstet 153:561–569.
84. Rosen A, Korobkin M, Silverman PM, et al. 1984. Mesenteric vein thrombosis: CT identification. AJR 143:83–86.
85. Williams LF Jr. 1988. Mesenteric ischemia. Surg Clin North Am 68:331–353.
86. Grim CE, Luft FC, Yune HY, et al. 1981. Percutaneous transluminal dilatation in the treatment of renal vascular hypertension. Ann Intern Med 95:439–442.
87. Goldblatt H, Lynch J, Hanzal RF and Summerville WW. 1934. Studies on experimental hypertension: production of persistent elevation of systolic blood pressure by means of renal ischemia. J Exp Med 59:347–379.
88. Smith HW. 1956. Unilateral nephrectomy in hypertensive disease J Urol 76:685–701.
89. Holley KE, Hunt JC, Brown AL Jr, et al. 1964. Renal artery stenosis: a clinical-pathologic study in normotensive and hypertensive patients. Am J Med 37:14–22.
90. Dustan HP, Humphries AW, deWolfe VG and Page IH. 1964. Normal arterial pressure in patients with renal arterial stenosis. JAMA 187:1028–1029.
91. Connor TB, Thomas WC Jr, Haddock L and Howard JE. 1960. Unilateral renal disease as a cause of hypertension: its detection by ureteral catheterization studies. Ann Intern Med 52:544–559.
92. Stamey TA, Nudelman IJ, Good PH, et al. 1961. Functional characteristics of renovascular hypertension. Medicine 40:347–394.
93. Marks LS, Maxwell MH, Varady PD, et al. 1976. Renovascular hypertension: does the renal vein renin ratio predict operative results? J Urol 115:365–368.
94. Mackay A, Boyle P, Brown JJ, et al. 1983. The decision on surgery in renal artery stenosis. QJ Med 207:363–381.
95. Skeggs LT, Dorer FE, Kahn JR, et al. 1976. The biochemistry of the renin-angiotensin system and its role in hypertension. Am J Med 60:737–748.
96. Muller FB, Sealey JE, Case DB, et al. 1986. The captopril test for identifying renovascular disease in hypertensive patients. Am J Med 80:633–644.
97. Wilcox CS, Williams CM, Smith TB, et al. 1988. Diagnostic uses of angiotensin-converting enzyme inhibitors in renovascular hypertension. Am J Hypertens 1:344S–349S.
98. Svetkey LP, Himmelstein SI, Dunnick NR, et al. 1989. Prospective analysis of strategies for diagnosing renovascular hypertension. Hypertension 14:247–257.
99. Rosenthal JT, Libertino JA, Zinman LN, et al. 1981. Predictability of surgical cure of renovascular hypertension. Ann Surg 193:448–452.
100. Genest J, Cartier P, Roy P, et al. 1983. Renovascular hypertension. In J Genest, O Kuchel, P Hamet and M Cantin (eds), Hypertension: Physiopathology and Treatment, 2nd ed. New York: McGraw-Hill, pp 1007–1034.
101. Foster JH, Maxwell MH, Franklin SS, et al. 1975. Renovascular occlusive disease: results of operative treatment. JAMA 231:1043–1048.
102. Foster JH, Dean RH, Pinkerton JA and Rhamy RK. 1973. Ten years experience with the surgical management of renovascular hypertension. Ann Surg 177:755–766.
103. Simon N, Franklin SS, Bleifer KH and Maxwell MH. 1972. Clinical characteristics of renovascular hypertension. JAMA 220:1209–1218.
104. Stanley JC and Fry WJ. 1977. Surgical treatment of renovascular hypertension. Arch Surg 112:1291–129.
105. Perloff D, Sokolow M, Wylie EJ and Palubinskas AJ. 1967. Renal vascular hypertension: further experiences. Am Heart J 74:614–631.

106. Moser RJ Jr and Caldwell JR. 1962. Abdominal murmurs: an aid in the diagnosis of renal artery disease in hypertension. Ann Intern Med 56:471–483.
107. Havey RJ, Krumlovsky F, delGreco F and Martin HG. 1985. Screening for renovascular hypertension: is renal digital-subtraction angiography the preferred noninvasive test? JAMA 254:388–393.
108. Buonocore E, Meaney TF, Borkowski GP, et al. 1981. Digital subtraction angiography of the abdominal aorta and renal arteries: comparison with conventional aortography. Radiology 139:281–286.
109. Nally JV Jr, Gupta BK, Clarke HS, et al. 1988. Captopril renography for the detection of renovascular hypertension: a preliminary report. Clev Clin J Med 55:311–318.
110. Sfakianakis GN, Bourgoignie JJ, Jaffe D, et al. 1987. Single-dose captopril scintigraphy in the diagnosis of renovascular hypertension. J Nucl Med 28:1383–1392.
111. Meier GH, Sumpio B, Black HR, et al. 1990. Captopril renal scintigraphy: an advance in the detection and treatment of renovascular hypertension. J Vasc Surg 11:770–777.
112. Dean RH, Burko H, Wilson JP, et al. 1974. Deceptive patterns of renal artery stenosis. Surgery 76:872–881.
113. Sheps SG, Osmundson PJ, Hunt JC, et al. 1965. Hypertension and renal artery stenosis: serial observations on 54 patients treated medically. Clin Pharmacol Ther 6:700–709.
114. Hricik DE, Browning PJ, Kopelman R, et al. 1983. Captopril-induced functional renal insufficiency in patients with bilateral renal-artery stenoses or renal-artery stenosis in a solitary kidney. N Engl J Med 308:373–376.
115. Meaney TF, Dustan HP and McCormack LJ. 1968. Natural history of renal arterial disease. Radiology 91:881–887.
116. Wollenweber J, Sheps SG and Davis GD. 1968. Clinical course of atherosclerotic renovascular disease: review. Am J Cardiol 21:60–71.
117. Libertino JA, Zinman L, Breslin DJ, et al. 1980. Renal artery revascularization: restoration of renal function. JAMA 244:1340–1342.
118. Ying CY, Tifft CP, Gavras H and Chobanian AV. 1984. Renal revascularization in the azotemic hypertensive patient resistant to therapy. N Engl J Med 311:1070–1075.
119. Beebe HG, Chesebro K, Merchant F, et al. 1988. Results of renal artery balloon angioplasty limit its indications. J Vasc Surg 8:300–306.
120. Hayes JM, Risius B, Novick AC, et al. 1988. Experience with percutaneous transluminal angioplasty for renal artery stenosis at the Cleveland Clinic. J Urol 139:488–492.
121. Stoney RJ. 1984. Transaortic renal endarterectomy. In RB Rutherford (ed), Vascular Surgery, 2nd ed. Philadelphia: W.B. Saunders, pp 1130–1135.
122. Franklin SS, Young JD Jr, Maxwell MH, et al. 1975. Operative morbidity and mortality in renovascular disease. JAMA 231:1148–1153.
123. Stanley JC and Graham LM. 1984. Renal artery fibrodysplasia and renovascular hypertension. In RB Rutherford (ed), Vascular Surgery, 2nd ed. Philadelphia: W.B. Saunders, pp 1145–1162.
124. Libertino JA and Selman FJ Jr. 1982. Alternatives to aortorenal revascularization. J Cardiovasc Surg 23:318–322.
125. Hypertension Detection and Follow-up Program Cooperative Group. 1982. Five-year findings of the hypertension detection and follow-up program. III. Reduction in stroke incidence among persons with high blood pressure. JAMA 247:633–638.
126. Carter AB. 1963. Strokes: natural history and prognosis. Proc R Soc Med 56:483–486.
127. David NJ and Heyman A. 1960. Factors influencing the prognosis of cerebral thrombosis and infarction due to atherosclerosis. J Chron Dis 11:394–404.
128. Dyken ML, Wolf PA, Barnett HJM, et al. 1984. Risk factors in stroke: a statement for physicians by the subcommittee on risk factors and stroke of the stroke council. Stroke 15:1105–1161.
129. Kirkendall WM and Hammond JJ. 1980. Hypertension in the elderly. Arch Intern Med 140:1155–1161.
130. Kannel WB, Dawber TR, Sorlie P and Wolf PA. 1976. Components of blood pressure and risk of atherothrombotic brain infarction: The Framingham study. Stroke 7:327–331.
131. Kannel WB, Wolf PA, McGee DL, et al. 1981. Systolic blood pressure, arterial rigidity, and risk of stroke: The Framingham study. JAMA 245:1225–1229.

132. Soltero I, Liu K, Cooper R, et al. 1978. Trends in mortality from cerebrovascular diseases in the United States, 1960 to 1975. Stroke 9:549–558.

133. Cressman MD and Gifford RW Jr. 1983. Hypertension and stroke. J Am Coll Cardiol 1:521–527.

134. The Management Committee. 1980. The Australian therapeutic trial in mild hypertension. Lancet 1:1261–1267.

135. Veterans Administration Cooperative Study Group on Antihypertensive Agents. 1967. Effect of treatment on morbidity in hypertension: results in patients with diastolic blood pressures averaging 115 through 125 mm Hg. JAMA 202:1028–1034.

136. Black DG, Heagerty AM, Bing RF, et al. 1984. Effects of treatment for hypertension on cerebral haemorrhage and infarction. Br Med J 289:156–159.

137. Whisnant JP, Fitzgibbons JP, Kurland LT and Sayre GP. 1971. Natural history of stroke in Rochester, Minnesota, 1945 through 1954. Stroke 2:11–22.

138. Cerebral Embolism Task Force. 1986. Cardiogenic brain embolism. Arch Neurol 43: 71–84.

139. Predictors of thromboembolism in atrial fibrillation: II. Echocardiographic features of patients at risk. The stroke prevention in atrial fibrillation investigators. 1992. Ann Intern Med 116:4–12.

140. Adams HP Jr, Kassell NF and Mazuz H. 1984. The patient with transient ischemic attacks: Is this the time for a new therapeutic approach? Stroke 15:371–375.

141. Fisher CM, Gore I, Okabe N and White PD. 1965. Atherosclerosis of the carotid and vertebral arteries—extracranial and intracranial. J Neuropathol Exp Neurol 24:455–476.

142. Martin MJ, Whisnant JP and Sayre GP. 1960. Occlusive vascular disease in the extracranial cerebral circulation. Arch Neurol 3:530–538.

143. Fields WS and Lemak NA. 1976. Joint study of extracranial arterial occlusion. X. Internal carotid artery occlusion. JAMA 235:2734–2738.

144. Javid H, Ostermiller WE Jr, Hengesh JW, et al. 1970. Natural history of carotid bifurcation atheroma. Surgery 67:80–86.

145. Roederer GO, Langlois YE, Jager KA, et al. 1984. The natural history of carotid arterial disease in asymptomatic patients with cervical bruits. Stroke 15:605–613.

146. Moneta GL, Taylor DC, Nicholls SC, et al. 1987. Operative versus nonoperative management of asymptomatic high-grade internal carotid artery stenosis: improved results with endarterectomy. Stroke. 18:1005–1010.

147. Chambers BR and Norris JW. 1984. The case against surgery for asymptomatic carotid stenosis. Stroke 15:964–967.

148. Podore PC, DeWeese JA, May AG and Rob CG. 1980. Asymptomatic contralateral carotid artery stenosis: a five-year follow-up study following carotid endarterectomy. Surgery 88:748–752.

149. Committee on Cerebrovascular Diseases. 1975. A classification and outline of cerebrovascular diseases II. Stroke 6:564–616.

150. Sandok BA, Furlan AJ, Whisnant JP and Sundt TM Jr. 1978. Guidelines for the management of transient ischemic attacks. Mayo Clin Proc 53:665–674.

151. Millikan CH. 1978. Cerebral circulation. JAMA 239:1313–1315.

152. Millikan CH. 1965. The pathogenesis of transient focal cerebral ischemia. Circulation 32:438–450.

153. Marshall J and Wilkinson IMS. 1971. The prognosis of carotid transient ischaemic attacks in patients with normal angiograms. Brain 94:395–402.

154. Kendell RE and Marshall J. 1963. Role of hypotension in the genesis of transient focal cerebral ischaemic attacks. Br Med J 2:344–348.

155. Reed RL, Siekert RG and Merideth J. 1973. Rarity of transient focal cerebral ischemia in cardiac dysrhythmia. JAMA 223:893–895.

156. Pessin MS, Duncan GW, Mohr JP and Poskanzer DC. 1977. Clinical and angiographic features of carotid transient ischemic attacks. N Engl J Med 296:358–362.

157. Whisnant JP. 1983. The role of the neurologist in the decline of stroke. Ann Neurol 14:1–7.

158. Easton JD and Sherman DG. 1983. Carotid endarterectomy (editorial). Mayo Clin Proc 58:205–207.

159. Whisnant JP, Matsumoto N and Elveback LR. 1973. Transient cerebral ischemic attacks in a community: Rochester, Minnesota, 1955 through 1969. Mayo Clin Proc 48:194–198.

160. Matsumoto N, Whisnant JP, Kurland LT and Okazaki H. 1973. Natural history of stroke in Rochester, Minnesota, 1955 through 1969: an extension of a previous study, 1945 through 1954. Stroke 4:20–29.
161. Estol C, Caplan LR. 1990. Therapy of acute stroke. Clin Neuropharmacol 13:91–120.
162. David TE, Humphries AW, Young JR and Bevin EG. 1973. A correlation of neck bruits and arteriosclerotic carotid arteries. Arch Surg 107:729–731.
163. Wolf PA, Kannel WB, Sorlie P and McNamara P. 1981. Asymptomatic carotid bruit and risk of stroke: The Framingham study. JAMA 245:1442–1445.
164. Hollenhorst RW. 1961. Significance of bright plaques in the retinal arterioles. JAMA 178:23–29.
165. Russell RWR. 1968. The source of retinal emboli. Lancet 2:789–792.
166. Pfaffenbach DD and Hollenhorst RW. 1973. Morbidity and survivorship of patients with embolic cholesterol crystals in the ocular fundus. Am J Ophthalmol 75:66–72.
167. Savino PJ, Glaser JS and Cassady J. 1977. Retinal stroke: Is the patient at risk? Arch Ophthalmol 95:1185–1189.
168. Poole CJ and Ross RW. 1985. Mortality and stroke after amaurosis fugax. J Neurol Neurosurg Psychiatry 48:902–905.
169. Yao JST and Bergan JJ. 1974. Application of ultrasound to arterial and venous diagnosis. Surg Clin North Am 54:23–38.
170. Cebul RD and Ginsberg MD. 1982. Noninvasive neurologic tests for carotid artery disease. Ann Intern Med 97:867–872.
171. Johnson JM, Kennelly MM, Decesare D, et al. 1985. Natural history of asymptomatic carotid plaque. Arch Surg 120:1010–1012.
172. Fish PJ, Kakkar VV, Corrigan T and Nicolaides AN. 1972. Arteriography using ultrasound. Lancet 1:1269–1270.
173. Keagy BA, Pharr WF, Thomas D and Bowes DE. 1982. Comparison of oculoplethysmography/carotid phonoangiography with duplex scan/spectral analysis in the detection of carotid artery stenosis. Stroke 13:43–45.
174. Gee W, Oller DW, Amundsen DG and Goodreau JJ. 1977. The asymptomatic carotid bruit and the ocular pneumoplethysmography. Arch Surg 112:1381–1388.
175. Kartchner MM, McRae LP, Crain V and Whitaker B. 1976. Oculoplethysmography: an adjunct to arteriography in the diagnosis of extracranial carotid occlusive disease. Am J Surg 132:728–732.
176. Weisberg LA and Nice CN. 1977. Intracranial tumors simulating the presentation of cerebrovascular syndromes: early detection with cerebral computed tomography (CCT). Am J Med 63:517–524.
177. Barnett HJM. 1980. Progress towards stroke prevention: Robert Wartenberg lecture. Neurology 30:1212–1225.
178. Millikan CH and McDowell FH. 1980. Treatment of progressing stroke. Prog Cardiovasc Dis 22:397–414.
179. McDowell FH, Millikan CH and Goldstein M. 1980. Treatment of impending stroke (editorial). Stroke 11:1–3.
180. Barnett HIM, Plum F and Walton JN. 1984. Carotid endarterectomy: an expression of concern (editorial). Stroke 15:941–943.
181. Thompson JE, Patman RD and Talkington CM. 1978. Asymptomatic carotid bruit: long term outcome of patients having endarterectomy compared with unoperated controls. Ann Surg 188:308–316.
182. Mohr JP. 1982. Asymptomatic carotid artery disease. Stroke 13:431–433.
183. Javid H, Ostermiller WE, Hengesh JW, et al. 1971. Carotid endarterectomy for asymptomatic patients. Arch Surg 102:389–391.
184. NASCET Investigators. 1991. Clinical alert: benefit of carotid endarterectomy for patients with high-grade stenosis of the internal carotid artery. Bethesda, MD: Public Health Service, National Institutes of Health, National Institute of Neurological Disorders and Stroke.
185. The Boston Area Anticoagulation Trial for Atrial Fibrillation Investigators. 1990. The effect of low-dose warfarin on the risk of stroke in patients with nonrheumatic atrial fibrillation. N Engl J Med 323:1505–1511.
186. The Canadian Cooperative Study Group. 1978. A randomized trial of aspirin and sulfinpyrazone in threatened stroke. N Engl J Med 299:53–59.

187. Bousser MG, Eschwege E, Haguenau M, et al. 1983. "AICLA" controlled trial of aspirin and dipyridamole in the secondary prevention of athero-thrombotic cerebral ischemia. Stroke 14:5–14.

188. Bengtsson BA and Malmvall BE. 1981. The epidemiology of giant cell arteritis including temporal arteritis and polymyalgia rheumatica: incidences of different clinical presentations and eye complications. Arthritis Rheum 24:899–904.

189. Huston KA, Hunder GG, Lie JT, et al. 1978. Temporal arteritis: a 25-year epidemiologic, clinical, and pathologic study. Ann Intern Med 88:162–167.

190. Hauser WA, Ferguson RH, Holley KE and Kurland LT. 1971. Temporal arteritis in Rochester, Minnesota, 1951 to 1967. Mayo Clin Proc 46:597–602.

191. Malmvall BE, Bengtsson BA, Alesting K, et al. 1980. The clinical picture of giant cell arteritis: temporal arteritis, polymyalgia, and fever of unknown origin. Postgrad Med 67:141–148.

192. Bengtsson BA and Malmvall BE. 1981. Prognosis of giant cell arteritis including temporal arteritis and polymyalgia rheumatica: a follow-up study on ninety patients treated with corticosteroids. Acta Med Scand 209:337–345.

193. Jonasson F, Cullen JF and Elton RA. 1979. Temporal arteritis: a 14-year epidemiological, clinical and prognostic study. Scott Med J 24:111–117.

194. Nordborg E and Bengtsson B-A. 1989. Death rates and causes of death in 284 consecutive patients with giant cell arteritis confirmed by biopsy. Br Med J 299:549–550.

195. Säve-Söderbergh J, Malmvall BE, Andersson R and Bengtsson BA. 1986. Giant cell arteritis as a cause of death: report of nine cases. JAMA 255:493–496.

196. Barrier J, Potel G, Renaut-Hovasse H, et al. 1982. The use of Doppler flow studies in the diagnosis of giant cell arteritis: selection of temporal artery biopsy site is facilitated. JAMA 248:2158–2159.

197. Hall S and Hunder GG. 1984. Is temporal artery biopsy prudent? Mayo Clin Proc 59: 793–796.

198. Fernandez-Herlihy L. 1989. Temporal arteritis: clinical aids to diagnosis. J Rheumatol 15:1797–1801.

199. Hunder GG, Bloch DA, Michel BA, et al. 1990. The American College of Rheumatology 1990 criteria for the classification of giant cell arteritis. Arthritis Rheum 33:1122–1128.

200. Healey LA and Wilske KR. 1978. The Systemic Manifestation of Temporal Arteritis. New York: Grune & Stratton.

201. Bengtsson BA and Malmvall BE. 1981. An alternate-day corticosteroid regimen and maintenance therapy of giant cell arteritis. Acta Med Scand 209:347–350.

202. Hunder GG, Sheps SG, Allen GL and Joyce JW. 1975. Daily and alternate-day corticosteroid regimens in treatment of giant cell arteritis: comparison in a prospective study. Ann Intern Med 82:613–618.

203. Fernandez-Herlihy L. 1980. Duration of corticosteroid therapy in giant cell arteritis. J Rheumatol 7:361–364.

204. Haimovici H. 1967. Patterns of arteriosclerotic lesions of the lower extremity. Arch Surg 95:918–933.

205. Lindbom A. 1950. Arteriosclerosis and arterial thrombosis in the lower limb: roentgenological study. Acta Radiol Suppl 80:1–80.

206. Mavor GE. 1956. The pattern of occlusion in atheroma of the lower limb arteries: the correlation of clinical and arteriographic findings. Br J Surg 43:352–364.

207. Kempczinski RF. 1981. The differential diagnosis of intermittent claudication. Pract Cardiol 7:53–61.

208. Kempczinski RF and Bernhard VM. 1984. The management of chronic ischemia of the lower extremities: introduction and general considerations. In RB Rutherford (ed), Vascular Surgery, 2nd ed. Philadelphia: W. B. Saunders, pp 547–558.

209. Spittell JA Jr. 1981. Recognition and management of chronic atherosclerotic occlusive peripheral arterial disease. Mod Conc Cardiovasc Dis 50:19–23.

210. Barnes RW. 1980. Hemodynamics for the vascular surgeon. Arch Surg 115:216–223.

211. Raines JK, Darling RC, Buth J, et al. 1976. Vascular laboratory criteria for the management of peripheral vascular disease of the lower extremities. Surgery 79:21–29.

212. Strandness DE Jr. 1979. The use and abuse of the vascular laboratory. Surg Clin North Am 59:707–717.

213. Fairbairn JF II. 1980. Clinical manifestations of peripheral vascular disease. In JL Juergens, JA Spittell Jr, and JF Fairbairn II (eds), Peripheral Vascular Diseases. Philadelphia: W. B. Saunders, pp 3–49.

214. Imparato AM, Kim G-E, Davidson T and Crowley JG. 1975. Intermittent claudication: its natural course. Surgery 78:795–799.

215. Juergens JL, Barker NW and Hines EA. 1960. Arteriosclerosis obliterans: review of 520 cases with special reference to pathogenic and prognostic factors. Circulation 21:188–195.

216. Schersten Y. 1982. Indications and methods of exercise training of patients with intermittent claudication. Pract Cardiol 8:45–59.

217. Radack K and Wyderski RJ. 1990. Conservative management of intermittent claudication. Ann Intern Med 113:135–146.

218. Lipid Research Clinics Program. 1984. The Lipid Research Clinics coronary primary prevention trial results. I. Reduction in incidence of coronary heart disease. JAMA 251:351–364.

219. Duffield RGM, Lewis B, Miller NE, et al. 1983. Treatment of hyperlipidaemia retards progression of symptomatic femoral atherosclerosis: a randomised controlled trial. Lancet 2:639–642.

220. Blankenhorn DH, Kramsch DM. 1988. Reversal of atherosis and sclerosis: the two components of atherosclerosis. Circulation 79:1–7.

221. LoGerfo FW and Coffman JD. 1984. Vascular and microvascular disease of the foot in diabetes: implications for foot care. N Engl J Med 311:1615–1619.

222. Maddison FE. 1984. Arteriography for lower extremity ischemia. In RB Rutherford (ed), Vascular Surgery, 2nd ed. Philadelphia: W. B. Saunders, pp 559–563.

223. Health and Public Policy Committee, American College of Physicians. 1983. Percutaneous transluminal angioplasty. Ann Intern Med 99:864–869.

224. Gallino A, Mahler F, Probst P, et al. 1984. Percutaneous transluminal angioplasty of the arteries of the lower limbs: a 5 year follow-up. Circulation 70:619–623.

225. Greenfield AJ. 1980. Femoral, popliteal, and tibial arteries: percutaneous transluminal angioplasty. AJR 135:927–935.

226. Martin EC, Frankuchen EI, Karlson KB, et al. 1981. Angioplasty for femoral artery occlusion: comparison with surgery. AJR 137:915–919.

227. Krepel VM, van Andel GJ, van Erp WF, et al. 1985. Percutaneous transluminal angioplasty of the femoropopliteal artery: initial and long-term results. Radiology 156:325–328.

228. Eagle KA, Coley CM, Newell JB, et al. 1989. Combining clinical and thallium data optimizes preoperative assessment of cardiac risk before major vascular surgery. Ann Intern Med 110:859–866.

229. Hertzer NR, Young JR, Kramer JR, et al. 1979. Routine coronary angiography prior to elective aortic reconstruction: results of selective myocardial revascularization in patients with peripheral vascular disease. Arch Surg 114:1336–1344.

230. Cutler BS, Wheeler HB, Paraskos JA and Cardullo PA. 1979. Assessment of operative risk with electrocardiographic exercise testing in patients with peripheral vascular surgery. Am J Surg 137:484–490.

231. Boucher CA, Brewster DC, Darling RC, et al. 1985. Determination of cardiac risk by dipyridamole-thallium imaging before peripheral vascular surgery. N Engl J Med 312:389–394.

232. Rutherford RB. 1984. Lumbar sympathectomy: indications and technique. In RB Rutherford (ed), Vascular Surgery, 2nd ed. Philadelphia: W. B. Saunders, pp 651–660.

233. Martin M. 1979. Thrombolytic therapy in arterial thromboembolism. Prog Cardiovasc Dis 21:351–374.

234. Totty WG, Gilula LA, McClennan BL, et al. 1982. Low-dose intravascular fibrinolytic therapy. Radiology 143:59–69.

235. McNamara TO and Fischer JR. 1985. Thrombolysis of peripheral arterial and graft occlusions: improved results using high-dose urokinase. AJR 144:769–775.

236. Kazmier FJ, Sheps SG, Bernatz PE and Sayre GP. 1966. Livedo reticularis and digital infarcts: a syndrome due to cholesterol emboli arising from atheromatous abdominal aortic aneurysms. Vasc Dis 3:12–24.

237. Wagner RB and Martin AS. 1973. Peripheral atheroembolism: confirmation of a clinical concept, with a case report and review of the literature. Surgery 73:353–359.

238. Rosansky SJ and Deschamps EG. 1984. Multiple cholesterol emboli syndrome after angiography. Am J Med Sci 288:45–48.
239. Drost H, Buis B, Hann D and Hillers JA. 1984. Cholesterol embolism as a complication of left heart catheterisation: report of seven cases. Br Heart J 52:339–342.
240. Karmody AM, Powers SR, Monaco VJ and Leather RP, 1976. "Blue toe" syndrome: an indication for limb salvage surgery. Arch Surg 111:1263–1268.
241. Smith MC, Ghose MK and Henry AR. 1981. The clinical spectrum of renal cholesterol embolization. Am J Med 71:174–180.
242. Kassirer JP. 1969. Atheroembolic renal disease. N Engl J Med 280:812–818.

16. CARDIAC MANIFESTATIONS OF NONCARDIAC DISEASE

DAVID W. SNYDER

In the elderly population, the heart may be involved secondarily by disease elsewhere in the body or may be affected by a systemic disorder. Thus, renal disease, lung disease, and hypertension may place excessive demands on the heart that can lead to cardiac decompensation. Direct involvement in a systemic process may be seen in some endocrine abnormalities, collagen-vascular diseases, or infiltrative processes such as amyloidosis. In this chapter we will review some of the more common extracardiac diseases that lead to cardiac dysfunction in the aged.

CHRONIC LUNG DISEASE
Cardiac abnormalities are commonplace among patients with advanced pulmonary disease. Right ventricular failure may be prominent and, when due solely to the pulmonary hypertension of lung disease, is referred to as *cor pulmonale*. Disturbances of cardiac rhythm represent another common and significant complication of lung disease. Potentially, both the arrhythmias and pulmonary hypertension can be prevented or reversed through an understanding of their pathogenesis.

Franz H. Messerli (ed.), CARDIOVASCULAR DISEASE IN THE ELDERLY (Third Edition). Copyright © 1993 Kluwer Academic Publishers. ISBN 0-7923-1859-5. All rights reserved.

Table 16-1. Conditions that produce cor pulmonale

Pulmonary artery occlusive disease
Primary pulmonary hypertension
Drug induced, i.e., aminorex
Recurrent pulmonary emboli
Pulmonary vasculitis
Intrinsic lung disease
Chronic obstructive pulmonary disease
Pulmonary fibrosis
Chronic alveolar hypoventilation
Thoracic deformity
Neuromuscular disease of respiratory muscles
Sleep apnea syndrome
Pickwickian syndrome

Cor pulmonale

Cor pulmonale is a secondary form of heart disease wherein right ventricular failure is precipitated by acute or chronic pressure overload due to pulmonary arterial hypertension. After age 50, cor pulmonale is the third most common form of heart disease, following coronary heart disease and hypertensive cardiovascular disease. Causes of pulmonary hypertension may include intrinsic lung disease, pulmonary arterial occlusive diseases, chronic alveolar hypoventilation, or idiopathic (primary) pulmonary hypertension. Excluded from the definition of cor pulmonale are conditions in which right ventricular pressure overload results from left ventricular failure or valvular or congenital heart disease. Conditions frequently complicated by cor pulmonale are listed in table 16-1.

Pathophysiology

In the elderly population, chronic obstructive pulmonary disease (COPD) is the predominant cause of cor pulmonale. Patients with asthma or predominantly emphysema develop pulmonary hypertension only very late in the course of their illness, which contrasts with the relatively early onset of pulmonary hypertension in chronic bronchitis. Pulmonary vascular resistance is increased due to the vasoconstriction triggered by hypoxia and acidosis [1]. In acute respiratory decompensation, successful treatment will produce improved gas exchange with reversal of hypoxia and acidosis, thus ameliorating pulmonary hypertension. When hypoxia becomes persistent, elevated pulmonary artery pressures lead to intimal and smooth muscle hyperplasia, which contribute to augmented pulmonary vascular resistance. Even very late in its course, however, hypoxic pulmonary hypertension will improve in response to improved ventilation and arterial oxygen saturation.

Both asthmatics and patients with emphysema have relatively normal arterial oxygenation at rest. On the other hand, ventilation and perfusion inequalities promote arterial desaturation and hypercapnia early in the course

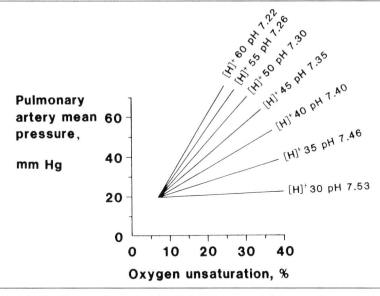

Figure 16-1. Graphic representation of the relationship among pulmonary artery mean pressure, arterial blood oxyhemoglobin saturation, and hydrogen ion concentration. (Reproduced with permission from Enson Y, Giuntini C, Lewis ML, et al. 1964. The influence of hydrogen ion concentration and hypoxia on the pulmonary circulation. J Clin Invest 43:1146–1162.)

of chronic bronchitis, with resultant pulmonary vasoconstriction. Right ventricular failure first occurs with the acute elevations of pulmonary resistance that accompany respiratory decompensation and becomes chronic if arterial desaturation persists.

Clinical findings

The usual patient with cor pulmonale has chronic bronchitis with evidence of airway obstruction and right heart failure. Neck vein distention, hepatic enlargement, edema, and often ascites are present without signs of left ventricular dysfunction. Arterial blood gases show oxygen desaturation and, generally, respiratory acidosis. The electrocardiogram may show right precordial T-wave inversions, a rightward shift in the frontal plane QRS axis, S-T depression in the inferior leads, or incomplete right bundle branch block. Late in cor pulmonale, electrocardiographic evidence of right ventricular hypertrophy may be found.

Figure 16-1 [2] depicts the relationship between pulmonary pressures, arterial pH, and oxygen saturation. For any degree of desaturation, the pulmonary artery pressure will be elevated in proportion to the degree of acidosis. Furthermore, even at a normal pH, oxygen saturation less than 80% precipitates pulmonary vasoconstriction. When significant oxygen desaturation is present, minor changes in pH will dramatically affect pulmonary pressures [2].

Additional factors in addition to hypoxic pulmonary vasoconstriction may further increase pulmonary artery pressures in chronic obstructive pulmonary disease. There may be an anatomic reduction in the pulmonary vascular bed due to intimal hyperplasia and capillary loss with loss of pulmonary parenchyma. Elevated cardiac output increases pulmonary pressure for any degree of pulmonary vascular resistance. Polycythemia may increase viscosity, and increased intrathoracic pressure during expiration is transmitted into the pulmonary circulation. While left heart failure is not a cause for cor pulmonale, right heart failure can shift the interventricular septum leftward, impeding left ventricular filling and increasing pulmonary venous back pressure by 5 to 6 mmHg [3].

Therapy

Effective therapy of acute cor pulmonale begins with efforts to reduce pulmonary vasoconstriction through improved gas exchange. Oxygen supplementation is required, with close monitoring of arterial blood gases to judge treatment response. In general, low-flow oxygen administration (1/2 to 2 L/min) is sufficient to improve oxygenation without depressing respiration. However, if hypoxia or respiratory acidosis persists in the acute setting, short-term mechanical ventilation may be necessary.

Improved alveolar ventilation can be achieved through the use of antibiotics to counter any acute infectious process, through postural drainage to help clear large airways, and through the use of catecholamines, anticholinergic agents, or methylxanthines to dilate constricted bronchioles and perhaps improve mucocilliary transport.

The role of theophylline relative to other therapeutic modalities is somewhat controversial. In acute exacerbations of COPD, controlled trials of theophylline have shown no added benefit to ongoing therapy with inhaled beta-agonists, steroids, and antibiotics as measured by spirometry, blood gases, or clinical improvement [4]. Nausea and vomiting are more common in the aminophylline-treated patients. Similarly, there is little evidence that maintenance theophylline therapy adds anything but expense and toxicity to a tailored regimen of inhaled bronchodilators [5].

However, when used acutely in patients with cor pulmonale, aminophylline has been demonstrated to decrease pulmonary vascular resistance and pressure, with little change in cardiac output or PaO_2 [6]. Short-term improvement in both right and left ventricular ejection fractions have also been found, independent of effects on airways or PaO_2 [7], and right ventricular diastolic (central venous) pressure is reduced [8]. Long-term theophylline treatment produces a sustained improvement in right and left ventricular function [9]. Sustained-release theophylline appears to reduce subjective dyspnea even in nonreversible obstructive airway disease [10].

Aminophylline is generally administered by the intravenous route in the acutely ill patient. In the elderly, the volume of distribution is slightly contracted, and clearance is slow. An initial loading dose of 5 mg/kg is used, with a maintenance infusion rate of 0.4 mg/kg per hour. Plasma levels should be determined during prolonged treatment, and will be affected by factors such as liver function, cardiac decompensation, smoking, and concurrent drugs. Clearance is slowed by concomitant use of erythromycin, propranolol, cimetidine, allopurinol, or oral contraceptives and is accelerated by rifampin, phenytoin, or phenobarbital. As a first approximation, oral theophylline therapy can be initiated using the same total daily dose as was established with intravenous aminophylline, or by starting with 400 mg per day.

Sympathomimetic drugs may be used alone or in combination with theophylline. Hemodynamic improvement in patients with cor pulmonale is similar to that seen with theophylline [11]. Subcutaneous terbutaline lowers pulmonary vascular resistance and results in an increase in cardiac output, improved oxygen delivery, and improved right and left ventricular ejection fractions [12]. Arterial PO_2 remains stable. It is unclear whether the addition of theophylline would augment the beneficial effects of optimal beta-agonist therapy. In the elderly, inhaled beta-two selective agents are preferred over nonselective or oral agents to reduce unwanted cardiac effects. Terbutaline, metaproterenol, or albuterol can be given by inhalation (or orally), beginning in low doses. Optimal doses in some patients will exceed the standard recommended dose. In elderly patients with coexistent heart disease, sympathomimetics may cause excessive tachycardia, and theophylline may be better tolerated.

If bronchospasm persists despite an adequate trial of theophylline plus a beta-agonist, corticosteroids should be added. Acutely, hydrocortisone 3 mg/kg can be given every three hours intravenously. Effects are delayed, however, with onset of action about six hours after initiation of therapy. Once the patient has recovered, steroids can be tapered rapidly over 7 to 10 days.

With improved ventilation and oxygenation, the pulmonary hypertension accompanying acute respiratory failure is readily reversible. Maintenance therapy for stable COPD is designed to maintain adequate ventilation, generally utilizing chronic bronchodilator therapy. Theophylline and/or inhaled beta-agonists have been used extensively and with good clinical results. Ipratropium bromide, an atropine derivative, is another effective bronchodilator. This inhaled anticholinergic agent does not affect intraocular pressure or bowel or bladder function. In a large controlled trial in COPD, ipratropium bromide was at least as effective as inhaled metaproterenol as measured by clinical response and spirometry [13].

Chronic steroids may be effective for patients with reactive airways, but their utility in COPD is less clear. A recent review of clinical trials [14],

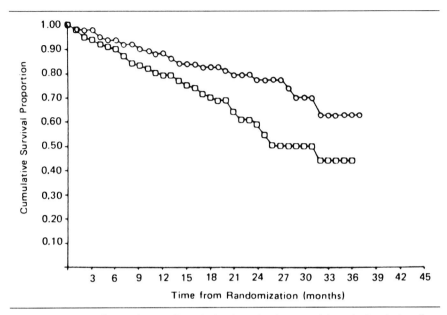

Figure 16-2. Overall mortality. Ordinate is fraction of patients surviving; abscissa is time from randomization or duration of treatment. Open circles represent continuous oxygen therapy group; open squares represent nocturnal oxygen therapy group. Of the total group, 80 patients were followed for 12 months, and 29 nocturnal oxygen and 37 continuous oxygen therapy patients were followed for 24 months. (Reproduced with permission from Nocturnal Oxygen Therapy Trial Group. 1980. Continuous nocturnal oxygen therapy in hypoxemic chronic obstructive lung disease: a clinical trial. Ann Intern Med 93:391–398.)

using a meta-analysis of those studies with adequate trial design, showed modest benefit. A 20% improvement in FEV_1 was achieved in only 10% more patients using steroids than in the placebo group. There were no clinical factors that could predict which patients would respond, and it was very difficult in any one patient to know if improved spirometry reflected steroid benefit or simply random fluctuation in the course of their disease. With the complication rate to be expected in an aging population, steroid therapy should generally be avoided.

In a minority of patients, hypoxia eventually becomes persistent, and worsening pulmonary hypertension with chronic right heart failure supervenes. In the setting of chronic cor pulmonale, home oxygen is essential and should be administered for at least 15 hours daily, especially during sleep. The resultant improvement in arterial oxygenation will reduce pulmonary vascular resistance and can reverse the electrocardiographic abnormalities and some of the arrhythmias associated with COPD [15]. Furthermore, mortality is markedly reduced by the use of oxygen at home, with the extent of protection increasing with more continuous oxygen supplementation (see figure 16-2) [16,17]. Patients likely to benefit from home oxygen include all those with documented PaO_2 less than 55 mmHg while clinically compensated, and those with a PaO_2 between 55 and 59 mmHg plus signs of right heart failure, pulmonary hypertension, or polycythemia [18].

Home oxygen and bronchodilator therapy will ameliorate pulmonary hypertension somewhat, but further efforts must be directed toward improving right ventricular performance and hemodynamics. Digitalis glycosides have been widely used for this purpose despite a paucity of evidence as to their efficacy. With acute digitalization, a small improvement in right ventricular contractility can be documented, although at the expense of further elevation of pulmonary artery pressure and an occasional fall in arterial oxygen saturation [19]. With chronic digitalis therapy it is difficult to demonstrate any improvement in right ventricular ejection fraction except in patients with concomitant left ventricular dysfunction [20,21]. On the other hand, elderly patients with chronic lung disease are predisposed to digitalis cardiotoxicity even at low serum levels. Thus, digoxin should be used cautiously, if at all, in cor pulmonale, and serum levels should be maintained in the lower therapeutic range. The principal indications for digoxin include coexisting left ventricular failure and the presence of supraventricular arrhythmias amenable to digitalis therapy.

Diuretics are also widely used in cor pulmonale to reduce central venous pressure and thus edema, hepatomegaly, and ascites. Care must be taken, however, to avoid excessive volume contraction with a resultant decrease in cardiac output. Particularly in elderly patients, fatigue, postural hypotension, prerenal azotemia, and alkalosis may result. Marked hyponatremia may also complicate therapy with potent diuretics when coupled with sodium restriction, forced hydration, and the high circulating levels of antidiuretic hormone seen in patients with lung disease.

Occasionally, marked hypoxia-induced erythrocytosis may contribute to pulmonary hypertension because of increased blood viscosity. A gradual reduction in the hematocrit through repeated phlebotomy can decrease pulmonary arterial pressure, but little change in central venous pressure or resting cardiac output is achieved, and total oxygen carrying capacity is reduced [22]. Several recent studies have shown that more beneficial effects of phlebotomy are evident during exercise. Thus, exercise capacity and oxygen consumption increase after lowering the hematocrit from the baseline of over 55% to 50% [22]. Venesection to reduce blood viscosity should be restricted to patients with marked erythrocytosis (hematocrit greater than 55% to 60%), and then only a modest hematocrit reduction is indicated (to 50% to 55%). Improving arterial oxygenation would be a preferable route to reverse erythrocytosis.

Areas of continued interest include the application of respiratory stimulants in COPD and the potential for reducing pulmonary vascular resistance pharmacologically with vasodilating drugs. Progesterone has been advocated by some as a useful ventilatory stimulant, but controlled studies demonstrating benefit are few. Doxapram may be useful for short-term intravenous therapy in patients with COPD and hypercarbia. Respiratory stimulation is thought to occur via peripheral carotid chemoreceptors and perhaps also through the central medullary respiratory centers. Both tidal volume and respiratory rate are augmented, and cardiac output may also increase. Doxapram has been recommended for short-term use in hopes that acute respiratory insufficiency can be reversed without resorting to mechanical ventilation. Infusions should be limited to no more than two hours.

Almitrine bismesylate has also been used as a ventilatory stimulant, working through peripheral chemoreceptors, especially the carotid body. In the usual clinical doses, however, almitrine has little effect on minute ventilation. Arterial oxygenation improves without change in $PaCO_2$. This improvement in oxygenation is due to reduced intrapulmonary shunting as a result of augmented hypoxic pulmonary vasoconstriction [23]. In a randomized trial, almitrine treatment reduced hospitalizations and episodes of right heart failure in patients with COPD [24]. On the other hand, almitrine treatment causes a significant increase in pulmonary artery pressures, both at rest and with exercise. Oxygen therapy produces similar improvements in oxygenation but with a decline in pulmonary pressures [25]. The role of this novel agent in the chronic treatment of cor pulmonale is not established.

Vasodilators, including hydralazine, nifedipine, and diltiazem, lower pulmonary vascular resistance acutely and improve cardiac output. Long-term treatment with calcium-channel antagonists produces sustained hemodynamic improvement in some patients, but with a fall in arterial oxygen saturation in some and no evidence as yet of clinical improvement [26,27]. Tolerance may develop during long-term use, reversing the initial effects of nifedipine [28]. Prazosin, a postsynaptic alpha-blocker, has been shown to increase cardiac output and decrease pulmonary artery pressure in some COPD patients, and similar results have been achieved with the alpha-blocker urapidil [29,30]. There is no evidence to date that any vasodilator will affect prognosis in cor pulmonale.

Arrhythmias in chronic lung disease

Both supraventricular and ventricular arrhythmias are commonplace in COPD. In acute respiratory failure, up to 70% of patients will experience clinically significant and sustained arrhythmias, including frequent ventricular ectopy, ventricular tachycardia, multifocal or paroxysmal atrial tachycardia, or atrial fibrillation [31]. In the stable outpatient with COPD, Holter-monitor findings resemble those seen in patients with coronary artery disease. Ventricular arrhythmias are frequent, commonly including multiform ventricular beats, couplets, and salvos [32]. Ventricular ectopy

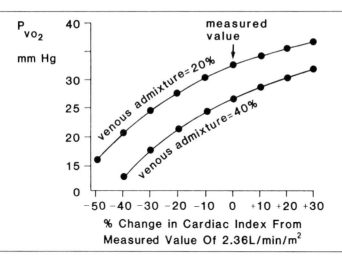

Figure 16-3. The effect of a change in cardiac output on mixed venous oxygen tension (PvO_2) in one patient studied whose pulmonary dysfunction had produced 20% venous admixture (upper curve). The lower curve shows the calculated change in PvO_2 that would accompany a change in cardiac output in a patient with similar hemoglobin concentration but more severe pulmonary disease (venous admixture = 40%). (Reproduced with permission from Holford FD and Mithoefer JC. 1973. Cardiac arrhythmias in hospitalized patients with chronic obstructive pulmonary disease. Am Rev Respir Dis 108:879–885.)

frequent enough to be recorded on a brief routine electrocardiogram in patients with acute respiratory failure predicts an in-hospital mortality rate of up to 70% and a poor long-term prognosis [33]. The 30% incidence of sudden death in survivors of acute respiratory failure, as well as the 10% incidence in stable COPD, underscores the significance of cardiac arrhythmias.

Furthermore, even ostensibly benign arrhythmias may have profound physiologic impact in the hypoxic patient. When appropriately timed atrial contraction is lost, as in atrial fibrillation or junctional rhythms, the cardiac output may fall as much as 30%. Frequent ventricular premature beats may have a similar effect and thus markedly curtail oxygen delivery to the tissues (see figure 16-3) [31].

Pathophysiology

Many factors contribute to the frequent occurrence of arrhythmias in COPD. Hypoxia and acid-base disturbance are certainly important, and improved pulmonary gas exchange may markedly improve cardiac dysrhythmia. Hypokalemia is common due to diuretics, steroid therapy, and loss of body mass in elderly patients with pulmonary cachexia. Even with normal serum levels, cellular potassium depletion should be assumed; and potassium chloride supplementation is indicated to help manage arrhythmias. If diuretics are required, use of potassium-sparing agents such as triamterene or amiloride should be considered, and serum potassium levels monitored.

Bronchodilators, including theophylline and sympathomimetic agents, are commonly implicated in arrhythmogenesis. Both have been shown to lower the ventricular fibrillation threshold in animals. Clinically, both can directly promote sinus tachycardia, accelerate conduction in atrial fibrillation, or induce ventricular arrhythmias in predisposed individuals. Theophylline clearance is delayed in the elderly, making cardiotoxicity more likely. Low doses of nonselective beta-adrenoceptor agonists like epinephrine or isoproterenol will cause cardioacceleration or arrhythmia. Only partial protection against cardiac effects is afforded by β-two selective agonists like terbutaline or albuterol, either of which can induce arrhythmia at high doses. The combination of theophylline plus a beta-two agonist, as commonly prescribed, is more apt to induce arrhythmia than either agent alone.

Digoxin may also precipitate ventricular or supraventricular dysrhythmias. Patients with pulmonary disease are prone to digitalis toxicity even at plasma levels well within the usual therapeutic range [34]. Paroxysmal atrial tachycardia with atrioventricular block is common and easily overlooked due to the relatively normal ventricular rate, the characteristically small size of the P-waves, and the superimposition of P-waves on the preceding T-waves. When unrecognized, atrial tachycardia with block will progress to lethal ventricular arrhythmia in up to 50% of cases. Treatment consists of withholding digoxin and suppressing ventricular arrhythmia with lidocaine or phenytoin.

Finally, intrinsic heart disease is common in this population, with approximately 30% of COPD patients having significant coronary artery disease. The scarred or ischemic myocardium is sensitive to metabolic perturbation, hypoxia, and drug effects, rendering the coronary patient prone to frequent and sustained arrhythmias. Rapid heart rates are poorly tolerated, causing an increase in myocardial oxygen demand. Tachycardia also foreshortens diastolic coronary perfusion time, thereby limiting oxygen delivery and aggravating ischemia.

Therapy

The major objective in both the acute and chronic management of arrhythmias complicating COPD should be to optimize pulmonary function. Reversal of hypoxia and acid–base disturbance may be all that is required to control otherwise refractory dysrhythmias. Awareness of drug effects on the heart and judicious compromise between the need for bronchodilators and the danger of cardioacceleration and precipitation of arrhythmia should help guide pharmacotherapy. Without such considerations, the empiric use of antiarrhythmic drugs is often unnecessary and generally unsuccessful.

When arrhythmias persist despite optimal pulmonary compensation, however, specific antiarrhythmic therapy may be indicated. Intravenous lidocaine is the agent of choice for serious ventricular arrhythmias. However, lidocaine toxicity is particularly common in the elderly and may depress respiration as well as induce central nervous system and cardiac toxicity. Lower initial and maintenance doses should be used. If arrhythmias persist, procainamide can be administered via the oral or intravenous route.

Management of acute reentrant supraventricular arrhythmias (paroxysmal atrial tachycardias) requires termination of the presenting arrhythmia and often maintenance therapy to prevent recurrences. Verapamil or adenosine can be given intravenously and will interrupt paroxysmal atrial tachycardia in almost all cases. Adenosine is usually preferred over verapamil because it will not cause hypotension and its brief duration of action limits the duration of any side effects to less than 30 seconds. When the arrhythmia is frequent or poorly tolerated, either digoxin, verapamil, or diltiazem can be given to prevent recurrences. Intravenous verapamil will promptly slow the ventricular rate in atrial fibrillation and atrial flutter, though hypotension may complicate its use. Intravenous calcium chloride will partially blunt the fall in pressure without reversing the effect of verapamil on the atrioventricular (A-V) node. Digoxin or calcium antagonists can be given to maintain rate control. In the hemodynamically unstable patient, electrical cardioversion of atrial flutter or fibrillation may be indicated.

Multifocal atrial tachycardia (MAT) is a particularly vexing arrhythmia seen in acutely ill, generally elderly patients. It is associated with a short-term mortality rate of 50%, which reflects the severity of the underlying illness rather than the direct consequences of the arrhythmia. MAT is generally tolerated well but can lead to myocardial ischemia or hemodynamic deterioration when the ventricular rate is rapid. Reductions in the dose of bronchodilator drugs or their discontinuation may slow the rate of MAT, occasionally allowing the return of sinus rhythm. Digoxin and membrane-active antiarrhythmic agents such as procainamide and quinidine have not been helpful. The most useful pharmacologic intervention has been the institution of beta-adrenoceptor blockade with propranolol or metoprolol, generally given intravenously [35]. Beta-blockade will slow the rate of MAT and frequently restore sinus rhythm. Bronchoconstriction may be aggravated, however, so that beta-blockade must be used with caution in patients with acute respiratory decompensation. On the other hand, beta-blockade is surprisingly well tolerated in many patients with COPD, with little change in airway resistance or ventilation. In fact, improved arterial oxygenation has been seen, probably as a result of reduced ventilation-perfusion mismatch [36]. Metoprolol should be used in preference to propranolol because it is relatively selective for blockade of beta-one receptors and has less effect on bronchial beta-two receptors. The ultra-short-acting, cardioselective beta-blocker esmolol may provide a safer means of titrating beta-blockade in pulmonary patients and has also been effective for MAT [37].

Because beta-blockers are usually avoided in the setting of respiratory failure, verapamil has been more widely used for the treatment of MAT. Though not as predictably effective as beta-blocker therapy, verapamil generally slows the atrial and ventricular rates in MAT [35,38]. Intravenous magnesium sulfate has also been effective in controlling MAT in small series of patients, even when pretreatment serum magnesium levels are normal [39].

The management of chronic arrhythmias in COPD does not differ significantly from arrhythmias in other settings. Ideally, atrial fibrillation should be reverted to sinus rhythm to maximize cardiac efficiency and reduce the risk of atrial thrombus formation and systemic embolization. Quinidine, disopyramide, or procainamide may bring about conversion chemically and should be continued after chemical or electrical cardioversion to maintain sinus rhythm. Flecainide or encainide can also be used, and either is occasionally effective when quinidine has failed. The recent reports of serious ventricular arrhythmias occurring after treatment with these drugs should discourage their routine use. Propafenone is also effective in the control of atrial fibrillation but has significant beta-blocker activity, possibly leading to bronchoconstriction.

When atrial fibrillation recurs despite adequate doses of antiarrhythmic agents, it is generally preferable to accept chronic atrial fibrillation as the rhythm of choice. Treatment with digoxin alone may be sufficient to control the ventricular rate. If rate control is inadequate, oral verapamil, diltiazem, or a cardioselective beta-blocker can be added. In the exceptional case in which refractory atrial fibrillation is poorly tolerated, amiodarone is often effective in maintaining sinus rhythm. However, toxicity of this drug includes severe pulmonary fibrosis, which is particularly worrisome in patients with preexisting lung disease [40].

Suppression of frequent ventricular ectopy is indicated in patients with concomitant cardiac disease or sustained ventricular tachycardia. Adequate therapy has been shown to reduce the risk of sudden death in this high-risk group, but no such data exist in patients with COPD or with lower grades of ventricular ectopy. Arbitrary recommendations, then, would include treatment of COPD patients with symptomatic arrhythmia or with sustained or accelerating ventricular tachycardia. Regardless of which antiarrhythmic drug is selected for the suppression of arrhythmia, treatment results must be rigorously assessed to document efficacy and avoid aggravation of arrhythmia. Serial electrophysiologic testing is recommended for patients with sustained arrhythmia or for survivors of cardiac arrest.

RENAL DISEASE

A gradual decline in renal function is an anticipated consequence of aging and has little effect on cardiac function. However, advanced renal disease may

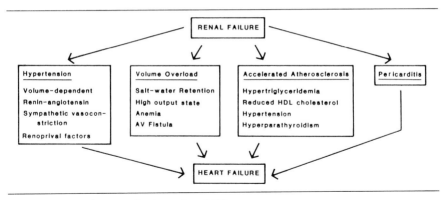

Figure 16-4. Cardiac complications of renal failure.

result from chronic hypertension, diabetes, recurrent kidney infections, lower urinary tract obstruction, or occlusive vascular disease, all common afflictions of the elderly. Once renal insufficiency is present, cardiac complications are the rule; they constitute the principal immediate cause of death in the uremic population [41]. Cardiac complications include congestive heart failure, accelerated coronary artery disease (CAD), and pericarditis.

Congestive heart failure

Congestive heart failure in uremia is generally the result of many factors (figure 16-4). Hypertension imposes a pressure load on the left ventricle; volume overload due to salt and fluid retention, anemia, and A-V shunting is common; and other factors including uremic toxins, electrolyte imbalance, and intrinsic heart disease may play a role [42]. Each of these factors must be considered for the optimal management of cardiac decompensation.

The hypertension seen in renal failure may be multifactorial. Salt and water retention, with resultant volume overload, may be primarily responsible. Such volume-dependent hypertension will respond to salt restriction and diuretic therapy, or to dialysis in the oliguric patient.

A second major cause of hypertension in renal insufficiency is augmented renin release, especially in patients with renal artery obstruction. If plasma volume contraction does not reverse hypertension, renin-dependent hypertension should be considered. Renin secretion can be partially suppressed by alpha-methyldopa or propranolol. Angiotensin-converting enzyme (ACE) inhibitors may be particularly effective, blocking the renin-angiotensin-aldosterone vasopressor cascade. However, these agents may also cause a precipitous deterioration of renal function, especially in patients with renal artery stenosis, so renal function should be monitored when beginning treatment with ACE inhibitors.

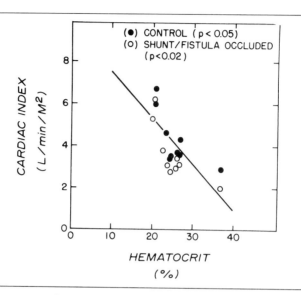

Figure 16-5. Inverse correlation between cardiac index and hematocrit demonstrable before and after arteriovenous occlusion(s). Cardiac index control = −0.187 hematocrit +9.11; cardiac index occlusion = −0.205 hematocrit +8.91. (Reproduced with permission from Capelli JP and Kaspian H. 1977. Cardiac work demands and left ventricular function in end-stage renal disease. Ann Intern Med 86:261–267.)

Other possible mechanisms leading to hypertension in chronic renal failure include sympathetically mediated vasoconstriction, production or delayed clearance of as yet unidentified vasopressor substance, or reduced production of vasodepressor substances. Regardless of the cause, sustained hypertension is a major factor precipitating left ventricular failure in chronic renal disease. Control of hypertension through volume manipulation, blockade of the renin-angiotensin-aldosterone axis, or treatment with vasodilators is of paramount importance.

Salt and water retention, with resulting volume overload, can further tax cardiac performance. Even in patients with normal left ventricular function, marked expansion of plasma volume can lead to edema formation or pulmonary congestion. Venodilating drugs, such as nitroprusside or nitroglycerine, will acutely improve left ventricular overload by pooling blood in venous capacitance vessels. However, long-term therapy depends on restricting sodium intake and on the use of diuretics.

Another stress on diminished left ventricular reserve is the demand for increased cardiac output. Severe anemia probably accounts for the characteristically high cardiac output seen despite clinical congestive heart failure in uremic patients, as suggested by the return of cardiac output to normal after acute transfusion [43]. Additional high output stress is imposed on patients on hemodialysis in whom 12% to 28% of the cardiac output is detoured through a single arteriovenous access shunt (figure 16-5) [42,44].

Finally, a uremic cardiomyopathy has been proposed. Cardiodepressant uremic toxins have not been identified, but their presence is suggested by the improvement in left ventricular function seen with chronic dialysis [45]. Additional negative inotropic effects may result from electrolyte imbalance, with hyperkalemia, hypermagnesemia, and hypocalcemia all being common in renal insufficiency.

It is important to realize that congestive heart failure among the uremic population can result from different mechanisms. Among nondiabetic dialysis patients studied with echocardiography and gated blood pool scanning, clinical heart failure was present in 10%. Eighteen percent of the patients had symptomatic coronary artery disease. Eighteen percent had a congestive cardiomyopathy, while 11% had a hypertrophic cardiomyopathy [46]. The latter two populations could not be distinguished on clinical grounds, though all patients with hypertrophic cardiomyopathy were hypertensive. Treatment and response are dramatically different. Heart failure due to hypertrophic cardiomyopathy may improve with beta-blockers or verapamil. Volume depletion by dialysis will relieve pulmonary congestion, but with a greater risk of hypotension and low cardiac output in patients with hypertrophic cardiomyopathy. Thus, an assessment of left ventricular systolic and also diastolic performance is essential for optimal treatment.

Coronary artery disease

CAD commonly accompanies renal insufficiency. Centers performing routine cardiac catheterization on dialysis patients report a 30% incidence of significant CAD [47]. Hypertension, hypertriglyceridemia, and reduced high-density lipoprotein cholesterol levels probably play a role in accelerated atherosclerosis [41]. Concomitantly, left ventricular mass and chamber size both increase as a result of pressure and volume overload. These changes lead to increased wall stress and myocardial oxygen demand and also limit coronary blood flow to the subendocardium [42]. Subendocardial ischemia is aggravated by anemia and CAD, setting the groundwork for angina, arrhythmias, and myocardial infarction.

Pericarditis

A final cardiac complication of renal failure is uremic pericarditis. Pericarditis occurs late in the course of chronic renal failure, generally as a preterminal event. However, it is also common among the otherwise stable dialysis population. The cause of pericarditis is unknown, though indirect evidence points to the presence of uremic toxins as one predisposing factor. Intensive dialysis often will reverse pericardial inflammation, and pericarditis among the chronic dialysis population has become less frequent with more effective modern dialysis [48,49]. Other factors, such as secondary hyperparathyroidism, circulating immune complexes, or toxic effects of drugs, may play a role in some patients [50]. Uremic pericarditis may be clinically silent but more often involves typical acute pericarditis, with pain, fever, cardiomegaly, and diagnostic electrocardiographic changes [51]. Documentation is usually straightforward by auscultatory detection of a rub or by demonstration of the presence of fluid by echocardiography. Hemodynamic compromise may occur, often first noted as hypotension during dialysis. Overt cardiac tamponade may occur spontaneously or after anticoagulation for dialysis. Late pericardial constriction is rare.

Therapy

Management of the cardiac complications of uremia centers on correction of precipitating factors. Thus, volume manipulation, blood pressure control, and meticulous attention to electrolytes and dialysis regimens will usually alleviate congestive heart failure. Inotropic support with digoxin may be helpful, but this drug must be administered cautiously. The daily percent clearance of body digoxin stores can be estimated to equal 14 + 0.2 X creatinine clearance (in millilites per minute) [52]. The anephric patient thus clears about 14% of digoxin stores daily. Since the loading dose is 0.01 to 0.015 mg/kg lean body mass, daily maintenance digoxin dose for the 70-kg anephric patient should be 14% of this, or approximately 0.10 to 0.125 mg. Actual clearance may vary, however, and plasma levels should be measured.

Digitoxin clearance is unchanged with renal insufficiency, which has been considered an advantage. However, in end-stage renal disease, the plasma half-life of digoxin is about the same as for digitoxin. The ready availability of plasma assays for digoxin makes it the preferred drug. Because of extensive plasma protein binding, neither digoxin nor digitoxin is removed by hemodialysis. However, dialysis often results in rapid alterations in plasma potassium and calcium levels, increasing the danger of digitalis cardiotoxicity even when digoxin plasma levels are well within the "therapeutic" range.

Treatment of uremic pericarditis generally involves intensive hemo- or peritoneal dialysis [53]. This is predictably effective in patients with end-stage uremia, but pericarditis in patients on chronic dialysis responds to more intensive dialysis in only 50% [50]. For patients not considered dialysis candidates, or those refractory to dialysis, a pericardial window or pericardiectomy should be performed. Systemic or intrapericardial steroids have been effective, although each approach has inherent dangers.

ENDOCRINE DISEASE

Cardiovascular disorders accompany many hormonal imbalances, as noted in table 16-2. Most of these endocrine diseases are relatively uncommon and more likely to occur in the younger population. Diabetes mellitus, on the

Table 16-2. Endocrine abnormalities of the heart

Acromegaly
  Hypertension, accelerated atherosclerosis, cardiomegaly, intraventricular conduction defects
Adrenal insufficiency
  Hypotension, shock
Cushing's syndrome
  Hypertension, accelerated atherosclerosis
Diabetes mellitus
  Accelerated atherosclerosis, cardiomyopathy
Hyperaldosteronism
  Hypertension, hypokalemia, arrhythmia
Hyperthyroidism
  Arrhythmia, heart failure, hypertension
Hypothyroidism
  Pericardial effusion, accelerated atherosclerosis, hypertension
Pheochromocytoma
  Hypertension, arrhythmia, hypotension, myocarditis

other hand, is commonplace in the elderly and is a major cause for accelerated vascular disease and cardiac dysfunction. Diabetes is easily recognized, and its complications and management are familiar to most physicians. In this chapter, then, discussion will be limited to abnormalities of thyroid function, since thyroid disease is a frequent cause of cardiac problems in the elderly and may be difficult to recognize.

Hyperthyroidism

In hyperthyroidism, the commonly associated signs of hyperactivity, heat intolerance, tremor, and weight loss may not be conspicuous in the elderly; only the cardiac manifestations of excessive thyroxine stimulation may be present [54]. Older patients with hyperthyroidism tend to have variable biochemical presentations, including elevations of only T3 or only T4, or normal absolute thyroid hormone levels that are nonetheless excessive in the individual. Thus, sinus tachycardia, frequent ventricular premature beats, or paroxysmal or sustained atrial fibrillation may be due to occult hyperthyroidism. Biventricular enlargement may occur, along with high-output congestive heart failure. Any elderly patient with unexplained arrhythmia, cardiomegaly, or congestive heart failure should be evaluated for thyrotoxicosis.

The cause of tachyarrhythmias and sustained high cardiac output in thyrotoxicosis is uncertain. While the peripheral metabolic rate is accelerated, the augmentation of cardiac output exceeds that needed to meet tissue oxygen demand. Thyoxine directly increases the rate of sinus-node discharge and accelerates conduction through the A-V node. Furthermore, the gratifying response to propranolol suggests that increased sympathetic stimulation may be another factor. Although circulating levels of catecholamines are not elevated, the cardiac response to exogenous catecholamines is enhanced. This may in part be due to the increased density or affinity of myocardial beta-receptors found in hyperthyroidism.

Atrial fibrillation is particularly common, occurring in 10% to 22% of hyperthyroid patients, with the frequency increasing with age [55]. Among patients without obvious predisposing cardiac causes for atrial fibrillation, occult hyperthyroidism is found in 5% to 20% [56,57]. A blunted thyroid-stimulating hormone (TSH) response to TRH stimulation is the most widely used screening test for subclinical hyperthyroidism, though the specificity of this test can be influenced by nonthyroid illnesses [58,59]. The newer ultrasensitive TSH measurements can document true suppression of TSH without the need for a TRH stimulation test. When occult hyperthyroidism is promptly treated with radioiodine, reversion to sinus rhythm is the rule [60].

In hyperthyroidism, atrial fibrillation occurs with a rapid ventricular rate that is often poorly tolerated by the elderly patient. Digoxin is of limited utility and must be administered in high doses to slow the heart rate. Absorption is diminished and renal digoxin clearance is accelerated in hyperthyroidism, but even when high doses result in adequate serum drug levels, digoxin does not fully counter the effects of thyrotoxicosis on A-V conduction [56]. The addition of propranolol or another beta-blocker is useful in this instance for adequate rate control. Calcium-channel antagonists are less effective in this setting. Cardioversion of atrial fibrillation should be deferred until a euthyroid state has been achieved, at which time spontaneous or quinidine-induced conversion to sinus rhythm often occurs. Persistent atrial fibrillation at that point is an indication for electrical cardioversion [61].

There is evidence suggesting predisposition to peripheral emboli, occurring in 10% to 40% of thyrotoxic patients with atrial fibrillation [62]. Anticoagulation has been recommended prior to pharmacologic or electrical cardioversion [63]. In the elderly population, the somewhat increased risks of bleeding must be weighed against the risk of stroke; but most patients can be safely anticoagulated. If anticoagulation is planned in a thyrotoxic patient, a low warfarin dose is required due to the accelerated turnover of clotting factors.

Congestive heart failure is seen relatively infrequently now, since the diagnosis of hyperthyroidism can be made early. In the thyrotoxic patient, heart failure most often reflects preexistent heart disease. Congestive heart failure is precipitated by the inability of the compromised heart to meet the accelerated demands placed upon it. Diuretics help relieve the congestive symptoms, though definitive treatment requires restoration of a euthyroid state. Digoxin and vasodilators are not indicated given the ongoing inotropic and vasodilator effects of thyrotoxicosis. When rapid atrial fibrillation aggravates heart failure, propranolol may produce hemodynamic improvement.

Hypothyroidism

Hypothyroidism may also be difficult to recognize, since its symptoms, including cold intolerance, weakness, constipation, and dyspnea, are non-specific and may be confused with the "normal aging process." Cardiovascular manifestations of hypothyroidism include eletrocardiographic changes, anginalike chest pains, cardiomegaly, and pericardial effusion. The electro-cardiographic alterations frequently consist of sinus bradycardia with low QRS and P-wave voltage and a prolonged Q-T interval. Atrioventricular and intraventricular conduction disturbances are common, but complete heart block is rare.

Cardiomegaly may be related to increased diastolic filling due to bradycardia, to pericardial effusion, or to cardiac decompensation. Thyroxine has been shown to stimulate contractility directly, while insufficient production of the hormone leads to depressed contractility [64]. Histologically, the myocardium in severe myxedema is edematous, with infiltration by mucopolysaccharides and with areas of necrosis and fibrinoid degeneration. Clinical studies have revealed phonocardiographic evidence of impaired contractility and echocardiographic evidence of left ventricular hypertrophy and diminished ejection fraction [65,66]. In some patients, a picture similar to obstructive hypertrophic cardiomyopathy is seen, with asymmetric interventricular septal hypertrophy and dynamic outflow tract obstruction [66]. Despite these findings, congestive heart failure is usually not a direct consequence of hypothyroidism, and its presence suggests concomitant intrinsic heart disease. The reduced cardiac output seen at rest reflects diminished peripheral oxygen demand, and cardiac output increases appropriately with exercise. Replacement thyroxine therapy results in reversal of the electrocardiographic changes and improved resting systolic function, with return of the heart size to normal. If digoxin therapy is needed, it should be initiated at half the usual dose because of retarded clearance, and plasma levels should be measured.

Atherosclerosis is common in hypothyroidism, probably because of the elevated cholesterol levels and blood pressure that occur with thyroid deficiency [67]. Perhaps due to decreased myocardial oxygen demand, however, myocardial infarction and true angina are relatively infrequent in myxedema [68]. Once thyroxine replacement is initiated, angina may then be precipitated. Accordingly, replacement therapy should be introduced at a low dose (0.025 mg daily) and slowly advanced over a period of months to full maintenance. Suppression of TSH release is a useful guide to physiologic replacement therapy. In elderly patients, maintenance thyroxine dose tends to be relatively low (average 120 mg daily) compared with that used for the middle-aged population [69].

When angina does occur in hypothyroidism, its management can be difficult. Beta-adrenergic blocking agents can precipitously slow the heart rate and must be used cautiously. Similar precautions should apply to verapamil and diltiazem, while the safety of nifedipine is uncertain. Thyroid hormone administration will increase heart rate and contractility—effects that are in part offset by a decline in heart size and peripheral resistance. The net effect on myocardial ischemia is variable. Thyroid replacement therapy should be initiated cautiously, using T4 rather than T3 or a mixture. In 70% of cases, no change in angina pattern is seen with hormonal replacement, and in some cases angina seems to improve [69,70]. However, worsening of angina or acute myocardial infarction may also be precipitated with injudicious hormonal supplementation. If chest pain is refractory to medical efforts, or in the presence of severe three-vessel or left main CAD, surgery is required. Aortocoronary bypass can be performed safely, even in the face of uncorrected hypothyroidism, as long as the anesthesiologist, surgeon, and internist remain aware of the patient's increased sensitivity to anesthetics, analgesics, and digitalis [71]. In the event of prolonged chest pain, interpretation of plasma enzyme results can be confusing. Blood levels of CK, LDH, and SGOT are all elevated in uncomplicated myxedema, and the isoenzyme pattern of LDH may match that of cardiac origin. Only when CK levels are extremely high, however, is the MB isoenzyme detectable.

Finally, pericardial effusion is common and generally asymptomatic, occurring in one third of patients with myxedema. This reflects increased capillary permeability with transudation of fluid. Tamponade may occur but is rare. The effusion subsides within 2 to 12 months after initiation of thyroid replacement.

COLLAGEN-VASCULAR DISEASES

While cardiac involvement is a prominent feature of many systemic collagen-vascular diseases (table 16-3), most of these diseases affect predominantly younger populations. Exceptions include temporal arteritis, a predominantly geriatric disorder, and rheumatoid arthritis, which is common in all age groups.

Temporal arteritis

Temporal arteritis, or giant-cell arteritis, occurs with increasing frequency with advancing age. There is a nearly 1% prevalence in patients over 80 years old [72]. Segmental inflammatory lesions may involve any large- or medium-sized artery, leading to focal narrowing or occlusion. Presenting symptoms are often directly related to the affected vessels, with temporal headaches commonly reflecting inflamed temporal arteries. Facial artery involvement leads to jaw claudication, and occlusion of the opthalmic or central retinal artery can result in blindness. The carotids, vertebrals, and aorta are commonly affected but infrequently produce symptoms.

Other manifestations of giant-cell arteritis are due to systemic illness, with fever, arthralgias, weight loss, anemia, hepatocellular dysfunction, and a markedly elevated erythrocyte sedimentation rate. Polymyalgia rheumatica

Table 16-3. Collagen-vascular disease and the heart

Acute rheumatic fever
  Pancarditis, valvular deformity
Ankylosing spondylitis
  Myocarditis, pericarditis, aortic regurgitation, conduction block
Giant-cell arteritis
  Cerebrovascular events, blindness, coronary occlusion
Periarteritis nodosa
  Coronary involvement, pericarditis
Rieter's disease
  Myocarditis, pericarditis, aortic regurgitation, conduction block
Rheumatoid arthritis
  Pericarditis, myocarditis, endocarditis
Scleroderma
  Small-vessel disease, cardiomyopathy, pericarditis
Systemic lupus
  Pericarditis, myocarditis, endocarditis
Systemic vasculitis
  Pericarditis, myocarditis

may accompany temporal arteritis; it causes marked tenderness and stiffness of the muscles of the shoulder girdle, hips, and thighs. Muscle enzymes, electromyograms, and muscle biopsy are normal.

The diagnosis of giant-cell arteritis is critical, since its complications are unpredictable and catastrophic; treatment with steroids is highly effective in preventing those complications. Unfortunately, the presentation is often atypical or nonspecific. A high index of suspicion is important for early recognition of the illness. Any elderly patient with malaise or fever is suspect, especially if there are signs or symptoms of vascular insufficiency. An elevated sedimentation rate is a supportive finding, although the definitive diagnosis generally depends on biopsy of one or both temporal arteries. Except in the most classic cases, histologic documentation should be obtained before submitting the elderly patient to the consequences of prolonged corticosteroid therapy. Yet a delay in the diagnosis runs the risk of blindness, opthalmoplegia, stroke, or, rarely, aortic dissection or coronary occlusion [73]. Steroids can be administered before the biopsy is obtained and will not alter histology for several days.

Prednisone therapy should be initiated at a dosage of 60 to 80 mg daily for the first four weeks. Thereafter, it is slowly tapered to the lowest effective dose, monitoring a low sedimentation rate and clinical response. Steroid therapy in low doses should continue for at least two years [74]. Alternate-day therapy is usually ineffective. If steroids alone do not control clinical manifestations of arteritis, or if steroid side effects are excessive, the adjunctive use of cyclophosphamide, methotrexate, or azathioprine should be considered.

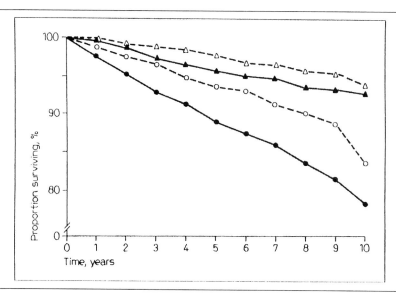

Figure 16-6. Survival (%) for cardiac deaths by the Lee and Desu (80) algorithm in patients with rheumatoid arthritis (closed circles represent men, closed triangles represent women) and controls (open circles represent men, open triangles represent women). (Reproduced with permission from Mutru O, Laakso M, Isomaki H, et al. 1989. Cardiovascular mortality in patients with rheumatoid arthritis. Cardiology 76:71–77.)

Rheumatoid arthritis

The cardiovascular complications of rheumatoid arthritis are common but generally clinically silent. Their recognition is important, though, in excluding more serious forms of heart disease. Pericarditis has been documented in 30% to 50% of patients by echocardiographic methods, although it is clinically evident in no more than 10% [75,76]. Many of these patients are asymptomatic, but the disease is recognized because of a pericardial rub and echocardiographic documentation of an effusion. When the cause of the effusion is in doubt, examination of pericardial fluid is helpful. Expected findings include elevated protein and cholesterol levels, depressed hemolytic complement, and often the presence of rheumatoid factor. Extremely low glucose levels are sometimes found, attributable to active phagocytosis carried out in polymorphonuclear leukocytes. The neutrophils themselves have large cytoplasmic inclusion bodies (RA cells), composed of immune complexes [77].

Pericardial tamponade and constriction may complicate the course of rheumatoid pericarditis. Treatment consists of aggressive therapy for the underlying disorder. Nonsteroidal anti-inflammatory drugs generally suffice to control symptoms. Corticosteroids are also effective, but there is no evidence that such therapy will prevent adhesive or constrictive disease. When signs of right heart failure develop, pericardial constriction is likely. Pericardiectomy in these individuals is usually curative [78].

Rheumatoid myocarditis and endocarditis are commonly seen at autopsy, although rarely recognized clinically. Only in severe systemic rheumatoid vasculitis is significant myocardial dysfunction likely to result. In occasional patients, though, rheumatoid granulomas may cause conduction abnormalities or may produce significant scarring of the mitral or aortic valve. Insufficiency of these valves has resulted, requiring surgical correction. Coronary arteritis is also common, documented histologically in 20% of rheumatoid patients at autopsy. This rarely leads to angina or infarction, however, and ischemic heart disease is the result of coexistent atherosclerotic involvement. Amyloidosis may complicate long-standing rheumatoid arthritis, but in this setting it rarely affects the heart. The cumulative burden of these cardiac effects results in an increased rate of cardiac mortality in patients with rheumatoid arthritis, commonly from congestive heart failure (figure 16-6) [79,80].

REFERENCES

1. Ferrer MI. 1979. Management of patients with cor pulmonale. Med Clin North Am 63:251–265.
2. Enson Y, Giuntini C, Lewis ML, et al. 1964. The influence of hydrogen ion concentration and hypoxia on the pulmonary circulation. J Clin Invest 43:1146–1162.
3. Bove AA and Santamore WP. 1981. Ventricular interdependence. Prog Cardiovasc Dis 23:365–388.
4. Rice KL, Leatherman JW, Duane PG, et al. 1987. Aminophylline for acute exacerbation of chronic obstructive pulmonary disease: a controlled trial. Ann Intern Med 107:305–309.
5. Dullinger D, Kronenberg R and Niewoehner DE. 1986. Efficacy of inhaled metaproterenol and orally-administered theophylline in patients with chronic airflow obstruction. Chest 89:171–173.
6. Parker JO, Kelkar K and West RO. 1966. Hemodynamic effects of aminophylline in cor pulmonale. Circ 33:17–25.
7. Matthay RA, Berger HJ, Loke J, et al. 1978. Effects of aminophylline on right and left ventricular performance in chronic obstructive pulmonary disease. Am J Med 65:903–910.
8. Parker JO, Ashekian PB, DiGiorgi S, et al. 1967. Hemodynamic effects of aminophylline in chronic obstructive pulmonary disease. Circulation 35:365–372.
9. Matthay RA, Berger HJ, Davies R, et al. 1982. Improvement in cardiac performance by oral long-acting theophylline in chronic obstructive pulmonary disease. Am Heart J 104:1022–1029.
10. Mahler DA, Matthay RA, Snyder PE, et al. 1985. Sustained-release theophylline reduces dyspnea in nonreversible obstructive airway disease. Am Rev Respir Dis 131:22–25.
11. Winter RJD, Langford JA and Rudd RM. 1984. Effects of oral and inhaled salbutamol and oral pirbuterol on right and left ventricular function in chronic bronchitis. Br Med J 288:324–325.
12. Brent BN, Mahler D, Berger HJ, et al. 1982. Augmentation of right ventricular performance in chronic obstructive pulmonary disease by terbutaline. A combined radionuclide and hemodynamic study. Am J Cardiol 50:313–319.
13. Tashkin DP, Ashutosh K, Blecker E, et al. 1985. Comparison of the anticholinergic bronchodilator ipratropium bromide with metaproterenol in chronic obstructive lung disease: a 90 day multicenter study. Am J Med 81 (Suppl 5A):81–89.
14. Callahan CM, Dittus RS and Katz BP. 1991. Oral corticosteroid therapy for patients with

stable chronic obstructive pulmonary disease: a meta-analysis. Ann Intern Med 114:216–223.

15. Tirlapur VG and Mir MA. 1982. Nocturnal hyopoxemia and associated electrocardiographic changes in patients with chronic obstructive airways disease. N Engl J Med 306:125–130.

16. Anthonisen NR. 1983. Long-term oxygen therapy. Ann Intern Med 99:519–527.

17. Nocturnal Oxygen Therapy Trial study group. 1980. Continuous or nocturnal oxygen therapy in hypoxemic chronic obstructive pulmonary disease: a clinical trial. Ann Intern Med 93:391–398.

18. Levin DC, Neff TA, O'Donohue WJ Jr, et al. 1988. Further recommendations for prescribing and supplying long-term oxygen therapy. Am Rev Respir Dis 138:745–747.

19. Green LH and Smith TW. 1977. The use of digitalis in patients with pulmonary disease. Ann Intern Med 87:459–465.

20. Mathur PN, Powles P, Pugsley SO, et al. 1981. Effect of digoxin on right ventricular function in severe chronic airflow obstruction. Ann Intern Med 95:283–288.

21. Brown SE, Pakron FJ, Milne N, et al. 1984. Effects of digoxin on exercise capacity and right ventricular function during exercise in chronic airflow obstruction. Chest 85:187–191.

22. Weisse AB, Moschos CB, Frank MJ, et al. 1975. Hemodynamic effects of staged hematocrit reduction in patients with stable cor pulmonale and severely elevated hematocrit levels. Am J Med 58:92–98.

23. Gothe B, Cherniack NS, Bachand RT Jr, et al. 1988. Long-term effects of almitrine bimesylate on oxygenation during wakefulness and sleep in chronic obstructive pulmonary disease. Am J Med 84:436–444.

24. Voisin C, Howard P and Ansquer JC. 1987. Vectarian International Multicenter Study. Bull Eur Pathophysiol Respir 23 (Suppl):169S–182S.

25. MacNee W, Connaughton JJ, Rhind GB, et al. 1986. A comparison of the effects of almitrine or oxygen breathing on pulmonary arterial pressure and right ventricular ejection fraction in hypoxemic chronic bronchitis and emphysema. Am Rev Respir Dis 134:559–565.

26. Sturani C, Bassein L, Schiavina M, et al. 1983. Oral nifedipine in chronic cor pulmonale secondary to severe chronic obstructive pulmonary disease (COPD). Chest 84:135–142.

27. Kennedy TP, Michael JR and Summer W. 1985. Calcium channel blockers in hypoxic pulmonary hypertension. Am J Med 78 (Suppl 2B):18–26.

28. Agostoni P, Doria E, Galli C, et al. 1989. Nifedipine reduces pulmonary pressure and vascular tone during short- but not long-term treatment of pulmonary hypertension in patients with chronic obstructive pulmonary disease. Am Rev Respir Dis 139:120–125.

29. Adnot S, Anrivet P, Piquet J, et al. 1988. The effects of urapidil therapy on hemodynamics and gas exchange in exercising patients with chronic obstructive pulmonary disease and pulmonary hypertension. Am Rev Respir Dis 137:1068–1074.

30. Adnot S, DeFouilloy C, Brun-Buisson C, et al. 1987. Hemodynamic effects of urapidil in patients with pulmonary hypertension: a comparative study with hydralazine. Am Rev Respir Dis 135:288–293.

31. Holford FD and Mithoefer JC. 1973. Cardiac arrhythmias in hospitalized patients with chronic obstructive pulmonary disease. Am Rev Respir Dis 108:879–885.

32. Kleiger RE and Senior RM. 1974. Long-term electrocardiographic monitoring of ambulatory patients with chronic airway obstruction. Chest 65:483–488.

33. Hudson LD, Kurt TL, Petty TL, et al. 1973. Arrhythmias associated with acute respiratory failure in patients with chronic airway obstruction. Chest 63:661–665.

34. Goldberg LM, Bristow JD, Parker BM, et al. 1960. Paroxysmal atrial tachycardia with atrioventricular block. Circulation 21:499–504.

35. Arsura E, Lefkin AS, Scher DL, et al. 1988. A randomized, double-blind, placebo-controlled study of verapamil and metoprolol in the treatment of multifocal atrial tachycardia. Am J Med 85:519–524.

36. Nordstrom LA, MacDonald F and Gobel F. 1975. Effect of propranolol on respiratory function and exercise tolerance in patients with chronic obstructive lung disease. Chest 67:287–292.

37. Esmolol Multicenter Research Group. 1985. Efficacy and safety of esmolol vs propranolol in the treatment of supraventricular tachyarrhythmias: a multicenter double-blind clinical trial. Am Heart J 110: 913–920.

38. Levine JM, Michael JR and Guarnieri T. 1985. Treatment of multifocal atrial tachycardia with verapamil. N Engl J Med 312:21–25.
39. Iseri LT, Fairshter RD, Hardemann JL, et al. 1985. Magnesium and potassium therapy in multifocal atrial tachycardia. Am Heart J 110:789–794.
40. Zipes DP, Prystowsky EN and Heger JJ. 1984. Amiodarone: electrophysiologic actions, pharmacokinetics, and clinical effects. J Am Coll Cardiol 3:1059–1071.
41. Lindner A, Charra B, Sherrard DJ, et al. 1974. Accelerated atherosclerosis in prolonged maintenance hemodialysis. N Engl J Med 290:697–701.
42. Capelli JP and Kasparian H. 1977. Cardiac work demands and left ventricular function in end-stage renal disease. Ann Intern Med 86:261–265.
43. Neff MS, Kim KE, Persoff M, et al. 1971. Hemodynamics of uremic anemia. Circulation 43:876–883.
44. Menno AD, Zizzi J, Hodson J, et al. 1967. An evaluation of the radial arteriovenous fistula as a substitute for the Quinton shunt in chronic hemodialysis. Trans Am Soc Artif Intern Organs 8:62–67.
45. Huug J, Harris PJ, Uren RF, et al. 1980. Uremic cardiomyopathy—effect of hemodialysis on left ventricular function in end-stage renal failure. N Engl J Med 302:547–551.
46. Parfrey PS, Harnett TD, Griffiths SM, et al. 1980. Congestive heart failure in dialysis patients. Arch Intern Med 148:1519–1525.
47. Ikram H, Lynn KL, Bailey RR, et al. 1983. Cardiovascular changes in chronic dialysis patients. Kidney Int 24:371–376.
48. Bailey GL, Hampers CL, Hager EB, et al. 1968. Uremic pericarditis: clinical features and management. Circulation 38:582–591.
49. Drueke T, LePailleur C, Zingraff J, et al. 1980. Uremic cardiomyopathy and pericarditis. Adv Nephrol 9:33–70.
50. Becker RC. 1988. Cardiovascular disease in patients with chronic renal failure. Cleve Clin J Med 55:521–530.
51. Comty CM, Cohen SL and Shapiro FL. 1971. Pericarditis in chronic uremia and its sequela. Ann Intern Med 75:173–183.
52. Jelliffe RW. 1971. Factors to consider in planning digoxin therapy. J Chronic Dis 24:407–416.
53. Silverberg S, Oreopoulos DG, Wise DJ, et al. 1977. Pericarditis in patients undergoing long-term hemodialysis and peritoneal dialysis. Am J Med 63:874–880.
54. Tibaldi JM, Barzel US, Albin J and Surks M. 1986. Thyrotoxicosis in the very old. Am J Med 81:619–622.
55. Forfar JC and Caldwell GC. 1985. Hyperthyroid heart disease. Clin Endocrinol Metab 14:491–508.
56. Symons C. 1979. Thyroid heart disease. Br Heart J 41:257–262.
57. Rohmer V, Hocq F, Galland F, et al. 1984. Occult thyrotoxicosis revealed by atrial arrhythmia. Presse Med 13:145–148.
58. Sulimani RA. 1989. Diagnostic algorithm for atrial fibrillation caused by occult hyperthyroidism. Geriatrics 44:61–69.
59. Fagerberg B, Lindstedt G, Stromblad SO, et al. 1990. Thyrotoxic atrial fibrillation: an underdiagnosed or overdiagnosed condition? Clin Chem 36:620–627.
60. Forfar JC, Miller HC and Toft AD. 1979. Occult thyrotoxicosis: a correctable cause of "idiopathic" atrial fibrillation. Am J Cardiol 44:9–12.
61. Nakazawa AK, Sakurai K, Hamada N, et al. 1982. Management of atrial fibrillation in the post-thyrotoxic state. Am J Med 72:903–906.
62. Bar-sela S, Ehrenfeld M and Eliakim M, 1981. Arterial embolism in thyrotoxicosis with atrial fibrillation. Arch Intern Med 141:1191–1192.
63. Staffurth JS, Gibberd MC and Ng Tang Fui S. 1977. Arterial embolism in thyrotoxicosis with atrial fibrillation. Br Med J 2:688–690.
64. Buccino RA, Spann JF Jr, Pool PE, et al. 1967. Influence of the thyroid state on the intrinsic contractile properties and energy stores of the myocardium. J Clin Invest 46:1669–1682.
65. Crowley WF Jr, Ridgway EC, Bough EW, et al. 1977. Noninvasive evaluation of cardiac function in hyperthyroidism. N Engl J Med 296:1–6.
66. Santos AD, Miller RP, Mathew PK, et al. 1980. Echocardigraphic characterization of the reversible cardiomyopathy of hypothyroidism. Am J Med 68:675–682.

67. Steinberg AD. 1968. Myxedema and coronary artery disease—a comparative autopsy study. Ann Intern Med 68:338–344.
68. Bastenie PA, Bonnyns M and Vanhaelst L. 1985. Natural history of primary myxedema. Am J Med 79:91–100.
69. Rosenbaum RL and Barzel US. 1982. Levothyroxine replacement dose for primary hypothyroidism decreases with age. Ann Intern Med 96:53–55.
70. Keating FR, Parkin TW, Selby JB, et al. 1960. Treatment of heart disease associated with myxedema. Prog Cardiovasc Dis 3:364–386.
71. Hay ID, Duick DS, Vlietstra RE, et al. 1981. Thyroxine therapy in hypothyroid patients undergoing coronary revascularization: a retrospective analysis. Ann Intern Med 95:456–457.
72. Goodman BW. 1979. Temporal arteritis. Am J Med 67:839–852.
73. Klein RG, Hunder GG, Stanson AW, et al. 1975. Large artery involvement in giant cell (temporal) arteritis. Ann Intern Med 83:806–812.
74. Kyle V and Hazelman BL. 1989. Treatment of polymyalgia rheumatica (PMR) and giant cell arteritis (GCA). II. The relationship between steroid dose and steroid-associated side effects. Ann Rheum Dis 48:662–666.
75. Bacon PA and Gibson DG. 1974. Cardiac involvement in rheumatoid arthritis. An echocardiographic study. Ann Rheum Dis 33:20–24.
76. Kirk J and Cosh J. 1969. The pericarditis of rheumatoid arthritis. Q J Med 38:397–423.
77. Hara KS, Ballard DJ, Ilstrup DM, et al. 1990. Rheumatoid pericarditis: clinical features and survival. Medicine 69:81–91.
78. Kelly CA, Bourke JP, Malcolm A, et al. 1990. Chronic pericardial disease in patients with rheumatoid arthritis: a longitudinal study. Q J Med 75:461–470.
79. Mutru O, Laakso M, Isomaki H, et al. 1989. Cardiovascular mortality in patients with rheumatoid arthritis. Cardiology 76:71–77.
80. Lee E, Desu M. 1972. A computer program for comparing k samples with right-censored data. Comput Programs Biomed 2:315–321.

17. PSYCHOLOGICAL ADAPTATION TO CARDIOVASCULAR DISEASE

RICHARD V. MILANI
ANDREW B. LITTMAN
CARL J. LAVIE

Every affection of the mind that is attended with either pain or pleasure, hope or fear, is the cause of an agitation whose influence extends to the heart.
—William Harvey, 1628 [1]

In elderly Americans, the most rapidly growing population group in the United States, cardiovascular disease represents the major cause of death and disability. In 1988, greater than 55% of all myocardial infarctions (MI) were in persons older than 65 years of age [2], and infarcts in this group are typically more severe and associated with increased complications, thus prolonging hospitalization with its attendant deconditioning. With the advent of improved technology and increasing survival following MI, the incidence of congestive heart failure has rapidly increased, with an eightfold increase among men in the seventh decade of life as compared to those in the fifth decade. Congestive heart failure is now the leading hospital discharge diagnosis in the United States in persons older than age 65 [3]. Depending on the severity of these cardiovascular disorders and the presence of comorbid conditions, elderly persons often have to make significant life-style modifications that impact a variety of daily functions, including social and recreational activities, occupational demands, relations with spouse and

Franz H. Messerli (ed.), CARDIOVASCULAR DISEASE IN THE ELDERLY (Third Edition). Copyright © 1993 Kluwer Academic Publishers. ISBN 0-7923-1859-5. All rights reserved.

family, sexual function, activities of daily living, and mood [4–6]. These modifications can be accompanied by constructive behavioral change, such as cessation of smoking or compliance with medication, or by maladaptive behavior such as denial of symptoms or the illness itself, which can lead to further deterioration of the primary condition.

The life-style demands imposed by cardiovascular disease must be recognized by health care providers as well as by the person who exhibits maladaptive change. As part of our coronary risk assessment, evaluating behavioral function may reduce the risk of future coronary events and foster constructive adaptive change. This chapter will discuss the role of psychological factors in the development of coronary heart disease (CHD) and in adaptive change. We will also discuss the impact of cardiovascular disease on functional status and well-being in the elderly.

GENERAL ISSUES

In the elderly, as in the general population, there is wide variance in behavioral, emotional, and cognitive functioning. Individual characteristics such as culture, sex, ethnicity, prior health status, and personality are more likely than chronologic age to influence the psychosocial and disability status of an elderly person [6]. Chronologic age does not predict morale or emotional lability following MI [7]. Consequently, elderly persons who have experienced coronary events should not be stereotyped as psychosocially impaired. Physicians, when asked to rate their elderly patients' psychosocial functions including global quality of life, physical comfort, mobility, depression, anxiety, and family relationships, are more likely to score them significantly worse than do patients themselves, thus demonstrating a natural bias [8]. Health care providers and patients should therefore guard against these negative stereotypes, which can stifle constructive change and by lack of adequate intervention lead to further deterioration of the patient's overall condition. This important interplay between the emotions and health of the individual was articulated by Dr. Viktor Frankl in his memoirs of the holocaust:

Those who know how close the connection is between the state of mind of a man—and his courage and hope, or lack of them—and the state of immunity of his body will understand that the sudden loss of hope and courage can have a deadly effect [9].

PSYCHOLOGICAL IMPAIRMENT

Psychological impairment may limit the recovery of coronary patients [10]. Major psychological problems of coronary patients include anxiety, depression, hostility, denial, and dependency. Initial in-hospital anxiety is realistic and appropriate and is related to fear of dying. "Appropriate" denial, generally characterized by confidence in a favorable outcome, is an effective coping strategy associated with an improved prognosis [11].

Depression

Depressive symptoms and major depressive disorder are prevalent among patients with coronary artery disease (CAD) and have been reported to occur in 20% to 30% of patients following MI and up to 40% of patients with stable CAD [5,12–14]. In patients with CAD, the presence of major depressive disorder has been shown to be a powerful independent predictor of future cardiac events including death, MI, angioplasty, and bypass surgery [15]. Depression may be a contributing factor in the pathogenesis and progression of CAD [16]. Following MI, patients with depression have the tendency to remain out of work, to experience sexual difficulties, to have higher hospital readmission rates, and to have a lower rate of adherence to treatment regimens [5,13].

Depression and depressive symptoms are associated with limitations in multiple aspects of patient well-being and functioning and may be additive to the medical condition. In fact, the combination of depressive symptoms and advanced CAD is associated with roughly twice the reduction in social functioning associated with either condition alone [17]. The presence of depressive symptoms has been shown to markedly impair physical functioning and is associated with more bodily pain and more days in bed [17].

Inappropriate delays in the recognition, evaluation, and treatment of patients with depression can result in life-style changes and "sick" role behaviors that frequently limit the success of treatment interventions such as coronary surgery because of postoperative psychological complications [18]. Depression is the major emotional disorder during convalescence following MI or bypass surgery, and its symptoms are often not recognized because of its similarity to organic illness [11]. These symptoms include fatigue, insomnia, headache, memory impairment, and vague chest and bodily discomfort. Although depression resolves spontaneously in many persons, 70% of patients who are depressed following MI continue to be depressed after one year [5]. In many of these patients, depression leads to long-term invalidism with fear of returning to prior life-style, inappropriate early retirement, and withdrawal from social interactions. Following hospitalization, the presence of depressive symptoms in persons enrolling in cardiac rehabilitation programs predicted lack of functional improvement following exercise training [19]. These data suggest that it is important to assess and treat depressive symptoms as well as major depressive disorder in patients with cardiovascular disease. Treatment of depressive disorder can be accomplished with short-term psychotherapy and/or pharmacotherapy (probably best done cojointly), but specifics of treatment strategies are beyond the scope of this chapter. It is important to be aware that although depressive symptoms are an important source of morbidity in cardiac patients, little is known about the most effective forms of treatment.

Hostility

. . . the outstanding feature was the incessant treadmill of practice; and yet if hard work—that badge of our tribe—was alone responsible, would there not be a great many more cases? Every one of these men had an additional factor—worry; in not a single case under 50 years of age was that feature absent. . . .
—Sir William Osler [20], 1910 Lumlein lecture, commenting
on physicians in his practice with angina pectoris

Persons who exhibit an emotional syndrome characterized by a continuously harrying sense of time urgency, aggressiveness, ambitiousness, competitive drive, and easily aroused free-floating hostility have been defined by Friedman and Rosenman [21] as having type A behavior. Persons with this behavior trait have been associated with a 2 to 7 times greater incidence of clinical CAD than persons not exhibiting this behavior (type B behavior) [21–25]. Further analysis of the components of type A behavior suggests that hostility and unexpressed anger are the features of type A behavior most frequently associated with significant CAD, and that competitiveness and job involvement are less reliable predictors of CAD and merely represent manifestations of hostility [26,27]. The association of this behavior trait with CAD was strengthened in 1981, when a review panel of the National Heart, Lung, and Blood Institute concluded that type A behavior was an independent coronary risk factor of the same order of pathogenetic magnitude as that of previously accepted risk factors (i.e., hypertension, hypercholesterolemia, etc.) [28].

The presence of hostility is associated with an increased incidence of reinfarction in patients following MI [29], and therapy directed at altering this behavior is associated with a greater than 50% reduction in the rate of nonfatal reinfarction as well as an overall decrease in mortality [25]. Patients with this behavior trait, whose life-style involves control, adapt poorly to a dependent role in an intensive care unit. These patients also respond poorly to sedation, which decreases their external perception and augments anxiety. By involving the patient in the planning for recovery and teaching self-monitoring of the heart rate response to activity, one can return control to the patient and therefore encourage adherence.

Type A subjects have been observed quite consistently to respond to laboratory stressors with a greater sympathetic nervous system response than type B subjects. There also seems to be a trend toward hyperactivity of the hypothalamic–pituitary–adrenocortical axis in type A persons [30–32]. The clinical relevance of these findings lies in the fact that an increasing body of evidence demonstrates the pathogenetic role of catecholamines and platelet aggregation in CAD. These neuroendocrine correlates may be responsible for the increased risk of CAD conferred by the type A behavior pattern [33]. Stressed animals have been shown to have higher rates of platelet aggregability than nonstressed animals [34], and spontaneous platelet aggregability in humans has been shown to be highly predictive of future coronary events [35]. Finally, dehydroepiandrosterone-sulfate (DHEA-S), a weak adrenal androgen that is inversely correlated with the degree of type A behavior, has been shown to be an independent predictor of death from CHD and all-cause mortality. In addition, exogenous administration of DHEA-S has been shown to lower aggressiveness and may ultimately prove to be one of the biologic links between behavior and CHD [33,36].

In patients entering cardiac rehabilitation and exercise programs, the presence of hostility symptoms has been shown to predict functional improvement following completion of the program [37]. In fact, the degree of hostility symptoms was directly proportional to the degree of improvement in functional status following cardiac rehabilitation, and this correlated with a proportional diminution in hostility scores. This type of exercise program therefore may be a useful method for treating patients with hostility and type A behavior.

Hostility symptoms have also been shown to relate to the presence of social isolation and loneliness. In laboratory animals, social deprivation is associated with increased atherosclerosis, and in population studies, social isolation has emerged as a strong independent predictor of future coronary events and all-cause mortality [38–41]. Factors related to social isolation include older age and low socioeconomic status.

Although the presence of hostility is less prevalent in elderly persons entering cardiac rehabilitation programs than in their younger counterparts, the presence of hostility symptoms should nevertheless be recognized in order to provide appropriate therapy. Friedman and colleagues [42] demonstrated that therapy aimed at reducing type A behavior in patients following MI was successful in as many as 35% of subjects, and this was associated with an almost 50% reduction in the rate of nonfatal reinfarction as well as a significant decrease in mortality. In a recent meta-analysis of controlled trials on psychotherapeutic treatments for type A behavior [43], the three-year incidence of death and MI was reduced by 50% in treated patients versus controls. In addition, treated patients had a reduction in the frequency of angina pectoris compared to controls. Data also suggest that treatment may lower the risk of recurrent ventricular arrhythmias [44]. Treatment generally consists of a combination of techniques including educational, cognitive, behavioral, or supportive approaches. Evidence is also accumulating that certain pharmacologic interventions may be effective. Beta-blockers have been demonstrated to reduce certain components of type A behavior [45,46], and alprazolam can reduce circulating catecholamines as well as blood pressure and cortisol responses to mental stress in type A men [47]. Finally, low levels of serotonin have been associated with the potential for hostility in normal subjects, and treatment with the serotonergic anxiolytic, buspirone, in type A patients has been shown to result in a significant reduction of hostility behavior [48].

Stress

The role of emotional stress has long been suspected in the pathogenesis of CHD [20]. *Stress* is an amorphous term that does not apply to a specific abnormality of behavior but rather a reaction to a constellation of life events. Frasure-Smith [49] demonstrated in the Ischemic Heart Disease Life Stress Monitoring Program that a high stress score was associated with nearly a threefold increase in risk of cardiac mortality over a period of five years and an approximately 1.5-fold increase in reinfarction over the same period. In addition, a simple treatment program aimed at monitoring and treating symptoms of stress resulted in a reduction in cardiac morbidity and mortality similar to that of the nonstressed control group. These data and others verify the importance of stress in the development of CHD. Ornish and others [50] utilized diet and stress modification techniques in a group of patients with known CAD, which led to marked reduction in coronary symptoms as well as significant regression of atherosclerotic lesions. Although the pathobiologic correlates of stress are probably similar to those related to type A behavior, the importance of evaluating and treating patients with high levels of stress following coronary events must be considered in view of recent studies.

ASSESSMENT AND TREATMENT

Following MI and other major cardiac events, patients who develop psychological difficulties usually demonstrate clinically evident symptoms before hospital discharge. Physicians and health care providers must therefore look for signs of these behavioral abnormalities. Various validated questionnaires can be helpful in assessing behavioral disorders. Use of instruments such as the SCL-90, the Symptom Questionnaire, the Jenkins Activity Survey, and the General Health Questionnaire can qualitatively and quantitatively measure stress, anxiety, depression, and hostility. More and more, cardiac rehabilitation programs are routinely utilizing behavioral assessment via questionnaire as part of their overall risk-factor assessment. These types of instruments are especially useful to the busy clinician who is not trained or does not have the time to personally assess these factors.

The three major strategies that appear to limit psychological complications in patients with cardiovascular disease are education/counseling, medications, and physical activity [51]. Cardiac rehabilitation facilitates the individual in attaining the behaviors and capacities to meet life demands by acquisition of skills, techniques, and knowledge. Many patients unnecessarily remain psychologically impaired because of misperceptions about their future vulnerability. Via rehabilitation, the patient learns that modest physical activity can be performed safely, which restores self-confidence and emotional stability [52]. We have found that rehabilitation and exercise programs can lead to a diminution in hostility scores. Finally, patients identified as having abnormal behavior patterns can be referred to a psychologist/psychiatrist, who can intervene through individual counseling, group therapy, or medications. These measures, when combined, can assist the patient in resuming active vocational, familial, and social pursuits, obtaining a healthier life style, and achieving a higher functional status [53,54].

RETURN TO WORK
As a group, elderly patients are much less likely to return to work following a major coronary event than their younger counterparts. Age has been shown to be a more significant indicator than other factors, including severity of illness, of the likelihood of returning to work in patients with cardiovascular disease [55]. Elderly patients often seek early retirement after a major CAD event [56]. They are also more likely than their younger counterparts to have expectations of disability following cardiac events, thus strengthening their belief that they are functionally disabled.

Disability after MI appears more dependent on psychological than on physiologic abnormalities. Factors that negatively influence return to work include older age, adequate nonwork income, anxiety or depression, occurrence of symptoms with effort, lower socioeconomic class, physically active jobs, and the perception that illness is job related [11]. Patients who do not return to work within six months are unlikely ever to do so [57].

Many patients also fail to return to work because of unwarranted medical restrictions or lack of professional assurance that they can do so safely. Cardiac rehabilitation can provide a mechanism for giving patients these assurances, and it has been shown independently to increase the chances that patients will return to work.

Finally, a number of nonmedical factors may influence the decision whether a person should return to work. These include financial and social concerns, degree of disability, and possible remunerative benefits of not returning to work.

SEXUAL FUNCTION
Between 22% and 42% of post-MI patients develop cardiac symptoms during intercourse, predominantly palpitations, dyspnea, and angina [58,59]. Such patients are slower to resume sexual activity or may avoid sex altogether. In up to two thirds of patients following MI, the frequency of sexual intercourse decreases by 24% to 75%. Impotence is much less frequent, with a reported incidence of between 0% and 14% [58–60]. There are no data to suggest that sexual dysfunction is more or less likely in elderly patients than in their younger counterparts following CHD events, and

methods used to assess and treat sexual dysfunction should not be withheld from elderly persons.

When determining the cause of a sexual problem in a post-MI patient, it is important to take premorbid factors into account. The rate of sexual dysfunction in the normal population is quite high, and the incidence of erectile or ejaculatory difficulties has been reported to be as high as 40% in "happily married, normal couples" [61]. In addition, in men who subsequently developed an MI, two thirds had reported a sexual difficulty before their MI, and most of these patients were impotent or had intercourse infrequently [62].

The incidence of impotence increases with age, from 40% in men in their 60s to between 80% and 90% in men over 80 years of age [63]. Moreover, any physical illness can be associated with sexual dysfunction. In addition to chronic illnesses such as diabetes, mental disorders can also lead to impairment of sexuality. Depression is especially associated with a loss of libido and primary marital discord.

Many pharmacologic agents frequently used in the treatment of cardiovascular disorders can have profound effects on sexual function. These include a variety of antihypertensive agents such as guanethidine, methyldopa, and propranolol, as well as other agents including digoxin and clofibrate [64]. The physician should also be aware of the potent effects of alcohol in reducing sexual function.

Many patients and their spouses fear sexual intercourse following major cardiac events. These fears are frequently not addressed by health care providers because sexual function is a topic that rarely surfaces in doctor–patient relationships. Patients are often too embarrassed to bring up the subject, and physicians often feel uncomfortable in broaching the subject with patients, especially elderly ones. These fears, which are frequently present both in the patient and the spouse, often go unaddressed.

For the most part, however, CHD patients return to their normal level of sexual activity within four months following major cardiac events [58]. Return to sexual function can be facilitated by assurances from physicians regarding the safety of returning to an active sex life, especially when the patient has exhibited safe responses to low workloads of up to 5 and 6 METS (the energy requirement of sexual intercourse). Further assessment and workup of sexual dysfunction in a minority of patients is required before return of normal sexual function can be expected.

INDECISION AND DELAY IN SYMPTOM RECOGNITION

The most important psychological danger to the patient with acute MI is delay, the time interval from symptom onset to arrival at a medical facility. The importance of this delay is underlined when one realizes that about 60% of all MI-related deaths occur each year within the first 60 minutes following the onset of symptoms. Approximately half of all patients with acute MI wait more than two hours before getting help. Elderly persons are more apt than younger persons to delay seeking medical attention for symptoms. The decision time, defined as the time between the onset of symptoms of acute MI and reaching a decision to seek medical help, is four times greater in persons aged 60 to 69 years than it is for persons younger than age 50; the decision time for patients over age 70 is more than six times greater than for the younger group [65]. This may be particularly true if the elderly person has a prior history of angina pectoris. Elderly persons with known angina should be counseled about the importance of symptom recognition and avoidance of delay in seeking medical attention.

SUMMARY

The incidence of cardiovascular disease in the U.S. population increases with age. Although the frequency of psychosocial disability increases with disease complexity and coexisting comorbid conditions, age appears to have little effect on psychological adaptation to acute or chronic cardiovascular disease. Psychological factors, including hostility, depression, anxiety, social isolation, and stress have been shown to play an important role in the development and progression of CHD. These factors should be evaluated routinely in patients with CHD and are frequently assessed in patients enrolling in outpatient cardiac rehabilitation programs. Treating these factors has been shown to reduce the rate of future cardiac events, including nonfatal MI and death. In addition, treatment can improve overall quality of life and can assist the patient in resuming active vocational, familial, and social pursuits as well as achieving a higher functional status.

By increasing one's awareness of these factors, the physician can recognize psychological problems in coronary patients as well as the presence of maladaptive behavior patterns. With the assistance of validated question-naires, the physician can screen patients for psychological disease and refer for intervention those who are subsequently identified. Group and individual psychotherapy, techniques that employ basic patient education and social support, and also more recent innovative psychopharmacologic techniques have proved highly effective in producing positive change for depressive symptoms or depressive disorder and excessive "stress."

REFERENCES

1. Harvey W. 1628. Exercitatio de motu et sanguinis. Cited in Hackett TP, Rosenbaum JF. 1984. Emotion, psychiatric disorders, and the heart. In Braunwald E (ed), Heart Disease. Philadelphia: W.B. Saunders, pp 1826–1946.
2. American Heart Association. 1991. Heart and Stroke Facts.
3. Parmley WW. 1989. Pathophysiology and current therapy of congestive heart failure. J Am Coll Cardiol 13:771–785.
4. Miller P, Wikoff R, McMahon M, et al. 1989. Personal adjustments and regimen compliance 1 year after myocardial infarction. Heart Lung 18:339–346.
5. Stern MJ, Pascale L and Ackerman A. 1977. Life adjustment postmyocardial infarction: determining predictive variables. Arch Intern Med 137:1680–1685.

6. Gentry WD, Aronson MK, Blumenthal J, et al. 1987. Behavioral, cognitive and emotional considerations. J Am Coll Cardiol 10:38A–41A.
7. Crooz SH and Levine S. 1982. Life After a Heart Attack: Social and Psychological Factors Eight Years Later. New York: Human Sciences Press, pp 176–201.
8. Uhlmann RF and Pearlman RA. 1991. Perceived quality of life and preferences for life-sustaining treatment in older adults. Arch Intern Med 151:495–497.
9. Frankl VE. 1963. Man's Search for Meaning. New York: Washington Square Press.
10. Razin AM. 1982. Psychosocial intervention in coronary artery disease: a review. Psychosom Med 44:363–387.
11. Wenger NK and Fletcher GF. 1990. Rehabilitation of the patient with atherosclerotic coronary heart disease. In JW Hurst, RC Schlant, CE Rackley, et al. (eds), The Heart: Arteries and Veins, 7th ed. New York: McGraw-Hill Information Services, pp 1103–1118.
12. Kurosawa H, Shimizu Y, Nishimatsu Y, et al. 1983. The relationship between mental disorders and physical severities in patients with acute myocardial infarction. Jpn Circ J 47:723–728.
13. Cay EL, Vetter NJ, Philip AE, et al. 1972. Psychological status during recovery from an acute heart attack. J Psychosom Res 16:425–435.
14. Carney RM, Rich MW, Tevelde A, et al. 1987. Major depressive disorder in coronary artery disease. Am J Cardiol 60:1273–1275.
15. Carney RM, Rich MW, Freedland KE, et al. 1988. Major depressive disorder predicts cardiac events in patients with coronary artery disease. Psychosom Med 50:627–633.
16. Friedman HS and Booth-Kewley S. 1987. The "disease-prone personality": a meta-analytic view of the construct. Am Psychol 42:539–555.
17. Wells KB, Stewart A, Hays RD, et al. 1989. The functioning and well-being of depressed patients: results from the Medical Outcomes Study. JAMA 262:914–919.
18. Oakley CM. 1987. Is there life after coronary artery surgery? (Editorial.) Q J Med 62: 181–182.
19. Milani RV, Littman AB and Lavie CJ. 1991. Simplified depression index predicts functional improvement following cardiac rehabilitation and exercise program (abstract). Clin Res 39:414A.
20. Osler W. 1910. The Lumlein lectures on anginal pectoris. Delivered before the Royal College of Physicians of London. Lancet 1:939.
21. Friedman M and Rosenman RH. 1959. Association of specific overt behavior pattern with blood and cardiovascular findings. Blood cholesterol level, blood clotting time, incidence of arcus senilis, and clinical coronary artery disease. JAMA 169:1286–1296.
22. Rosenman RH, Brand RJ, Jenkins CD, et al. 1975. Coronary heart disease in the Western Collaborative Group Study. Final follow-up experience of 8 1/2 years. JAMA 233:872–877.
23. Jenkins CD. 1976. Recent evidence supporting psychologic and social risk factors for coronary disease. (First of two parts.) N Engl J Med 294:987–994.
24. Haynes SG, Feinleib M and Kannel WB. 1980. The relationship of psychosocial factors to coronary heart disease in the Framingham Study. III. Eight-year incidence of coronary heart disease. Am J Epidemiol 111:37–58.
25. Friedman M, Thoresen CE, Gill JJ, et al. 1986. Alteration of type A behavior and its effect on cardiac recurrences in post myocardial infarction patients: summary results of the recurrent coronary prevention project. Am Heart J 112:653–665.
26. Matthews KA, Glass CD, Rosenman RH, et al. 1977. Competitive drive, pattern A, and coronary heart disease: a further analysis of some data from the Western Collaborative Group Study. J Chronic Dis 30:489–498.
27. Dembroski TM, MacDougall JM, Williams RB, et al. 1985. Components of type A, hostility, and anger-in: relationship to angiographic findings. Psychosom Med 47:219–233.
28. The Review Panel on Coronary-prone Behavior and Coronary Heart Disease. 1981. Coronary-prone behavior and coronary heart disease: a critical review. Circulation 63: 1199–1215.
29. Jenkins CD, Zyzanski SJ and Rosenman RH. 1976. Risk of myocardial infarction in middle-aged men with manifest coronary heart disease. Circulation 53:342–347.
30. Friedman M, Byers SO, Diamant J, et al. 1975. Plasma catecholamine response of coronary-prone subjects (type A) to a specific challenge. Metabolism 24:205–210.
31. Simpson MT, Olewine DE, Jenkins CD, et al. 1974. Exercise-induced catecholamines and platelet aggregation in the coronary-prone behavior pattern. Psychosom Med 36:476–487.

32. DeQuattro V, Loo R and Foti A. 1985. Sympathoadrenal responses to stress: the linking of type A behavior pattern to ischemic heart disease. Clin Exp Hypertens A7:469–481.

33. Fava M, Littman A and Halperin P. 1987. Neuroendocrine correlates of the type A behavior pattern: a review and new hypotheses. Int J Psychiatry Med 17:289–307.

34. Haft JI and Fani K. 1973. Intravascular platelet aggregation in the heart induced by stress. Circulation 47:353–358.

35. Trip MD, Cats VM, van Capelle FJL, et al. 1990. Platelet hyperreactivity and prognosis in survivors of myocardial infarction. N Engl J Med 322:1549–1554.

36. Barrett-Connor E, Khaw K-T and Yen SSC. 1986. A prospective study of dehydroepiandrosterone sulfate, mortality, and cardiovascular disease. N Engl J Med 315:1519–1524.

37. Milani RV, Littman AB and Lavie CJ. 1990. Simplified hostility index predicts improvement in functional capacity following cardiac rehabilitation (abstract). J Cardiopulmon Rehab 10:364.

38. Shively CA, Clarkson TB and Kaplan JR. 1989. Social deprivation and coronary artery atherosclerosis in female cynomolgus monkeys. Atherosclerosis 77:69–76.

39. Welin L, Tibblin G, Svardsudd K, et al. 1985. Prospective study of social influences on mortality. The study of men born in 1913 and 1923. Lancet 1:915–918.

40. Broadhead WE, Kaplan BH, James SA, et al. 1983. The epidemiologic evidence for a relationship between social support and health. Am J Epidemiol 117:521–537.

41. Ruberman W, Weinblatt E, Goldberg JD, et al. 1984. Psychosocial influences on mortality after myocardial infarction. N Engl J Med 311:552–559.

42. Friedman M, Thoresen CE, Gill JJ, et al. 1986. Alteration of type A behavior and its effect on cardiac recurrences in post myocardial infarction patients: summary results of the Recurrent Coronary Prevention Project. Am Heart J 112:653–665.

43. Nunes EV, Frank KA and Kornfeld DS. 1987. Psychologic treatment for the type A behavior pattern and for coronary heart disease: a meta-analysis of the literature. Psychosom Med 49:159–173.

44. Reich P and Gold PW. 1983. Interruption of recurrent ventricular fibrillation by psychiatric intervention. Gen Hosp Psychiatry 5:255–257.

45. Krantz DS, Durel LA, Davia JE, et al. 1982. Propranolol medication among coronary patients: relationship to type A behavior and cardiovascular response. J Hum Stress 8:4–12.

46. Krantz DS, Contrada RJ, Durel LA, et al. 1988. Comparative effects of two beta-blockers on cardiovascular reactivity and type A behavior in hypertensives. Psychosom Med 50:615–626.

47. Stratton JR and Halter JB. 1985. Effect of benzodiazepine (alprazolam) on plasma epinephrine and norepinephrine levels during exercise stress. Am J Cardiol 56:136–139.

48. Littman AB, Fava M, Lamon-Fava S, et al. 1990. Treatment of type A behavior in cardiac patients with buspirone (abstract NR340). Presented at the American Psychiatric Association, 143rd Annual Meeting, New York City.

49. Frasure-Smith N. 1991. In-hospital symptoms of psychological stress as predictors of long-term outcome after acute myocardial infarction in men. Am J Cardiol 67:121–127.

50. Ornish D, Brown SE, Scherwitz LW, et al. 1990. Can lifestyle changes reverse coronary heart disease? Lancet 336:129–133.

51. Stern MJ and Cleary P. 1981. National Exercise and Heart Disease Project. Psychosocial changes observed during a low-level exercise program. Arch Intern Med 141:1463–1467.

52. Ewart CK, Taylor CB, Reese LB, et al. 1983. Effects of early postmyocardial infarction exercise testing on self-perception and subsequent physical activity. Am J Cardiol 51:1076–1080.

53. Wenger NK. 1973. Benefits of a rehabilitation program following myocardial infarction. Geriatrics 28:64–67.

54. Giese H and Schomer HH. 1986. Lifestyle changes and mood profile of cardiac patients after an exercise rehabilitation program. J Cardiopulmon Rehab 6:30–37.

55. Nagle R, Gangola R and Picton-Robinson I. 1971. Factors influencing return to work after myocardial infarction. Lancet 2:454–456.

56. Gentry WD. 1979. Psychological concerns and benefits in cardiac rehabilitation. In ML Pollack and DH Schmidt (eds), Heart Disease and Rehabilitation. Boston: Houghton Mifflin, pp 690–700.

57. Almeida D, Bradford JM, Wenger NK, et al. 1983. Return to work after coronary bypass surgery. Circulation 63(3, part 2):II205–II213.
58. Hellerstein HK and Friedman EH. 1970. Sexual activity and the postcoronary patient. Arch Intern Med 125:987–999.
59. Kolman PBR. 1984. Sexual dysfunction and the post-myocardial infarction patient. J Cardiac Rehabil 4:334–340.
60. Bloch A, Maeder J-P and Haissly J-C. 1975. Sexual problems after myocardial infarction. Am Heart J 90:536–537.
61. Frank E, Anderson C and Rubinstein D. 1978. Frequency of sexual dysfunction in "normal" couples. N Engl J Med 299:111–115.
62. Wabrek AJ and Burchell RC. 1980. Male sexual dysfunction associated with coronary heart disease. Arch Sex Behav 9:69–75.
63. Verwoerdt A, Pfeiffer E and Wang HS. 1951. Sexual behavior in senescence—patterns of sexual activity and interest. Geriatrics 6:304–308.
64. Papadopoulos C. 1980. Cardiovascular drugs and sexuality. A cardiologist's review. Arch Intern Med 140:1341–1345.
65. Moss AJ, Wynar B and Goldstein S. 1969. Delay in hospitalization during the acute coronary period. Am J Cardiol 24:659–665.

18. ETHICAL CONSIDERATIONS

K. DANNER CLOUSER
DWIGHT DAVIS

Avoiding in-depth discussion of moral matters, this chapter will present practical guidelines for dealing with moral issues frequently encountered in caring for the elderly. What follows is not intended as legal advice, but many cases at law seem to have turned on the soundness of the moral reasoning exemplified in the situation in question. The main focus here will be on the question: to treat or not to treat? There are, however, several related issues in the final section of this chapter that must be briefly addressed.

GENERAL CONSIDERATIONS

The elderly have usually thought a great deal about dying. Many, and perhaps most, of their friends and family have died. They are emotionally prepared for death in a way that is difficult for a young person to imagine. Even in good health, the elderly can be very weary of what they have come to see as a constant uphill battle. And if they have been in poor health, so much the worse. In good health or poor, they have all generally suffered sufficiently that the thought of death is not nearly as unacceptable as it is to someone considerably younger. These observations become relevant for physicians when they must assess the rationality of a patient's desire to live or die.

Franz H. Messerli (ed.), CARDIOVASCULAR DISEASE IN THE ELDERLY (Third Edition). Copyright © 1993 Kluwer Academic Publishers. ISBN 0-7923-1859-5. All rights reserved.

If the patient is **critical** (and there is no time for talk) → treat first and ask questions later at the earliest next decision point.

If the patient is **competent** → obtain **valid consent** from the patient → and treat accordingly.

\ if the competent patient refuses treatment, reexamine his understanding of his situation and his reasons. If his decision is not **irrational**, do as the patient says.

If the patient is not competent → look for an **advanced directive** ("living will") or a **durable power of attorney**.

\ if none exists → obtain a **substituted judgment**.

\ if no substituted judgment is possible → determine by "**best interests**" or "**reasonable person**" criterion.

Figure 18-1. A decision flow chart

The import of these experiences and perspectives of the elderly for their medical decision making is that the balance shifts—the balance between risk of harms and chances of good outcomes. That is, given the relatively short life that remains to elderly patients in any case, most of them are not willing to risk its quality for a procedure that has a significant probability of leaving them in pain, disabled, demented, or permanently unconscious. They may well still prefer life, but what they are willing to risk for that life has changed. Thus it becomes reasonable to refuse life-saving treatment if success is a long shot and these other harms have a high probability.

The elderly generally know themselves to be frail. They are aware that even after minor injuries and illness it has taken them a long time to come back. Their appearances of health and alertness frequently belie their general lack of stamina and reserve. The younger observer can easily be misled by external appearances and should take seriously the claims of the elderly about what they are and are not able to endure.

Of course, these generalities are only generalities. They do not apply to every individual. Naturally each elderly person must be seen as an individual with all his or her particular characteristics. These generalities are only meant as reminders of what things are typical, relevant, and often overlooked.

TO TREAT OR NOT TO TREAT

A decision flow chart would look something like the one depicted in figure 18-1.

Underlying all these maneuvers and deliberations is one basic principle: the right of the patient to self-determination. Therefore, everything is designed to discover the patient's will in the matter or to come as close to it as possible. There are conceptual pitfalls along the way to this discovery. These are discussed below in the order of their appearance in the flow chart (figure 18-1).

Critical

In many emergencies there is no time to determine the desires of the patient. Physicians are justified in responding so as to save the patient's life, stabilize the patient, or otherwise maximize the patient's subsequent options. An exception would be a situation wherein the physician knew the patient desired not to be treated in an anticipated crisis. Many chronically ill patients can reasonably predict such crises and should be able to make their desires known to their physicians in advance. Residents of nursing homes present a problem if advance determinations have not been made. Even though the resident/patient might be severely demented, in a coma, or in the final stages of a fatal disease, in the absence of any advance directives or information concerning the will of the patient or his family, the attending physician probably has no choice but to treat. (For possible exceptions, see "Best Interests" below.)

Competent

This concept is very elastic. It has different meanings in different contexts and seems to mean different things to different people. It is not a medical term, though most frequently medical professionals are the ones who, in order to act appropriately, must decide whether or not a person is competent. Competence is not a global appraisal so much as a highly specific one. One is or is not competent to do this or that particular task. Here the question must be whether the patient is competent specifically to make decisions regarding his or her own health care.

How does the physician know if the patient can do this? Ultimately it is a judgment call. The physician tries to assess whether the patient understands the situation—not just that he can recite the facts, but whether he *appreciates* that these facts concern him and that his decision will affect his own life in ways he also understands and appreciates. The patient's understanding is judged by the appropriateness of his or her responses, questions, and reasoning concerning the situation [1].

A word of caution: It is inappropriate to use the patient's actual decision in the instant case as the sole evidence of his or her competence. Since that decision is the very point in question, one should first determine a patient's competence on customary grounds, such as understanding and appreciating the facts and being able to reason about them. Otherwise, one runs the risk of deciding the patient's competence on the basis of his concurring with the physician's treatment plan.

Valid consent

To be valid, a consent must be freely and voluntarily given, without explicit or implicit coercion. Morever, the consent must be informed. That is, the patient must be informed of the probability of harms and benefits that might result from the treatment as well as from the withholding of treatment. A patient must also be provided with the same details about all alternative treatments. Particularly with the elderly, *it is important to present "comfort care only" as one of the alternatives.* The patient should never be led to see his options as simply treatment or abandonment. That would be tantamount to coercion for treatment. The alternative of *modified care* or *comfort care only* should always be assured. And just because the patient requests *Do-Not-Resuscitate (DNR)* status does not mean he or she wants to die. Rather, the patient desires that for certain specifiable crises the possibility of significant harm outweighs the likelihood of benefit, but meanwhile he or she would like to be kept alive and comfortable.

Irrational decision

An irrational decision in this context is a patient's refusal of treatment when such treatment is associated with few or no adverse consequences for the patient and significant benefits can be expected. This is an instance in which the physician is justified in going against the decision of an otherwise competent patient. (One might be tempted to label the patient incompetent because of the irrational decision, but that would involve making the mistake of using the actual decision as the sole evidence of incompetence.) An irrational decision is one that, if acted on, would bring harm to oneself for no adequate reason [2]. For example, a patient may otherwise be in good health and need only temporary noninvasive therapy to correct an arrhythmia.

One must be very careful in using the "irrational" label. It applies only to a decision by a patient that will result in unnecessary harm to that patient without adequate reason and without any compensating gain. On the other hand, in many situations it is not irrational for an elderly person to choose no treatment even though this will result in death. The person might well have adequate reasons, that is, reasons that would be accepted by most persons in similar circumstances of age and condition. Treatment may involve intense suffering and pain over a period of time or it may put the patient at risk of permanent unconsciousness, severe disability, or dementia. Those would be examples of adequate reasons for refusing treatment in certain circumstances. In the context of balancing reasons for refusing treatment against the benefits of treatment, the physician is reminded how important it is to minimize the side effects of therapy by fine-tuning the medications in order to make the balance favorable in the eyes of the patient. This balance can affect everything from daily compliance to patient decisions in life-threatening crises.

Advance directive

This has been commonly known as a "living will." It is a statement signed by a person while competent that goes into effect when he or she is no longer competent to make health care decisions. Specifically, the declaration describes medical interventions that the person refuses under certain specified conditions. However, advance directives can vary from two lines to many pages, and thus from terribly imprecise generalities to hopelessly minute details. The norm is approximately 1 or 2 pages in length containing the statement that life-sustaining treatment is to be withheld or withdrawn under certain conditions, usually when there is little hope of returning to a normal cognitive, sapient life. Advanced directives also typically state which therapies are to be withdrawn or withheld—for example, antibiotics, CPR, renal dialysis, and even nutrition and hydration. At this writing, more than half of the states have legislated one or another version of advance directives, ensuring that such a document has some authority and that physicians who comply with them are not legally at risk on that account. Indeed, in some places, physicians are at risk if they *do not* comply with an advance directive. If they cannot in good conscience comply, they should refer the case to someone who will.

Durable power of attorney

Detailing in an advance directive what one wants done in every conceivable circumstance is extremely difficult, if not ultimately self-defeating. Consequently, an increasingly used method is for competent persons to grant power of attorney to a friend or family member who will make health care decisions for them in the event that they become incompetent to make such decisions for themselves. This can be accomplished in a brief paragraph properly signed and witnessed. Often guidelines are attached making known to the appointee the general preferences and values of the person executing the durable power of attorney. The sense of *durable* in this context is that it is a power of attorney that *endures* beyond the competency of the person executing the power of attorney. Bestowing power of attorney and durable power of attorney is a well-established legal practice. The extension of this power to health care decision making is relatively new, but there is a general consensus that it will hold up. Some states have passed legislation specifically allowing its use for health care decisions.

Substituted judgment

If a patient is not competent and has not executed an advance directive or durable power of attorney, then one must turn to those best situated to speak on behalf of the patient. Typically these persons are members of the patient's family, but it is not unusual for close friends to know more about the patient's desires for treatment or nontreatment than the family. It must be clear that the patient's family or friends are not being asked what *they* would want done for the patient, but rather what they have reason to believe that the *patient* would want done.

The best kind of evidence is remembered conversations on the topic when the patient at an earlier time stated what he would want done in such an eventuality. Ideally, the statement should not have been simply an expression of dismay at visiting a relative or seeing a movie portraying someone suffering a questionable quality of life but rather should show evidence of having been a thoughtful decision that the patient made concerning himself. Much weaker and more questionable as evidence are those guesses at the patient's wishes by "deducing" them from observations of the patient's life-style. Does the statement, "He avoided going to doctors all his life" mean that surely he would not want to be sustained on life supports now? Does "He was always an out-of-doors type, who enjoyed hiking, hunting, and camping" mean that therefore he would never want to be maintained on dialysis?

Though courts have preferred the evidence of documented or remembered conversations in which the patient at an earlier time seemed to have made a decision, a good case can be made for simply trusting families to speak on behalf of patients. Family members, after all, are typically best positioned to know what the patient would have wanted. Whether or not they can remember specific conversations or explicit decisions on the part of the patient, through many years of interaction they are surely in a better position than most to know the will of the patient in these matters. And if the patient is suffering from a chronic condition, surely he could have predicted that there would come a time when a crisis decision would have to be made. Ordinarily the family is better acquainted than anyone else with what the patient has suffered and what his anticipations and hopes are [3].

In effect, it is being suggested that the family should be considered the "default" authority for representing the patient's wishes and values, since generally they are in the best position to possess such knowledge. This is the assumption *unless the physician has a reason to believe otherwise*. For example, if a patient is in a condition for which there is the possibility of a good outcome, the physician certainly should be suspicious of a family that the patient says that would not want treatment. Appropriately, the physician should not follow the family's instructions in this instance. However, in cases in which it is reasonable not to want treatment because of the high probability of "fates worse than death" and a best possible outcome that is not very desirable anyway, it is a reasonable practice to allow the family to speak on behalf of the patient. In cases of disagreement between equally close family members, the physician probably has no choice but to opt for full treatment until an agreement can be reached within the family.

Best interests

This is the last (and the least) in the flow chart's serial lineup of appeals for determining the patient's desires. If the patient has not executed an advance directive or durable power of attorney and if there is no one who can testify to the expressed wishes of the patient, then as a last resort there has been some precedent for turning to the patient's "best interests" as objectively determined by the physician. This is conceptually muddy territory.

Naturally, a physician who does not know the patient's desires must act in what he or she believes to be to the best interests of the patient, erring on the side of life and a chance for recovery. However, this situation usually arises when the patient is in a persistent vegetative state, and the question is whether to sustain life (e.g., with respirator or nourishment) and whether to rescue the patient in a crisis (e.g., with CPR or antibiotics). In this situation, the balance of benefits and burdens (as *best interests* is frequently interpreted) is difficult if not impossible to determine. It is doubtful that the patient is experiencing either pleasure or pain. If the patient appears to be experiencing constant, unalleviated pain, the balance of benefits and burdens seems to be clear. On the other hand, the situation of a severely demented person who appears to experience occasional sensations of pleasure and pain is problematic, and consequently—until there is further guidance from society—that patient's life should be sustained.

The authors believe that *best interests* should be interpreted more broadly, that is, beyond benefits and burdens, which are typically thought of as sheer sensations of pleasure or pain, and beyond the patient's current conscious desires, which in fact are nil. *Best interests* should include those interests strongly held during the patient's lifetime. For example, these interests might have been to conserve money for important family ventures, to relieve the anxiety and suffering of his family, to use limited medical resources efficiently, and not to have his grandchildren remember him lying in a persistent vegetative state, etc. It would seem that honoring these best interests is far more important and appropriate than merely assessing the existence and balance of pleasurable and painful sensations.

Another way to think about best interests would be the *reasonable person* criterion. This is a helpful fiction frequently used in legal deliberations. It leads one to consider what a reasonable person would do in relevantly similar circumstances. In the context of this discussion, one would want to know what a reasonable, elderly person would choose to do if he were in a persistent vegetative state, or if he were facing surgery that had a 5% chance of cure but a 95% chance of causing significant brain damage. This method has a somewhat empirical flavor to it because, in fact, real people can be asked what they would choose. This could be helpful when the choice is practically universal—such as a person's desire to be allowed to die if he is in a persistent vegetative state.

Best interests, *balancing benefits and burdens*, and *reasonable person* are concepts that, as used in these circumstances, are something of a legal quagmire. As yet there are no legal certainties. Yet they are appropriate *moral* consider- ations and, as such, they are sound formulations of relevant concerns that may help familes think through what it is that the patient would have wanted. Therapies can become torture, and if they hold no promise of regaining any desirable human function and if they affront every significant interest the patient ever had in the matter, it would seem that striving assiduously to maintain life would be contrary to a physician's traditional duty to act in the best interest of the patient and to do no harm.

OTHER RELEVANT CONSIDERATIONS

Bargaining with the patient

Although the premise of this chapter has been the patient's right to self-determination, it should be clear that the physician ought not immediately and without question capitulate to the patient's apparent decision. The example of disregarding irrational decisions was discussed earlier. But there is another type of case in which the patient's false beliefs, irrational fears, misperceptions, or current condition leads to a decision that does not seem to be in the patient's best interests. Here the physician should temporize and bargain with the patient—for example, by taking one therapeutic step that is painless and noninvasive, with the promise to reevaluate the patient's condition before continuing treatment. For example, a patient refusing treatment for atrial fibrillation might be convinced to let the physician get the tachycardia under control through easy and noninvasive means, at which time the next stages of diagnosis and treatment (say, long-term anticoagulation therapy) would be considered. Frequently when a patient is reluctant to undergo treatment, it is the condition speaking rather than the patient's real self, so if the patient can be "normalized" before making crucial decisions, so much the better. Sometimes an alternative therapeutic method, even one that is outmoded or less efficacious, may alleviate the patient's fears (for example, placement of an arterial line). Bargaining takes time and involves the physician in the process of ferreting out hidden factors blocking the patient from making rational decisions.

Physician as gatekeeper

The physician should not be a gatekeeper. With the constant national concern over our dwindling resources and skyrocketing costs, an individual physician may be tempted to protect society's interests by rationing these limited resources as he or she sees fit. Very likely, the elderly would be among the first to be deprived through rationing. It is generally believed that they use up the greatest amount of medical resources and have less to show for it in terms of quality of life over time. Whether or not this is true, it is irrelevant to the point concerning gatekeeping. To have each physician tacitly rationing care according to how he or she interprets society's resources, needs, and merits would be to create havoc. Furthermore, it is the traditional duty of a physician to do everything necessary for each patient. To do less would be to betray that patient's trust and expectation.

In a sense, good medicine necessarily involves some rationing. One does not order every conceivable test or therapy, nor spend every conceivable moment with the patient. Good medicine must deal with probabilities and what is most likely. However, the rationing implicit in good medicine is practiced toward everyone equally and not just toward one selected group. There are times when the physician should cease and desist medical interventions, but, as seen above, the decision to do so should be made in response to other factors, especially including consideration of the patient's wishes, and not simply because the patient is elderly.

The dangers of ambiguity

There are two key situations in which this problem is particularly evident. The first is in the writing of DNR orders. In this case, it is not always clear precisely which medical interventions are supposed to be withheld. Originally, DNR meant that only efforts to resuscitate following cardiac arrest were ruled out. Later it came to be understood more generically and thus included all means of rescue in a crisis—antibiotics, renal dialysis, ventilator, etc. It is important in writing orders to specify precisely what is to be withheld, as determined by the patient's desires and his particular malady [4].

The other situation in which ambiguity is dangerous concerns the patient's own statements of his desires for his future care should he become incompetent. Such statements are often general and imprecise, and it is up to the physician to clarify them. Statements such as, "I never want to live like *that*," "Please just shoot me if *that* ever happens to me," or "Just let me die if I end up in *that* state" do not specify exactly what aspect of *that* condition they refer to: is it dementia, unrelieved pain, inability to communicate, unconsciousness, or need for a feeding tube or respirator? And what is the patient asking: that feeding be stopped? That infections not be treated? That cardiac resuscitation be avoided? These matters can be clarified in a relatively brief conversation with the patient, the results of which should be documented. This conversation should focus uniquely and explicitly on the matter of treatment limitations. The physician should have in mind several paradigm scenarios to present to the patient. Such examples facilitate the patient's grasp of the clinical possibilities and sharpen his awareness of the variables about which he must decide [5]. The patient should always be assured that whatever he chooses, his physician will keep him as pain free and comfortable as possible.

The trial run

A matter closely related to clarifying the patient's wishes is the frequently overlooked option of trying a course of treatment, even life-sustaining treatment, to see if it will succeed in bringing the patient to an acceptable quality of life. Elderly patients who are gravely ill tend to agree to this course of action only when the physician promises that if it does not work, the patient's request to be allowed to die will be honored. One reason why elderly patients are apt to forgo treatment before they have to is because they want to make treatment decisions while they are still in control. But if they are assured that their wishes to cease and desist treatment will be honored if therapy does not succeed to their specifications, then they are more willing to attempt treatment.

Some situations of ambiguity will be partially alleviated by the Self-Determination Act passed by the United States Congress for implementation in December 1991. Among a number of provisions is the requirement that all persons being admitted to any institution that receives Medicare funds must be told of their state laws regarding advance directives and be helped to formulate and record their own wishes for treatment in the event that they should become incompetent. Their directive will then be placed in their patient/resident file.

REFERENCES

1. Chell B. 1987. Competency: what it is, what it isn't and why it matters. In JF Monagle (ed), Medical Ethics: A Guide for Health Professionals. Rockville: Aspen Publications, pp 99–110.
2. Culver CM and Gert B. 1990. The inadequacy of incompetence. Milbank Q 68:619–644.
3. Rhoden NK. 1988. Litigating life and death. Harvard Law Rev 102:375–446.
4. Council on Ethical and Judicial Affairs—American Medical Association. 1991. Guidelines for the appropriate use of do-not-resuscitate orders. JAMA 265:1868–1871.
5. Emanuel LL and Emanuel EJ. 1989. The medical directive: a new comprehensive advance care document. JAMA 261:3288–3293.

SUGGESTED READING

Adams J and Wolfson AB. 1990. Ethical issues in geriatric emergency medicine. Emerg Care Elderly 8:183–192.
Barondess JA, Kalb P, Weil WB, et al. 1988. Clinical decision-making in catastrophic situations: the relevance of age. J Am Geriatr Soc 36:919–937.
Cassel CK, Meier DE, and Traines ML. 1986. Selected bibliography of recent articles in ethics and geriatrics. J Am Geriatr Soc 35:399–409.
Clouser KD. 1977. Allowing or causing: another look. Ann Intern Med 87:622–624.
Clouser KD. 1983. Life-support systems: some moral reflections. Bull Am Coll Surg 68:12–17.
Jonsen AR, Siegler M, and Winslade WJ. 1992. Clinical Ethics, 3rd ed. New York: McGraw-Hill.

19. RISK MODIFICATION

JAMES A. SCHOENBERGER

The epidemiology of the atherosclerotic diseases has recently been comprehensively reviewed [1]. The many studies reported in this chapter underscore the concept that there are easily identified characteristics (risk factors) in the elderly that place individuals and whole populations at increased risk of developing premature atherosclerosis. The major risk factors that can be altered by intervention are elevated blood pressure, elevated serum cholesterol, and cigarette smoking [2]. Such factors as physical inactivity, obesity, excess alcohol consumption, and psychosocial factors are also susceptible to intervention, but their importance is less certain. Factors associated with an increased risk, such as age, sex, and family background, are not susceptible to intervention. Implicit in the risk-factor concept is the hope that reduction of the level of risk will result in an improved outlook not only for the individual but also for whole populations treated by public health measures.

Currently, Americans over age 65 constitute 12% of the population. In 50 years it is estimated that 21% of the population will be "elderly." At age 65 these people have a life expectancy of over 14 years for men and nearly 19 years for women [1]. Hypertension and hypercholesterolemia are very prevalent in the elderly, and the elderly consume a disproportionally high

Franz H. Messerli (ed.), CARDIOVASCULAR DISEASE IN THE ELDERLY (Third Edition). Copyright © 1993 Kluwer Academic Publishers. ISBN 0-7923-1859-5. All rights reserved.

Table 19-1. Ten-year probability (%) of a 65- to
67-year-old man developing coronary heart disease

Cholesterol level mg/dl	Systolic blood pressure (mmHg)									
	121–129		130–139		140–149		150–160		161–172	
	NS	S	NS	S	NS	S	NS	S	NS	S
200–219	14	19	16	23	18	25	19	27	21	29
220–239	16	23	18	25	19	27	21	29	23	31
240–269	18	25	19	27	21	29	23	31	25	33
263–288	19	27	21	29	23	31	25	36	27	36

Note: NS = nonsmoking; S = smoking; nondiabetic, LVH absent, HDL = 47–50 mg/dl.
Data from American Heart Association: Risk Factor Prediction Kit (#64–9590). 1990.

volume of health care. The very large number of elderly people who are at increased risk of atherosclerotic diseases constitutes a challenge to physicians to employ effective methods of risk-factor modification with the goal of prolonging life and preventing coronary heart disease (CHD) and stroke.

Aside from prospective clinical trials demonstrating the benefit of risk reduction, the most convincing supporting evidence that atherosclerosis is preventable comes from the decline in CHD and cardiovascular disease (CVD) mortality observed in the United States in the past 20 years. From 1969 to 1981, CHD deaths declined 31.8% and stroke deaths declined 45.9% [3]. These reductions in mortality benefited all age, sex, and race groups to a comparable degree.

The impact of these trends is striking. Heart disease mortality is no longer the major cause of death below age 65, but it continues to be the predominant cause of death in those age 65 and older. In people younger than age 65, malignant neoplasms are now the major cause of death. In people aged 65 to 74, the death rates for cancer and heart disease are nearly equal [4].

The reasons for these declines are not clear [5]. It has been reasoned, however, that a substantial proportion of the decline can be accounted for by changes in life-style leading to a reduction in serum cholesterol levels and cigarette smoking and improved control of high blood pressure [6].

The risk factors, although independent, act together synergistically when more than one factor are present to greatly increase the risk of developing CHD or stroke. With increasing age, the relative influence of the risk factors changes. The interrelations between systolic blood pressure, smoking status, and serum cholesterol at ages 65 to 67 are shown in table 19-1 for men and at ages 61 to 67 in table 19-2 for women [7].

It can be seen that for any given level of systolic blood pressure, in either men or women, elevation of serum cholesterol from 200 to 288 mg/dl increases the risk by only a modest degree, approximately 30%. On the other

Table 19-2. Ten-year probability (%) of a 61- to
67-year-old woman developing coronary heart disease

Cholesterol level mg/dl	Systolic blood pressure (mmHg)									
	121–129		130–139		140–149		150–160		161–172	
	NS	S	NS	S	NS	S	NS	S	NS	S
200–219	7	12	8	13	9	14	10	16	12	18
220–239	8	13	9	14	10	16	12	18	13	19
240–269	9	14	10	16	12	18	13	19	14	21
263–288	10	16	12	18	13	19	14	21	16	23

Note: NS = nonsmoking; S = smoking; nondiabetic, LVH absent, HDL = 47–50 mg/dl.
Data from American Heart Association: Risk Factor Prediction Kit (#64–9590). 1990.

Table 19-3. Ten-year probability (%) of a 66- to 68-year-old man developing a stroke

	Systolic blood pressure (mmHg)				
	127–137	138–148	149–159	160–170	171–181
LVH absent	6.3	7.3	8.4	9.7	11.2
LVH present	14.8	17.0	19.5	22.4	25.5

Note: LVH = left ventricular hypertrophy.
Data from American Heart Association: Risk Factor Prediction Kit (#64–9590). 1990.

Table 19-4. Ten-year probability (%) of a 66- to 68-year-old woman developing a stroke

	Systolic blood pressure (mmHg)				
	125–134	135–144	145–154	155–164	165–174
LVH absent	6.3	7.3	8.4	9.7	11.2
LVH present	11.2	12.9	14.8	17.0	19.5

Note: LVH = left ventricular hypertrophy.
Data from American Heart Association: Risk Factor Prediction Kit (#64–9590). 1990.

hand, an increase in systolic blood pressure from 121 to 172 mmHg increases the risk approximately 50% at any given cholesterol level. For any combination of systolic blood pressure and serum cholesterol, cigarette smoking adds significantly to the risk in women and men, by approximately 50%.

Similar data on the risk factors for stroke are shown in tables 19-3 and 19-4 [7]. The major risk factor for stroke in elderly men and women is elevated blood pressure. There is a twofold increase in the 10-year risk comparing systolic blood pressure of 171 to 181 mmHg to that of 127 to 137 mmHg. Increasing levels of serum cholesterol do not increase the risk of stroke [7].

Cigarette smoking adds modestly to the risk of stroke in men. The presence of left ventricular hypertrophy (LVH) on the electrocardiogram nearly doubles the risk of stroke at any given level of systolic blood pressure.

From a practical standpoint, then, the greatest potential benefit from risk reduction in the elderly should come from a comprehensive program lowering elevated blood pressure, reducing serum cholesterol, and quitting cigarette smoking. These considerations must be kept in mind when one attempts risk modification in the elderly. Drastic reductions in life-style with too many interventions introduced at the same time cannot be supported if the price to be paid is an overall reduction in the patient's quality of life and pleasurable life-styles. Before physicians interfere, they must be reasonably certain that the patient will benefit.

Recent studies of atherosclerosis in the coronary and peripheral vessels using quantitative arteriography and ultrasound have confirmed that the atherosclerosis is a dynamic, usually progressive process [8]. There is no reason to suppose that progression stops at any age. It is likely that it continues throughout life, and that the rate of progression is influenced in part by the level of risk factors, which are statistically and probably causally related to the process. Spontaneous regression is uncommon, but retardation of progression has been demonstrated in a number of studies by a number of methods, including diet and drugs [9].

Delayed evidence of benefit from reduction of the level of risk has been demonstrated in the 10.5-year follow-up of the Multiple Risk Factor Intervention Trial (MRFIT) [10] and in the 15-year follow-up of the Coronary Drug Project (CDP) [11]. These results suggest that intervention is possible and beneficial provided it is maintained for a long period. The failure of the MRFIT and CDP to show benefit of the intervention at the end of the original study period can be explained by too few cardiovascular events at that point. Reduction of the level of risk sustained for 5 to 8 years was ultimately shown to yield a reduction in cardiovascular events, even though the study participants did not necessarily continue the risk reduction regimen after the studies ended.

In this chapter, the role of risk modification in the elderly will be reviewed, with major emphasis on control of elevated blood pressure, reduction of serum cholesterol by diet and drugs, and cessation of cigarette smoking. The evidence from clinical trials that reduction of risk in the elderly is of proven benefit will be evaluated, and recommendations for physicians treating the elderly will be offered.

ELEVATED BLOOD PRESSURE

Average blood pressure rises with age in both men and women in the United States. Average diastolic pressure plateaus at around 90 mmHg, but systolic blood pressure continues to rise with age [12]. However, the prevalence of elevated blood pressure is very high in the elderly [13]. About 44% of white

Table 19-5. Prevalence of hypertension among noninstitutionalized men and women, black and white, aged 65 to 74 years, 1976 to 1980

	Blood pressure ≥160/95 mm Hg, %[a]	Blood pressure ≥140/90 mm Hg, %[b]
Black women	72.8	82.9
Black men	42.9	67.1
White women	48.3	66.2
White men	37.5	59.2
Total blacks	59.9	76.1
Total whites	43.7	63.1
Total (all races)[c]	45.1	64.3

[a] Defined as the average of three blood pressure measurements 160 mmHg or greater (systolic) and/or 95 mmHg or greater (diastolic) taken on a single occasion or the self-reported taking of antihypertensive medication.
[b] Defined as the average of three blood pressure measurements 140 mmHg or greater (systolic) and/or 90 mmHg or greater (diastolic) taken on a single occasion or the self-reported taking of antihypertensive medication.
[c] Includes races in addition to blacks and whites.
From The Working Group on Hypertension in the Elderly, 1986. Statement on hypertension in the elderly. JAMA 256:70–74. Copyright 1986, American Medical Association. With permission.

men and women and 60% of blacks aged 65 to 74 have definite hypertension (≥160 mmHg systolic and/or ≥95 mmHg diastolic). Hypertension defined as systolic blood pressure of ≥140 mmHg and diastolic blood pressure of ≥90 mmHg is even more prevalent. These rates are shown in table 19-5 [13].

The prevalence of isolated systolic hypertension, usually defined as ≥160 mmHg systolic and ≤90 mmHg diastolic in persons aged 60 to 69 years, has been estimated to be 5.3% in white men, 7.4% in white women, 6.4% in black men, and 8.3% in black women [14].

Elevation of either the systolic or diastolic blood pressure increases the risk of coronary heart disease and stroke [1]. This relationship has been demonstrated in many prospective studies, such as the Framingham Study [15]. Table 19-6 shows the risk relationships associated with blood pressure levels in elderly men and women. The risk of all-cause mortality associated with isolated systolic hypertension has also been shown to be doubled in both men and women aged 55 to 74. The risk for cardiovascular morbidity and mortality is increased 2 to 4 times [15].

Treatment of hypertension in the elderly has been shown to be beneficial in several large clinical trials. In the Veterans Administration Cooperative Study Group Trial [16], a reduction of 50% in terminating plus nonterminating cardiovascular events in men over age 60 was associated with active treatment compared to placebo. In the Australian Therapeutic Trial in Mild Hypertension [17], fatal and nonfatal events were reduced by 26% in treatment of the elderly with diastolic blood pressure of 95 to 109 mmHg. The Hypertension Detection and Follow-up Program demonstrated a 16.4% reduction in mortality in participants aged 60 to 69 with elevated blood

Table 19-6. Risk of cardiovascular disease
in elderly persons according to hypertension status

	Average annual incidence/1000	
Hypertension status	Men 65–74 years	Women 65–74 years
140/90 mmHg	17.1	8.6
140–159/90–94 mmHg	32.7	22.5
160/95 mmHg	51.0	35.6

Data From Kannel WB. 1981. Implications of Framingham study data for treatment of hypertension: impact of other risk factors. In Laragh JH, Buhler FR, Seldin DW (eds), Frontiers in Hypertension Research. New York: Springer-Verlag, pp 17–21.

pressure ≥90 mmHg [18]. In this study there was no placebo group. The experimental group received stepped care, and the reference group received currently available care from community sources. Since both groups received treatment, the reduction in mortality understates the benefit that would have been seen if the reference group received placebo.

In the European Working Party on High Blood Pressure in the Elderly Trial, patients over age 60 with a baseline blood pressure of 90 to 119 mmHg were randomized to treatment or placebo [19]. Although total mortality was not significantly reduced (26%), the cardiovascular mortality rate was reduced by 38%, mainly as a reduction in cardiac mortality of 47% and in myocardial infarction of 60%. This study confirmed the benefit of treating hypertension in the elderly and was the first trial to report a reduction in death from coronary heart disease as a result of treatment. All other trials have consistently demonstrated that the treatment benefit was especially relevant to stroke mortality.

Isolated systolic hypertension has also been associated with an increased risk of cardiovascular disease and may even be a more useful index of risk assessment [1,20]. Preliminary studies have revealed that blood pressure can be lowered with treatment [21]. The benefit of treating isolated systolic hypertension in the elderly has recently been documented [22]. The incidence of stroke was reduced by 36% with low-dose medication (chlorthalidone). The incidence of nonfatal myocardial infarction plus coronary death was reduced by 27%.

In a review of several hypertension trials in the elderly [23], it was concluded that antihypertensive drug treatment can decrease cardiovascular mortality, mainly through a decrease in fatal and nonfatal cerebrovascular events. The evidence that treatment reduces coronary heart disease or total mortality was not demonstrated in these trials. There are no data on the value of treating asymptomatic hypertension in individuals over age 80. Concern regarding the risk of excessive reduction of elevated blood pressure has been

Table 19-7. Population distribution of plasma cholesterol levels in whites

| Age | Percentiles | | | | | |
| | 50 | | 75 | | 90 | |
	Men	Women	Men	Women	Men	Women
55–59	214	229	236	251	260	278
60–64	215	226	237	251	262	282
65–59	213	233	250	259	275	282
70+	214	226	236	249	253	268

From The Lipid Research Clinics Population Studies Data Book, Vol I. The Prevalence Study. 1956. Lipid Metabolism Branch, Division of Heart and Vascular Diseases, National Heart, Lung and Blood Institute. NIH Publication 80–1527.

raised, and a so-called J-curve in benefit from blood pressure reduction has been postulated [24]. Although the concept is controversial, it would appear to be prudent to lower elevated blood pressure slowly in elderly patients, particularly if there is evidence of cerebral or coronary insufficiency.

In the management of hypertension in the elderly, diastolic blood pressure should be lowered to less than 90 mmHg and systolic blood pressure to less than 160 mmHg [13]. Side effects such as orthostatic hypotension and adverse changes in the quality of life should be avoided by careful dose titration. A diuretic has commonly been recommended for initiation of treatment [25]. Other drugs recommended in the past as second-step drugs, such as clonidine, angiotensin-converting enzyme inhibitors, and alpha-blockers, may also be appropriate as initial therapy. Calcium antagonists have been tested extensively and found to be effective as monotherapy of hypertension in the elderly. The best drugs for the treatment of hypertension in the elderly have not yet been established. That treatment is beneficial is clearly established, and widespread treatment of elderly hypertensives may account, in part, for the decline in cardiovascular mortality in the elderly [26].

ELEVATED BLOOD CHOLESTEROL
As in the case of hypertension, mean cholesterol levels rise with age, reaching a plateau at 213 to 215 mg/dl in men and at 226 to 233 mg/dl in women over age 55. However, 25% of elderly men and women have cholesterol levels of 250 mg/dl or more, and 10% have levels well above 250 mg/dl. These population distributions are shown in table 19-7 [27].

The relationship of elevated cholesterol to the development of atherosclerosis has been clearly established by many studies at the molecular, animal, experimental, and human epidemiologic levels [1,28,29]. Yet the inability to establish by clinical trials the benefit in humans with regard to total mortality of cholesterol reduction by dietary or pharmacologic means has resulted in resistance by many to acceptance of the relationship of dietary cholesterol and fat consumption to heart disease.

Recently, the results of the Lipid Research Clinics Coronary Primary Prevention Trial have convincingly demonstrated that reduction in serum cholesterol by dietary and pharmacologic means significantly reduces the incidence of coronary heart disease [30]. This study of middle-aged men (aged 35 to 59 years) followed for an average of 7.4 years demonstrated that the benefit of treatment was proportional to the amount of fall in serum cholesterol. There are no published studies regarding intervention for elevated blood cholesterol in the elderly. It is possible that the atherosclerotic lesions have become complex and fibro-calcific in the elderly and are no longer amenable to regression. On the other hand, the major etiologic factor associated with atherosclerosis, namely, low-density lipoprotein (LDL), probably continues to play a role in the progression of atherosclerosis at all ages. The relationship between high levels of total and LDL cholesterol and the risk of CHD has been shown to be present at all ages through age 82 [31]. Although the relative risk of CHD seems to decline with age, the attributable risk increases, and the potential benefit of cholesterol reduction in the elderly is great. Therefore, even in the absence of evidence to support intervention, prudent dietary recommendations in the elderly seem justified [32,33].

A recent Consensus Development Statement of the National Institutes of Health [34] recommends a reduction of saturated fat and cholesterol for the general population as well as more aggressive intervention for hyperlipidemic patients. A systematic approach to the patient with hyperlipidemia has been devised [35]. Employment of dietary and pharmacologic measures in the elderly beyond the phase I diet recommended by the American Heart Association [32] (30% of total calories as fat, equally distributed between saturated, monosaturated and polyunsaturated fat, and cholesterol intake below 300 mg/day) cannot be supported by existing data. In severely hyperlipidemic patients, more aggressive intervention with harsher dietary restrictions and drugs has not been shown to be beneficial. Employment of these more drastic interventions may have adverse effects on the patient's quality of life but yield no effective protection.

CIGARETTE SMOKING

Cigarette smoking has been consistently related to morbidity and mortality of cardiovascular disease. Many studies have been carried out and have been extensively reviewed [36,37]. The smoking habits of elderly men have changed over the past few decades. The percentage of smokers has declined and the percentage of former smokers has increased. For women, the percentage of smokers continues to rise at the same time that the percentage of former smokers increases. These findings are shown in table 19-8 [36].

The relatively low impact of smoking on increased risk of CHD and stroke in the elderly [7] may indicate that people susceptible to the effects of

Table 19-8. Percentage distribution of
current and former smokers over age 65

	Current smokers			Former smokers		
	1965	1976	1980	1965	1976	1980
Men	28.5	23.0	17.9	28.1	44.4	47.4
Women	9.6	12.8	16.8	4.5	11.7	14.2

Data From Report of the Surgeon General. The health consequences of smoking: cardiovascular disease. Rockville, MD: U.S. Department of Health and Human Services, Office on Smoking and Health, 1983.

Table 19-9. Relative risk[a] for death attributable to smoking for current and former smokers

	Men		Women	
	Current	Former	Current	Former
Hypertensive disease	1.9	1.3	1.7	1.2
Ischemic heart disease				
Age 35–64	2.8	1.8	3.0	1.4
Age 65	1.6	1.3	1.6	1.3
Cerebrovascular disease				
Age 35–64	3.7	1.4	4.8	1.4
Age 65	1.9	1.3	1.5	1.0

[a] Relative to never smokers.
From Centers for Disease Control. 1991. MMWR. Smoking—attributable mortality and years of potential life lost—United States, 1988.

smoking have expired and that the survivors have a relative resistance. The risk of cigarette smoking, determined by comparing current and former smokers to people who have never smoked, is shown in table 19-9 [38]. The relative risk for CHD is higher in those under age 65 but is still evident in elderly smokers. Former smokers have a 50% reduction in risk. There have been no controlled clinical trials of the benefit of quitting smoking. Those who do quit appear to benefit, and cessation of smoking at any age can be recommended. This would appear to be equally applicable to elderly smokers, especially those with other risk factors such as known CHD, hypercholesterolemia, hypertension, or diabetes. Despite the fact that cessation may deprive elderly patients of a life-long pleasurable (but addictive) habit, its recommendation must be made in the strongest terms.

OTHER RISKS

A number of other characteristics have been associated with an increased risk of CHD. The greatest interest on the part of the general public has focused on physical activity. Prospective and retrospective studies appear to confirm a relationship between low levels of physical activity and increased risk of CHD. No adequately controlled clinical trial of the benefit of regular exercise has been carried out, even in young to middle-aged people. In the absence of supportive data, recommendations to exercise regularly can be justified in the elderly, since overall physical and cardiovascular fitness will be benefited. Caution must be observed to avoid musculoskeletal injury. Such exercises as walking and swimming are ideal.

Psychosocial factors in CHD have also received a great deal of attention. The relationships remain controversial, but diffuse hostility does appear to be a more sensitive index than the type A behavior pattern [1]. There is little evidence that modification of behavior will reduce the risk, especially in elderly patients whose behavior patterns are deeply ingrained.

Alcohol consumption appears to have a quadratic or J-shaped relationship to CHD [1]. Abstainers and heavy users both have a greater risk of CHD. Moderate consumption may afford some protection, possibly through the mechanism of increased levels of high-density lipoprotein (HDL) cholesterol.

The identification of obesity as an independent risk factor for CHD remains controversial, and those who are above ideal weight may be at increased risk. For many reasons, weight reduction can be recommended for elderly patients even though patients of all ages are often resistant to intervention in this respect. Central obesity is a more important risk factor than overall obesity.

CONCLUSIONS

Despite the absence of clinical trials to establish the value of all risk-factor reductions in the elderly, physicians can still take an active role in advising their elderly patients. Treatment of hypertension has been established as beneficial and should be offered to all elderly patients. Modest restriction of fat and cholesterol consumption, cessation of cigarette smoking, regular physical exercise, moderation in alcohol consumption, and control of excess weight are all prudent, hygienic measures that are equally applicable to the elderly. In view of the increasing proportion of elderly people with substantial life expectancy, there is a great opportunity for physicians and patients to reduce the risk of both CHD and stroke and make these years as healthy as possible.

REFERENCES

1. Atherosclerosis Study Group. 1984. Optimal resources for primary prevention of atherosclerotic diseases. Circulation 70:157A–205A.
2. American Heart Association. 1980. Risk factors and coronary disease: statement for physicians (abstract). Circulation 62 (Suppl 2):455A.
3. National Heart, Lung and Blood Institute. 1982. Fact Book for Fiscal Year 1982. Washington, DC: Department of Health and Human Services, U.S. Public Health Service.
4. Sutherland JE, Persky VW and Brody JA. 1990. Proportionate mortality trends: 1950 through 1986. JAMA 264:3178–3184.
5. National Heart, Lung and Blood Institute. 1979. Proceedings of the Conference on the

Decline in Coronary Heart Disease Mortality. Washington, DC: NIH Publication No. 79–1610, Department of Health and Human Services, Public Health Service.

6. Goldman L and Cook F. 1984. The decline in ischemic heart disease mortality rates. An analysis of the comparative effects of medical interventions and changes in lifestyle. Ann Intern Med 101:825–836.

7. American Heart Association. 1990. Risk Factor Prediction Kit (#64–9590). Dallas: American Heart Association.

8. Blankenhorn DH, Johnson RL, Mack WJ, et al. 1990. The influence of diet on the appearance of new lesions in human coronary arteries. JAMA 263:1646–1652.

9. Brown BG. 1991. Regression of atherosclerosis: what does it mean? Am J Med 90 (Suppl 2A):53S–55S.

10. Multiple Risk Factor Intervention Trial Research Group. 1990. Mortality rates after 10.5 years for participants in the Multiple Risk Factor Intervention Trial. JAMA 263:1795–1801.

11. Canner PL, Berge KG, Wenger NK, et al. 1986. Fifteen year mortality in the Coronary Drug Project patients. Long-term benefit with niacin. J Am Coll Cardiol 8:1245–1253.

12. American Heart Association. 1985. Risk Factors in Stroke. A Statement for Physicians By the Subcommittee on Risk Factors and Stroke of the Stroke Council. Dallas: American Heart Association.

13. The Working Group on Hypertension in the Elderly. 1986. Statement on hypertension in the elderly. JAMA 256:70–74.

14. Curb JD, Borhani NO, Entwisle G, et al. 1985. Isolated systolic hypertension in 14 communities. Am J Epidemiol 121:362–370.

15. Kannel WB. 1981. Implications of Framingham study data for treatment of hypertension: impact of other risk factors. In JH Laragh, FR Buhler, and DW Seldin (eds): Frontiers in Hypertension Research. New York: Springer-Verlag, pp 17–21.

16. Veterans Administration Cooperative Study Group on Antihypertensive Agents. 1972. Effects of treatment on morbidity in hypertension, III. Influence of age, diastolic pressure and prior cardiovascular disease. Further analysis of side effects. Circulation 45:991–1004.

17. Report of the Management Committee: The Australian therapeutic trial in mild hypertension. Treatment of mild hypertension in the elderly. 1981. Med J Aust 68:396–402.

18. Hypertension Detection and Follow-up Program Cooperative Study Group. 1979. Five-year findings of the Hypertension Detection and Follow-up Program. II. Mortality by race, sex and age. JAMA 242:2572–2577.

19. Mortality and Morbidity Results from the European Working Party on High Blood Pressure in the Elderly Trial. 1985. Lancet 1:1349–1354.

20. Abernathy J, Borhani NO and Hawkins CM. 1986. Systolic blood pressure as an independent predictor of mortality in the hypertension detection and follow-up program. Am J Prev Med 2:123–132.

21. Hulley SB, Furburg CD, Gurland B, et al. 1985. Systolic Hypertension in the Elderly Program (SHEP): antihypertensive efficacy of chlorthalidone. Am J Cardiol 56:913–920.

22. Prevention of stroke by antihypertensive drug treatment in older persons with isolated systolic hypertension. 1991. Final results of the Systolic Hypertension in the Elderly Program (SHEP). JAMA 265:3255–3264.

23. Staessen J, Fagard R, Lijnen P, et al. 1990. Review of the major hypertension trials in the elderly. Cardiovasc Drugs Ther 4:1237–1248.

24. Cruickshank JM, Thorpe JM and Zacherissis FJ. 1987. Benefits and potential harm of lowering high blood pressure. Lancet 1:581–584.

25. The 1988 Report of the Joint National Committee on Detection, Evaluation, and Treatment of High Blood Pressure. 1988. Arch Intern Med 148:1023–1038.

26. Schoenberger JA. 1986. Epidemiology of systolic and diastolic systemic blood pressure elevation in the elderly. Am J Cardiol 57:45C–51C.

27. The Lipid Research Clinics Population Studies Data Book, Vol I. The Prevalence Study. 1956. NIH Publication 80–1527. Washington, DC: Lipid Metabolism Branch, Division of Heart and Vascular Diseases, National Heart, Lung and Blood Institute.

28. Joint Statement of the Nutrition Committee and the Council in Arteriosclerosis of the American Heart Association. 1984. Recommendations for the treatment of hyperlipidemia in adults. Arteriosclerosis 4:445A–468A.

29. Tyroler HA. 1985. Total serum cholesterol and ischemic heart disease risk in clinical trials and observational studies. Am J Prev Med 1:18–24.

30. The Lipid Research Clinics Coronary Primary Prevention Trial Results. 1984. I. Reduction in incidence of coronary heart disease. JAMA 251:351–364.
31. Castelli WP, Wilson PW, Levy D and Anderson K. 1989. Cardiovascular risk factors in the elderly. Am J Cardiol 63:12H–19H.
32. A Joint Statement by the American Heart Association and the National Heart, Lung and Blood Institute. 1990. The cholesterol facts. A summary of the evidence relating dietary fats, serum cholesterol, and coronary heart disease. Circulation 81:1721–1727.
33. Grundy SM. 1990. Cholesterol and coronary heart disease: future directions. JAMA 264:3053–3059.
34. National Institutes of Health Consensus Development Conference Statement: lowering blood cholesterol to prevent heart disease. Vol 5, No 7, 1985.
35. Hoy JM, Gregg RE and Brewer HB. 1986. An approach to the management of hyperlipoproteinemia. JAMA 255:512–521.
36. Report of the Surgeon General. 1983. The health consequences of smoking: cardiovascular disease. Rockville, MD: U.S. Department of Health and Human Services, Office on Smoking and Health.
37. Ravenholt RT. 1985. Tobacco's impact on twentieth-century U.S. mortality patterns. Am J Prev Med 1:4–17.
38. Centers for Disease Control. 1991. MMWR. Smoking—attributable mortality and years of potential life lost—United States, 1988.

20. DIETARY CONSIDERATIONS IN THE ELDERLY: NUTRITION AND CARDIOVASCULAR DISEASE

JOYCE P. BARNETT

Nutrition intervention has been identified as an important component in prevention and treatment of cardiovascular disease requiring different approaches in each phase of the life span. To effectively intervene in the elderly, we must first identify how they differ from younger adults and how these differences influence needs. These steps will help us interpret and apply current knowledge appropriately when caring for our growing elderly population.

NUTRITION NEEDS

Age-related changes

While the Recommended Dietary Allowances (RDA) are our standard for evaluating nutrition needs for all healthy persons [1], there are some significant limitations in applying these guidelines to elderly people [2]. One factor is age itself. In the RDA, the first 50 years of life are divided into nine age categories, while a single category is designated for the remainder of the life span. Chronologic age is not always a good indicator of physiologic or functional status, especially in people over 65 years of age. Very different needs may exist among individuals in the same age group. Unfortunately there are limited data to identify these diverse needs. Requirements for older

Franz H. Messerli (ed.), CARDIOVASCULAR DISEASE IN THE ELDERLY (Third Edition). Copyright © 1993 Kluwer Academic Publishers. ISBN 0-7923-1859-5. All rights reserved.

Table 20-1. Nutrient-poor and nutrient-dense 1400 kcal menus

Menu I	Menu II
1 cinnamon roll 2 cups coffee/cream and sugar	1 oz bran flake cereal 1 cup 1% low-fat milk 1 slice wheat toast 1/2 cup orange juice 1 cup coffee
1 cup chicken noodle soup 6 saltine crackers 1 cup tea/1 tsp sugar	1/2 cup low-fat cottage cheese 1/2 cup juice packed peaches 1 slice raisin bread 1 cup tea
1 small hamburger on bun with condiments 1 oz processed cheese 1 oz potato chips 12 oz cola drink	2 oz lean roast beef 1 small potato 1/2 cup broccoli 3/4 cup tossed salad 2 tsp olive oil/vinegar 1 tsp corn oil margarine 1/2 cup vanilla pudding 1 cup tea
2 chocolate chip cookies 1/2 cup vanilla ice cream	2 graham crackers 1 tbsp peanut butter 1 cup 1% low-fat milk

people are often extrapolated from research with younger subjects [2,3]. The high incidence of chronic disease among the elderly complicates assessment of needs. The RDA are designed for "healthy persons," but the presence of disease, and sometimes treatment as well, can have a negative effect on nutrition status. With these limitations in mind, there are still significant age related changes to consider.

Although many physiologic changes occur with increasing age, the decrease in energy requirement is one of profound significance from a nutrition standpoint [4]. As lean body mass begins to decline with aging, caloric requirements also decrease [1,5]. Caloric intake of men exceeds that of women throughout the life span. It peaks during early adulthood and then gradually declines [6]. Men experience a 21% decrease in energy needs, from 2900 kcal for 21- to 50-year-olds to 2200 kcal for the over-age-50 reference man. For the reference woman, there is a 14% decrease from 2200 kcal to 1900 kcal for the 21–50 and over-50 age categories, respectively. In determining the RDA for energy for those over age 50, a normal variation of ±20% is possible and a marked decline in activity is not assumed. Those over age 75 are likely to have somewhat reduced needs due to decreased body size, activity, and resting energy expenditure [1]. Although the decrease in recommended energy requirement is greater for men, the decrease for women is of more concern because intake of many nutrients is linked to total caloric intake. To meet recommended levels of vitamin and mineral intake,

Table 20-2. Comparison of selected nutrients in table 20-1 menus

Nutrient	Recommended intake[a]	Nutrient analysis[b]	
		Menu I	Menu II
Protein (gm)[c]	50	35	73
Total fat[d] (percent of kcal)	30	39	28
Saturated fatty acids (percent of kcal)[d]	<10	17	9
Cholesterol (mg)[d]	<300	172	93
Vitamin A (IU)[c]	4000	1828	4698
Ascorbic acid (mg)[c]	60	15	120
Vitamin B-6 (mg)[c]	1.6	0.3	1.6
Folacin (mcg)[c]	180	80	321
Iron (mg)[c]	10	5.9	15.9
Calcium (mg)[c]	800	422	1007
Zinc (mg)[c]	12	4.9	12.8

[a] For 65-year-old reference female, 65 kg, 160 cm.
[b] Nutrient analysis using Computrition™ Nutritional Software Library, Computrition, Inc., Chatsworth, CA.
[c] Recommended Dietary Allowances.
[d] National Cholesterol Education Program.

there is little room for nutrient-poor, calorie-dense foods if less than 1500 kcal (RDA for energy less 20%) per day are needed to meet energy requirements. A comparison of two 1400 kcal menus in table 20-1 illustrates this point. Menu I represents a combination of easy-to-prepare and fast-food/convenience items of calorie-dense but nutrient-poor foods. It provides approximately 50% or less of the RDA for 8 of 10 vitamins and minerals. Menu II, on the other hand, includes carefully selected nutrient-dense foods, which provide 100% of the RDA for the same 10 nutrients. Table 20-2 compares the quality of nutrition provided by the two menus in relation to the recommended intake of selected nutrients for the 65-year-old reference female weighing 65 kg who is 160 cm in height. Some elderly women may not consume as much as 1400 calories per day [7], and probably very few are able to consistently choose a menu with the nutrient density of menu II. If foods such as those in menu I are eaten preferentially, nutrition status will suffer. In elderly men, because of their higher total caloric intake, this is less critical; but even so, consistently poor food choices can lead to marginal intake of essential nutrients.

With the decrease in lean body mass and the increase in body fat that accompany aging, it might seem that protein requirements would decrease. However, some studies suggest that there may be decreased protein utilization, especially if caloric intake is limited [8–11]. The recommended intake of 0.75 gm/kg is felt to be adequate for elderly adults and represents a protein intake of 63 gm and 50 gm, respectively, for the reference man and woman 51 years of age or older. This level of intake is usually not difficult to obtain in the average American diet with approximately 15% of calories from protein [1].

The data are limited to support recommendations for specific vitamin and mineral requirements. A wide range of vitamin intake among the elderly has been found in surveys [12,13]. Intake of vitamins A, D, C, B-6, and folate are often less than recommended levels. Some minerals are also at risk for less than recommended intake, especially iron, calcium, and zinc [14]. A low energy requirement in conjunction with poor food choices can contribute to less than recommended levels of intake. Smoking and alcohol intake can alter vitamin requirements, as well as intake and utilization of other nutrients [1,15].

Nutrition–drug interactions

The body's ability to metabolize some drugs is altered with the physiologic changes of aging [16]. As an increasing number of prescription and nonprescription medications are taken, the possibility of adverse reactions increases. Medications commonly used in treatment of cardiovascular diseases can affect appetite and thus nutrition status. Nausea, vomiting, anorexia, diarrhea, constipation, dry mouth, and decreased taste acuity are recognized side effects of a number of these drugs and thus have obvious potential for a negative effect on food intake [16,17]. Other gastrointestinal side effects, such as flatulence, can also influence intake. Gastrointestinal blood loss as a result of anti-inflammatory drugs for arthritis or as preventive anticoagulant therapy is a recognized cause of iron deficiency anemia [18]. Other drugs may also have significant nutritional and metabolic effects, such as diuretics leading to mineral loss [17].

INFLUENCE OF NUTRITION IN CARDIOVASCULAR DISEASE

There is convincing evidence that nutrition plays a significant role in a number of problems associated with the elderly population [19]. The nutritional status of mature adults is a product of genetic predisposition affected by lifelong eating habits and influenced by culture and environment. With increasing age it becomes more difficult to separate the various influences and determine cause and effect, but in industrialized countries dietary excesses rather than deficiencies are likely to be the problem. Cardiovascular disease, the leading cause of death in the United States, can be the result of such dietary excesses. The susceptibility to and severity of cardiovascular disease can be influenced by other diseases, such as diabetes and hypertension, which are also associated with obesity and caloric excesses [20,21]. Although the predictive power of elevated serum cholesterol levels for coronary heart disease is less than at younger ages [22], the incidence of cardiovascular disease increases significantly with age [23–25]. Serum cholesterol levels rise with age [22,26], and excess caloric intake and a high intake of cholesterol and saturated fat are among the factors known to

Table 20-3. Dietary therapy of high blood cholesterol level

Nutrient	Recommended intake	
	Step-one diet	Step-two diet
Total fat	Less than 30% of total calories	Less than 30% of total calories
Saturated fatty acids	Less than 10% of total calories	Less than 7% of total calories
Polyunsaturated fatty acids	Up to 10% of total calories	Up to 10% of total calories
Monounsaturated fatty acids	10% to 15% of total calories	10% to 15% of total calories
Carbohydrates	50% to 60% of total calories	50% to 60% of total calories
Protein	10% to 20% of total calories	10% to 20% of total calories
Cholesterol	Less than 300 mg/dl	Less than 200 mg/dl
Total calories	To achieve and maintain desirable weight	To achieve and maintain desirable weight

Source: Archives of Internal Medicine 1988;148:36–69

influence serum lipid levels and thus incidence of cardiovascular disease [27–29]. Hypertriglyceridemia can also be aggravated by obesity, intake of alcohol, and high intake of carbohydrate, especially simple sugars [30,31].

Obesity is one risk factor for coronary heart disease that is directly related to nutrition. Approximately 24% to 31% of the adult men and women in our country, respectively, are overweight (body mass index 25 to 30 kg/m^2), and approximately 12% of men and women have a body mass index greater than 30 [32–34]. The incidence of overweight increases in men to approximately 50 years of age, but continues to rise in women until after age 60 [33]. Middle-aged women seem to be at risk for weight gain associated with increased cardiovascular risk factors such as total serum cholesterol, triglyceride, and blood pressure, as well as elevated fasting insulin levels [35,36]. When excess adipose tissue is concentrated in the abdominal area in either men or women, it poses a significantly greater risk for cardiovascular disease [37–39].

NUTRITION MANAGEMENT OF CARDIOVASCULAR DISEASE

The recommendations of the National Cholesterol Education Program Adult Treatment Panel Report in table 20-3 can be applied to elderly as well as younger adults [31,40]. Dietary modification is the treatment of choice at any age, but it is especially important in the elderly, who may already be taking several prescription medications. Diet modification may be less burdensome and have fewer adverse effects than medical therapy [31,41].

The physician and patient should have realistic expectations of the results to be achieved by dietary changes. Changing from the typical American diet to the step-one diet (i.e., a decrease from 38% to 30% of calories from fat) can reduce serum cholesterol on average by 30 to 40 mg/dl. Following the step-two diet can decrease serum cholesterol by an additional 15 mg/dl [31]. Normal fluctuations in serum lipid levels should be explained, so that the anxious 70-year-old is not overly frightened when the cholesterol level is slightly higher than it was at the previous reading.

Fat does serve essential functions in the body, and "zero" fat in a normal mixed diet is neither obtainable nor desirable. If dietary fat is severely limited, carbohydrate intake usually increases to compensate. If hypertriglyceridemia exists, the increased carbohydrate intake may hinder efforts to control it [30,31]. It is not difficult to obtain adequate amounts of essential fatty acids when consuming a mixed diet, but certain amounts (approximately 2% of total energy) must be ingested [14,42]. In addition, dietary fat aids in absorption and utilization of fat-soluble vitamins. Because dietary fat adds flavor and contributes to the texture of foods, high-fat foods remain popular despite recent negative publicity.

Limiting total fat to approximately 30% of calories and limiting cholesterol to less than 300 mg per day are desirable changes and not unrealistic goals. People seem to be more aware of the importance of limiting dietary cholesterol than of limiting total fat and saturated fat intake. With moderate intake of egg yolks (three per week), it is possible to achieve an average cholesterol intake of less than 300 mg per day, provided that other foods high in cholesterol such as meats and whole-milk dairy products are limited [31].

The importance of limiting both total fat to control caloric intake and saturated fat to lower serum lipids deserves greater emphasis. Regarding selection of dietary fat, scientific evidence supports limiting saturated fat to less than 10% of calories and allowing polyunsaturated fat up to 10% of calories with the remainder coming from monounsaturated fats [31]. Attempting to eliminate added fat entirely can make weight maintenance difficult for some patients because they are unable to consume enough high-carbohydrate, high-fiber foods for energy balance. An alternate strategy is to include certain amounts of monounsaturated fat to help meet energy needs. Monounsaturated fat must be used in place of saturated fat, not in addition to fat already in the diet [43]. Patient education is very important here. Lean meats, poultry, fish, and low-fat dairy products must be selected. Hidden fat in baked products and some meats may not be recognized as a significant source of fat and calories. Increased intake of monounsaturated fats can be accomplished by use of olive or canola oil, olives, and avocados. Other good sources of monounsaturated fats include almonds, pecans, peanuts, and peanut oil [44–46].

Achieving and maintaining an acceptable body weight is very important in management of hyperlipidemia [31]. Fat is a major nutrient affecting caloric intake, and high levels of fat intake, especially saturated fat, are not desirable for a number of reasons. Excess fat and caloric intake leads to weight gain and obesity. In addition to increased cardiovascular risk, this also increases risk for hypertension and diabetes. Excess weight usually contributes to decreased mobility and increasing likelihood of additional weight gain.

Weight loss is extremely difficult for the elderly sedentary obese person, who may not be consuming large quantities but is eating calorically dense foods.

Because the level of physical activity influences caloric requirements, it is important to encourage some form of exercise to whatever extent is feasible [47]. Even with no dietary restrictions, sedentary elderly people may find it difficult to meet vitamin and mineral requirements because they have decreased caloric needs [48]. Dietary deficiencies and excess weight gain are less likely with increased physical activity because more energy and thus more food are needed. Even the risk of certain chronic diseases seems to be reduced in persons who are more physically active [49].

Intake of whole-grain products, fruits, and vegetables should be encouraged in place of high-fat foods, but budget constraints may limit consumption of these low-calorie, nutrient-dense foods. Digestive disorders may also influence intake of fresh fruits and vegetables, again limiting nutrients and fiber in the diet.

Limiting salt intake to 6 gm (~2400 mg sodium) or less per day is appropriate for most individuals [50]. This can be accomplished by avoiding high-sodium processed foods and limiting added salt. Because elderly people have reduced energy needs, this level of limitation allows use of a variety of grain products, fruit, vegetables, fresh meats, poultry, and fish and selected dairy products. When physical limitations decrease ability to prepare foods, compromise on sodium intake may be necessary to allow greater use of convenience foods. Many manufacturers are beginning to recognize a need for reasonably priced products appropriate for modified diets. This change is now making it possible to use some convenience foods and still maintain moderate dietary modifications. Elderly patients with heart disease often need a more severe sodium restriction, and each case must be individually evaluated. Severe levels of sodium restriction (less than 2000 mg) are difficult to achieve in an outpatient situation.

APPROACH TO THE ELDERLY PATIENT

Effective nutrition intervention can improve treatment outcome and contribute to overall improved health and quality of life. The degree of success achieved in any intervention depends upon recognition that each person is an individual with specific needs. Perhaps more so than in any other age group, individual variation must be considered as we work with the elderly who represent such a wide range of physical capability and function.

Assessing nutrition status

Assessing nutrition status is an important step in planning the course of treatment. Initial assessment of nutrition-related concerns in the physician's office can help focus treatment and determine whether referral is needed. Table 20-4 lists suggestions for pertinent questions during the initial evaluation. The responses to these questions can identify areas of concern and

Table 20-4. Questions for initial assessment of nutrition status

Is weight appropriate for height?
Has there been any dramatic weight loss/gain in the past six months? If so, what conditions
   contributed to this?
Does the person live alone and eat alone?
How many meals are eaten per day? Is a hot meal eaten once a day?
Is there any physical condition that impairs ability to shop, prepare food, or eat? If so, is there
   adequate social support to provide for good nutrition?
Are there adequate storage and preparation facilities (i.e., a refrigerator and a stove that work)?
What is the status of dentition?
Do any medications, prescription or over-the-counter, interfere with food intake, nutrient
   absorption, and/or utilization?
Are any dietary restrictions being followed?
Are there dietary intolerances?

point to the type of intervention needed. While excesses are often the root of chronic diseases, one should always keep in mind the possibility of nutritional inadequacies when evaluating the elderly [51].

One important factor to determine is appropriate weight for height, using age-adjusted height–weight tables [52]. A recent gain or loss of weight can be an indicator of adequacy of intake. Nutritional care of the underweight elderly person can be as challenging as achieving weight loss in the obese. Because significant unexplained weight loss can be an indicator of a serious problem, obtaining a weight history is vital [53,54]. A loss of 10% of body weight in a six-month period is significant and requires investigation. In addition to medical problems, nutrition-related factors are often involved [55]. Severe dietary restriction, self-imposed or prescribed, may lead to unwarranted weight loss unless suitable substitutes are found to replace calories eliminated from the diet. Anorexia often develops in response to illness. In an underweight person, a few days of not eating can quickly deplete already marginal reserves. In situations such as cardiac cachexia, malnutrition occurs as a result of interaction of the disease process and treatment. Gorbien [56] recently reviewed the mechanisms and management of this complex and challenging problem.

Before recommendations for change in diet are made, present intake should be evaluated both quantitatively and qualitatively [57,58]. Appropriate fluid intake must be considered as well. The 24-hour recall and/or dietary history can be helpful, but these tools have some limitations for use with the elderly [59–61].

Periodic reassessment of nutrition needs, including determination of the dietary restrictions currently followed, is essential. Problems arise when a patient continues a dietary modification beyond its appropriate limit. A 65-year-old woman, advised to eat liver because of anemia during her child-bearing years, will significantly increase her cholesterol intake if she continues to follow this advice.

Table 20-5. Suggestions to facilitate dietary change

Reinforce existing positive habits
Encourage gradual change rather than drastic dietary restriction and food elimination
Encourage moderation
Avoid concept of good/bad food
Identify alternative choices when imposing limitations
Enlist family support
Utilize food assistance programs when possible

Physical limitations must be noted, such as status of dentition and any impairment of mobility and dexterity. Referral to the physical therapist or occupational therapist may lead to improved food intake by alleviation of some of the physical impediments to eating. Dental care to insure proper fit of dentures and correction of other problems of the oral cavity have obvious benefits. Changes in taste and smell can be more difficult to identify, but these problems also have implications for decreased intake. In addition, xerostomia has also been noted to limit food intake, thus increasing the risk of malnutrition [62].

Use of dietary supplements among the elderly must be considered. Caution is needed because of the risks related to excessive intake of supplements [50,63] and the possibility of adverse nutrient interaction with use of unbalanced supplements. Often the patients most likely to take supplemental vitamins and minerals are those least likely to need them [50]. We recommend that patients obtain their nutrients from food because imbalances and excesses are less likely from a varied diet. However, in the elderly, it is easy to see that the limiting effect of reduced energy needs can significantly affect intake of other nutrients. The comparison of nutrient content in the menus in table 20-2 shows that it is possible to obtain recommended amounts of vitamins and minerals from food, but it is also possible to fall far short. The need for supplements in an elderly patient should be based upon assessment of the individual situation. Nutrition counseling about better food choices may resolve some problems, but for others supplementation may be appropriate.

Facilitating dietary change

Assessment of the patient's current food intake to evaluate what has to be changed and what does not is an essential first step in modifying dietary habits. Positive reinforcement of existing good habits is beneficial. Because dietary habits are not easy to change, frequent follow-up and encouragement are important to achieve the desired results. Some suggestions for facilitating dietary change are outlined in table 20-5.

Among the elderly, as among younger adults, some are more health conscious and receptive to change in diet. Others seemingly have no desire whatsoever to make dietary changes, no matter what the consequences. Successful dietary intervention is highly unlikely in the latter case unless a motivating factor can be found.

Benefits versus risks of nutrition intervention

The benefits of dietary modification should be evaluated in view of the difficulty of the required change and the severity of the risks. We must consider the nutritional implications of dietary restrictions for elderly individuals likely to have marginal intake [64]. Appropriate counseling about overall improvement of diet in light of existing medical problems may facilitate a better response than emphasizing further dietary restrictions.

The healthy, active elderly person with hyperlipidemia is likely to experience greater benefit from aggressive dietary treatment than someone of advanced age with several problems who is already burdened by multiple dietary restrictions and poor appetite [31,65]. The effects of a lifetime of high saturated fat and cholesterol intake will not be reversed in a short period. At least six months of dietary modification should be allowed to effectively evaluate the patient's response to the diet [31].

Severity of the restrictions recommended must be evaluated against the patient's existing dietary habits. An elderly person who is at an acceptable weight and who already limits fat and cholesterol intake may not benefit from further restriction. This person may, however, need information about appropriate alternate food choices to maintain weight and good nutrition status. On the other hand, an obese patient who adopts a low-fat, low-cholesterol diet is likely to reduce serum cholesterol and triglycerides and may also experience some weight loss secondary to decreased caloric intake.

Inappropriate implementation or inadequate supervision of dietary prescriptions can have unforseen negative results. Periodic follow-up and review are needed to evaluate how well the patient is following the dietary recommendations. For example, sodium restriction is frequently indicated in management of congestive heart failure and hypertension. For persons used to a high level of sodium in the diet, a sodium-restricted diet may be totally unacceptable, leading to severe restriction of food intake. An explanation of appropriate alternate seasonings may be sufficient to help some resume eating. Others may refuse to eat unless some salt is allowed. If high-sodium foods are avoided, a measured small amount of salt per day for cooking or adding at the table may allow decreased sodium intake and encourage intake of necessary nutrients and energy.

Inadequate patient education on dietary modifications can lead to some peculiar and often ineffective choices for meeting the objectives of the prescribed diet. One example is using low-sodium bread (~20 mg sodium/slice) and margarine (1 mg sodium/teaspoon) while continuing to use regular or even "reduced-sodium" canned soup. One cup of regular soup (~1000 mg sodium) or reduced-sodium soup (~500 mg sodium) provides considerably more sodium than one slice of regular bread (~150 mg sodium) and one teaspoon of margarine (~50 mg sodium) [66]. Another example of the need for patient education involves ability to correctly apply nutrition information from food labels. A nondairy creamer that is "low cholesterol, low saturated fat" (but not low in fat or calories) is not an appropriate or equivalent substitute for skim milk on cereal. From a nutrient-density standpoint, 2% milk would be a better choice, because along with some cholesterol and saturated fat one also gets protein, vitamins, and minerals.

Nutrients of special concern

In addition to the possibility of inadequate energy intake when fat is severely restricted, some other risks of dietary intervention in the elderly require further exploration. These risks include inadequate intake of protein, fat-soluble vitamins, and some minerals. Certain precautions can improve the likelihood that overall nutrition status is not compromised as a result of intervention.

Several factors can influence protein intake in the diet. Sources of protein are usually expensive, so economic issues may determine the quantity available when income is limited. Dental problems often limit meat intake as well. Less expensive alternate protein sources should be encouraged. Even though eggs are high in cholesterol, they provide an excellent source of protein and are much less expensive than meats. Inclusion of lean meats, poultry, fish, low-fat dairy products, peanut butter, dried beans and peas, and even eggs in moderation can help assure adequate protein intake.

When limiting total fat and especially added fat, adequate intake of fat-soluble vitamins must be considered. Less than recommended levels of vitamin A and D intake among some groups of elderly people have been noted [13,14]. Fortified low-fat milk can contribute to intake of both of these vitamins. Encouraging intake of fruits and vegetables should allow for increased opportunity to obtain adequate amounts of vitamin A.

Potential for decreased mineral intake as a result of dietary restrictions is of concern. Suboptimal intake of several minerals has been documented in a number of surveys of the elderly [14]. Another consideration is that high-fiber, complex carbohydrate foods are encouraged in place of high-fat foods. There is concern that a high-fiber diet may interfere with absorption of some minerals [67]. Iron, zinc, and calcium are of particular importance in the elderly and will be discussed in greater depth.

Iron-deficiency anemia can be a problem among the elderly, most often as a result of blood loss [18]. Inadequate intake of iron, though, is the most common nutritional cause of iron-deficiency anemia. Some of the best sources of iron are red meats, which unfortunately are often high in saturated fat and cholesterol; however, the heme iron in meat is more readily absorbed than the nonheme iron from vegetable sources. With help to identify leaner cuts and use of low-fat preparation techniques, people can consume red meat in moderation. The average American diet contains approximately 6 mg of iron per 1000 kcal [68]. With the limited caloric intake of many elderly people, it can be difficult to meet the RDA for iron (10 mg) if good sources are not included in the diet. Some substances, such as large amounts of tea and phytates in grain products, interfere with absorption of iron. In addition, limited intake of recognized enhancers of iron absorption, such as meat and ascorbic acid, may further limit iron availability [69]. Encouraging other sources of iron such as dried beans and peas and dried fruits can supplement a diet that may otherwise be limited in iron.

The elderly, especially women, are at risk for osteoporosis. Increased intake of calcium is one strategy to help compensate for the increased bone loss of aging; however, the usual intake of calcium by women (450 to 550 mg) is less than the RDA (800 mg) and declines with age [50,70,71]. Some authorities recommend as much as 1500 mg of calcium per day for postmenopausal women [72]. Because dairy products are a major source of calcium, the high saturated fat and cholesterol content is of concern. Use of low-fat or skim milk products can resolve this problem, but some may find skim milk unacceptable, leading to total elimination of dairy products. Changing from whole milk to 2% milk may be a compromise from a cholesterol and saturated-fat standpoint, but it is preferable to eliminating milk entirely.

As with iron, some of the best sources of zinc are meat, poultry, and fish. The zinc in meat is more readily absorbed than that from plant sources [69]. The dietary intake of zinc by elderly men and women is marginal in comparison to the RDA (12 mg), indicating the need for caution when recommending dietary changes that might limit good sources [73]. Even though other factors may be involved, zinc deficiency in humans and animals has been linked to depressed immune function [74]. For the elderly this is of particular concern, because the aging process itself results in decreased efficacy of the immune system [75–77]. In addition, altered taste acuity and behavioral disturbances in human subjects have been attributed to zinc deficiency, and these could have a negative impact on food intake [74]. Limiting zinc intake inadvertently via dietary restriction for another problem, such as severely restricting meat intake to treat hypercholesterolemia, may be detrimental to overall health status.

Socioeconomic and psychological impact on nutrition

The frequency and degree with which personal losses are experienced is often magnified with increasing age. Emotional losses, such as death of a spouse or friends, can have great impact and lead to negative responses [78]. Loss of physical capability may limit one's ability to procure, prepare, and consume the foods normally eaten. Familiar foods become comfort foods in times of stress, making it difficult to change lifelong eating habits. Because of increasing physical problems, the elderly are more vulnerable to food fads and quackery, which can adversely affect nutrition.

Those who have experienced economic deprivation over a lifetime are particularly vulnerable as they age. Minority and lower socioeconomic groups are more likely to suffer from cumulative effects of poverty and a lifetime of marginal nutrition [79–82]. Even more privileged persons may suffer if their income decreases following retirement. This may necessitate a change in living arrangements affecting quantity and types of foods available. The availability of storage and preparation facilities also influences the types of foods eaten. If there is no refrigerator, use of fresh perishable foods is severely limited. A hot plate obviously limits the methods of food preparation.

The degree of socialization influences the quality and quantity of food consumed [83]. Recognizing that the elderly in the United States often live alone and are nutritionally vulnerable led to establishment of the Title III-C nutrition services as a part of the Older Americans Act of 1965 [84,85]. This program offers a meal that meets one third of the RDA (usually five days per week) to at-risk elderly in a community setting to ameliorate the social isolation that can occur with aging. Meals can be delivered to the home for nonambulatory persons, providing them with needed nourishment and contact with people that otherwise might not occur [86]. Program participants have better dietary intake than do their nonparticipating peers [87–90].

Although elderly women more often live alone than men, a woman may adapt more readily from a nutritional standpoint because of her previous role as provider of nourishment for her family. An elderly man whose spouse dies or becomes incapacitated is especially at risk. He suddenly finds himself responsible for providing his own meals. His options include 1) eating out on a regular basis if he can afford it, 2) relying on convenience foods, or 3) learning to plan and prepare meals. His adaptation to this challenge may lead to less than optimal nutrition, depending upon which option he chooses [91,92]. Timely referral to an appropriate agency along with encouraging participation in available support programs can truly make a difference in outcome for such a person.

SUMMARY

Dietary modification for cardiovascular health can be beneficial in the elderly because it may extend active, useful life. As with other forms of intervention, benefits and risks exist that must be evaluated based upon circumstances in each individual case. The elderly patient often has multiple problems, but effective management of nutrition issues can contribute to overall improved quality of life.

REFERENCES

1. Recommended Dietary Allowances. 1989. Committee on Dietary Allowances, Food and Nutrition Board, Committee on Life Sciences, National Research Council, 10th ed. Washington, DC: National Academy Press.
2. Andres R and Hallfrisch J. 1989. Nutrient intake recommendations needed for the older American. J Am Diet Assoc 89:1739–1741.
3. Zheng JJ and Rosenberg IH. 1989. What is the nutritional status of the elderly? Geriatrics 44:57–64.
4. Watkin DM. 1982. The physiology of aging. Am J Clin Nutr 36:750–758.
5. Steen B. 1988. Body composition and aging. Nutr Rev 46:45–51.
6. Bray GA. 1982. The energetics of obesity. Med Sci Sports Exerc 15:32–40.
7. Carroll MD, Abraham S and Dresser CM. 1983. Dietary Intake Source Data: United States, 1976–1980. Vital and Health Statistics, Series 11, No. 231. DHHS Publ No. (PHS) 83-1681. Hyattsville, MD: National Center for Health Statistics, Public Health Service, U.S. Dept Health and Human Services.
8. Uauy R, Winterer JC, Bilmazes C, et al. 1978. The changing pattern of whole body protein metabolism in aging humans. J Gerontol 33:663–671.
9. Uauy R, Scrimshaw NS and Young VR. 1978. Human protein requirements: nitrogen balance response to graded levels of egg protein in elderly men and women. Am J Clin Nutr 31:779–785.
10. Cheng AHR, Gomez A, Bergan JG, et al. 1978. Comparative nitrogen balance study between young and aged adults using three levels of protein intake from a combination wheat–soy–milk mixture. Am J Clin Nutr 31:12–22.
11. Gersovitz M, Motil K, Munro HN, et al. 1982. Human protein requirements: assessment of the adequacy of the current Recommended Dietary Allowance for dietary protein in elderly men and women. Am J Clin Nutr 35:6–14.
12. Betts NM and Vivian VM. 1985. Factors related to the dietary adequacy of noninstitutionalized elderly. J Nutr Elderly 4:3–14.
13. Suter PM and Russell RM. 1987. Vitamin requirements of the elderly. Am J Clin Nutr 45:501–512.
14. Bidlack WR and Smith CH. 1988. Nutritional requirements of the aged. Crit Rev Food Sci Nutr 27:189–218.
15. Iber FL. 1990. Alcoholism and associated malnutrition in the elderly. Prog Clin Biol Res 326:157–173.
16. Smith CH. 1990. Drug–food/food–drug interaction. In JE Morley, Z Glick, LZ Rubenstein (eds), Geriatric Nutrition. New York: Raven Press, pp 371–396.
17. Roe DA. 1987. Drugs and nutrition in the elderly. In Geriatric Nutrition, 2nd ed. Englewood Cliffs, NJ: Prentice Hall, pp 176–200.
18. Herbert V. 1990. Nutritional anemias in the elderly. Prog Clin Biol Res 326:203–227.
19. Nissinen A and Stanley K. 1989. Unbalanced diets as a cause of chronic diseases. Am J Clin Nutr 49:993–998.
20. Kannel WB. 1988. Nutrition and the occurrence and prevention of cardiovascular disease in the elderly. Nutr Rev 46:68–78.
21. Grundy SM and Barnett JP. 1990. Metabolic and health complications of obesity. Dis Mon 36:643–696.
22. Kannel WB, Castelli WP and Gordon T. 1979. Cholesterol in the prediction of atherosclerotic disease. New perspectives based on the Framingham Study. Ann Intern Med 90:85–91.
23. The Lipid Research Clinics Programs Epidemiology Committee. 1979. Plasma lipid distributions in selected North American populations: the Lipid Research Clinics Program Prevalence Study. Circulation 60:427–439.
24. National Center for Health Statistics. 1986. Total Serum Cholesterol Levels of Adults 20–74 years of Age: United States, 1976–1980. Hyattsville, MD: U.S. Department of Health and Human Services, Public Health Service, National Center for Health Statistics; Vital and Health Statistics. Series II, No. 236, DHHS Publication No. (PHS) 86-1686.
25. Wilson PWF, Christiansen JC, Anderson KM and Kannel WB. 1989. Impact of national guidelines for cholesterol risk factor screening. The Framingham offspring study. JAMA 262:41–44.

26. Heiss G, Tamir I, Clarence ED, et al. 1980. Lipoprotein cholesterol distributions in selected North American populations: The lipid research clinic prevalence study. Circulation 61: 302–315.
27. Kesaniemi YA, Beltz WF and Grundy SM. 1985. Comparisons of metabolism of apoliproprotein B in normal subjects, obese patients, and patients with coronary heart disease. J Clin Invest 76:586–595.
28. Egusa G, Beltz WF, Grundy SM, et al. 1985. Influence of obesity on the metabolism of apolipoprotein B in man. J Clin Invest 76:596–603.
29. Spady DK and Dietschy JM. 1985. Dietary saturated triacylglycerols suppress hepatic low density lipoprotein receptors in the hamster. Proc Natl Acad Sci USA 82:4526–4530.
30. Grundy SM and Vega GL. 1988. Hypertriglyceridemia: causes and relation to coronary heart disease. Semin Thromb Hemost 14:149–164.
31. The Expert Panel. 1988. Report of the National Cholesterol Education Program Expert Panel on Detection, Evaluation and Treatment of High Blood Cholesterol in Adults. Arch Intern Med 148:36–69.
32. Abraham S and Johnson CL. 1980. Prevalence of severe obesity in adults in the United States. Am J Clin Nutr 33:364–369.
33. Van Itallie TB. 1985. Health implication of overweight and obesity in the United States. Ann Intern Med 103:983–988.
34. Gray DS. 1989. Diagnosis and prevalence of obesity. Med Clin North Am 73:1–13.
35. Manson JE, Colditz GA, Stampfer MJ, et al. 1990. A prospective study of obesity and risk of coronary heart disease in women. N Engl J Med 322:882–889.
36. Wing RR, Matthews KA, Kuller LH, et al. 1991. Weight gain at the time of menopause. Arch Intern Med 151:97–102.
37. Krotkiewski M, Bjorntorp P, Sjostrom L, et al. 1983. Impact of obesity on metabolism in men and women: importance of regional adipose tissue distribution. J Clin Invest 72: 1150–1162.
38. Larsson B, Svardsudd K, Welin L, et al. 1984. Abdominal adipose tissue distribution, obesity and risk of cardiovascular disease and death: 13-year follow-up of participants in the study of men born in 1913. Br Med J 288:1401–1404.
39. Bjorntorp P. 1985. Obesity and the risk of cardiovascular disease. Ann Clin Res 17:3–9.
40. Stamler J. 1988. Risk factor modification trials; implications for the elderly. Eur Heart J 9 (Suppl D):9–53.
41. Denke MA and Grundy SM. 1990. Hypercholesterolemia in elderly persons: resolving the treatment dilemma. Ann Intern Med 112:780–792.
42. Grundy SM. 1989. Monounsaturated fatty acids and cholesterol metabolism: implications for dietary recommendations. J Nutr 119:529–533.
43. Grundy SM. 1987. Monounsaturated fatty acids, plasma cholesterol, and coronary heart disease. Am J Clin Nutr 45:1168–1175.
44. USDA. 1979. Composition of Foods—Raw, Processed and Prepared. Agriculture Handbook 8-4: Fats and Oils. Agriculture Research Service, U.S. Department of Agriculture. Washington, DC: U.S. Government Printing Office.
45. USDA. 1984. Composition of Foods—Raw, Processed and Prepared. Agriculture Handbook 8-12: Nut and Seed Products. Agriculture Research Service, U.S. Department of Agriculture. Washington, DC: U.S. Government Printing Office.
46. Gebhardt SE and Matthews RH. 1988. Nutritive Values of Foods. USDA Home and Garden Bulletin, No 72. Washington, DC: U.S. Government Printing Office.
47. Karvonen MJ. 1988. Prevention of cardiovascular disease among the elderly. Bull WHO 66:7–14.
48. Evans WJ and Meredith CN. 1989. Exercise and nutrition in the elderly. In HN Munro and DE Danford (eds), Nutrition, Aging, and the Elderly. New York: Plenum Publishing, pp 89–126.
49. Powell KE, Caspersen CJ, Koplan JP and Ford ES. 1989. Physical activity and chronic diseases. Am J Clin Nutr 49:999–1006.
50. National Research Council. 1989. Diet and Health. Committee on Diet and Health, Food and Nutrition Board, Commission on Life Sciences. Washington, DC: National Academy Press, pp 16–17, 69, 347–352.
51. Gupta KL, Dworkin B and Gambert SR. 1988. Common nutritional disorders in the elderly: atypical manifestations. Geriatrics 43:87–97.

52. Master AM, Lasser RP and Beckman G. 1960. Tables of average weight and height for Americans aged 65 to 94 years. JAMA 114:658–62.
53. Verdery RB. 1990. "Wasting away" of the old: can it—and should it—be treated? Geriatrics 45:26–31.
54. Fischer J and Johnson MA. 1990. Low body weight and weight loss in the aged. J Am Diet Assoc 90:1697–1706.
55. Silver AJ. 1988. Anorexia of aging. Ann Intern Med 109:890–904.
56. Gorbien MJ. 1990. Cardiac cachexia. In JE Morley, Z Glick, LZ Rubenstein (eds), Geriatric Nutrition. New York: Raven Press, pp 315–323.
57. Fanelli MT and Abernethy MM. 1986. A nutritional questionnaire for older adults. Gerontologist 26:192–197.
58. Simko MD, Cowell C and Hreha MS. 1989. Practical Nutrition. A Quick Reference for the Health Care Practitioner. Appendix A, Dietary Assessment Tools. Rockville, MD: Aspen Publishers, pp 281–286, 291–297.
59. Campbell VA and Dodds ML. 1967. Collecting dietary information from groups of older people. J Am Diet Assoc 51:29–33.
60. Madden JP, Goodman SJ and Guthrie HA. 1976. Validity of the 24-hour recall: analysis of data obtained from elderly subjects. J Am Diet Assoc 68:143–147.
61. Dwyer JT, Krall EA and Coleman KA. 1987. The problem of memory in nutritional epidemiology research. J Am Diet Assoc 87:1509–1512.
62. Rhodus NL and Brown J. 1990. The association of xerostomia and inadequate intake in older adults. J Am Diet Assoc 90:1688–1692.
63. Alfin-Slater RB. 1988. Vitamin use and abuse in elderly persons. Ann Intern Med 109:896–898.
64. Ludman EK and Newman JM. 1986. Frail elderly: assessment of nutrition needs. Gerontologist 26:198–202.
65. Myrianthopoulos M. 1987. Dietary treatment of hyperlipidemia in the elderly. Clin Geriatr Med 3:343–359.
66. Pennington JAT (ed). 1989. Bowes & Church's Food Values of Portions Commonly Used, 15th ed. Philadelphia: J.B. Lippincott.
67. Sandstead HH, Dintzis FR, Bogyo TP, et al. 1990. Dietary factors that can impair calcium and zinc nutriture of the elderly. Prog Clin Biol Res 326:241–262.
68. Hallberg L. 1984. Iron. In RE Olson, HB Broquist, CO Chichester, et al. (eds), Nutrition Reviews' Present Knowledge in Nutrition, 5th ed. Washington, DC: The Nutrition Foundation, pp 459–478.
69. Hunt SM and Groff JL. 1990. Microminerals. In Advanced Nutrition in Human Metabolism. St. Paul, MN: West Publishing, pp 286–306.
70. Wardlaw G. 1988. The effects of diet and life-style on bone mass in women. J Am Diet Assoc 88:17–25.
71. Brickman AS. 1990. Calcium, vitamin D, and osteopenia in the elderly. In JE Morley, Z Glick, LZ Rubenstein (eds), Geriatric Nutrition. New York: Raven Press, pp 149–160.
72. National Institutes of Health. 1984. Statement of the Consensus Development Conference on Osteoporosis. DHHS Publication No. (PHS) 421-132, vol 5, no. 3. Washington, DC: U.S. Government Printing Office.
73. Pennington JAT, Young BE, Wilson DB, et al. 1986. Mineral content of foods and total diets: the Selected Minerals in Foods Survey, 1982 to 1984. J Am Diet Assoc 86:876–891.
74. Cousins RJ and Hempe JM. 1990. Zinc. In ML Brown (ed), Present Knowledge in Nutrition, 6th ed. Washington, DC: International Life Sciences Institute-Nutrition Foundation, pp 251–260.
75. Goodwin JS and Burns EL. 1991. Aging, nutrition, and immune function. Clin Appl Nutr 1:85–94.
76. Goodwin JS, Searles RP and Tung KSK. 1982. Immunological responses of a healthy elderly population. Clin Exp Immunol 48:403–410.
77. Roe DA. 1990. Geriatric nutrition. Clin Geriatr Med 6:319–334.
78. Natow AB and Heslin J. 1980. Psychosocial forces that affect nutrition and food choices. In Geriatric Nutrition. Boston: CBI Publishing, pp 197–224.
79. Davies L. 1984. Nutrition and the elderly: identifying those at risk. Proc Nutr Soc 43:295–302.

80. Norton L and Wozny MC. 1984. Residential location and nutritional adequacy among elderly adults. J Gerontol 39:592–595.
81. Davis MA, Randall E, Forthofer RN, et al. 1985. Living arrangements and dietary patterns of older adults in the United States. J Gerontol 40:434–442.
82. Bianchetti A, Rozzini R, Carabellese C, et al. 1990. Nutritional intake, socioeconomic conditions, and health status in a large elderly population. J Am Geriatr Soc 38:521–526.
83. McIntosh WA, Shifflet PA and Picou JS. 1989. Social support, stressful events, strain, dietary intake, and the elderly. Med Care 27:140–153.
84. Watkin DM. 1977. The Nutrition Program for Older Americans: a successful application of current knowledge in nutrition and gerontology. World Rev Nutr Diet 26:26–40.
85. Greene JM, 1981. Coordination of Older Americans Act programs. J Am Diet Assoc 78:617–620.
86. Posner BE, Smigelski CG and Krachenfels MM. 1987. Dietary characteristics and nutrient intake in an urban homebound population. J Am Diet Assoc 87:452–456.
87. Kohrs MB, O'Hanlon P and Ecklund D. 1978. Title VII—Nutrition Program for the Elderly I. Contribution to one day's dietary intake. J Am Diet Assoc 72:487–492.
88. Kohrs MB, O'Hanlon P, Krause G and Nordstrom J. 1979. Title VII—Nutrition Programs for the Elderly II. Relationship of socioeconomic factors to one day's nutrient intake. J Am Diet Assoc 75:537–542.
89. Kohrs MB, Nordstrom J, Plowman EL, et al. 1980. Association of participation in a nutritional program for the elderly with nutritional status. Am J Clin Nutr 33:2643–2656.
90. United States Department of Health and Human Services: longitudinal evaluation of the national Nutrition Program for the Elderly. Report on First-wave Findings. 1979. Washington, DC: U.S. Government Printing Office. DHEW Publication No. (OHDS) 80-20249.
91. Ries CP, Kline K and Weaver SO. 1987. Impact of commercial eating on nutrient adequacy. J Am Diet Assoc 87:463–468.
92. Davis MA, Murphy SP, Neuhaus JM and Lein D. 1990. Living arrangements and dietary quality of older U.S. adults. J Am Diet Assoc 90:1667–1672.

21. EXERCISE AND REHABILITATION IN ELDERLY CARDIAC PATIENTS

NANETTE K. WENGER

The altered functional status of the elderly cardiac patient reflects both the anatomic and physiologic cardiovascular changes that occur with aging and the dysfunction that results from the specific cardiovascular disorder or disorders. The changes of aging decrease the reserve capacity of the heart; problems become manifest at times of cardiovascular stress, as occurs with a variety of cardiac disease states. Both of these limitations must be considered when making activity recommendations for the elderly cardiac patient, and variable components of each are amenable to therapeutic interventions.

Additionally, cardiac disease rarely occurs in isolation in the elderly; there are typically additive impairments of multiple systemic illnesses that may directly or indirectly impair cardiovascular performance. More than 40% of persons over age 65 years have some limitation of activity due to chronic disease. Psychologic factors, particularly depression and loss of motivation, may exacerbate functional losses and disability. Because of these variables, chronologic age among the elderly poorly predicts physiologic age and functional capabilities. The rehabilitative approach must encompass attention to this combination of medical, psychological, and social problems encountered in elderly patients, many of whom have chronic multisystem disease. Goals should include enhancement and maintenance of physical

Franz H. Messerli (ed.), CARDIOVASCULAR DISEASE IN THE ELDERLY (Third Edition). Copyright © 1993 Kluwer Academic Publishers. ISBN 0-7923-1859-5. All rights reserved.

function (including mobility and self-sufficiency), preservation of mental function (including self-image, self-respect, and alertness), limitation of anxiety and depression, and attainment of reasonable independence with return to community and social roles.

ALTERATIONS IN THE NORMAL RESPONSE TO EXERCISE WITH AGING

The decrement in maximal oxygen consumption, maximal exercise heart rate, exercise stroke volume, and exercise cardiac output with aging decreases the capacity to exercise, to work, and to tolerate a variety of cardiovascular stresses. However, the age-associated decrease in maximal aerobic capacity is less than was previously described when the values for maximal oxygen uptake are corrected for the decreased lean body mass that is characteristic of aging [1]. The extent of the decrease in muscle mass due to aging and that due to inactivity remains uncertain. Preservation of cardiac output with aging appears predominantly due to an increased stroke volume enabled by an increase in end-diastolic volume [2]. Because of the dependence on late diastolic filling to maintain the exercise cardiac output, the atrial contribution to ventricular filling of sinus rhythm assumes great importance, and exercise capacity may deteriorate with loss of sinus rhythm. Elderly people have a decreased response to beta-adrenergic stimulation; as a result, the increased cardiac output with exercise depends less on the catecholamine-mediated increase in heart rate and decrease in end-systolic volume than on the Frank–Starling mechanism. Changes in ventilatory function with aging appear not to limit physical work capacity in elderly persons in the absence of lung disease, but limited data are available about peripheral factors such as muscle mass, muscle blood flow, cellular mitochondrial changes, and so forth.

In contrast to training of young persons, the usual modest-intensity exercise training of older people does not significantly increase maximal heart rate or aerobic capacity. Even with a comparable initial aerobic capacity, exercise training produces less improvement in elderly individuals. Training in the elderly usually produces little or modest increase in maximal oxygen uptake; the major physiologic effect of training that enhances function is the decrease in the heart rate response to any submaximal workload. In one report of short-term exercise training of elderly men, although the aerobic capacity (maximal oxygen uptake) did not increase, improvement in work efficiency was evidenced by a decrease in heart rate. The decrease in heart rate increased the oxygen pulse, the amount of oxygen removed from the blood per heartbeat. In another study, three months of endurance training significantly increased both maximal workload (16%) and maximal oxygen uptake (11%) [3]. However, elderly subjects who volunteer for exercise training studies are likely to be more fit than the general aged population; thus the improvement described may underestimate the potential benefits of training. Even with these limitations, more intensive and prolonged training can modestly increase the maximal oxygen uptake (about 10% to 15%), as well as decrease the heart rate response, in the subset of elderly persons suitable for this demanding exercise regimen [3–5]. Although a significant increase in endurance and in work capacity can be achieved by many elderly persons as a result of physical training [6,7], there is no evidence that longevity is altered by exercise training.

As with younger people, exercise training results in predominantly peripheral hemodynamic adaptations. Trained skeletal muscle extracts increased oxygen from its perfusing blood, with a resultant decrease in cardiac work. The aerobic requirement for any submaximal task is decreased by the skeletal muscle, autonomic nervous system, and peripheral vascular resistance adaptations that lessen the rate–pressure product. Trained elderly coronary patients thus require a lesser percentage of their increased physical capacity to perform daily activities, and thereby perceive an improvement in endurance; they also function farther from their ischemic threshold, so that activity-induced angina is less likely to limit their usual tasks.

Static or isometric strength and endurance (as measured by handgrip) decrease more from age 60 to 80 than from age 30 to 60. The heart rate response to static exercise decreases with age, while the systolic blood pressure response increases; diastolic blood pressure response is essentially unchanged.

More time is needed for the heart rate to return to normal after exercise in elderly people [8]. The exaggerated exercise-induced rise in systolic blood pressure characteristic of elderly patients can be reduced by training. However, skin blood flow remains decreased, limiting the ability to sweat efficiently with exercise and compromising temperature regulation with heat stress and/or exercise.

EXERCISE REHABILITATION OF THE ELDERLY CARDIAC PATIENT [8–10]

A variety of medical problems may predispose elderly patients to relative inactivity and resultant physical deconditioning, causing cardiovascular disability by potentiating the decreased physical work capacity of aging or exacerbating underlying cardiovascular disease. Even before illness, many elderly patients often unintentionally decrease their habitual level of physical activity owing to combinations of musculoskeletal instability, peripheral vascular disease, decreased muscle mass and contractile strength, anxiety, loss of motivation, depression, and inappropriate admonitions from physicians, friends, and family members [11]. Maximal oxygen uptake in sedentary elderly individuals is 10% to 20% less than that of their physically active counterparts. Because of the decrease in aerobic capacity with aging, any submaximal task is perceived to require increased work, because it entails a greater percentage of the lowered functional capacity; this increase in relative energy cost further contributes to restriction of activity [12]. Even at low intensities of exercise, exercise-induced dyspnea may occur, owing to the decreased compliance of the aged ventricle; this further contributes to the overestimation of activity intensity in the elderly. The resultant decrease in physical work capacity and functional status threatens continuation of an independent life-style, which potentiates the anxiety and depression that may engender a further decrease in activity.

Physicians know little about the exercise habits of their elderly patients and typically underestimate their habitual activity level. Unfortunately, physicians may potentiate the problems of illness by prescribing excessive bed rest or activity limitation for elderly cardiac patients and by overmedicating them in an attempt to assure comfort and adequate rest. Complications of immobilization and bed rest are accentuated in the elderly. Physical work capacity decreases rapidly with prolonged inactivity or bed rest; thrombophlebitis and pulmonary embolism are common complications. Other prominent problems associated with inactivity include relative hypovolemia, with resulting reflex tachycardia and orthostatic hypotension when activity is initiated; a decrease in lung volume and vital capacity; and a generalized decrease in muscle mass and muscular contractile strength. Anxiety and depression are common sequelae, since elderly patients fear deterioration of function as a threat to their independent life-style [13]. Although the physical and emotional benefits of regular exercise have been known for many years, physical activity is inadequately recommended for the elderly population because of inappropriate physician concern about risk and due to overcautious attitudes of family, friends, and community. Dr. Paul D. White emphasized that "exercise of almost any kind, suitable in degree and duration . . . can and does play a useful role in the maintenance of both physical and mental health of the aging individual" [14]. However, only limited information is available about the optimal activity levels and regimens for elderly patients with cardiovascular disease.

Functional capacity can be preserved and often improved with the institution or reinstitution of physical activity, even in old age [15,16]. Exercise maintains the work efficiency of both the musculoskeletal and the cardiovascular systems. As a result, the usual daily activities of older individuals are not curtailed by an excessive decrease in physical work capacity, and moderate episodic increased work demands can be tolerated.

REHABILITATION OF THE ELDERLY PATIENT WITH CORONARY HEART DISEASE

Twelve percent of the U.S. population is currently older than 65 years of age. About one half of these 26 million people have some cardiac disorder, and coronary atherosclerotic heart disease is the preponderant clinical problem. Despite the decreased cardiovascular mortality in the U.S. in recent years, there has been less impact in the elderly population owing to the dramatic increase in the number of individuals in this age group. In addition to mortality, cardiovascular disease is a major contributor to disability among elderly patients, as well as to their needs for hospital, ambulatory, and custodial care, since the majority of patients with clinical manifestations of coronary disease in the U.S. are currently older than age 65.

Many features of coronary disease in the elderly are less activity dependent than in younger populations [17–19]. For example, angina pectoris in the aged is less often reported as typical effort angina, in part because of the relatively sedentary life-style of many older patients, or because arthritis, other musculoskeletal problems, or claudication limits their activity before the onset of anginal pain. The frequent precipitation or accentuation of angina by the increased myocardial oxygen demand of a complicating illness such as uncontrolled hypertension, arrhythmia, pneumonia, anemia, and so forth enables an improved prognosis for rehabilitation by correction of these problems.

The hospital stay for elderly patients with a coronary event is almost twice that of their younger counterparts, owing to increased anatomic severity of the coronary disease, greater comorbidity, and an excess of complications including heart failure, arrhythmias, conduction abnormalities, and cardiogenic shock. These extend the period spent at bed rest or at limited activity as well, with resultant greater residual impairment and posthospitalization invalidism.

Although myocardial infarction in the elderly is commonly characterized by increased morbidity and mortality and a more protracted hospital stay among survivors, a substantial number of elderly patients with myocardial infarction have an essentially uncomplicated clinical course and a normal response to predischarge exercise testing; these people have an excellent prognosis for recovery and rehabilitation despite their older age [17–20].

Rehabilitation is a learning process for the patient and often requires the help of multidisciplinary specialists for effective care. Since limitation of physical work capacity is the predominant cause of disability in the elderly, resumption of activity is emphasized.

Early ambulation after myocardial infarction [21]

Ambulation and gradually progressive physical activity should be initiated in the hospital as soon as feasible following a coronary event. Early ambulation helps prevent cardiovascular deconditioning of elderly patients, who are particularly susceptible to the deleterious effects of prolonged immobilization, which include an excess of pulmonary atelectasis and thromboembolic complications. Such low-level activities as sitting in a chair for several hours each day can obviate the orthostatic intolerance that occurs with protracted bed rest; exposure to gravitational stress, rather than the intensity of the activity, appears to be the determining feature to prevent these problems.

The gradual progression of physical activity during the hospitalization is comparable to that recommended for younger patients (table 21-1) [22]. In the coronary care unit, patients are typically permitted to feed themselves,

Table 21-1. Inpatient rehabilitation: Myocardial infarction seven-step program

Step	Date	M.D. initials	Nurse/P.T. notes	Supervised exercise	CCU/ward activity	Educational/recreational activity
CCU						
1		—		Active and passive ROM all extremities, in bed Teach pt ankle plantar and dorsiflexion—repeat hourly when awake	Partial self-care Feed self Dangle legs on side of bed Use bedside commode Sit in chair 15 min 1–2 times a day	Orientation to CCU Personal emergencies, social service aid as needed
2		—		Active ROM all extremities—sitting on side of bed	Sit in chair 15–30 min 2–3 times a day Complete self-care in bed	Orientation to rehab team, program Smoking cessation Educational literature if requested Planning transfer from CCU
Ward						
3		—		Warm-up exercises, 2 METS —stretching —calisthenics Walk 50 ft and back at slow pace	Sit in chair ad lib To ward class in wheelchair Walk in room	Normal cardiac anatomy and function Development of atherosclerosis What happens with myocardial infarction 1-2 MET craft activity

Step		Exercise	Ward Activity	Educational, Recreational, and Diversional Activity
4	—	ROM and calisthenics, 2.5 METS Walk length of hall (75 ft) and back, average pace Teach pulse counting	OOB as tolerated Walk to bathroom Walk to ward class, with supervision	Coronary risk factors and their control
5	—	ROM and calisthenics, 3 METS Check pulse counting Practice walking few stairsteps Walk 300 ft bid	Walk to waiting room or telephone Walk in ward corridor prn	Diet Energy conservation Work simplification techniques (as needed)
6	—	Continue above activities Walk down flight of steps (return by elevator) Walk 500 ft bid Instruct on home exercise	Tepid shower or tub bath, with supervision To Cardiac Clinic teaching room, with supervision	Heart attack management —medications —exercise —surgery —response to symptoms —family, community adjustments on return home
7	—	Continue above activities Walk up flight of steps Walk 500 ft bid Continue home exercise instruction—present information re outpatient exercise program	Continue all previous ward activities	Discharge planning: Medications, diet, activity Return appointments Scheduled tests Return to work Community resources Educational literature Medication cards

Source: Reproduced with permission from Wenger NK and Fletcher GF. 1990. Rehabilitation of the patient with atherosclerotic coronary heart disease. In JW Hurst (ed), The Heart, 7th ed. New York: McGraw-Hill, p 1110.

bathe, and perform other personal care activities, use a bedside commode, and sit in bed or in a bedside chair. Selected arm and leg exercises, designed primarily to maintain muscle tone and joint mobility, entail an energy expenditure of 1 to 2 METS (one to two times the resting metabolic rate).

After transfer from the coronary or intensive care unit, the goal of rehabilitative ambulation is to achieve a functional level that will permit self-care and homebound activities at the time of discharge from the hospital. Household tasks generally require a work intensity of 2 to 3 METS. Patients continue to perform personal care, sit in a chair for increasing periods, and perform supervised selected predominantly isotonic (dynamic) exercises involving the arms, legs, and trunk. These activities are characterized by rhythmic, repetitive movements of large muscle groups. Subsequent to these "warm-up" exercises, the major prescriptive component of physical activity is walking, with a gradual increase in both the pace and distance walked. Patients who will have to climb steps at home should practice this before discharge from the hospital by walking down a flight of stairs one day, usually returning by elevator, and walking slowly up a flight of steps on a subsequent day. The safe accomplishment of this activity at the end of the hospital stay decreases the anxiety of the patient and family when stair-climbing is attempted on return home.

Surveillance of early ambulation activities by health care professionals identifies any disproportionate response to these low-level activities. An appropriate response to in-hospital physical activity is characterized by the absence of chest pain, dyspnea, undue fatigue, or palpitations; undue tachycardia or arrhythmia; S-T-segment displacement on the electrocardiogram (ECG) suggestive of ischemia; and/or inadequacy of the blood pressure response to activity (a fall in systolic blood pressure in excess of 10 to 15 mmHg). An appropriate response to activity indicates that the patient can safely tolerate that workload and may be gradually advanced to an activity of slightly greater intensity.

Demonstration that self-care and other low-level physical activities produce no cardiac symptoms is reassuring to both patient and family. The performance of personal care and other daily activities on return home is facilitated; this may avert or delay functional dependency and the need for institutional care. However, subsequent maintenance of appropriate activity levels at home so as to sustain physical and mental independence by elderly patients often requires reinforcement and encouragement from the physician and other health professionals, as well as from family and friends.

Exercise training [8,23]

Exercise training can increase endurance and physical work capacity in elderly patients. Additional benefits include the maintenance of joint mobility and neuromuscular coordination, which often deteriorate with age, and improvement in general coordination and flexibility. Exercise increases muscle mass and muscle and tendon strength; this enhances joint stability and enables an appropriate response to occasional, unexpected, sudden activity demands. Modest intensity training of elderly patients results both in replacement of fat by lean tissue and in arrest or reversal of mineral loss from bone [24,25]; this is of particular importance for women, given the increased occurrence of myocardial infarction among women in the seventh and eighth decades, with an occurrence comparable to that in men. Although in the early years of exercise rehabilitation coronary patients older than age 65 were arbitrarily excluded from participation in supervised exercise programs following a coronary event, they now constitute an increasing percentage of the coronary patients in such programs. In general, coronary patients aged 65 to 75 years are more comparable to their younger counterparts; for patients older than age 75, chronologic age poorly predicts their very variable functional, behavioral, cognitive, emotional, and social status. The intensity and duration of exercise required to achieve a training effect are within the capabilities of most elderly coronary patients.

Exercise enhances self-confidence and the sense of well-being. This, added to the improved physical work capacity, encourages the patient to renounce sick role behavior and to continue participation in tasks of daily living and in recreational and social activities. Conversely, sedentary, inactive aged individuals may progressively deteriorate owing to a combination of psychologic and physiologic depression, precipitating the need for institutional care. Institutionalization further accelerates the decline in physical and emotional status because physical activity is seldom encouraged in residential facilities for the aged, and both physical and emotional stimuli are limited. However, even among frail elderly nursing home residents, resistance exercise training improved muscle mass, muscle strength, and functional mobility [26]; rapid regression of the improved status followed cessation of exercise training. Evaluation of family and community support systems is therefore part of the rehabilitative assessment.

The energy expenditure of walking represents a large percentage of the lessened aerobic capacity that occurs with aging; walking provides an effective physical conditioning stimulus in the elderly—even walking as slowly as 3 or 3½ miles per hour [15]. The physical activity regimen recommended after leaving the hospital is typically a walking program, with progressive increases in the pace and distance walked. Walking requires no specific skills, equipment, or facilities and enables socialization with a walking companion. Because improvement in the exercise response to arm work depends on arm muscle training, an exercise regimen also should include arm exercise. Strength training, which can increase muscle mass and function, can result in a further improvement in aerobic capacity.

Exercise testing, performed for risk stratification after myocardial infarction, can also be used to prescribe the appropriate intensity of activity to be undertaken [23]. At times the exercise test is "therapeutic" as well; the patient (and spouse or family) discover the level of activity that can be performed without symptoms. When patients are tested to a sign- or symptom-limited endpoint, the heart rate achieved prior to this endpoint is characterized as the highest heart rate safely attained at exercise testing. The exercise prescription identifies a target heart rate range for exercise training of between 60% and 75% of this rate. As in younger patients, this heart rate range engenders greater comfort and enjoyment of exercise, as well as fewer musculoskeletal complications than the 70% to 85% heart rate range advocated in prior years. This lower level of exercise intensity also ensures greater safety when exercise is unsupervised, yet remains a safe and effective range to stimulate aerobic metabolism and improved endurance. Initially a heart rate range as low as 40% to 60% may be effective. The absence of exercise-induced angina cannot be assumed to indicate the absence of myocardial ischemia, given the increased likelihood of painless ischemia in an elderly population, with dyspnea often occurring as an anginal equivalent [27]. Patients with coronary disease should never exercise at a level higher than that documented to elicit an appropriate cardiovascular response at exercise testing.

The other two components of the exercise "dosage" in prescriptive physical activity (in addition to the intensity, as described) are exercise frequency and duration. In general, patients are advised to exercise 2 or 3 times weekly, preferably on nonsuccessive days. Exercise sessions should be at least 30 to 45 minutes in duration, including warm-up and cool-down periods, a duration adequate to stimulate aerobic metabolism. In the initial days of exercise at home, shorter sessions can be undertaken more frequently if patients become fatigued. Aerobic exercise of low intensity (2 to 3 METS) should initially be recommended, with increases in intensity and duration as gradual as necessary to limit discomfort and injury.

The design of an exercise program for an individual elderly patient may vary with the person's initial level of fitness, cardiovascular impairment from disease, impairment due to other disorders, and the patient's skills, likes, and dislikes [22]. An exercise regimen should be enjoyable, easily accessible, and without adverse consequences, and should involve predominantly dynamic exercise. As noted above, patients initially often walk in and around the home, walking outdoors when they can avoid extremes of temperature and humidity. In large communities, enclosed shopping malls are ideal level sites for walking, in a temperature- and humidity-controlled environment, and also allow for the companionship of other exercisers. At times, exercise "groups" walk the corridors of high-rise dwellings for the elderly. Because patients should be taught, while in the hospital, to monitor their pulse rate response to exercise, they can ascertain whether walking elicits an appropriate heart rate response. Use of the rating of perceived exertion [28] can also guide the intensity of exercise. Alternatively, a "talk test" may provide effective guidance, when elderly patients are instructed to exercise only to an intensity that permits them to continue to talk with an exercising companion. Patients also must be taught inappropriate symptomatic responses to exercise, for example, chest pain, palpitations, undue breathlessness, or fatigue; these symptoms indicate that exercise should be discontinued and the physician notified. Patients who resume exercise after a hiatus of days to weeks, whether due to illness or other reasons, should be cautioned to do so at lower intensity and to progress gradually to higher exercise levels.

Several distinctive features of an elderly person's response to exercise are of importance in the design of a physical activity program. Warm-up or limbering-up exercises are valuable in enabling musculoskeletal and cardiorespiratory readiness for exercise and in allowing effective training to occur. Because a prolonged time is required for the exercise heart rate to return to resting levels, the activity regimen design should incorporate longer intervals of rest or low-intensity activity between periods of exercise training [8]. More protracted cool-down allows gradual dissipation of the heat load of exercise and subsidence of exercise-related peripheral vasodilatation. Avoidance of running, jumping, and other high-impact activities can limit serious musculoskeletal complications. Because older individuals sweat less efficiently and thus have a less effective thermal regulation and a lower tolerance for heat stress than younger people, even moderate physical activity should be limited in hot and humid environments.

It takes older people longer than young people to attain a training effect; only after more prolonged training will an older person's heart rate and blood pressure response decrease for any level of submaximal work. This appears in part due to the appropriately low-level training intensity initially undertaken and in part to their slower adaptation to and acceptance of an exercise regimen. Nevertheless, this intervention is likely to prove cost-effective because it increases the patient's ability to maintain and prolong independent community living, and improves quality of life.

The National Council on Fitness and Aging classified physical activities for the elderly as follows:

1. Activities with little energy expenditure that occur too intermittently to promote endurance: light housework, walking at 1 to 2 mph on level ground, playing golf using a powered cart, or bowling
2. Activities that build moderate endurance if carried out continuously for 15 to 30 minutes: cleaning windows, mopping floors, walking 3 mph on level ground, cycling at 6 mph, and playing golf pulling a cart
3. Activities that promote good endurance if carried out for 15 to 30 minutes: walking at 3½ to 4 mph, cycling at 8 to 10 mph, playing golf carrying clubs, skating (ice or roller), aerobic dancing, and swimming at less than 20 yards/min

In addition, because elderly patients are likely to manifest the deconditioning effects of immobilization even after a few days of inactivity, sustained low-intensity activity should become a lifetime pattern if benefits are to be maintained. Any illness-enforced rest may require a fairly intensive rehabilitative approach to restore physical fitness during convalescence. Nevertheless, even elderly coronary patients with a medically complex course, including those with ventricular systolic dysfunction, can attain a substantial improvement in physical work capacity from a low-intensity, long-duration exercise training regimen [16].

Education and counseling

Elderly patients often have more disorientation and cerebral dysfunction in the coronary or intensive care unit, in part reflecting the increased occurrence of hypotension, heart failure, and arrhythmias as complications of myocardial infarction and in part related to adverse responses to medications, particularly narcotics, analgesics, and sedatives. Problems related to unfamiliar surroundings, complex monitoring devices, the multiplicity of personnel and procedures, and so forth generate anxiety. Brief and repeated explanations and reassurance, with attention to ensuring time and place orientation, are vital.

Coronary risk modification is appropriate [20], since 1983 statistics identify a life expectancy of 14.5 years for U.S. men aged 65 years and an 18.6-year life expectancy for their female counterparts. Classic coronary risk factors remain predictive at least through the eighth decade; because of the high incidence of recurrent coronary events in the elderly, the benefits of risk factor modification can be substantial. These interventions are designed to retard atherosclerotic progression. Advice should be given to discontinue cigarette smoking [29], which is associated with an increased risk of coronary death and reinfarction at all ages. Blood pressure regulation, as in younger patients, helps control angina pectoris and congestive heart failure. Dietary sodium and fat restriction should be encouraged; recommendations for identification and management of hyperlipidemia are the same as for younger patients. The increased energy expenditure of exercise is an adjunct to dietary therapy in weight control, for the prevention or management of obesity.

Weight control poses a problem in elderly patients when physical activity is limited, because the secondarily restricted diet necessary to maintain ideal body weight may provide inadequate nutrients. Difficulties in food purchase and preparation, dental problems that impair chewing of food, lack of interest in eating when alone, depression, and financial constraints often further impair the protein-calorie nutritional status of elderly patients.

The male preponderance of myocardial infarction decreases with age, until it has an approximately equivalent incidence in both sexes beyond age 70. Teaching energy-conserving techniques in performing household tasks is an important rehabilitative component for both elderly women and men with myocardial infarction. The frequently increased severity of infarction in the elderly, with more residual functional impairment, renders this approach valuable. The National Council on Fitness and Aging has also emphasized the need for elderly women to participate in physical exercise as much as men. Emphasis should be on the return to preinfarction life-style, in which regular physical activity and intervening rest are both important. Continued involvement in social and recreational activities should be encouraged, as should return to a light job if appropriate. Return to the prior pattern of sexual activity is also recommended.

Restoration of preillness physical activity level and life-style can be a major deterrent against anxiety and depresson [30], both of which pose therapeutic problems in elderly cardiac patients. Many psychotropic drugs are contraindicated after myocardial infarction because of their undesirable effects on heart rate, blood pressure, and cardiac rhythm. Benzodiazepine drugs appear to offer the greatest safety.

Clear and specific instructions should be repeated as necessary about diet, activity, medications, etc. Information should be provided in a manner that is supportive of the patient's self-image and conforms with the patient's sociocultural background; this permits adaptations of life-style to conform with the cardiovascular impairment.

Special considerations regarding cardiovascular drug therapy [20,31]

An excess of adverse drug reactions occurs in the elderly, particularly reactions to cardiovascular and psychotropic drugs. Changes of aging in other organ systems, with resultant diminution of hepatic, renal, gastrointestinal, and central nervous system functions, increase the incidence of drug sensitivity. Variations in drug absorption, metabolism and half-life, distribution, excretion, and receptor sensitivity are common with advancing age. There is a decreased lean body mass for drug distribution. Visual and memory impairments may complicate medication-taking, as may the combined medical, psychological, and social problems that often occur in patients with multisystem degenerative diseases.

For example, the decreased glomerular filtration rate (even with a normal BUN) and diminished creatinine clearance prolong the half-life of digoxin, predisposing to toxicity, particularly in the presence of the frequently associated hypokalemia. Digitalis toxicity in the elderly is often manifest by cardiac arrhythmias in the absence of systemic symptoms other than decreased appetite.

Excessive diuresis with potent drugs may result in hypovolemic hypotension, azotemia, and confusion. Orthostasis may occur even with milder diuretic drugs; and thiazide-associated potassium depletion may potentiate muscle weakness and increase digitalis-related arrhythmias; thiazide-induced hyperglycemia may aggravate preexisting diabetes mellitus or glucose intolerance.

Particularly in hypovolemic patients, vasodilator drugs are more likely to produce unacceptable postural hypotension, dizziness, and syncope; similarly, nitroglycerin taken while standing may cause syncope. Compromised baroreceptor function limits compensatory tachycardia, as may frequent conduction system disease and decreased efficacy of stretch receptors in the rigid aortic wall. Thus vasodilator drugs, including calcium blocking drugs, and beta-adrenergic blocking agents, both of which are major therapeutic advances for coronary patients, are generally administered in lower dosage.

A further problem is that the multiple, vague, multisystem, somatic complaints commonly described by elderly patients (often a manifestation of otherwise unrecognized depression) are often inappropriately palliated and managed with a variety of pharmacologic agents rather than with reassurance and counseling.

Psychosocial factors assume great importance in the prescription of medication for elderly patients. Hearing or visual impairment may limit the patient's ability to follow a prescribed regimen, as may cognitive impairment. Elderly patients often have difficulty opening safety caps on medicine bottles or measuring accurately the dosage of liquid medications. Medication cards or daily medication charts for use at home may serve as reminders. Fixed incomes and limited insurance benefits may discourage the purchase of expensive medications. Also, living alone, without reinforcement of medication-taking from family and friends, may limit adherence to medication regimens [32]. Written instructions can enable family members, friends, or community health aides to help the aged patient adhere to recommendations for care.

Coronary bypass surgery and coronary angioplasty [33–36]
Because of the unfavorable long-term outcome in many elderly coronary patients, coronary bypass surgery and coronary angioplasty have increasingly become therapeutic options for symptomatic elderly patients with significant coronary obstructive lesions and adequate residual ventricular function. In the U.S., more than one third of all cardiovascular diagnostic procedures (including coronary arteriography) and coronary bypass surgical operations are performed in patients older than 65 years of age. Although symptomatic relief and improvement of functional status are comparable to that achieved by younger patients, the increased morbidity and mortality of coronary bypass surgery in elderly patients must be considered when recommending surgery, despite the improved symptomatic status and long-term survival after operation as compared with medical therapy alone. Coronary bypass surgery is associated with an excess of perioperative complications and a greater requirement for ventilatory support, temporary pacemakers, and aortic balloon counterpulsation; these entail a longer time spent at bed rest. A five-year event-free survival at age 65 and older of 47% was described in the Coronary Artery Surgery Study (CASS) Registry [34]. The advisability and feasibility of surgery are often determined by noncardiac features: cerebrovascular insufficiency, atherosclerotic changes in the aorta and large

arteries, peripheral vascular insufficiency, pulmonary and renal insufficiency, prostatic obstruction, debilitation, and malnutrition. Nevertheless, excellent functional improvement and survival are described among octogenarians [35]. Postoperatively, early ambulation and progressive resumption of activity should be instituted as soon as feasible; these lessen complications and improve functional capacity at the time of discharge from the hospital. Recent reports suggest that the risk and success of coronary angioplasty in the elderly are comparable to the risk and success in younger patients, with excellent functional improvement and long-term survival described even among octogenarians [36].

When previously sedentary elderly patients initiate a more active life-style, as may occur after successful coronary bypass surgery or angioplasty, they perceive a limited tolerance for physical work. The deleterious effects of long-term continuous bed rest are often magnified by the relative immobilization, physical deconditioning, and emotional stress of the hospitalization. If not forewarned, patients may misinterpret these physical limitations as indicative of excessively severe coronary disease or inadequate surgical correction. This problem is magnified in previously active elderly coronary patients. Fortunately, appreciable improvement in physical work capacity and activity performance often occurs within a few weeks of beginning exercise training. Physiologic adaptations to exercise training are comparable among elderly patients recovering from myocardial infarction and from myocardial revascularization procedures, despite the greater clinical stability and lesser ischemia among the latter group.

Associated cerebrovascular accident

Both young and elderly patients with residual neurologic deficits resulting from a cerebrovascular accident require increased energy expenditure for self-care and other daily living tasks. Transfer and ambulation activities are important considerations. This is particularly evident in patients whose cerebrovascular accident is a sequel to myocardial infarction or coronary surgery, an occurrence more common in the elderly. Less difficulty is encountered by elderly patients with an acute coronary event whose disability is due to a remote cerebrovascular accident; these patients have already acquired the skills needed to perform daily activities, which can be accomplished without excessive energy cost.

REHABILITATION OF ELDERLY PATIENTS WITH OTHER CARDIOVASCULAR PROBLEMS

Hypertension

Much of the cardiovascular morbidity and mortality in the elderly is related to hypertension, a condition present in about 40% of white persons and over 50% of black persons over age 65 in the U.S. Hypertension increases the risk of myocardial infarction, stroke, and congestive heart failure comparable to the increased risk in younger individuals [37]. Conversely, control of even modest diastolic hypertension reduces substantially both cardiovascular and total morbidity and mortality [38]. Control of isolated systolic hypertension in the elderly may limit cardiovascular morbidity and mortality [39].

Current recommendations are for drug therapy to achieve goal blood pressure levels of 140/90 to 160/90 mmHg [32]. However, complications of antihypertensive therapy are frequent in elderly patients; decreased renal function increases the likelihood of drug toxicity, and the aged patient with diminished baroreceptor sensitivity is more susceptible to the orthostatic complications of volume depletion. Teaching patients who receive anti-hypertensive drugs to assume upright posture gradually may limit dizziness and syncope.

Dosage of antihypertensive drugs should be increased gradually in elderly patients. When the response to therapy is assessed, blood pressure should be measured both in the sitting and standing postures because of the frequent orthostatic decrease in blood pressure. Supplementary potassium is generally warranted when a thiazide diuretic is used because dietary inadequacies in the elderly increase the likelihood of hypokalemia. Reserpine should be avoided in patients with associated depression. Dietary sodium restriction is helpful in limiting the dosage of drugs and the complicating hypokalemia.

Aortic valve disease

Heart valves increase in thickness and rigidity with age, have an increased collagen content, and may undergo degenerative calcification. Alternatively, myxomatous valvular degeneration may occur.

A short, early-peaking basal systolic murmur is the most common murmur in the elderly, occurring in as many as one third to one half of patients. A frequently associated S_4 reflects the reduced compliance of the aged ventricle. It typically is asymptomatic, without hemodynamic consequence, and probably reflects aortic sclerosis, although turbulent blood flow in a dilated aorta has also been proposed as an explanation. Education is appropriate regarding the need for endocarditis prophylaxis.

This entity must be differentiated from hemodynamically significant aortic stenosis, characteristically with valvular calcification, the most common anatomic cause of syncope in the elderly and the major valvular disease of the elderly patient amenable to surgical correction [17,20,40,41]. Because the clinical examination may be misleading, with a rigid arterial wall masking the diagnostic slow-rising carotid pulse abnormality, the late-peaking character of the murmur should be sought. Echocardiography with Doppler study can estimate the severity of aortic outflow obstruction, but cardiac catheterization is necessary before surgery in a symptomatic patient—that is, one with exertional syncope, congestive heart failure, or angina pectoris—since coronary arterial status must be known to define the need for concomitant coronary bypass surgery. Exercise testing is hazardous if critical aortic stenosis is suspected because it may precipitate sudden death. Left ventricular function is typically well preserved, and aortic valve replacement is the indicated procedure. It significantly increases survival, and the relief of symptoms is often spectacular even in old age [17,20,40,41]. Gradually progressive ambulation is appropriate after successful surgery and decreases postoperative complications.

Hypertrophic obstructive cardiomyopathy

Hypertrophic obstructive cardiomyopathy (idiopathic hypertrophic subaortic stenosis) is a common problem in the elderly population and predominates in women; it is often either unrecognized or confused with valvular aortic stenosis or atherosclerotic coronary heart disease with papillary muscle dysfunction [20,42].

Following diagnosis by echocardiography, the discontinuation of drugs such as nitroglycerin, cardiac glycosides, diuretic agents, and so forth, which may exacerbate outflow tract obstruction, and the institution of therapy with beta-adrenergic blocking agents or verapamil typically cause remission of symptoms. Hypovolemia should be avoided, and education is needed about antibiotic prophylaxis against infective endocarditis.

Management of the elderly cardiac patient with congestive heart failure [20,43,44]

The initial approach to the management of heart failure in the elderly cardiac patient is the search for remediable precipitating factors: anemia, infection with fever and tachycardia, pulmonary embolism, thyrotoxicosis, etc. Dietary sodium indiscretion may be a precipitating factor. The cornerstones of therapy are physical and emotional rest, decrease of sodium and water retention, reversal of excessive compensatory peripheral vasoconstriction, and improvement of myocardial contractility. The term *heart failure*, often frightening to the patient, should be explained as signifying only limitation of the heart's pumping ability, a feature that can be improved by therapy.

Although the elderly patient with congestive cardiac failure is often restless and agitated, these symptoms respond better to control of heart failure than to sedation or tranquilizers. Gradual diuresis is indicated, with avoidance of hypovolemia and hypokalemia. Transient elevation of the blood urea nitrogen and, at times, confusion are common when diuresis is excessively brisk.

The patient with severe heart failure may, initially, breathe more easily and be more comfortable sitting in a chair than recumbent in bed. Once the heart failure is controlled, gradual mobilization is indicated; the patient should be closely observed for fatigue, breathlessness, edema, or weight gain as activity is increased. Dietary alterations may prove difficult for elderly patients, and repeated explanations, including specific instructions about food purchase and preparation, may be needed; the help of family members may be enlisted. The preprocessed "convenience foods," often a significant component of the diet of elderly individuals, have high sodium content and should be avoided. At times, asking patients to weigh themselves daily demonstrates the weight gain caused by excess sodium intake and may encourage adherence to sodium restriction.

Psychologic rehabilitation, with an optimistic attitude that the patient need not be a cardiac cripple, is important. Newer vasodilator drugs have greatly improved the symptomatic status and prognosis for patients with severe congestive heart failure. However, these drugs must be administered judiciously, since the compromised baroreceptor function of elderly patients may result in symptomatic hypotension if vasodilator therapy is excessive. Before discharge from the hospital, maintenance drug therapy should be simplified, using as few drugs and as limited a dosage schedule as are feasible.

In elderly patients with preserved systolic function (and usually with normal heart size), pulmonary congestion and other typical manifestations of heart failure may be due to diastolic dysfunction [45]. Differentiation from systolic dysfunction has important therapeutic implications; the patient with abnormal ventricular compliance and often a hypertrophied left ventricle often responds adversely to digitalis and diuretic drugs that reduce ventricular filling volume.

The elderly patient with a cardiac pacemaker [20,46]
The cardiac skeleton becomes increasingly dense with age. An increase in fibrous and elastic tissue, sclerosis of collagen, and often subsequent calcification of the conduction system underlie the increased occurrence of conduction disturbances and atrioventricular block. Atherosclerotic coronary heart disease is a further contributor. Sinoatrial node disease may result in symptomatic bradyarrhythmias and tachyarrhythmias.

Patients with symptomatic complete heart block and the sick sinus syndrome have had an improvement both in survival and in life quality when treated with permanent cardiac pacemakers. Dual-chambered pacemakers are preferrable for reasonably active elderly patients, despite their increased cost and more complex requirements for implantation and surveillance. Atrial synchrony contributes importantly to late diastolic ventricular filling and adequacy of the cardiac output in the poorly compliant aged ventricle. However, elderly patients tend to be excessively concerned about failure of life-sustaining equipment such as cardiac pacemakers, because they more readily appreciate their importance than understand the features of their electromechanical performance. Education regarding pacemaker surveillance is an important rehabilitative component; teaching elderly patients to check the function of their pacemaker and instructing them in the use of telephone pacemaker surveillance systems can provide the needed reassurance.

ACKNOWLEDGEMENT

With appreciation to Julia Wright and Jeanette Zahler for help in the preparation of the manuscript.

REFERENCES

1. Fleg JL and Lakatta EG. 1988. Role of muscle loss in the age-associated reduction in VO_2 max. J Appl Physiol 65:1147–1151.
2. Rodeheffer RJ, Gerstenblith G, Becker LC, et al. 1984. Exercise cardiac output is maintained with advancing age in healthy human subjects: cardiac dilatation and increased stroke volume compensate for a diminished heart rate. Circulation 69:203–213.
3. Haber P, Honiger B, Klicpera M and Niederberger M. 1984. Effects in elderly people 67–76 years of age of three-month endurance training on a bicycle ergometer. Eur Heart J 5 (Suppl E):37–39.
4. Skinner JS. 1970. The cardiovascular system with aging and exercise. In D Brunner and E Jokl (eds), Physical Activity and Aging. Baltimore: University Park Press, pp 100–108.
5. Adams GM and DeVries HA. 1973. Physiological effects of an exercise training program upon women 52 to 79. J Gerontol 28:50–55.
6. DeVries HA. 1971. Exercise intensity threshold for improvement of cardiovascular respiratory function in older men. Geriatrics 26:96–101.
7. Blumenthal JA, Emery CF, Madden DJ, et al. 1989. Cardiovascular and behavioral effects of aerobic exercise training in healthy older men and women. J Gerontol 44:M147–M157.
8. Wolfel EE and Hossack KF. 1989. Guidelines for the exercise training of elderly healthy individuals and elderly patients with cardiac disease. J Cardiopulmon Rehabil 9:40–45.
9. Williams MA, Maresh CM, Esterbrooks DJ, et al. 1985. Early exercise training in patients older than age 65 years compared with that in younger patients after acute myocardial infarction or coronary atery bypass grafting. Am J Cardiol 55:263–266.
10. Wenger NK. 1992. Populations with special needs for exercise rehabilitation; elderly coronary patients. In NK Wenger and HK Hellerstein (eds), Rehabilitation of the Coronary Patient, 3rd ed. New York: Churchill Livingstone, pp 415–420.
11. Bassey EK. 1978. Age, inactivity and some physiological responses to exercise. Gerontology 24:66–77.
12. Shephard RJ. 1989. Habitual physical activity levels and perception of exertion in the elderly. J Cardiopulmon Rehabil 9:17–23.
13. Peach H and Pathy J. 1979. Disability in the elderly after myocardial infarction. J R Coll Phys Lond 13:154–157.
14. White PD. 1957. The role of exercise in the aging. JAMA 165:70–71.
15. Larson EB and Bruce RA. 1987. Health benefits of exercise in an aging society. Arch Intern Med 147:353–356.
16. Ades PA and Grunvald MH. 1990. Cardiopulmonary exercise testing before and after conditioning in older coronary patients. Am Heart J 120:585–589.
17. Wenger NK. 1989. The elderly patient with cardiovascular disease. In WW Parmley and K Chatterjee (eds), Cardiology. Philadelphia: JB Lippincott, pp 1–18.
18. Semple T and Williams BO. 1976. Coronary care for the elderly. In FI Caird, JLC Dall, and RD Kennedy (eds), Cardiology in Old Age. New York: Plenum Press, pp 297–313.
19. Chaturvedi NC, Shivalingappa G, Shanks B, et al. 1972. Myocardial infarction in the elderly. Lancet 1:280–282.
20. Wenger NK, Marcus FI and O'Rourke RA (eds). 1987. 18th Bethesda Conference. Cardiovascular disease in the elderly. J Am Coll Cardiol 10 (Suppl A):2A–87A.
21. Wenger NK. 1992. In-hospital exercise rehabilitation after myocardial infarction and myocardial revascularization: physiologic basis, methodology, and results. In NK Wenger and HK Hellerstein (eds), Rehabilitation of the Coronary Patient, 3rd ed. New York: Churchill Livingstone, pp 351–365.
22. Wenger NK and Fletcher GF. 1990. Rehabilitation of the patient with atherosclerotic coronary heart disease. In JW Hurst (ed), The Heart, 7th ed. New York: McGraw-Hill, pp 1103–1118.

23. Shephard R. 1990. The scientific basis of exercise prescribing for the very old. J Am Geriatr Soc 38:62–70.
24. Fentem PH, Jones PRM, MacDonald IC and Scriven PM. 1976. Changes in the body composition of elderly men following retirement from the steel industry. J Physiol 258: 29P–30P.
25. Sidney KH, Shephard RM and Harrison JE. 1977. Endurance training and the body composition of the elderly. Am J Clin Nutr 30:326–333.
26. Fiatarone MA, Marks EC, Ryan ND, et al. 1990. High-intensity strength training in nonagenarians. Effects on skeletal muscle. JAMA 263:3029–3034.
27. Gottlieb SO, Gottlieb SH, Achuff SC, et al. 1988. Silent ischemia on Holter monitoring predicts mortality in high-risk postinfarction patients. JAMA 259:1030–1035.
28. Borg G. 1982. Psychophysical bases for perceived exertion. Med Sci Sports Exerc 14: 377–381.
29. Jajich CL, Ostfeld AM and Freeman DH. 1984. Smoking and coronary heart disease mortality in the elderly. JAMA 252:2831–2834.
30. Pathy MS and Peach H. 1980. Disability among the elderly after myocardial infarcton: a 3-year follow-up. J R Coll Phys Lond 14:221–223.
31. Ouslander JG. 1981. Drug therapy in the elderly. Ann Intern Med 95:711–722.
32. The Working Group on Hypertension in the Elderly. 1986. Statement on hypertension in the elderly. JAMA 256:70–74.
33. Gersh B. 1983. Coronary arteriography and coronary artery bypass surgery: morbidity and mortality in patients ages 65 years or older. Circulation 63:483–491.
34. Gersh BJ, Kronmal RA, Schaff HV, et al. 1983. Long-term (5 year) results of coronary bypass surgery in patients 65 years old or older: a report from the Coronary Artery Surgery Study. Circulation 68 (Suppl II):II-190–II-199.
35. Naunheim KS, Kern MJ, McBride LR, et al. 1987. Coronary artery bypass surgery in patients aged 80 years or older. Am J Cardiol 59:804–807.
36. Jeroudi MO, Kleiman NS, Minor ST, et al. 1990. Percutaneous transluminal coronary angioplasty in octogenarians. Ann Intern Med 113:423–428.
37. Whelton PK. 1985. Hypertension in the elderly. In R Andres, EL Bierman, and WR Hazzard (eds), Principles of Geriatric Medicine. New York: McGraw-Hill, pp 536–551.
38. Amery A, Birkenhager W, Brixko P, et al. 1985. European Working Party on High Blood Pressure in the Elderly: mortality and morbidity results from the European Working Party on High Blood Pressure in the Elderly Trial. Lancet 1:1349–1354.
39. SHEP Cooperative Research Group. 1991. Prevention of stroke by antihypertensive drug treatment in older persons with isolated systolic hypertension: final results of the Systolic Hypertension in the Elderly Program (SHEP). JAMA 265:3255–3264.
40. Craver JM, Goldstein J, Jones EL, et al. 1984. Clinical, hemodynamic, and operative descriptors affecting outcome of aortic valve replacement in elderly vs young patients. Ann Surg 199:733–741.
41. Levinson JR, Akins CW, Buckley MJ, et al. 1989. Octogenarians with aortic stenosis. Outcome after aortic valve replacement. Circulation 80 (Suppl I):I-49–I-56.
42. Lever HM, Karam RF, Currie PJ, et al. 1989. Hypertrophic cardiomyopathy in the elderly. Distinctions from the young based on cardiac shape. Circulation 79:580–589.
43. Fleg JL. 1988. Congestive heart failure in the elderly. J Geriatr Drug Ther 3:5–22.
44. Jessup M, Lakatta EG, Leier CV, et al. 1990. Managing CHF in the older patient. Patient Care 24:55–75.
45. Wong WF, Gold S, Fukuyama O, et al. 1989. Diastolic dysfunction in elderly patients with congestive heart failure. Am J Cardiol 63:1526–1528.
46. Report of the Joint American College of Cardiology/American Heart Association Task Force on Assessment of Cardiovascular Procedures (Subcommittee on Pacemaker Implantation). 1984. Guidelines for permanent cardiac pacemaker implantation, May 1984. J Am Coll Cardiol 4:434–442.

22. MEDICAL TREATMENT OF CARDIOVASCULAR DISEASE

LIONEL H. OPIE
T.A. MABIN
P. de V. MEIRING

Unique features of illness in the elderly may interfere with effective
drug therapy more than changed pharmacokinetics.

—J.G. Ouslander [1]

Elderly patients constitute a group in whom diseases are "creeping up."
These diseases may not be cardiovascular, but they do influence the general
level of activity of the patient and the general feeling of health or ill health.
Therefore, the patient may apparently present with a cardiovascular problem
when the real diagnosis lies elsewhere.

Among such conditions are anemia, whether caused by iron deficiency or
by a mitotic process; uremia presenting with anemia or a general lack of
energy; and infections, among which infective endocarditis (especially the
classical subacute variety) is important. The manifestations of all these
diseases may be atypical in the elderly.

In cardiac disease, there are important changes in the clinical presentation.
For example, the murmur of aortic stenosis may best be heard at the apex
and not at the base of the heart. A patient with a small nodular goiter or with
a retrosternal goiter unapparent in the neck may develop thyrocardiac
disease, which must be suspected and excluded. Similarly, a patient generally

Franz H. Messerli (ed.), CARDIOVASCULAR DISEASE IN THE ELDERLY (Third Edition). Copyright
© *1993 Kluwer Academic Publishers. ISBN 0-7923-1859-5. All rights reserved.*

"dropping off" in health and presenting with heart disease, especially with an enlarged heart, may be suffering from myxedema.

A disease not usually missed in the elderly, but misdiagnosed, is hypertension. The levels for normality vary greatly, and there are no conclusive data showing that treatment of mild hypertension without end-organ damage improves overall mortality in this age group, although cardiovascular events are lessened [2]. Systolic hypertension can be a serious problem because of the difficulty in assessing its significance and the difficulty in treating it successfully. Yet hypertension may present with cardiac or renal failure or with a cerebrovascular event.

INDIVIDUAL ASSESSMENT

Not only may disease present in an obscure way, but also the resistance of elderly people to disease varies greatly. It is common knowledge that some elderly patients retain mental and physical vigor, while others suffer severely from apparently minor disease. Especially critical is the retention of *cerebral function*: can the patient understand and carry out the doctor's instructions? Social factors, too, may play a critical role. A loving, alert family can give great personal support, even to a patient in an old-age home. Poverty cannot only rob the patient of optimal medical care but can also divert the patient's drive from attaining optimal health to simply staying alive.

Specific attention must be paid to *renal function*. Whereas cardiac failure, liver disease, and cerebrovascular accidents are usually not difficult to diagnose, renal impairment may be inapparent and only disclosed by measuring plasma creatinine and urea. Renal function critically governs the dose of commonly used drugs excreted by the kidneys and not metabolized by the liver: digoxin and atenolol. Renal impairment also governs the ultimate excretion of some drugs that undergo prior hepatic metabolism such as procainamide and methyldopa.

Compliance in the elderly

One significant factor in compliance of the elderly is that a failing mind, if present, would mean that complex instructions need simplification. Other factors that hinder compliance are multiple chronic illness with complex drug regimes, poor vision, poor hearing, and weakened arthritic hands, to which can be added sheer obstinacy or other psychological problems, perhaps the result of a small and inapparent stroke [1]. Remedies include clear instructions, tablet identification cards, tear-off calendars, and above all, careful supervision with repetitive checks on compliance. A useful procedure can be followed in patients taking digoxin among other drugs. Once the patient is stabilized under careful supervision and the correct dosage is found, any variations in the blood level are most likely to result from variable compliance.

Favoring good compliance is the relatively straightforward daily regimen of many elderly patients, especially those in nursing homes. Such elderly patients are among the few in whom thrice-daily medications are likely to be taken, whereas in younger patients the dose taken in the middle of the day is frequently missed. Bearing in mind the above factors, compliance in the elderly with good brain function is as good as in young patients.

Polypharmacy

Elderly patients are said to receive quite often between 3 and 12 medications, many of which are ineffective or inappropriate. Thus there are two dangers: multiple-drug interactions and failure of compliance. Physicians are often not rigorous enough in making exact diagnoses in the elderly and in limiting drugs to the minimum number needed. It is a real problem to decide which of the multiple antidepressants and analgesics that many elderly patients receive are really essential. Similarly, the physician attending the elderly patient for the first time may find that digoxin and antihypertensive drugs are being taken apparently for no reason. Nevertheless, the physician fears that removal of the drug will allow inapparant cardiac failure or hypertension to "creep back." In the case of digoxin, several studies have shown that the agent is overprescribed and unnecessary for many elderly patients. For example, Dall found that 75% of his elderly population did not need their digoxin [3]. Frequently, the dose was too high; more frequently, the dose was too low and compliance was poor.

Cautious withdrawal with a reversed therapeutic trial is essential; otherwise, polypharmacy will be perpetuated.

Drug interactions

Elderly patients are frequently treated with mood-altering drugs, which can interact with cardioactive drugs. For example, lithium can interact with diuretics, and tricyclic antidepressants can interact with cardiac and antihypertensive drugs. Multiple-drug therapy is not taken, not only because of problems of compliance but because of problems with cost. In every case the physician should consider whether any proposed new therapy is really essential, because for every additional tablet taken, the incidence of noncompliance arises.

PHARMACOKINETICS IN THE ELDERLY

Altered pharmacokinetics of normally used agents may also cause unusual manifestations of disease (tables 22-1, 22-2, and 22-3). For example, the low liver blood flow associated with age means that propranolol accumulates in the blood with the potential for serious central nervous side effects (figure 22-1). In a similar way, the decreased glomerular filtration rate of the elderly means that digitalis toxicity is more likely to occur when digoxin is used because it is excreted by the kidneys. Those elderly patients who are poorly nourished may have low plasma protein concentrations with altered

Table 22-1. Digoxin pharmacokinetics and effects in the elderly

Process	Effect of age	Reference
Absorption	Slightly delayed	[4]
Distribution to tissue	Decreased distribution volume	[5]
Protein binding (20%)	Unchanged	[6][a]
Binding to receptor	Probably normal	[7][a]
Inotropic effect	Decreased	[7,8][a]
Toxic arrhythmias	Unchanged	[8][a]
Plasma half-life	Increased	[9]
Renal excretion	May be decreased	[5]

[a] Animal studies.

Table 22-2. Propranolol pharmacokinetics and its effects in the elderly

Process	Effect of age	Reference
Absorption	Probably delayed	—
Hepatic metabolism	Diminished metabolism	[10]
Bioavailability	Increased	[11]
Receptor sensitivity	Decreased	[11]
Lymphocyte receptor density	Decreased	[12]

Table 22-3. Effects of aging on metabolism of ACE inhibitors

	Effect	Reference
1. *Captopril-like drugs*	Delayed renal clearance	[13]
2. *Enalapril-like drugs*	1. Delayed conversion to active form, e.g. enalaprilat	[14]
Enalapril	2. Delayed clearance of active form	[15]
Cilazapril		[16]
Perindopril		
Ramipril		[17]
3. *Lisinopril-like drugs*	Delayed renal clearance in relation to fall in glomerular	
Lisinopril	filtration rate	[18]

pharmacokinetics of plasma-bound beta-blockers (propranolol, alprenolol, pindolol) so that the lower doses are required for the same effective blood level. Because tissue sensitivity to beta-antagonists is decreased (table 22-2), the "average" dose of propranolol in younger subjects will also be about right for the elderly. It goes without saying that an initial small dose should be cautiously increased, especially in view of the impaired cardiovascular function found in the elderly [1]. Increasingly, changes in receptor density and signaling systems are being emphasized.

The general pharmacokinetic rule is that the tendency is toward decreased

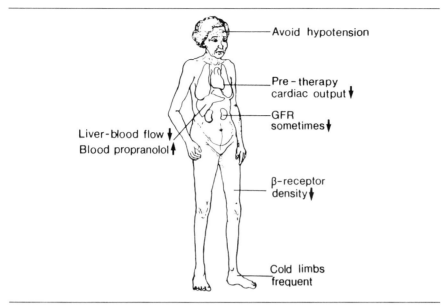

Figure 22-1. Beta-blockade in the elderly. Figure copyright: L.H. Opie.

clearance with higher effective blood levels and a greater chance of side effects (table 22-4) [1,7,20–26]. In the case of nitroprusside, increased sensitivity is explained by impaired reflex vasoconstriction. For beta-adrenoreceptor agonists, the decreased tissue beta-receptor density explains the decreased response to beta-stimulation, so a higher than normal dose should be required. This is, therefore, an exception to the general rule.

Angiotensin-converting enzyme (ACE) inhibitors are now being used increasingly in elderly patients both for the treatment of hypertension and congestive heart failure. Their pharmacokinetics are also altered by age (table 22-3). In general, there are three types of agents: those like captopril, those like enalapril, and those like lisinopril. For different reasons, the dose of each of these agents may have to be reduced in elderly patients, particularly in those in whom there is impairment of hepatic or renal blood flow.

HYPERTENSION

The picture, therefore, emerges of disease "creeping up" inadvertently in elderly patients and of unusual manifestations of common diseases, as well as problems with drug doses and compliance. Within this overall context, certain specific cardiovascular disease entities must be recognized and treated. Of these, hypertension is probably the most common. Although the blood pressure normally increases with age, there is some evidence that levels for therapy should be similar to those taken in younger patients, and in the

Table 22-4. Effects of aging on other cardiovascular agents

Drug	Effect of age	Reference
Beta-agonists	Decreased chronotropic response	[13,14]
	Decreased inotropic response	[14,15]
Beta$_2$ agonists	Increased vasodilator response	[19]
Lidocaine	Potentially decreased hepatic clearance if low cardiac output; otherwise normal	[16]
Nitroprusside	Greater fall in blood pressure during infusion	[1]
Procainamide and	Decreased renal clearance	[17]
N-acetyl-procainamide	Increased blood levels	[7]
Quinidine	Decreased renal and total clearance	[18]
Warfarin	Greater depression of clotting factors	[19]

Sources:
1. Ouslander, Ann Intern Med 95:711, 1981.
7. Gerstenblith et al., Circ Res 44:517, 1979.

European study, patients whose pressures exceeded 160/90 mmHg were treated with apparent benefit [2]. However, our view is that diastolic pressures should be higher, probably above 105 mmHg, to warrant treatment [27] and that initial treatment in the lower range should be nonpharmacologic. We recognize the importance of systolic hypertension, but await trials currently underway in the United States for specific guidance.

The benefits of treatment based on meta-analysis [28] include a 28% fall in cardiovascular mortality, largely a cerebrovascular effect with a significant fall of 41%, and little significant effect on coronary mortality. The total mortality, however, was not significantly reduced, with a fall of 14% ($p = 0.07$). Whereas in middle-aged patients large numbers must be treated to avoid one stroke, in the elderly only 34 patients need to be treated for one year to avoid one cerebrovascular event [29].

Diuretics

Traditionally, diuretics are the mainstay of hypertension therapy in elderly patients. Equally traditionally, it is the thiazide diuretics that are normally first chosen. Yet such diuretics can have unusual effects. For example, in a recent series described by Ashraf et al., a small number of elderly patients were in danger of developing severe hyponatremia, presenting indirectly with a change in mood and failure to concentrate mentally [30]. Patients sometimes collapsed within two weeks of the onset of thiazide treatment, and some developed permanent brain damage caused by cerebral edema. The basic cause was impaired ability to dilute urine, with consequent dilutional hyponatremia. Fortunately, this is clearly a rare complication; however, the message is that electrolytes should be checked within two weeks of starting thiazide therapy. This will also guard against the occasional patient developing hypokalemia, which usually occurs within a week of starting therapy if it is going to occur at all. A further potential problem is diuretic-induced hypotension, predisposed to by impaired renal mechanisms for conservation of salt and water [31].

The present trend with hypertension is away from the routine use of potassium supplements, especially because they require dosages of many tablets, which in turn lead to loss of compliance. Potassium-sparing diuretics used alone or in combination have an added theoretical danger in that impaired renal function in the elderly may predispose to hyperkalemia. It should be recalled that in hypertension the dose–response curve to diuretics is flat; hence, failure to respond to a diuretic calls for another agent rather than a higher dosage of diuretic. The optimal dose of hydrochlorothiazide is likely to be no more than 25 mg daily, as in the thiazide-triamterene (K^+ sparing) combination successfully used in the European trial [2].

In hypertensive patients with renal impairment, furosemide is thought to be the agent of choice, although strict data are missing. Again, potassium replacement is not routinely necessary; small doses of furosemide (no more than 20 mg) should be used at the start, because some of these patients will react adversely with marked volume loss and hemoconcentration. As in the case of thiazide diuretics, the best policy is to start the treatment with small doses and to bring the patient back soon to check for possible adverse effects and to check the electrolytes. Much higher doses may be needed in renal failure.

A mild diuretic recently introduced is indapamide. This is a thiazide-like agent that is effectively hypotensive at doses that do not cause a marked diuresis. Although it is claimed to have few side effects, hypokalemia has been reported.

Beta-blockade

Beta-blockade, although frequently held to be harmful in the elderly group, is in fact a permissible form of therapy for hypertension [32], and some authorities consider it a preferred form of treatment in patients with symptoms of ischemic heart disease. Beta-blockade may be used as initial monotherapy and, if needed, a diuretic added [33], despite conventional wisdom opting for initial diuretic therapy. Propranolol has some problems with pharmacokinetics, stemming from a low cardiac output and poor renal perfusion—and hence an altered first-pass effect and an unexpected accumulation in the blood. Therefore, beta-blockers with simple pharmacokinetics and no first-pass metabolism, such as nadolol, sotalol, and atenolol, are preferred. In our practice, we routinely use atenolol because of the added advantage of cardioselectivity and because dose-ranging is usually not needed. In the United Kingdom and South Africa, the standard dosage of atenolol is 100 mg daily, irrespective of age. Hence, the American recommended standard dosage of 50 mg daily gives an added safety factor.

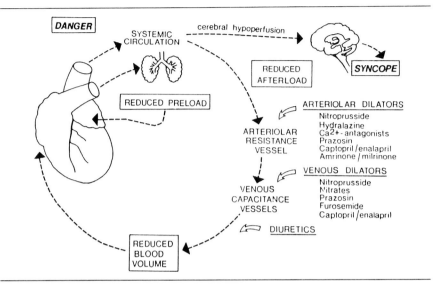

Figure 22-2. Vasodilator therapy in the elderly. A contraindication is aortic stenosis (frequently difficult to diagnose in the elderly), and a relative contraindication is a history of cerebral ischemia. Figure copyright: L.H. Opie.

Another promising agent is celiprolol, a vasodilating cardioselective beta-blocker [34].

Vasodilators

Vasodilators have been regarded as third-line therapy for hypertension in the elderly, with care taken to use small initial doses. Vasodilators frequently do not work satisfactorily because of rather rigid vessel walls. Furthermore, agents such as hydralazine can cause a very acute vasodilation with a marked drop in blood pressure and threatened cerebral vascular accident. After cautious introduction (10 mg twice daily), standard doses of hydralazine (up to 100 mg daily) can be used. Two new alternatives in therapy are the calcium antagonists and the converting enzyme inhibitors, which will be discussed later. Prazosin must be introduced at a low dosage of 0.5 mg at night to avoid first-pass syncope; progressive increases up to 20 mg in two divided doses per day are permissible. Side effects are common with vasodilators (figure 22-2).

The arterial blood pressure must never be decreased too abruptly in elderly patients: there is an ever-present risk of cerebral hypoperfusion with stroke [35]. Therefore, after thiazide diuretics and beta-blockade have failed to hold the day, we usually turn to a centrally acting agent such as reserpine or methyldopa. Methyldopa is contraindicated in the presence of liver disease and requires a check for blood hemolysis after starting. Because of possible effects on memory, we avoid using methyldopa whenever possible, although it was the second-line agent in the European trial [2]. Reserpine must be avoided in elderly patients who are depressed—and many of them are. In others, a low dosage of reserpine should be safe. Clonidine we avoid because of its side effects: sedation and mood depression, and the danger of withdrawal-rebound hypertension.

Calcium antagonists

Verapamil can be used in graded doses and is reported specifically to benefit hypertension of the elderly [36]. Side effects have thus far not been serious, although constipation is the most common. Other calcium antagonists such as nitrendipine [36] and nifedipine have also been used. Nifedipine is especially effective in systolic hypertension (next section); we usually first give a test dose of 5 mg in case of adverse, overvigorous vasodilation.

Angiotensin–converting enzyme inhibitors

Because many other vasodilators may precipitate hypoperfusion of organs in the elderly, the ACE inhibitors such as captopril and enalapril are now being used as vasodilators of choice, and even as first-line treatment in elderly patients [37,38]. There are seldom serious side effects, provided that bilateral renal artery stenosis is absent. These agents often seem to work best in the presence of an added diuretic [38]. When using an ACE inhibitor with a diuretic, any potassium-retaining compounds should be avoided because of the antialdosterone effect of the ACE inhibitors. This consideration may be particularly important in the elderly, in whom renal function is more likely to be depressed.

Systolic hypertension therapy

The therapy of systolic hypertension is generally difficult. A pragmatic approach is that a systolic level of about 170 mmHg may be accepted in an elderly patient, whereas higher values can be brought down; much depends on whether there is target organ involvement. In the United States, the tendency is to treat systolic hypertension more actively. Recent data show that calcium-antagonist agents such as nifedipine are usually effective in systolic hypertension in the elderly [39]. Trials recently published show that the treatment of isolated systolic hypertension is warranted and benefits the patient.

CONGESTIVE HEART FAILURE

The most common causes of congestive heart failure in the elderly are, as in middle age, ischemic heart disease, hypertensive heart disease, valvular heart disease, and cardiomyopathy [40].

The principles of treatment of congestive heart failure are the same as in other patients: diuretics first, then added digitalis, and then added afterload-reducing agents. The hazards of diuretics in the elderly have already been underlined in the section dealing with hypertension.

Diuretics

As far as diuretics are concerned, the care required has been outlined. Diuretics are frequently given to the elderly for a variety of reasons; in one study, about one third of elderly patients were receiving diuretic therapy. Elderly patients should be gently treated and not be "hammered" with diuretics, especially not with chlorthalidone, which is long-acting and may cause nocturia and insomnia. As the glomerular filtration rate falls with age, a loop diuretic such as furosemide becomes a particularly useful agent, and many elderly patients can be maintained on small doses. In addition, small further doses of thiazide diuretic appear to potentiate and maintain diuresis. A reasonable regimen is to alternate a low dosage of furosemide—the lowest required (say 20 mg daily)—with one tablet of thiazide diuretic. Such therapy is frequently effective once the edema of the heart failure has been controlled.

Although there may be risks to loop diuretic therapy in the elderly, the effects of furosemide are in fact delayed in this age group, and the tendency to excrete potassium [41,42] is less. Thus, the risks of potassium depletion in the average elderly treated with low-dose loop diuretic may be rather low, unless the dietary intake is poor.

The dangers of electrolyte disequilibrium are twofold. First, both thiazides and loop diuretics can occasionally cause substantial potassium and sodium loss. Hypokalemia sensitizes the patient to digitalis toxicity. As is the case when diuretics are used for hypertension, the plasma potassium level needs checking soon after starting diuretic therapy, and if low (below 3.5 mEq/L), a diuretic with added potassium-retaining qualities (Dyazide, Moduretic, Maxide) is indicated. Of these, Dyazide is best tested in the elderly [2]. Oral potassium supplements come in bulky packing and are frequently not taken. Hence, we frequently combine low-dose furosemide with low-dose combination thiazide-amiloride or thiazide-triamterene except in the presence of renal impairment. Such attention to the potassium balance may be required even in the elderly because of their lower estimated dietary potassium intake. Thus, some elderly patients may not like or cannot afford potassium-rich fruits, fruit juices, and milk. It was thought that the total body potassium drops as age proceeds [43], but the basic problem is a loss of potassium-rich tissue rather than a true action depletion [44].

A converse danger of diuretic therapy is that of hyperkalemia, resulting from the combination of a potassium-sparing diuretic with oral potassium supplements in the presence of even mild renal impairment. Thus, measurements of plasma potassium and creatinine before and soon after starting diuretic therapy are highly desirable, with further six-month measurements thereafter.

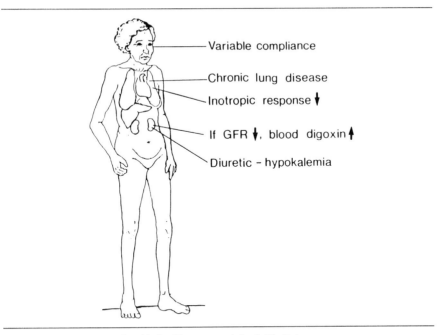

Figure 22-3. Digoxin in the elderly. Figure copyright: L.H. Opie.

Afterload reduction

Afterload reduction has not been well tested in elderly patients and needs special care because of, as already stressed, the danger of hypotension (figure 22-2). Hypotension may also develop in response to the converting enzyme inhibitors captopril and enalapril, so a low first dose is recommended (e.g., 6.25 mg captopril). Hospitalization for the introduction of the new therapy is sometimes advisable in trial patients. Otherwise, ACE inhibitors are probably the vasodilators of choice in elderly as in younger patients with congestive heart failure. Other vasodilators, such as hydralazine or the calcium antagonists, should also be used with care. An interesting afterload-reducing agent is the oral agent salbutamol, which because of its bronchodilating properties is frequently useful in the elderly patient with chronic obstructive airways disease. However, there are no specific reports commenting on the benefits of this preparation in elderly patients.

ATRIAL FIBRILLATION

Verapamil and/or digoxin

A very good indication for digitalis is atrial fibrillation combined with heart failure. Atrial fibrillation by itself in the absence of heart failure is now frequently treated by verapamil (Isoptin; Calan) instead of digitalis. Verapamil, being a calcium-antagonist agent, acts in a completely different way from digitalis, which inhibits the atrioventricular (A-V) node by increasing the cholinergic vagal tone. Digitalis is positively inotropic, whereas verapamil usually leaves the inotropic state unchanged or decreases it. Therefore, the contraindications are different, but these two agents can be combined provided that high doses of neither are used.

It is widely appreciated that digoxin is excreted by the kidneys; therefore, with the fall in glomerular filtration rate occurring with age, the blood level rises with increased risk of toxicity (figure 22-3). It is perhaps less well appreciated that some elderly patients can be extremely sensitive to the side effects of digitalis compounds and especially appear to develop nausea on low and apparently therapeutic doses. Because of these dangers, doses in the elderly have been generally thought to be about half-normal and sometimes even quarter-normal. However, such low doses frequently have no therapeutic benefit, and, in fact, elderly patients are frequently given digitalis when it is not needed. Therefore, the real need for digitalis should always be reassessed.

To establish the dose of digoxin, excellent nomograms are available. The critical factor is that renal function may be impaired so that the dose must be reduced. Even with normal renal function, a lower than normal body weight means that the maintenance dose is usually below the standard 0.25 mg digoxin given to younger patients; hence a frequent dose is somewhere between 0.125 and 0.25 mg daily. (Quinidine, verapamil, and a number of other drugs are now known to interact with digoxin pharmacokinetics and to raise serum digoxin levels. Extra caution should be taken when these drugs are used in combination, and the dose of digoxin should generally be halved.) The optimal dose can be known only by measuring the blood level and taking the clinical response into account. That response is easiest to assess when the endpoint is the ventricular rate in atrial fibrillation.

Anticoagulation

In patients with nonrheumatic atrial fibrillation, with an average age of 68 years, and about half of whom were hypertensive, anticoagulant therapy with long-term low-dose warfarin markedly reduced the rate of stroke and death [45]. The prothrombin time was about 1.2 to 1.5 times normal, corresponding to an International Normalized Ratio (INR) of 1.5 to 2.7. Whether aspirin is as good as warfarin remains an open question, since there are no really good direct comparisons. In the SPAF study [46], aspirin seems similar to warfarin in efficacy in patients under age 75. The choice between these two agents could in part be decided by coincident aspects of the health of the elderly patient, such as a history of a fall, which is a serious problem in elderly patients receiving warfarin therapy [47].

ANGINA PECTORIS

As stressed in the section on hypertension, beta-blockade should be given with care to the elderly patients. Nitrates remain standard, together with beta-blockade, in the management of angina of effort; overdose must be guarded against so that syncope does not develop. The use of calcium antagonists such as verapamil (Isoptin) is increasing in angina of effort and becoming extremely popular in angina at rest. Verapamil may be a better agent in elderly patients than nifedipine. The latter is a very powerful coronary dilator but also a very powerful afterload reducer, and the blood pressure can fall too abruptly.

An important point of differential diagnosis is that between esophageal spasm and coronary spasm. For a very long time, astute clinicians have appreciated that a cardiac-like pain can originate in the esophagus. The recent description of the syndromes of coronary spasm has also led to an expansion of our knowledge on esophageal spasm. Luckily, both forms of spasm respond to smooth muscle relaxants such as verapamil and nifedipine.

Coronary artery surgery

For severe relentless angina, operative intervention is now being undertaken. Coronary bypass operations are no longer contraindicated in the elderly, and spectacular results can be obtained on selected patients [48]. A heavily calcified aortic arch is a contraindication to cross-clamping of the aorta (and therefore to a bypass operation) because of the risk of atherosclerotic emboli [49].

PTCA

Percutaneous transluminal coronary angioplasty (PTCA) is now used increasingly in elderly patients, whenever possible, to avoid surgery.

ACUTE MYOCARDIAL INFARCTION

Myocardial infarction is almost a physiologic event because of the frequency of coronary atherosclerosis in this age group. Acute myocardial infarction is more likely to be silent in elderly patients than in the younger age groups and may present in unusual ways, such as confusion. These silent MIs frequently occur in diabetic patients; one should therefore specifically look for diabetes and determine whether the patient is experiencing a temporary diabetic state following acute myocardial infarction. The general picture is that of multiple small infarctions caused by the slow development of coronary artery disease. Elderly patients do not tolerate large infarcts well, and mortality and morbidity are generally high.

Once again, the principle of therapy in the acute state is clear: overly vigorous treatment should be avoided, and there should be careful selection of the drugs and dosages. Especially when morphine is given, it should be very carefully titrated, with the patient in the horizontal position, and care should be taken to avoid hypotension. Judging from studies in elderly patients with cancer, smaller doses of morphine are needed for an adequate analgesic effect in elderly patients [1].

Postinfarct anticoagulation

In the postinfarct follow-up period, clinicians usually avoid anticoagulant therapy in the geriatric population because of the hazards of cerebral vascular accident. A European double-blind trial on nearly 900 elderly patients confirmed the higher risk of definite intracranial hemorrhage in the anticoagulant group [50]. An unexpected finding was that the placebo group had a greater number of "intracranial events of unknown nature" (a diagnosis probably including transient ischemic attacks), so that in the placebo group there was an increased number of deaths and a greater number of days lost through neurologic disablement. The anticoagulant group did have the expected tenfold increase in extracranial bleeding episodes, and some required hospitalization; none died. Another problem with anticoagulation in the elderly is the risk of clinically inapparent gastrointestinal or urogenital lesions, benign or malignant, which increase the risk of hemorrhage. The conclusion that the hazards of anticoagulation do not outweigh the benefits when anticoagulation is clinically indicated [50] must be tempered, because patients in that study were a highly selective group and most had already been on anticoagulant therapy for years before the start of the trial. Clinical common sense suggests that anticoagulation should only be undertaken when very clearly required.

Postinfarct beta-blockade

Three recent trials with three different beta-blockers (timolol, metoprolol, propranolol) have shown a benefit for beta-blockade in patients followed after myocardial infarction. All three trials have been excellently designed, and in particular, the timolol trial has been very carefully analyzed without major faults being found thus far. There have been some questions raised by the earlier trials with alprenolol as to whether beta-blockade after infarction is also beneficial in the elderly. That doubt is dispelled by the positive results of the American B-HAT (Beta-Blocker Heart Attack Trial) in patients aged 60 to 69 years [51], timolol in patients aged 65 to 75 years [52], and metoprolol in patients over 65 years [53].

Postinfarct exercise training

Now that elderly patients are more actively treated during their acute infarct period, postinfarct exercise rehabilitation is becoming correspondingly more common. Little is known about the benefits and risks of this procedure in the elderly. In normal elderly subjects, exercise training can be achieved without reversing an exercise-induced fall in the left ventricular ejection fraction [54].

Postinfarct antiplatelet agents

In 1975 the Anturane (sulfinpyrazone) reinfarction trial was started in North America; in 1980 the results showed a reduction in total deaths and especially sudden deaths in the first six months [55]. The results were criticized and not accepted by the FDA. Very recently, the Italian Anturane reinfarction study on 700 patients followed for 1 to 4 years showed an impressive reduction in reinfarction rate with a dose of 400 mg twice daily, but did not show any alteration in total death or sudden death rate as demonstrated in the North American study [56].

The situation with other antiplatelet agents is even less clear. The AMIS (Aspirin Myocardial Infarction Study) found no benefit with a dose of 1 g daily—yet a lower dose, theoretically, could be much more effective [57]. The PARIS (Persantine-Aspirin Reinfarction Study) showed only suggestive benefit [58]. Nonetheless, low-dose aspirin is now routine even for elderly postinfarct patients.

VALVULAR HEART DISEASE

Aortic valve disease

There is a high incidence of systolic murmur in the elderly, and evaluation of such is vital. Aortic ejection murmurs are most commonly due to degenerative aortic sclerosis, but aortic stenosis does occur in about 5% of elderly people. Its severity is often difficult to assess, especially because of the frequency of associated systemic hypertension [59]. Symptoms such as syncope, dyspnea, or angina are attributed to coexisting conditions. Hardening of the arteries and systolic hypertension make evaluation of the character of the pulse unreliable. Isolated aortic stenosis is most commonly due to a congenital bicuspid valve, and this is invariably calcified. Fluoroscopic screening may also reveal calcification of coronary arteries or mitral annular calcification and assists toward the diagnosis and management of systolic murmurs. Critical aortic stenosis should be actively sought in all patients who present with congestive heart failure of unknown cause. The murmur is frequently soft and difficult to hear because of lowered cardiac output. Although classically best heard at the base of the heart and radiating to the neck, it is frequently maximal at the apex and misdiagnosed as mitral incompetence. Two-dimensional echocardiography is often valuable in differentiating aortic from mitral valve disease and in assessing left ventricular function.

Predominant aortic incompetence is less common and is due to degeneration of the aortic valve leaflets, chronic rheumatic heart disease, or rheumatoid valvular involvement.

Left untreated, patients with symptomatic aortic valve disease have a poor prognosis. They represent an urgent indication for investigation and valve replacement. Surgical techniques are now improved and results encouraging; aortic valve replacement therefore should not be denied to elderly patients who are otherwise unwell [59,60,61]. If surgery is not possible for whatever reason, then balloon valvuloplasty may be a viable option.

Mitral valve disease

Degenerative calcification of the mitral ring is common in patients over the age of 70, and the incidence rises with age. Moreover, it is the only degenerative heart condition more common in women. It is usually of no significance, but extensive involvement results in mitral incompetence, and mitral annular calcification is probably the most common abnormality seen in elderly patients with a systolic murmur. Mitral annular calcification is frequently associated with aortic valve calcification [62].

The incidence of chronic rheumatic heart disease is still relatively high in the older patient but is bound to decline in the future with reduction of the disease in the young age group. Less common causes of mitral incompetence in the elderly are papillary muscle dysfunction due to ischemic heart disease, mitral valve prolapse, and hypertrophic cardiomyopathy. Mitral valve prolapse may underlie arrhythmias, bacterial endocarditis [40], disabling chest pain, syncope, and mitral valve regurgitation [63]. Acute mitral incompetence, due to papillary muscle or chordal rupture, gives rise to enormous rises in left atrial pressure, and presents with acute severe dyspnea; it usually necessitates early mitral valve replacement.

Diastolic murmurs due to mitral stenosis from chronic rheumatic heart disease are often difficult to detect in elderly patients because of low cardiac output and hyperinflated lung fields. So-called "silent" mitral stenosis should always be considered in patients presenting in pulmonary edema of unknown cause.

Unlike symptomatic aortic valve disease, mitral valve disease is treated initially with medication. Diuretics should be the first line of treatment, with the addition of digoxin if atrial fibrillation or significant mitral incompetence is present. In patients with atrial fibrillation, anticoagulation or at least the use of aspirin should be considered. Cautious administration of vasodilator therapy in patients with predominant mitral incompetence may bring considerable relief to those elderly patients unable to have mitral valve replacement.

Mitral valve replacement should be considered if medical treatment fails to control the symptoms adequately. Valvotomy is rarely possible in the elderly because calcification of the valve is invariable, and mitral valve replacement is usually necessary. Once again, the results of surgery in the 70-to-80 age group have been most encouraging.

ACUTE PULMONARY EDEMA

In the therapy of acute pulmonary edema in the elderly, the possibility of sensitivity to diuretics and insensitivity to digitalis must be taken into account. Acute preload reduction may be achieved with sublingual nitroglycerine 0.5 mg or sublingual isosorbide dinitrate 5 mg, taking care to avoid hypotension. Effective preload reduction may also be achieved in the gravely ill patient with intravenous furosemide (dose, 40–80 mg); if necessary, nitroprusside is used, provided that intensive hemodynamic monitoring is available to avoid arterial hypotension (beware of rebound hypertension if nitroprusside is abruptly stopped).

INFECTIVE ENDOCARDITIS

In general, in elderly patients even mild septicemic states can cause great problems in diagnosis and treatment. Elderly patients can die with only a mild temperature despite a septicemia that is frequently gram-negative in origin. In recent years infective endocarditis has become predominantly a disease of the elderly, not only because of the availability of antibiotic prophylaxis and the decline in rheumatic fever but also because of the increased frequency with which the older population experiences infections, investigations, and surgical procedures likely to produce bacteremia. *Streptococcus viridans* remains the most common infecting organism, and, in the absence of positive identification of organisms, penicillin and aminoglycoside are still the most effective combination of antibiotics. Careful attention should be paid to the high sodium content in intravenous penicillin preparations, which may be sufficient to cause fluid overload and pulmonary edema. Because of the increased incidence of impaired renal function, the doses of aminoglycosides in the long-term treatment of infective endocarditis should be tailored accordingly.

Prophylaxis against infective endocarditis in the elderly is recommended for all patients with a valvular heart condition who undergo dental and surgical procedures. The current recommended regimen for dental procedure is amoxycillin 4 g (16 capsules), under supervision, one hour before the procedure. Penicillin-sensitive patients can receive erythromycin 1 g orally one half hour before procedure, followed by erythromycin 500 mg orally every eight hours for three doses. For all other procedures our regimen is ampicillin 1 g plus gentamicin 80 mg by intramuscular injection one half hour before the procedure, followed by two more doses at eight-hour intervals. All patients who have prosthetic valves and require dental attention should be covered by the ampicillin and gentamicin regime.

CARDIOMYOPATHIES

Just when the physiologic changes of age melt into those of cardiomyopathy remains a moot point. Already in 1923, Yandell Henderson [64] had written as follows: "If an old man's heart relaxes slowly, his capacity for physical exertion is thus limited; for the circulation rate would not be accelerated proportionately to the pulse rate during exertion, even though the systolic contractions were still those of youth."

All the standard cardiomyopathies can occur in elderly patients. For

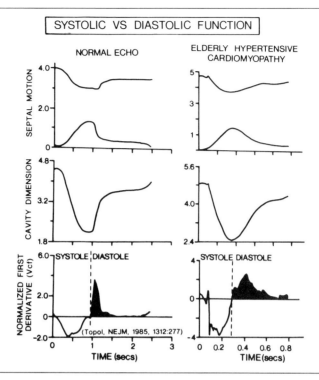

Figure 22-4. Echocardiographic changes in elderly hypertensive black females with cardiomyopathy. Note the impairment of the early phase of rapid diastole as well as prolonged relaxation when compared with the normal echocardiogram on the left. Figure redrawn from Topol et al. [67].

example, a hypertrophic obstructive cardiomyopathy may present for the first time in later years. Some other cardiomyopathies of special interest are 1) dilated cardiomyopathy on the basis of ischemic heart disease, 2) amyloidosis, and 3) hemochromatosis. Such diseases may develop slowly over many years or may present more acutely.

Hypertrophic cardiomyopathy of the elderly

A *specific hypertrophic cardiomyopathy of the elderly* is now increasingly being recognized. Besides the age-related decrease in contractile function, despite an increase in ventricular wall thickness with progressive stiffness of the ventricles [65], there appears to be a selective type of increase in left ventricular hypertrophy that differs in its contour from that found in hypertrophic cardiomyopathy in younger patients [66]. In the latter study, the hypertension was often mild and not thought to be a major etiologic factor. In the study by Topol et al. [67], the patients were predominantly hypertensive black females, and in them a prominent feature was diastolic dysfunction (figure 22-4). Accordingly, the authors recommended that beta-blockers or calcium antagonists were preferred therapy, whereas vasodilators including ACE inhibitors had potentially harmful effects.

Clinically, this disease frequently mimics mitral incompetence because it is often associated with some degree of mitral incompetence. Such cardiomyopathy is well described in the elderly and is often misdiagnosed as either aortic stenosis, mitral incompetence, hypertensive heart disease, or ischemic heart disease. Both in the series of Lever et al. [66] and Topol et al. [67], the patients were predominantly female. There is frequent atrial fibrillation with heart failure and a high risk of developing systemic emboli. Digoxin, normally contraindicated in hypertrophic cardiomyopathy, is useful when there is a dilated heart with atrial fibrillation. In a hypercontractile heart with atrial fibrillation, oral verapamil is preferable to digoxin to inhibit the A-V node. When anticoagulation is given, the risk of bleeding in the elderly needs careful evaluation.

Senile heart disease

This ill-defined term includes senile amyloidosis and the nonspecific cardiomyopathy of aging. Senile amyloidosis is rarely diagnosed before necropsy because it presents in nonspecific ways, causing unexplained heart failure, arrhythmias, or emboli. Amyloid changes are almost physiologic, being found in half the patients age 70 to 79 and in two thirds of patients age 90 or more [40]. Frequently, there is associated hypertension or ischemic heart disease. Hence, it may be doubted whether senile cardiac amyloidosis is of much clinical significance.

Nonspecific cardiomyopathy of aging

A nonspecific term, *cardiomyopathy of aging*, is used when heart failure or arrhythmias in elderly patients occur without a well-defined cause (such as ischemic heart disease or a specific cardiomyopathy). Its causes will include senile amyloidosis and ordinary types of cardiomyopathy presenting in the elderly. In addition, there is an age-related decrease in the contractile function (despite an increase in ventricular wall thickness) with progressive stiffness of the ventricles [65]. Hypocontractility could precipitate cardiac failure, especially in the presence of some additional features frequently found in the elderly, such as some degree of coronary artery disease or hypertension or calcified valves. Standard measures for congestive cardiac failure may be applied. Amyloidosis also has no specific treatment except to search for the underlying and associated conditions, which will usually be obvious (myeloma, chronic rheumatoid arthritis). Hemochromatosis may respond well to repeated venesection; occasionally, arrhythmias need more specific treatment.

ENDOCRINE HEART DISEASE

The hazards of thyrotoxicosis have already been stressed, as has the facility with which the diagnosis can be missed in myxedema. The principles of treatment are the same as in younger patients except that there is frequently associated non-thyroid heart disease. Therefore, the thyrocardiac patient is not simply treated with beta-blockade as in the younger patient. Indeed, beta-blockade should not be introduced until the thyroid state is under reasonable control; if urgent, one can use old-fashioned Lugol's iodine to obtain rapidly an euthyroid state. Digitalis and diuretics must also be used before beta-blockade is given because of the danger of exaggerating heart failure by beta-blockade. It should be noted that a true thyrotoxic heart is resistant to digitalis and that abnormally high doses may therefore be required, resulting in higher than usual blood levels of digoxin. Such abnormally high doses represent one clue in the possible diagnosis of thyrotoxic heart disease.

In the case of myxedema in the elderly patient, there is likely to be associated coronary artery disease and angina; even infarction may be precipitated as thyroid replacement therapy is started. Therefore, such therapy is begun cautiously with a low dosage of thyroxine (0.025 mg or less daily) and with medical vigilance all the time for possible angina. In patients with severe angina, even the addition of low doses may precipitate infarction. Frequently, coronary artery surgery with bypass grafting must be undertaken prior to such medical treatment.

ARRHYTHMIAS AND SICK SINUS SYNDROME

The principles of therapy of arrhythmias are the same as in younger patients, but the problems of chronic ischemic heart disease assume a preponderance. Therefore, the problem may well be how to manage postinfarct arrhythmias or how to manage apparently benign arrhythmias, such as chronic stable ectopic beats. There is as yet no evidence that the management of chronic stable ectopic beats leads to improved mortality in patients with ischemic heart disease, and the medical practitioner should not be pressured into therapy. This advice is especially pertinent because ectopic rhythms and tachyarrhythmias are frequent in apparently healthy elderly subjects [68]. When therapy is started, it should be borne in mind that disopyramide, as is now clear, has many of the same side effects as quinidine and in particular causes myocardial depression. Furthermore, by its parasympathetic effects, it can precipitate bladder neck obstruction and should particularly not be used in elderly males unless really indicated.

The hazards of combining digitalis and quinidine are now well appreciated. Hence, the blood digitalis level (digoxin) must be rechecked once quinidine has been started; frequently, the digoxin dose will be halved by quinidine addition. In the case of supraventricular tachycardias, as in the young patient, there is usually a gratifying response to verapamil.

Symptomatic atrioventricular block causing Stokes–Adams attacks or chronic heart failure are clear indications for permanent pacing. Other forms of bradycardia such as those seen in association with sick sinus syndrome, which is symptomatic, may also respond to pacing. Sick sinus syndrome is frequently seen in the elderly and should be borne in mind as frequently associated with added A-V node disease. The tachyarrhythmias may respond to treatment with digitalis or verapamil. Caution should be exercised with the use of verapamil in sick sinus syndrome, since the response is unpredictable, especially because of its inhibitory effect on the A-V node, which may also be diseased. Hence permanent cardiac pacing may be indicated. Drug therapy is needed, even in paced patients, to control the tachyarrhythmia part of the syndrome. There can be dramatic improvement in elderly patients when pacing is instituted, and it can be a most worthwhile procedure.

A frequently overlooked cause of syncope in the elderly, which occurs particularly in males, is carotid sinus hypersensitivity. Clinical assessment of the patient presenting with syncope should always include the application of carotid sinus pressure with concurrent electrocardiographic monitoring. When such hypersensitivity occurs and is responsible for symptoms, pacing may be required.

TRANSIENT ISCHEMIC ATTACKS

Transient ischemic attacks in the elderly patient call for a full cardiovascular examination because a potential source of embolus may be anywhere from the left atrium to the cerebral circulation. Structural abnormalities associated with mitral valve disease, cardiomyopathy or ischemic heart disease with mural thrombi, and enlargement of the left atrium from whatever cause can all give rise to peripheral emboli, particularly when associated with paroxysmal or established arrhythmias. Echocardiography may be extremely useful in the search for a potential source of a transient ischemic attack.

A variety of trials with antiplatelet agents such as acetyl salicylate, sulfinpyrazone, and dipyridamole, alone or in combination, have not shown any consistent benefits in the management of patients with transient ischemic attacks and underlying cardiac abnormalities. Full anticoagulation under careful supervision may be considered, especially when there is clear evidence for an intracardiac source. The major Canadian Cooperative Study on aspirin/sulfinpyrazone in threatened stroke (at least one transient ischemic attack) showed a specific benefit for aspirin (325 mg daily) in male patients who were, by the nature of the disease, mostly elderly. In contrast, patients did not benefit from sulfinpyrazone. It is not clear from the summary publication [69] how many of the patients had a cardiac source for the transient ischemic attacks. In another study (AITIA, Aspirin in transient ischemic attacks), most of the patients were over 55 and about one third were over 65 years of age. Once again, aspirin helped to prevent stroke or death in men more than in women [70]. However, the actual occurrence rate of transient ischemic attacks was equally dimished in men and women in the AITIA trial at a daily dose of 1300 mg. Therefore, aspirin may be considered as suitable therapy for all patients with transient ischemic attacks.

SUMMARY

In summary, there are several questions the physician considers when treating the elderly patient with cardiovascular disease. First, what is the correct diagnosis? Second, what are the particular problems specific to each patient that will alter drug pharmacokinetics or compliance? In considering such pharmacokinetics, it is important to evaluate carefully how renal function may critically influence the effects of digoxin and diuretics. Third, which is the best drug to give? Fourth, what side effects might occur in this particular patient? And, finally, is the prescribed drug really necessary, and if so, are there any other drugs that can be discontinued to avoid polypharmacy and help improve patient compliance?

REFERENCES

1. Ouslander JG. 1981. Drug therapy in the elderly. Ann Intern Med 95:711–722.
2. Amery A, Brixko P, Clement D, et al. 1985. Mortality and morbidity results from the European Working Party on High Blood Pressure in the Elderly Trial. Lancet 1:1349–1345.
3. Dall JLC. 1970. Maintenance digoxin in elderly patients. Br Med J 2:705–706.
4. Causack B, Kelly J, O'Malley K, et al. 1979. Digoxin in the elderly: pharmacokinetic consequences of old age. Clin Pharmacol Ther 25:772–776.
5. Ewy GA, Kapadia GG and Yao L. 1969. Digoxin metabolism in the elderly. Circulation 39:449–453.
6. Berman W Jr and Musselman J. 1979. The relationship of age to the metabolism and protein binding of digoxin in sheep. J Pharmacol Exp Ther 208:263–266.
7. Gerstenblith G, Spurgeon HA, Froehlich JP, et al. 1979. Diminished inotropic responsiveness to ouabain in aged rat myocardium. Circ Res 44:517–523.
8. Guarnieri T, Spurgeon H, Froehlich JP, et al. 1979. Diminished inotropic responses but unaltered toxicity to acetylstrophanthidin in the senescent beagle. Circulation 60:1548–1554.
9. Whiting B, Wandless I, Summer DJ and Goldberg A. 1978. Computer-assisted review of digoxin therapy in the elderly. Br Heart J 40:8–13.
10. Castleden CM, Kaye CM and Parsons RL. 1975. The effect of age on plasma levels of propranolol and practolol in man. Br J Clin Pharmacol 2:303–306.
11. Vestal RE, Wood AJ and Shand DG. 1979. Reduced beta-adrenoceptor sensitivity in the elderly. Clin Pharmacol Ther 26:181–186.
12. Schocken DD and Roth GS. 1977. Reduced beta-adrenergic receptor concentrations in ageing man. Nature 267:856–858.
13. Creasey WA, Funke PT, McKinstry DN and Sugerman AA. 1986. Pharmacokinetics of captopril in elderly healthy male volunteers. J Clin Pharmacol 26:264–268.
14. Hockings N, Ajayi LAA and Reid JL. 1985. The effects of age on the pharmacokinetics and dynamics of the angiotensin converting enzyme inhibitors enalapril and enalaprilat. Br J Clin Pharmacol 20:262P–263P.
15. Lees KR and Reid JL. 1987. Age and the pharmacokinetics and pharmacodynamics of chronic enalapril treatment. Clin Pharmacol Ther 41:597–602.
16. Williams PEO, Brown AN, Rajaguru S, et al. 1989. A pharmacokinetic study of cilazapril in elderly and young volunteers. Br J Clin Pharmacol 27:211S–215S.
17. Gilchrist WJ, Beard K, Manhem P, et al. 1987. Pharmacokinetics and effects on the renin-angiotensin system of ramipril in elderly patients. Am J Cardiol 59:28D–32D.
18. Gautam PC, Vargas E and Lye M. 1987. Pharmacokinetics of lisinopril (MK 521) in healthy

young and elderly subjects and in elderly patients with cardiac failure. J Pharm Pharmacol 39:929–931.

19. Kendall MJ, Woods KL, Wilkins MR and Worthington DJ. 1982. The effects of age are cardioselective. Br J Clin Pharmacol 14:821–826.

20. Yin FCP, Spurgeon HA, Raizes GS, et al. 1976. Age-associated decrease in chronotropic response to isoproterenol (abstract). Circulation 54:II:167.

21. Cokkinos DV, Tsartsalis GD, Heimonas ET and Gardikas CD. 1980. Comparison of the inotropic action of digitalis and isoproterenol in younger and older individuals. Am Heart J 100:802–806.

22. Guarnieri T, Filburn CR, Zitnik G, et al. 1980. Contractile and biochemical correlates of beta-adrenergic stimulation of the aged heart. Am J Physiol 239:H501–H508.

23. Nation RI, Triggs EJ and Selig M. 1977. Lignocaine kinetics in cardiac patients and aged subjects. Br J Clin Pharmacol 4:439–448.

24. Reidenberg MM, Camacho M, Kluger J and Drayer DE. 1980. Ageing and renal clearance of procainamide and acetylprocainamide. Clin Pharmacol Ther 28:732–735.

25. Ochs HR, Greenblatt DJ, Woo E and Smith TW. 1978. Reduced quinidine clearance in elderly persons. Am J Cardiol 42:481–485.

26. Shepherd AM, Hewick DS, Moreland TA and Stevenson IH. 1977. Age as a determinant of sensitivity to warfarin. Br J Clin Pharmacol 4:315–320.

27. Staessen J, Bulpitt C, Clement D, et al. 1989. Relation between mortality and treated blood pressure in elderly patients with hypertension: report of the European Working Party on High Blood Pressure in the Elderly. Br Med J 298:1552–1556.

28. Staessen J, Fagard R, Lijnen P, et al. 1990. Review of the major hypertension trials in the elderly. Cardiovasc Drugs Ther 4:1237–1248.

29. O'Malley K, Cox JP and O'Brein E. 1990. Further learnings from the European Working Party on High Blood Pressure in the Elderly (EWPHE) Study: focus on systolic hypertension. Cardiovasc Drugs Ther 4:1249–1252.

30. Ashraf N, Locksley R and Arieff AI. 1981. Thiazide-induced hyponatremia associated with death or neurologic damage in outpatients. Am J Med 70:1163–1168.

31. Epstein M and Hollenberg NK. 1976. Age as determinant of renal sodium conservation in normal man. J Lab Clin Med 87:411–417.

32. Zacharias FJ and Cruickshank JM. 1979. Treating the elderly hypertensive. Acta Ther 5:179–192.

33. Coope J and Warrender TS. 1986. Randomised trial of treatment of hypertension in elderly patients in primary care. Br Med J 293:1145–1148.

34. Lamon KD. 1990. Evaluation of celiprolol, a new cardioselective beta-adrenergic blocker with vasodilating properties, in the treatment of mild to moderate hypertension in the elderly. Cardiovasc Drugs Ther 4:1291–1296.

35. Strandgaard S. 1990. Cerebral blood flow in the elderly: impact of hypertension and antihypertensive treatment. Cardiovasc Drugs Ther 4:1217–1222.

36. Buhler FR, Bolli P, Erne P, et al. 1985. Position of calcium antagonists in antihypertensive therapy. J Cardiovasc Pharmacol 7 (Suppl 4):S21–S27.

37. Jenkins AC, Knill JR and Dreslinski GR. 1985. Captopril in the treatment of the elderly hypertensive patient. Arch Intern Med 145:2029–2031.

38. Perry IJ and Beevers DG. 1989. ACE inhibitors compared with thiazide diuretics as first-step antihypertensive therapy. Cardiovasc Drugs Ther 3:815–819.

39. Ben-Ishay D, Leibel B and Stessman J. 1986. Calcium channel blockers in the management of hypertension in the elderly. Am J Med 81 (Suppl 6A):30–34.

40. Harris R. 1980. The old heart. In G Bourne (ed), Hearts and Heart-like Organs, Vol 3. New York: Academic Press, pp 159–188.

41. Chaudhry AY, Bing RF, Castleden CM, et al. 1984. The effect of ageing on the response to frusemide in normal subjects. Eur J Clin Pharmacol 27:303–306.

42. Andreasen F, Hansen U, Husted SE, et al. 1984. The influence of age on renal and extrarenal effects of frusemide. Br J Clin Pharmacol 18:65–74.

43. Hamdy RC. 1978. Diuretic Therapy in the Older Patient. Philadelphia: Smith, Kline and French, pp 47–50.

44. Lye M. 1982. Body potassium content and capacity of elderly individuals with and without cardiac failure. Cardiovasc Res 16:22–25.

45. Boston Area Anticoagulation Trial for Atrial Fibrillation Investigators. 1990. The effect of low-dose warfarin on the risk of stroke in patients with nonrheumatic atrial fibrillation. N Engl J Med 323:1505–1511.
46. Stroke Prevention in Atrial Fibrillation Study Group Investigators. 1991. Preliminary report of the stroke prevention in atrial fibrillation study. Circulation 84:527–539.
47. Chesebro JH, Fuster V and Halperin JL. 1990. Atrial fibrillation—risk marker for stroke. N Engl J Med 323:1556–1558.
48. Gersh BJ, Kronmal RA, Schaff HV, et al. 1983. Long-term (5 year) results of coronary bypass surgery in patients 65 years old or older: a report from the Coronary Artery Surgery Study. Circulation 68 (Suppl II):II-190–II-199.
49. Knapp WS, Douglas JS, Craver JM, et al. 1981. Efficacy of coronary bypass grafting in elderly patients with coronary artery disease. Am J Cardiol 47:923–930.
50. Wintzen AR, Tijssen JGP, deVries WA, et al. 1982. Risk of long-term oral anticoagulant therapy in elderly patients after myocardial infarction. Second report of the sixty plus reinfarction study research group. Lancet 1:64–68.
51. Hawkins CM, Richardson DW and Vokonas PS. 1983. Effect of propranolol in reducing mortality in older myocardial infarction patients. The Beta-Blocker Heart Attack Trial experience. Circulation 67 (Suppl I):I-94-I-97.
52. Gundersen T, Abrahamsen AM, Kjekshus J and Ronnevik PK. 1982. Timolol-related reduction in mortality and reinfarction in patients aged 65–75 years surviving acute myocardial infarction. Circulation 66:1179–1148.
53. Olsson G, Rehnqvist N, Sjogren A, et al. 1985. Long-term treatment with metoprolol after myocardial infarction: effect on 3 year mortality and morbidity. J Am Coll Cardiol 5:1428–1437.
54. Schocken DD, Blumenthal JA, Port S, et al. 1983. Physical conditioning and left ventricular performance in the elderly: assessment by radionuclide angiocardiography. Am J Cardiol 52:359–364.
55. The Anturane Reinfarction Trial Research Group. 1980. Sulfinpyrazone in the prevention of sudden death after myocardial infarction. N Engl J Med 302:250–256.
56. Anturane Reinfarction Italian Study. 1982. Sulphinpyrazone in postmyocardial infarction. Lancet 1:237–242.
57. Aspirin Myocardial Infarction Study Research Group. 1980. A randomized controlled trial of aspirin in persons recovered from myocardial infarction. JAMA 243:661–669.
58. Persantine-Aspirin Reinfarction Study Research Group. 1980. Persantine and aspirin in coronary heart disease. Circulation 62:449–461.
59. Murphy ES, Lawson RM, Starr A, et al. 1981. Severe aortic stenosis in patients 60 years of age and older: left ventricular function and 10-year survival after valve replacement. Circulation 64 (Suppl II):II-184-II-188.
60. Commerford PJ, Curcio A, Albanese M and Beck W. 1981. Aortic valve replacement in the elderly. S Afr Med J 59:975–976.
61. De Bono AHB, English TAH and Milstein BB. 1978. Heart valve replacement in the elderly. Br Med J 2:917–919.
62. Waller BF and Roberts WC. 1983. Cardiovascular disease in the very elderly. Analysis of 40 necropsy patients aged 90 years or over. Am J Cardiol 51:403–421.
63. Kolibash AJ, Bush CA, Fotana MB, et al. 1983. Mitral valve prolapse syndrome: analysis of 62 patients aged 60 years and older. Am J Cardiol 52:534–539.
64. Henderson Y. 1923. Volume changes of the heart. Physiol Rev 3:165–208.
65. Templeton GH, Platt MR, Willerson JT and Weisfeldt MI. 1979. Influence of ageing on left ventricular hemodynamics and stiffness in beagles. Circ Res 44:189–194.
66. Lever HM, Karam RF, Currie PJ and Healy BP. 1989. Hypertrophic cardiomyopathy in the elderly. Distinctions from the young based on cardiac shape. Circulation 79:580–589.
67. Topol EJ, Traill TA and Fortuin NJ. 1985. Hypertensive hypertrophic cardiomyopathy of the elderly. N Engl J Med 312:277–283.
68. Camm AJ, Evans KE, Ward DE and Martin A. 1980. The rhythm of the heart in active elderly subjects. Am Heart J 99:598–603.
69. Canadian Cooperative Study Group. 1978. A randomized trial of aspirin and sulfinpyrazone in threatened stroke. N Engl J Med 229:53–59.
70. Fields WS, Lemak NA, Frankowski KF, et al. 1980. Controlled trial of aspirin in cerebral ischemia. Circulation 62 (Suppl V):V90–V96.

SUGGESTED READING

Anderson GJ. 1980. Clinical clues to digitalis toxicity. Geriatrics 35:57–65.

Harris R. 1970. The Management of Geriatric Cardiovascular Disease. Philadelphia: Lippincott.

Lowenthal DT and Affrime MB. 1981. Cardiovascular drugs for the geriatric patient. Cardiology 36:65–74.

Mitenko PA, Comfort A, and Crooks J (eds). 1983. Drugs and the Elderly. Proceedings of a symposium. J Chronic Dis 36:1–144.

O'Hanrahan M and O'Malley K. 1981. Compliance with drug treatment. Br Med J 283:298–300.

Swift CG. 1979. Clinical pharmacology in the elderly. Scott Med J 24:221–225.

Unverferth DV, Magorien RD, and Leier CV. 1980. Drug regimens for congestive heart failure. Geriatrics 35:26–33.

Vestal RE. 1978. Drug use in the elderly: a review of problems and special considerations. Drugs 16:358–382.

23. INTERVENTIONAL CARDIOLOGY

STEPHEN R. RAMEE
CHRISTOPHER J. WHITE

Interventional cardiology is an invasive subspecialty of cardiology that utilizes a wide array of percutaneous therapies for treating patients with coronary artery disease (CAD) and valvular stenosis. In patients with CAD, percutaneous interventions currently approved for clinical use in the United States include percutaneous transluminal coronary balloon angioplasty (PTCA) and directional coronary atherectomy. Newer approaches that are not yet approved but are undergoing clinical trials include the use of intravascular stents, laser angioplasty, and novel atherectomy devices. In patients with valvular stenosis, percutaneous balloon valvuloplasty is a clinically approved treatment for valvular pulmonic stenosis, and the procedure is under investigation for aortic and mitral stenosis. This chapter reviews the role of interventional cardiology in the management of cardiovascular disease in the elderly.

CORONARY ARTERY DISEASE

The population of the United States is aging, with 25.8 million people over age 65 in 1985. It is estimated that by the year 2020, 44.3 million Americans, or 17.3% of the population, will be over age 65 [1]. The prevalence of cardiovascular diseases increases with increasing age. It was estimated in 1984

Franz H. Messerli (ed.), CARDIOVASCULAR DISEASE IN THE ELDERLY (Third Edition). Copyright © 1993 Kluwer Academic Publishers. ISBN 0-7923-1859-5. All rights reserved.

that nearly one half of the 25 million Americans over age 65 had some form of cardiovascular disease, with atherosclerotic coronary heart disease being the most prevalent cardiac condition [2]. Postmortem studies reveal that 50% of autopsies in patients over age 70 have 75% or greater stenosis in one or more coronary arteries [1]. Furthermore, it has been estimated that nearly half of all deaths in Americans over age 65 can be attributed to CAD [3].

Since CAD is a disease of aging, many patients with CAD are over age 65. Unlike younger patients, the treatment goal in the geriatric population is more concerned with symptom relief than with longevity. It is important that all of the potential treatment options, including medical therapy, coronary artery bypass surgery, and angioplasty, are considered when evaluating the elderly patient with CAD. Although there are no randomized trials comparing these three treatments in the geriatric population, medical therapy is generally considered to be the initial treatment of choice in these patients unless they have very high-risk anatomy, such as significant left main CAD or critical stenosis in a major vessel with a large amount of myocardium in jeopardy. Revascularization is generally reserved for patients with high-risk anatomy and those who continue to have limiting symptoms despite medical therapy. The introduction of PTCA by Andreas Grüntzig in 1977 [4] has dramatically changed the management of patients with CAD, including that of the elderly.

Coronary artery bypass surgery in the elderly

As individuals age, the morbidity and mortality associated with all types of major surgery increase. This is especially true for coronary artery bypass surgery, which has markedly increased morbidity and mortality and often results in prolonged hospitalization in elderly patients [5–9]. This risk also increases substantially with advancing age (i.e., octogenarians) and female sex. Most investigators who have compared the surgical results of coronary revascularization in the geriatric population with those in younger patients have found that elderly patients are also more likely to have multivessel disease, impaired left ventricular function, and associated medical illnesses such as chronic lung disease and renal insufficiency. Undoubtedly, these conditions are major contributors to the increased morbidity and mortality in the elderly. In 1983, Faro and coworkers [5] reported the results of a 15-year experience with coronary artery bypass surgery in 2667 patients who had an overall mortality of 3.8%. For the 2562 patients under age 70, the in-hospital mortality was 3.2% (5.5% in women). In the 105 patients over age 70, the mortality was 10.5%, with a strikingly high 28.6% mortality rate in women over age 70. Significant morbidity was also encountered in the elderly patients, including cardiac complications (myocardial infarction (MI), arrhythmia, and congestive heart failure) in 45%, stroke in 8.6%, reoperation for bleeding in 8.5%, and renal failure in 5.7%.

Hochberg and associates [6] reported a higher mortality in 75 patients over

70 years of age (12% mortality) compared with a group of 75 patients under 70 years of age (4% mortality). Horneffer and colleagues [7] also reported a higher mortality in 228 patients over age 70 when compared to those under age 70 (9.3% versus 2.2%). In addition, the older patients suffered more complications, including stroke, wound infections, reoperation for bleeding, and prolonged ventilation. The average length of hospitalization was also longer in the older group (14 days versus 9 days). Horvath et al. [8] reported an overall mortality of 10.8% in 222 patients over age 75 who underwent coronary artery bypass surgery. Thirty-seven percent had significant complications. In this study population, the mortality risk increased with patient instability preoperatively, such that it was only 3.8% in elective procedures versus 14.9% in urgent operations and 35% in emergency operations.

The increased mortality risk of between 9% and 28% and increased morbidity with bypass surgery in patients over age 70 are not purely age-dependent phenomena, as several authors have pointed out. Elderly patients are more likely to have severe coronary disease, with a high incidence of unstable angina, prior MI, and longer cardiopulmonary bypass pump runs than younger patients. They are also more likely than younger patients to have concomitant cerebrovascular disease, peripheral vascular disease, and other medical illnesses [7–11]. Despite the increased acute morbidity and mortality in the elderly population, the long-term results with respect to freedom from angina and cardiovascular events in patients over age 70 are quite good. Horvath et al. [8] showed that 75% of patients over age 75 who survived bypass surgery survived four years, and 77% were angina free at six years. Therefore, despite the high initial risk, coronary artery bypass graft surgery does offer relatively good survival and excellent symptom relief in the elderly population.

Percutaneous coronary angioplasty in the elderly

The increased morbidity and mortality in elderly patients undergoing coronary artery bypass surgery, coupled with the high success and low morbidity of PTCA in younger patients, has provided the impetus for interventional cardiologists to offer angioplasty as an alternative method of revascularization in older patients with symptomatic coronary disease (figure 23-1). Coronary angioplasty has been performed in elderly patients with excellent results. A number of investigators have reported their experience with angioplasty in the elderly [12–20]. Some have compared the results of PTCA in older patients with those in younger patients [21–24]. A review of these data will provide some idea of the relative safety and efficacy of angioplasty in the older patient population.

The results of nine studies that reported the clinical success of PTCA, complications, restenosis rates, and follow-up of at least one year are summarized in table 23-1. The age groups evaluated in these studies vary,

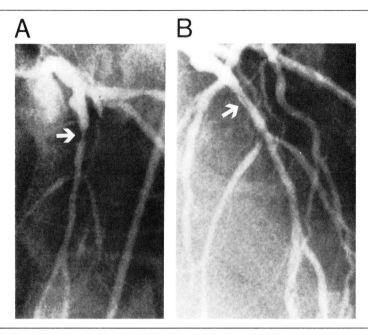

Figure 23-1. A. High-grade proximal left anterior descending artery stenosis (arrow) in a 76-year-old man with unstable angina. **B.** Same lesion (arrow) immediately after balloon angioplasty.

with some including patients 65 years and older and others including only patients over 70 years of age. One study looked at the results of PTCA in octogenarians [15]. Success was reported in these patients as either angiographic success or clinical success without a major complication. In-hospital mortality included death from cardiac as well as noncardiac causes. The major acute complications included Q-wave myocardial infarction (QMI) and emergency coronary artery bypass graft surgery (CABG). The restenosis rates were based on clinical follow-up rather than angiographic follow-up. Patients with restenosis generally had recurrent symptoms and underwent repeat angiography to confirm the presence of restenosis. The presence of silent restenosis was not evaluated angiographically. Survival data in these studies included mortality from all causes. Event-free survival was defined as freedom from death, myocardial infarction, and coronary artery bypass surgery at the time interval specified. Repeat angioplasty was required in a number of these patients for restenosis or progressive disease in non-dilated vessels; however, repeat angioplasty was not included as a cardiac event in table 23-1.

One of the most compelling clinical indications for coronary revascularization in older patients is unstable angina. The value of PTCA for

Table 23-1. PTCA for angina pectoris in the elderly

Study	Patient	Age	Success (%)[a]	Hospital deaths (%)	Complications (%)		Restenosis (%)	Survival (%)	Event[b] Free (%)
					QMI	CABG			
Mock et al. 1984 [21]	370	>65	53	2.2	5.6	6.8	9.9	96 at 1 yr	46
Holt et al. 1988 [12]	54	>70	80	0	3.7	5.5	12	91 at 3 yr	79
Simpfendorfer et al. 1988 [13]	336	>70	92	0.6	0.9	3.3	22	91 at 2 yr	68
Dorros et al. 1989 [14]	242	>70	86	3.3	2.1	1.2	35	85 at 1 yr	75
Cook and Hubner 1989 [22]	29	>65	76	6.9	6.9	3.4	23		
Jeroudi et al. 1990 [15]	54	>80	91	3.7	3.7	3.7	22	87 at 1 yr	81
Kelsey et al. 1990 [17]	486	>65	75	3	5.3	5.3	19	91 at 2 yr	65
Cannon and Dean 1991 [20]	213	>70	83	4	6	6		91 at 1 yr	
Bedotto et al. 1991 [24]	1373	>65	96	1.6	1.4	0.8	36	92 at 1 yr	81

[a] Immediate PTCA success without in-hospital death, MI, or CABG.
[b] Without death, MI, or CABG.
Note: CABG = Coronary artery bypass graft; PTCA = Percutaneous coronary angioplasty; QMI = Q-wave myocardial infarction.

elderly patients with unstable angina, defined by the authors as recent onset of exertional angina, rest angina, or worsening of class III or IV angina, was the subject of a paper by Holt and associates [12]. In 54 patients over 70 years of age (mean age 74, range 70 to 84 years), they reported an 80% immediate success rate with no in-hospital mortality, a 3.7% incidence of QMI, and a 5.5% incidence of emergency coronary artery bypass surgery. At a mean follow-up of 37 months (range 6 to 73 months), survival was 91%, and 72% of the patients were angina free. Nine patients required either repeat PTCA or CABG for recurrent symptoms. In this small, nonrandomized group of unstable angina patients over age 70, the results are really quite good in terms of initial success, long-term survival, and relief of symptoms.

The Cleveland Clinic experience with angioplasty in 336 patients over age 70, excluding patients with acute MI and PTCA of bypass grafts, was published by Simpfendorfer et al. [13]. These authors had a 92% primary success rate with a very low acute complication rate, including 0.6% mortality, 0.9% QMI, and 3.3% bypass surgery. At 28 months follow-up, there was a 91% survival rate, and 68% of the patients had not had MI, repeat angioplasty, or bypass surgery. Dorros et al. [14] reported similar morbidity and mortality results in 242 patients over age 70 (table 23-1) but encountered a higher clinical restenosis rate (35%). Jeroudi et al. [15] examined the short- and long-term outcome of PTCA in 54 octogenarians with a mean age of 82 years. The angiographic success rate of 91% mortality of 3.7%, and low complication rate (3.7% QMI, 3.7% CABG) compare favorably with the other studies cited previously and with the expected outcome from bypass surgery in this age group.

What is the role of coronary angioplasty in elderly patients with multivessel disease? One recently published retrospective study [24] suggests that multivessel PTCA is a safe and effective alternative to bypass surgery. The authors reviewed 1373 patients over age 65 who underwent multivessel angioplasty. Their angiographic success rate was 96%, with very low morbidity (1.4% QMI, 0.8% CABG) and only 1.6% in-hospital mortality. The clinical restenosis rate was reported to be 36%. A total of 1023 patients had been followed for more than one year, with a mean follow-up interval of 32.5 ± 21 months. The actuarial survival was 92% at one year, 86% at three years, and 78% at five years.

PTCA in the elderly: Comparison with PTCA in younger patients

The results of PTCA in the elderly population have been compared with results in younger patients in several studies. The first study to do so was the report of the National Heart, Lung, and Blood Institute (NHLBI) PTCA Registry in 1984 [21]. This study included 2790 patients under 65 years of age and 370 patients age 65 or older. It suggested that PTCA had a significantly lower primary success rate (53% versus 62%) in older patients than in younger patients. It also reported a significantly higher in-hospital mortality

(2.2% versus 0.7%) and a higher risk of elective coronary artery bypass surgery during the initial hospitalization (25.4% versus 8.1%) in the older patients. There was no difference between the older and younger patients in the rate of emergency bypass surgery (6.8% versus 6.5%), MI (5.6% versus 4.9%), or other nonfatal complications. At one-year follow-up, the older group had a slightly higher mortality (4.5% versus 2.2%) and need for CABG (41.5% versus 36.1%) but fewer repeat PTCA procedures (6.4% versus 10.8%) than the younger group.

Among patients in this initial report from the NHLBI PTCA Registry who had an initially successful angioplasty, the younger and older age groups were very similar in terms of mortality, MI, and need for repeat CABG at one year. The authors also noted that the older population included a larger percentage of women, more patients with severe angina, and more patients with multivessel disease than the younger patient group. Despite the slightly increased morbidity and mortality of PTCA in the elderly when compared to the younger patients, the authors noted that the elderly patients still did well based on comparison with published reports of morbidity and mortality in elderly patients undergoing CABG. The lower initial success rates in this initial report by the NHLBI PTCA Registry include patients undergoing PTCA between 1977 and 1981, a period when coronary angioplasty was in its infancy in terms of technology and operator experience. Subsequent studies more accurately reflect the success rates that can be expected with current equipment and experienced operators.

Mills et al. [23] compared the Mayo Clinic experience with PTCA in patients over age 65 with the experience of patients with PTCA who were under age 65. They subdivided the patients into groups undergoing elective and nonelective angioplasty. There were 971 patients under 65 years old and 546 patients over 65 years old in the elective angioplasty group. Initial success was similar in the younger and older age groups undergoing elective angioplasty (84% versus 83%), and the acute mortality was 0.3% for the younger patients compared with 0.9% for the elderly. In patients undergoing urgent or emergent angioplasty, the initial success rate was lower (66%) and the mortality rate slightly higher (3%) than in the elective group, but there was no difference between the age groups. The authors found no age-related differences in success rate or morbidity and suggested that PTCA can produce excellent results and may be the procedure of choice for elderly patients with symptomatic single-vessel disease or multivessel disease with a discrete "ischemia-producing" stenosis amenable to PTCA.

In 1990, a second report was published from the 1985–1986 NHLBI PTCA Registry comparing the results of PTCA in 486 patients over 65 years of age with the results in 1315 patients under age 65 [17]. Although the success rates for the two groups were similar and higher than those reported previously [21], patients over age 65 were more likely to require emergency bypass surgery (5.4% versus 2.8%) or elective bypass surgery (3.9% versus

1.6%). The hospital mortality was also higher for the older patients (3.1% versus 0.2%).

Cook and Hubner [22] reported the results of a low-volume catheterization laboratory that averaged only 54 angioplasties per year over a five-year period between 1982 and 1988. Of the 287 patients studied, 258 were under age 65 and 29 were over age 65. Only three patients were over age 70. Although there were no differences in the primary success rate, the rate of non-fatal complications, or the rate of restenosis, the acute mortality in the older patients (6.9%) was strikingly higher than in the younger patients (0.4%). This probably reflects the increased complexity of performing PTCA in elderly patients and suggests the need to consider performing such high-risk procedures in a large-volume catheterization laboratory where complex interventional procedures are commonly performed.

What kind of results can we expect from PTCA in patients over age 65 who are in need of revascularization (table 23-1)? Although angioplasty has a similar initial success rate and clinical results one year after angioplasty, whether it is performed in elderly or young patients, older patients are at increased risk of in-hospital mortality and complications. If we extrapolate from the results of these uncontrolled studies of PTCA in the elderly, excluding the small study, we can predict a clinical success rate of between 75% and 92%, a rate similar to that in younger patients. There is an increased in-hospital mortality rate of between 2% and 4% in patients over 65 years of age. The elderly also have an increased incidence of QMI (1% to 6%) and an increased likelihood of requiring emergency bypass surgery (1% to 6%). Restenosis rates in older patients can be expected to be similar to those reported in younger patients, roughly between 20% and 40%. One-year survival should be approximately 90%, and the event-free survival at one year should be between 65% and 80%.

PTCA in the elderly: Comparison with CABG

Although PTCA is a safe and effective treatment for selected patients with symptomatic CAD, its widespread use has never been supported by a randomized, prospective trial comparing PTCA with either medical therapy or coronary artery bypass surgery in patients of any age. Several ongoing trials, including the BARI Trial (Bypass surgery, Angioplasty Revascularization Investigation) and the EAST study (Emory Angioplasty versus Surgery Trial), are underway to help answer this question. Similarly, no randomized, prospective trials have compared angioplasty to bypass surgery or medical therapy in the elderly population. In fact, there are only two published retrospective reports comparing angioplasty to bypass surgery in patients over 70 years of age [24,25].

The Mid-America Heart Institute compared 68 patients over age 70 who underwent PTCA with 107 patients in the same age group who underwent CABG [26]. There was no difference in the in-hospital mortality rate (4.4%

PTCA versus 4.7% CABG); however, at follow-up of between 1 and 3 years, the CABG group had more patients who were asymptomatic (82% PTCA versus 90% CABG). Boston University [26] found an increased mortality in 102 CABG patients (7.8%) when compared with 104 angioplasty patients (1.9%); however, this difference was not statistically significant. This study also reported a higher incidence of minor complications (arrhythmias, bleeding, and infection) in the surgery patients (76% CABG versus 38.6% PTCA).

PTCA for acute myocardial infarction

The treatment of acute MI in the elderly is a far from settled issue. Thrombolytic therapy has been shown in numerous controlled studies to reduce mortality and improve left ventricular function in selected patients treated within six hours of the onset of symptoms. It is also a well-established fact that acute mortality is increased in the elderly with acute MI. In patients over age 70, 14% to 21% succumb acutely to MI, and the one-year mortality in survivors of acute MI is similarly increased (19% to 24%) in elderly patients [27–29]. Despite the high mortality in geriatric patients with MI, controversy remains regarding the value of thrombolytic agents in this population.

Four of five large, placebo-controlled trials of thrombolysis, utilizing three different thrombolytic agents and involving a total of 9984 patients over age 65 [30–34], showed reduced mortality in patients over age 65 who were given thrombolytic agents for acute MI. Although the benefit of thrombolytic therapy was not statistically significant in the elderly subsets in each individual study, in three of the trials [32–34] the mortality reduction was greatest in the older age groups, and the benefit relative to placebo was statistically significant in each trial. In pooled data from these five studies, the acute mortality in patients over age 65 was reduced from 20.7% in placebo-treated patients to 17.2% in patients treated with one of the three thrombolytic agents tested [35]. This lifesaving benefit was somewhat diminished but not offset by the increased incidence of bleeding complications in the older population.

Direct angioplasty without the use of thrombolytic agents has been shown to be very effective at opening the infarct vessel (figure 23-2) and reducing in-hospital mortality in patients with acute MI [36]. Furthermore, direct angioplasty is not associated with the hemorrhagic complications commonly seen in patients receiving thrombolytic agents. Data are limited regarding the use of direct angioplasty in patients over age 65 for treatment of acute MI. In a report by Lee and associates [37], PTCA was used as primary therapy in 105 patients over age 70 (mean age 75 years). Fifty percent had anterior wall MI, 67% had multivessel coronary disease, and 11% were in cardiogenic shock. The primary success rate was 91% and the in-hospital mortality was 18%. Predictors of early mortality were cardiogenic shock and multivessel

A   B

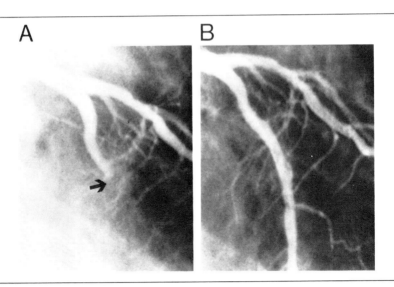

Figure 23-2. A. Proximal left circumflex occlusion in an elderly woman presenting with an acute myocardial infarction. **B.** Same vessel immediately after successful acute intervention with balloon angioplasty.

disease. The authors noted improvement in the global ejection fraction from 54% to 61%. Survival at one year, including in-hospital deaths, was 73%, and survival at five years was 67%.

A second, smaller series of 35 patients over age 70 who underwent PTCA for acute MI was reported by Holland et al. [19]. Seventeen (49%) had received thrombolytic therapy before angioplasty. They reported a primary success rate of only 66% and an in-hospital mortality of 34%. The in-hospital mortality in patients with an occluded infarct-related artery was extremely high—78% versus 19% in patients with a patent infarct vessel. Compared with 200 consecutive patients under age 70, the elderly patients had a lower primary success rate (66% versus 90%) and a higher early mortality rate (34% versus 6%).

It is difficult to reach conclusions regarding the role of angioplasty as primary therapy for acute MI in the elderly based on such limited data. However, both of these studies suggest that PTCA may be at least as effective as thrombolysis in restoring patency to the infarct vessel and in reducing mortality. One subset of patients with acute MI who have particularly high mortality are patients with cardiogenic shock. In a retrospective study from the University of Michigan [38], 24 patients (mean age 59 ± 12 years) who underwent emergent PTCA for acute MI were compared with 59 patients (mean age 62 ± 12 years) treated with conventional therapy without thrombolysis but including inotropic support, hemodynamic monitoring, and intra-aortic ballon counterpulsation. Thirty-day survival was better in the angioplasty group (50% versus 17%), and patients who had successful angioplasty had a survival of 77% (10 of 13 patients) versus 18% (2 of 11) in patients with unsuccessful PTCA. These findings suggest that angioplasty improves survival in patients with cardiogenic shock and acute MI, and that survival is dependent upon patency of the infarct vessel.

PTCA in the elderly: Summary

The treatment of CAD in the ever-growing geriatric population is primarily aimed at improving symptoms rather than prolonging survival, except in selected high-risk situations. Both coronary artery bypass surgery and coronary angioplasty are effective treatments, but they have a greater risk of morbidity and mortality in the elderly than in younger patients. Although no controlled trials have been performed to compare PTCA with CABG in the aged, the available data in comparable patient groups suggest that PTCA has an advantage over bypass surgery in terms of lower hospital morbidity and reduced acute mortality. The trials that have been presented here illustrate that single-vessel and multivessel angioplasty can be performed safely and effectively in the elderly population, with an excellent immediate result and substantial long-term benefit in terms of angina relief that rival results of the surgical series. The dilation of "culprit lesions" can provide sufficient relief of ischemia and significant clinical improvement. It may be possible to palliate symptoms and return an elderly patient to full function simply by dilating the culprit vessel in a patient with multivessel disease [14].

NEW PERCUTANEOUS TREATMENTS FOR CORONARY ARTERY DISEASE

A number of new percutaneous therapies are playing an expanding role in the treatment of patients with CAD. These have been developed to address the limitations of balloon angioplasty: abrupt reocclusion, restenosis rates of 20% to 40%, totally occluded vessels, and the need for hemodynamic support for unstable patients or patients with high-risk anatomy for PTCA. These include supported angioplasty, atherectomy, laser angioplasty, and intra-vascular stents. Although these devices are being used in geriatric patients, no studies have evaluated their efficacy in this specific population.

Supported angioplasty

One adjunctive measure reported to be beneficial in elderly patients with acute MI or unstable angina and cardiogenic shock is percutaneous cardiopulmonary support (CPS), or "supported" angioplasty [39]. Supported angioplasty uses a membrane oxygenator and circulatory pump that can generate flows up to 4 or 5 L/min through percutaneously inserted arterial and venous cannulae. This type of circulatory support allows safer

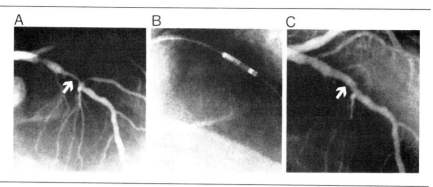

Figure 23-3. Directional atherectomy. **A.** Diffusely diseased left anterior descending artery in a 76-year-old woman with a high-grade eccentric stenosis proximal to the first septal perforator and diagonal branches (arrow). This type of lesion is unfavorable for balloon angioplasty. **B.** A 5 French Simpson Atherocath™ positioned across the lesion during directional atherectomy. **C.** Widely patent vessel after atherectomy at the atherectomy site (arrow).

angioplasty in patients with severe left ventricular dysfunction or in whom the culprit vessel supplies a very large amount of myocardium.

A second method of "supported angioplasty" recently reported uses intra-aortic balloon pump counterpulsation. It has had excellent initial results and no acute mortality in 28 elderly patients (mean age 66, 10 patients > age 70) undergoing high-risk angioplasty [40]. The main source of morbidity associated with both of these procedures is related to the vascular access site. Relatively large cannulae are required, so vascular compromise, bleeding, and pseudoaneurysm are more likely to occur during these procedures than with routine PTCA. These two methods of cardiac support make PTCA possible in patients who would otherwise be too hemodynamically unstable to undergo the procedure.

Coronary atherectomy

The term *coronary atherectomy* refers to the removal of atherosclerotic tissue from the coronary vessel wall. There are several types of atherectomy: directional coronary atherectomy, transluminal extraction, and rotational coronary atherectomy.

Directional coronary atherectomy (DCA) is a clinically approved method of percutaneous tissue removal that utilizes a cup-shaped cutter and housing that excises atherosclerotic tissue and stores it in a distal collection chamber for eventual removal (figure 23-3). DCA was performed in 52 lesions in the first 50 patients with a procedural success rate of 60% in the initial experience [41]. A higher success rate of 81% was achieved in the later patients. In one patient, abrupt occlusion necessitated emergency coronary bypass surgery. In a second series [42], directional coronary atherectomy was successfully

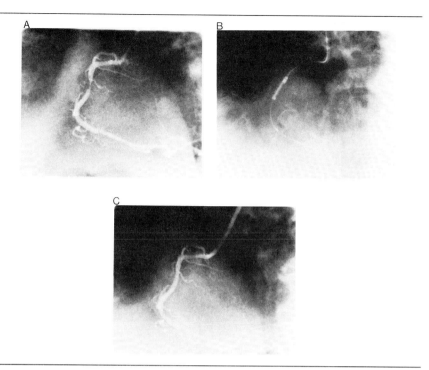

Figure 23-4. Directional atherectomy after failed PTCA. **A.** Mid-right coronary artery after balloon angioplasty. The PTCA result is suboptimal, and a high-grade residual stenosis remains after balloon angioplasty. **B.** Simpson Atherocath™ across the lesion during "salvage" atherectomy. **C.** Final angiographic result.

performed in 88% of the procedures attempted in 67 patients. One or more complications occurred in 9% of the patients. The six-month restenosis rate was 30% by life-table analysis. The four-year experience of Sequoia Hospital in Redwood City, California was recently published in abstract form [43]. The primary success rate in 502 procedures was 88.2%, with major complications observed in 4.2%, including death in 0.4%, CABG in 4.0%, and QMI in 1.0%. In a multicenter trial [44], directional coronary atherectomy was successful in 85% of 1069 lesions during 958 procedures. The mortality rate was 0.5%; emergency bypass surgery was required in 4.1%. Restenosis rates following directional atherectomy in the United States multicenter coronary trial [45] in native coronary vessels were 30% for de novo lesions and 46% for restenoses. Bypass graft atherectomy restenosis rates were 31% for de novo lesions and 68% for restenoses.

There is a growing body of evidence that DCA may be especially useful in certain patients with lesions that are unsuited for balloon angioplasty [46], and in patients with suboptimal balloon angioplasty results (figure 23-4)

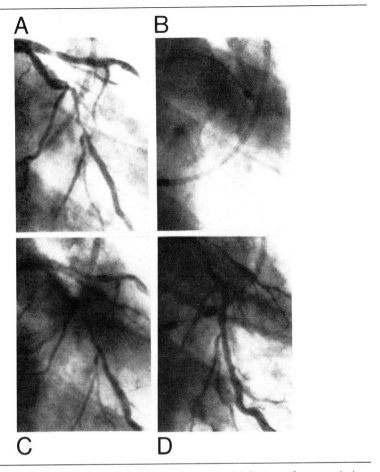

Figure 23-5. Rotational atherectomy. **A.** Long, complex mid-left circumflex stenosis in a patient with restenosis four months after PTCA. **B.** Rotablator™ during rotational atherectomy. **C.** Angiogram after rotational atherectomy alone. **D.** Final result after adjunctive balloon angioplasty. (Courtesy of Martin B. Leon, MD.)

[47,48]. This technique may provide a special benefit to elderly patients in whom the risk of emergency bypass surgery is increased if directional atherectomy can be used as a "bail-out" device for salvaging inadequate angioplasty results.

It appears from these preliminary reports that the success rates and complication rates for DCA approach those of conventional balloon angioplasty and that the restenosis rates are not necessarily superior to those achieved with PTCA; however, this technology is still in its infancy. Although the restenosis rate seems to be lower in the later cases, this should be substantiated. A randomized comparison of directional atherectomy with PTCA (the CAVEAT trial) will be starting soon. At this time, DCA is an appropriate treatment for patients who have discrete, proximal, eccentric stenosis in nontortuous vessels greater than 3.0 mm in diameter, provided that there are no contraindications, such as intracoronary thrombus, calcified coronary arteries, or severe peripheral vascular disease [49]. As mentioned previously, DCA may also be appropriate for patients with a suboptimal PTCA result in order to avoid emergency bypass surgery.

The percutaneous coronary rotational angioplasty (Rotablator^{TM}, Heart Technology, Inc., Bellevue, WA) and the transluminal extraction catheter (TEC^{TM}, Interventional Therapies, Danvers, MA) are two new atherectomy devices undergoing clinical trials in the coronary arteries. The Rotablator is a rotational atherectomy catheter with a diamond-studded tip that rotates at 150 to 180,000 rpm over a guidewire to selectively ablate inelastic tissue (figure 23-5). One hundred eighteen patients underwent rotational atherectomy with a 95% success rate [50]. Adjunctive PTCA was performed in 42% of patients. There were no deaths or Q-wave infarcts. Other complications included non-Q-wave MI (2.5%) and emergency CABG (0.8%). Although it is still relatively early to draw firm conclusions regarding the role of rotational atherectomy, the investigators believe the device may be particularly useful in treating lesions not amenable to PTCA, such as ostial stenosis, bifurcation lesions, calcified lesions, and long lesions in small-diameter arteries (<2.5 mm).

Transluminal extraction coronary atherectomy was performed in 147 patients in a multicienter trial with a 93% primary success rate and no deaths, strokes, or MIs. Emergency coronary bypass surgery was required in 5% of the patients because of dissection, vessel disruption, or thrombosis. Like rotational atherectomy, transluminal extraction atherectomy appears to be of value in patients with lesions that are unfavorable for balloon angioplasty [41], although restenosis rates appear to be no better than with PTCA.

Even if acute success and restenosis rates are not improved with coronary atherectomy, these types of treatments may be useful additions to the interventional cardiologist's percutaneous armamentarium because they expand the application of percutaneous angioplasty techniques to lesions that are not currently amenable to conventional balloon angioplasty. The final role of all types of atherectomy in our treatment of CAD in the elderly remains to be defined by further study.

Intracoronary stents

The development of percutaneously implantable endovascular prostheses, or stents, is intended to address two of the major problems associated with percutaneous ballon angioplasty: abrupt occlusion of the dilated vessel leading to emergency surgery, and restenosis or recurrence of the arterial stenosis or occlusion. The incidence of abrupt occlusion following balloon angioplasty of the dilated artery requiring emergency surgical revascularization ranges from 2% to 5% [51–54].

Early clinical trials [55,56] have suggested that stents can effectively reverse abrupt artery occlusion following coronary angioplasty, allowing elective surgical revascularization or continued medical therapy without concomitant MI. The clinical application of stents as effective "bail-out" devices would not only increase the overall safety and efficacy of routine coronary angioplasty but would expand the indications for percutaneous angioplasty to patients currently not considered candidates due to the high risk of death or limb loss should abrupt occlusion occur. The Palmaz–Schatz™ stent (Johnson & Johnson Interventional Systems, Warren, NJ) was successfully deployed in 72 patients for dissection following PTCA [57]. Four patients (5.6%) had abrupt reocclusions requiring either repeat PTCA or bypass surgery. At mean follow-up of 5.3 months (range 1 to 16 months), 58 patients (82%) were asymptomatic, 6 had stable angina, and 4 had unstable angina. The angiographic restenosis rate in 27 patients restudied was 33%. This suggests that stenting is an acceptable alternative to emergency bypass surgery for failed PTCA.

Restenosis of the dilated lesion occurs in approximately 30% of elective coronary angioplasty patients within six months [58,59]. A reduction of the restenosis rate would reduce the need for repeat procedures and, by sustaining the immediate benefits of angioplasty, reduce the overall costs of the procedure. A preliminary report from Sigwart et al. [60] suggested that, with use of a self-expanding stainless steel mesh stent, coronary restenosis of the stented artery did not occur in 12 patients with angiographic follow-up 3 to 6 months later. However, in a large series of patients followed for an average of six months [61], abrupt occlusion or restenosis of this coronary stent was a significant problem. Abrupt occlusion within the first two weeks occurred in 21 of 95 (22%) patients. Late restenosis, presumed to be due to intimal hyperplasia and smooth muscle proliferation, occurred in 32% of patients [61].

Restenosis following stent implantation also seems to be related to the number of stents deployed. In a recent report [62], the angiographic restenosis rate in 122 of 160 (67%) consecutive patients who underwent follow-up angiograms was 19% for single stents and 58% for multiple stents. Because of this finding, the placement of multiple stents to cover long stenoses or dissections should be avoided.

Human clinical trials of coronary and peripheral stents have indicated that stents have a bimodal failure curve [57,60,61]. The early failures, which occur within the first two weeks, appear to be due to thrombosis of the stents and should be preventable or significantly reduced with adequate systemic anticoagulation. The second group of stent failures, which occur after weeks to months, are due to stenosis of the lumen of the stented segment due to excessive intimal thickening. It has been suggested that

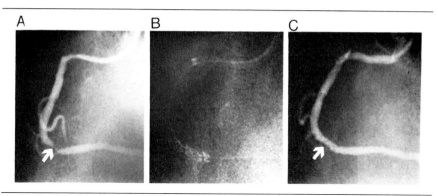

Figure 23-6. Stent implantation. **A.** Distal right coronary artery restenosis lesion (arrow) before stent implantation. **B.** Radiopaque tantalum Wiktor™ stent implanted in the lesion. **C.** Final angiographic result after stent deployment.

factors that promote this excessive intimal thickening include an excessive amount of thrombus deposited on the stent's surface due to the inherent thrombogenicity of electropositively charged metals, as well as repeated trauma to the endothelium of the artery from the stent, which stimulates a high turnover of collagen and smooth muscle cells.

We have begun clinical implantation of a new radiopaque balloon expandable coronary artery stent (Medtronic–Wiktor), which has been used successfully in a preliminary trial in Europe [63]. The stent is composed of a 0.005-inch tantalum wire in a coiled configuration, tightly crimped over an angioplasty delivery balloon. Patients are selected for the protocol if they have native coronary artery restenosis or abrupt reocclusion after balloon angioplasty and no contraindications to anticoagulation (figure 23-6). After the lesion is predilated, the balloon-mounted stent is advanced to the lesion through an angioplasty guiding catheter. After stent implantation, the patients reveive 325 mg of aspirin daily and intravenous heparin, which is continued until the patient is on a stable dose of coumadin. Anticoagulation is continued for three months.

To date we have implanted coronary stents in 14 patients for restenosis following balloon angioplasty. Stent diameters implanted have ranged in size from 3.0 mm to 4.0 mm. No patients have suffered abrupt occlusion or early stent failure. The length of follow-up has been too short to make any conclusions regarding restenosis rates. The major advantages of this balloon expandable device include its radiopacity, which facilitates accurate placement, and its coil configuration, which improves flexibilty and trackability over a guidewire in tortuous coronary vessels.

As experience with intracoronary stents grows, the indications for their use and their clinical efficacy should become better defined. At present, they are investigational tools only and should be used in elderly patients who are candidates for the investigational protocols and have no contraindications to chronic anticoagulation.

Coronary laser angioplasty

The generic term *laser angioplasty* encompasses a broad field of clinical applications that use the energy derived from laser light to remodel blood vessels. The primary applications of laser angioplasty are atherolysis, ablation or vaporization of intraluminal atherosclerotic material, and tissue welding, sealing of the layers of the artery wall after therapeutic disruption by balloon dilation. The explosion of basic research and clinical investigation directed over the past decade towards the development of a clinically useful laser angioplasty system is a direct result of the success and limitations of the percutaneous treatment of atherosclerotic occlusive vascular disease with balloon angioplasty. As with stents and atherectomy, it is hoped that a successful laser angioplasty system will improve the results and extend the indications for the percutaneous treatment of CAD.

Coronary angioplasty trials with three excimer laser multifiber delivery systems have been reported [64–70]. Only one laser system has been approved for use in the United States as a treatment for CAD (Advanced Interventional Systems (AIS), Irvine, CA). This system combines a unique, stretched-pulse, excimer (XeCl, 308 nm) laser with a 5 French multifiber catheter. Laser angioplasty was attempted with this device on 53 lesions (44 stenoses and 9 total occlusions), with successful recanalization occurring in 39 of 53 (74%) lesions [64]. Of the 39 successful cases, only six were performed without adjunctive balloon angioplasty. There were no laser-related perforations or deaths in this series; restenosis data are not yet available. The authors concluded that a larger catheter would be necessary to reduce the need for adjunctive balloon angioplasty to determine whether the restenosis rate following laser recanalization alone was improved over balloon angioplasty.

More recent data describing the results of 55 patients treated with a 1.6-mm-diameter multifiber catheter demonstrated an increase in the success rate to 84% [65]. This multicenter trial included patients in whom a guidewire could be passed across the coronary lesion, over which the laser catheter could then be advanced. Serious clinical complication, which occurred in 5% of patients, included abrupt coronary artery occlusion, arterial dissection, MI, and the need for emergency coronary bypass surgery.

A multicenter pilot study designed to test the safety and efficacy of laser balloon angioplasty to seal dissections following conventional balloon angioplasty was performed in 55 patients with native coronary artery lesions [71]. A successful result was obtained in each of the 55 treated patients, including salvage of an unsuccessful angiographic result after conventional angioplasty in 14 patients. Of the 14 unsuccessful conventional angioplasty

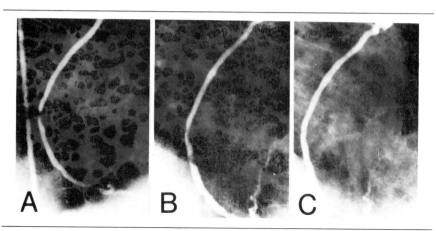

Figure 23-7. Laser angioplasty. **A.** Midbody lesion in a saphenous vein graft supplying the distal right coronary artery. **B.** Angiographic appearance after laser angioplasty alone. **C.** Final result after adjunctive balloon angioplasty.

procedures, eight were the result of dissection and three were related to occlusive thrombus. The mean diameter stenosis in these patients at baseline, $78 \pm 8\%$, was reduced by conventional balloon angioplasty to $43 \pm 18\%$ ($p < 0.001$), and was further reduced after laser balloon treatment to $26 \pm 11\%$ ($p < 0.001$). Complications associated with the procedure included severe pain at the higher energy levels during laser delivery, ventricular fibrillation in one patient, and mild elevation of myocardial enzymes in three patients without ECG evidence of infarction. Six-month follow-up demonstrated that a higher rate of recurrence (67%) was associated with the highest energy levels delivered. A higher restenosis rate also occurred, regardless of laser dosimetry, in patients with prior restenosis (67%). In patients without prior restenosis treated with the lowest laser dosimetry, a restenosis rate of 29% (6 of 21) was found. The overall restenosis rate for the entire series was 51%. The authors concluded that laser balloon angioplasty was effective in increasing the immediate post-PTCA luminal diameter, probably by overcoming elastic recoil of the artery. They believed that the laser balloon's ability to salvage unsatisfactory angioplasty results due to dissection could be attributed to successful tissue welding and that the improvement in arteries with thrombus may have been due to desiccation. Whether or not the laser balloon can improve the rate of restenosis following balloon angioplasty must await further refinements in laser dosimetry.

We have recently begun a clinical trial of a mid-infrared laser angioplasty system, holmium:YAG (Trimedyne, Tustin, CA), using multifiber catheters over a guidewire. Successful delivery of holmium:YAG laser energy and partial recanalization of the coronary stenoses was accomplished in all seven lesions in which it was attempted (figure 23-7). The baseline coronary stenosis averaged 96.6 ± 3.5% (mean ±SD) and was reduced to 38.6 ± 24.1% ($p = 0.0006$) after laser angioplasty. One patient with a 99% stenosis in a 2.5-mm artery was treated with laser alone and left with a residual stenosis of 10%. Following laser therapy, balloon angioplasty was used in two lesions and atherectomy (Simpson Atherocath[TM], Devices for Vascular Intervention, Santa Clara, CA) was used in the four remaining lesions to reduce the final mean stenosis to 12.9 ± 4.9%.

No complications were associated with laser energy delivery. The patients reported no sensations other than intermittent angina pectoris during laser treatment, presumably due to temporary occlusion of the artery when the laser catheter was engaged. No large dissections, coronary spasm, or emboli were identified on angiograms following laser recanalization. One patient underwent coronary angioscopy following laser treatment, which revealed evidence of numerous superficial intimal tears at the site of the lesion. There was no evidence of tissue charring, but the walls of the neolumen had a dull red appearance consistent with tissue removal by laser ablation. Four patients had tissue specimens removed for histologic examination with the atherectomy catheter. The samples showed no evidence of thermal charring, but there was evidence of thermal tissue effect.

The ultimate role of laser angioplasty in the treatment of CAD has not been established, and to date no conclusive data have been presented to support the presumption that laser angioplasty is any better than conventional balloon angioplasty. No randomized trials comparing laser angioplasty to conventional angioplasty have been undertaken. The preliminary data presented here show no particular advantage of laser angioplasty over conventional PTCA in terms of safety, efficacy, or long-term benefit, so further investigation is warranted before laser angioplasty becomes standard therapy for elderly patients with symptomatic CAD.

BALLOON VALVULOPLASTY FOR VALVULAR STENOSIS

Aortic stenosis

Aortic stenosis remains a significant problem in the elderly. The most common cause of aortic stenosis in adults is calcific aortic stenosis. In patients who are between 50 and 70 years of age, this is due to fibrosis and calcification of congenitally bicuspid aortic valves. In patients over age 70, the most common cause of aortic stenosis is senile calcific degeneration of congenitally normal tricuspid valves.

The prognosis in patients with aortic stenosis is related to the development of symptoms, and is quite poor once symptoms develop. In one third of patients, angina is the presenting symptom. Other significant symptoms include congestive heart failure and syncope. The survival rates in patients who do not undergo surgery for symptomatic aortic stenosis is 57% at one year, 37% at two years, and 25% at three years, compared with 93% at one year and 85% at two years in age-matched controls [72]. Therefore, intervention is indicated once symptoms develop in elderly patients with severe, symptomatic aortic stenosis.

The traditional therapy for aortic stenosis is aortic valve replacement. Like most other major surgical procedures, the risk of aortic valve replacement increases with increasing age. In one recent series, the in-hospital mortality in patients between 50 and 60 years of age was 5.1%; between ages 60 and 70 years it was 7.1%; and over age 70 it rose to 12% [73]. Survival in patients who undergo valve replacement for aortic stenosis is also related to the complexity of the operation performed. In octogenarians, there is a 94% acute survival for aortic valve replacement alone; however, the survival rate drops to 69% in patients who require concomitant coronary artery bypass surgery or mitral valve replacement [74].

Balloon aortic valvuloplasty is a new palliative treatment for patients with symptomatic aortic stenosis who are not good candidates for valve replacement. This includes patients at high risk who are over age 80 and patients who refuse surgery [75]. It also includes elderly patients with severe left ventricular dysfunction or severe underlying medical illnesses such as malignancy, uremia, and lung disease [75,76]. It also may be indicated in patients with severe aortic stenosis who have a small transvalvular gradient and severe left ventricular dysfunction. In these patients, "pseudo-aortic stenosis" may be present, meaning that moderate aortic stenosis in combination with cardiomyopathy on some other basis may lead to a situation in which the weakened ventricle cannot open the sclerotic but not stenotic aortic valve adequately, thus leading to a miscalculation of valve area [77]. Of note, these patients may not benefit from valve replacement, since the main problem is with left ventricular dysfunction due to CAD, viral cardiomyopathy, or some other primary muscle disorder, not severe aortic stenosis. Balloon valvuloplasty may also serve as a bridge to valve replacement in patients with severe aortic stenosis and severe left ventricular dysfunction with cardiogenic shock [78].

Balloon aortic valvuloplasty can be performed in extremely ill and moribund patients with severe aortic stenosis. The only contraindications to the procedure are severe aortic insufficiency and left ventricular thrombus. Balloon dilation of the aortic valve is accomplished by passing a guidewire and balloon across the stenotic aortic orifice. The balloon is then inflated quickly to its maximum diameter and rapidly deflated so that left ventricular outflow is restricted only briefly (figure 23-8). Valvuloplasty relieves calcific aortic stenosis, presumably by fracturing the calcified plates and nodules within the valve leaflets, causing microfractures within the leaflets [79,80] and stretching the wall of the aorta [81].

The acute results of balloon aortic valvuloplasty have been reported by a number of investigators [82–89]. The immediate benefits of aortic valvuloplasty include reduction of the transvalvular gradient and increase in

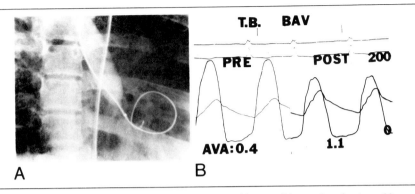

Figure 23-8. Balloon aortic valvuloplasty. **A.** Balloon dilation of the aortic valve in an 82-year-old man with severe aortic stenosis. **B.** Hemodynamic tracings before and after valvuloplasty. The aortic valve area was increased from $0.4\,cm^2$ to $1.1\,cm^2$ by balloon valvuloplasty.

Table 23-2. Aortic valvuloplasty: initial hemodynamic results

		Prevalvuloplasty			Postvalvuloplasty		
Study	Patients (N)	Peak gradient (mmHg)	Mean gradient (mmHg)	Valve area (cm^2)	Peak gradient (mmHg)	Mean gradient (mmHg)	Valve area (cm^2)
Cribier et al. [85]	302	72 ± 14		0.54 ± 0.18	28 ± 2		0.98 ± 0.32
Safian et al. [87]	170	71 ± 20	56 ± 19	0.60 ± 0.20	36 ± 14	31 ± 12	0.90 ± 0.30
Block and Palacios [88]	90		61 ± 2	0.40 ± 0.02		30 ± 2	0.80 ± 0.03

Modified from Banks AK and Laird JR. 1991. Balloon aortic valvuloplasty. In CJ White and SR Ramee (eds), Interventional Cardiology: Clinical Application of New Technologies. New York: Raven Press, pp 199–221. Used with permission.

the calculated aortic valve area. The majority of patients will be left with a valve area of between $0.7\,cm^2$ and $1.1\,cm^2$ after valvuloplasty (table 23-2) [90]. This modest improvement in valve area, generally 50% to 75% larger than the prevalvuloplasty measurement, is generally enough to lower the left ventricular filling pressure and pulmonary capillary pressure, resulting in acute improvement in symptoms in more than 90% of patients treated [91]. Immediate complications of aortic valvuloplasty include death in 3% to 10% and vascular complications in 7% to 13% [83–87]. In our experience, as well as the experience of others, deaths usually occur in patients who are already moribund at the time the procedure is performed. The incidence of stroke is approximately 1.5%. Other serious complications, including ventricular perforation, MI, and severe aortic insufficiency, occur less commonly.

Although the immediate symptomatic results of balloon valvuloplasty for aortic stenosis are very gratifying in the majority of patients, the long-term benefit is limited by a high restenosis rate. About 80% of patients have recurrent symptoms within two years of balloon aortic valvuloplasty that result in death, repeat balloon valvuloplasty, or valve replacement [91]. In four studies reporting follow-up data after balloon aortic valvuloplasty, one- to two-year survival was between 52% and 70% [85–88].

Because of the high restenosis rate with balloon valvuloplasty for calcific aortic stenosis, patients without contraindications for surgery should be referred for aortic valve replacement regardless of age. Patients who have contraindications to surgery or associated medical conditions that may negate the long-term benefit of valve replacement, or who refuse surgery, should be offered balloon valvuloplasty. Although there are no data to support improved longevity with this procedure, it certainly offers excellent short-term palliation of symptoms in the majority of patients.

Mitral stenosis
Mitral stenosis is generally considered to be a disease of the young; however, symptomatic mitral stenosis occasionally presents in the elderly patient. Although surgical commissurotomy and mitral valve replacement have long been the treatments of choice for symptomatic patients with mitral stenosis, Inoue and colleagues [91] pioneered the technique of balloon mitral commissurotomy in 1984. This technique, also known as balloon mitral valvuloplasty, is still considered to be investigational in the United States; however, the short- and long-term results have been excellent, and the procedure has gained broad acceptance worldwide and has become the procedure of choice in selected patients with mitral stenosis (figures 23-9–23-11) [92].

The mechanism of balloon mitral commissurotomy involves commissural splitting, including splitting of heavily calcified commissures [93] and fracture of calcium nodules within the leaflets [94] without gross fracturing of the tissue or tearing of the valve leaflets. In postmortem studies [93] and in clinical trials [94–105], the procedure generally doubles the mitral valve orifice size, increasing the mitral valve area to $>2.0\,cm^2$. The increase in valve area is accompanied by a decrease in the mean transvalvular pressure gradient, an increase in the cardiac output, and a reduction in pulmonary artery and pulmonary capillary wedge pressures acutely. This degree of improvement in valve area results in a substantial clinical benefit for most patients and usually renders them asymptomatic or minimally symptomatic [104,105].

In 219 patients between the ages of 19 and 76 years, balloon valvuloplasty was performed successfully, with clinical improvements in 97% [106]. Immediate complications included one death and three systemic emboli. Increase in mitral regurgitation was noted in 33%, with 3+ mitral

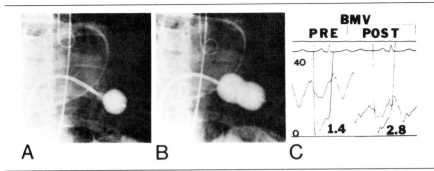

Figure 23-9. Balloon mitral valvuloplasty using the Inoue™ balloon. **A.** Partial inflation of balloon in left ventricle to assist positioning across the mitral valve. **B.** Maximal inflation to open the fused commissures. **C.** Hemodynamics before and after valvuloplasty. The mitral valve area was increased from 1.4 cm² to 2.8 cm² by balloon inflation. The increase in mitral valve area was accompanied by reduction in the left atrial pressure and the diastolic pressure gradient across the mitral valve.

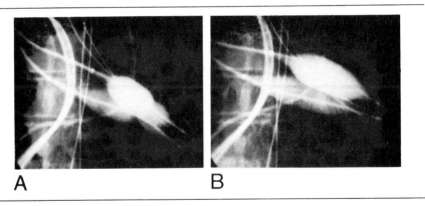

Figure 23-10. Double balloon technique of balloon mitral valvuloplasty. **A.** Both balloons partially inflated with "waisting" of the balloons across the stenotic mitral orifice. **B.** Balloon "waisting" eliminated by complete balloon inflation.

regurgitation in 6%. Fifteen percent had oximetry-detected atrial shunts from the transeptal puncture. Even patients with suboptimal gradient response to balloon valvuloplasty, and those with resultant mitral regurgitation had clinical improvement following the procedure. The more calcified valves responded less well to balloon dilation than the more pliable valves in this and in other series [107]. The cardiovascular event-free survival for patients with noncalcified valves was 100% at up to 42 months. In patients with calcified valves or severe subvalvular lesions, the cardiac event-free survival was 91% at 12 months and 76% at 31 months. These results compare

Pre   Post

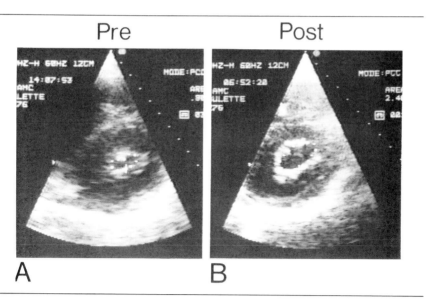

A   B

Figure 23-11. Two-dimensional echocardiography in the parasternal short-axis view before (**A**) and after (**B**) balloon mitral valvuloplasty. Note the increase in the valve orifice after valvuloplasty.

favorably with the best surgical results with open or closed commissurotomy [90,108–112].

The most important predictor of the immediate and long-term outcomes of balloon valvuloplasty for mitral stenosis is the morphology of the valve (table 23-3) [95] as characterized by its echocardiographic score [106–108]. Other predictors of suboptimal results with balloon dilation of the mitral valve include advanced age and the presence of atrial fibrillation or mitral regurgitation. Elderly patients are more likely to have atrial fibrillation, calcification of the leaflets and subvalvular apparatus, and worse echocardiographic scores. In the series by Block et al. [106] fewer than 50% of patients 65 years or older had postvalvuloplasty valve areas >1.5 cm^2 with less than a two-grade increase in mitral regurgitation and less than 1.5:1 left-to-right shunts.

In summary, balloon valvuloplasty can be performed safely in a variety of patients with mitral stenosis. The best short- and long-term results can be obtained with patients who have pliable, noncalcified leaflets in the absence of mitral regurgitation and atrial fibrillation. Patients who are not good surgical candidates may also be candidates for balloon valvuloplasty even in the presence of suboptimal valve morphology and mitral regurgitation, since they may still receive excellent symptomatic palliation with balloon mitral valvuloplasty.

Table 23-3. Mitral valve echocardiography score based on morphologic features

Score	Definition
	Mobility
1	High mobile valve with only leaflet tips restricted
2	Normal mobility of leaflet midportion and base
3	Valve continues to move forward in diastole, mainly from the base
4	No or minimal forward movement of leaflets in diastole
	Leaflet Thickening
1	Leaflet nearly normal in thickness (4–5 mm)
2	Midportion of leaflets normal; marked thickening of margins (5–8 mm)
3	Thickening extending through entire leaflet (5–8 mm)
4	Marked thickening of all leaflet tissue (>8–10 mm)
	Subvalvular Thickening
1	Minimal thickening just below mitral leaflets
2	Thickening of chordal structures up to one third of the chordal length
3	Thickening extending to distal third of the chords
4	Extensive thickening and shortening of all chordal structures extending down to papillary muscles
	Calcification
1	Single area of increased echo brightness
2	Scattered areas of brightness confined to leaflet margins
3	Brightness extending into midportion of leaflets
4	Extensive brightness throughout much of the leaflet tissue

Modified from Abascal VM, Wilkins GT, Choong CY, et al. 1988. Mitral regurgitation after percutaneous balloon mitral valvuloplasty in adults: evaluation by pulsed doppler echocardiography. J Am Coll Cardiol 11:257–263. Used with permission.

CONCLUSION

The interventional cardiologist has been playing an expanding role in the management of patients with CAD and valvular stenosis. This is especially true in elderly patients who are at increased risk for coronary artery bypass and valvular surgery. Numerous studies have demonstrated that coronary angioplasty is an excellent means of palliating symptoms in elderly patients with single or multivessel CAD, and PTCA may be the treatment of choice in patients who are at the highest risk for morbidity and mortality with coronary bypass surgery. Likewise, balloon valvuloplasty is an effective means of palliating symptoms in selected patients with mitral stenosis and patients with aortic stenosis who are not acceptable surgical candidates. Certain recommendations can be made based upon the available information summarized in this chapter. These recommendations should be considered as a general philosophy for approaching elderly patients with cardiovascular disease, rather than as strict guidelines.

Elderly patients with symptomatic CAD should be treated medically unless they have refractory symptoms or high-risk anatomy, such as critical proximal lesions with a large amount of myocardium in jeopardy. In patients who have unstable ischemic syndromes or who continue to be limited by symptoms despite medical therapy, revascularization with bypass surgery or angioplasty should be considered. Although coronary bypass surgery carries an increased risk in elderly patients, some septuagenarians and even octogenarians will certainly benefit from surgical revascularization. This includes patients with multivessel CAD, fair-to-good left ventricular function, and good distal vessels in the absence of other medical contraindications. Coronary angioplasty may be preferred in lieu of bypass surgery in patients with single or multivessel disease and discrete stenoses or in patients who are not good candidates for bypass surgery because of severe left ventricular dysfunction, distal disease, or associated medical illnesses. It may even be possible to palliate the elderly patient with multivessel disease and a "culprit" lesion with single-vessel angioplasty of that lesion alone. The addition of newer percutaneous devices, including stents, atherectomy, laser angioplasty, and supported angioplasty, may be appropriate in selected patients; however, investigational devices should be offered only to patients who are enrolled in experimental protocols.

Generally, elderly patients with aortic stenosis are best managed surgically if they are acceptable candidates for valve replacement. Patients with aortic stenosis who are not good candidates for surgery may still achieve excellent temporary symptomatic benefit from balloon valvuloplasty. This includes patients with aortic stenosis, severe left ventricular dysfunction and low cardiac output states, patients with severe underlying medical conditions, and patients who refuse surgery. Patients with rheumatic mitral stenosis and favorable valve morphology by echocardiography are candidates for balloon mitral valvuloplasty as an alternative to surgical commissurotomy, and can be offered enrollment in one of the ongoing investigational trials.

The future of interventional cardiology in the elderly depends upon the results of ongoing trials evaluating the safety and efficacy of balloon angioplasty and the impact of the newer percutaneous therapies on the short- and long-term results of catheter intervention. It is hoped that the ongoing investigations of intravascular stents, atherectomy devices, and lasers will lead to safer and more effective angioplasty and a reduction in the rate of restenosis after percutaneous intervention.

REFERENCES

1. Elveback L and Lie JT. 1984. Continued high incidence of coronary artery disease at autopsy in Olmsted County, Minnesota, 1950 to 1979. Circulation 70:345–349.
2. Glazer MD, Hill RD and Wenger NK. 1985. Dx and Tx of the elderly patient with atherosclerotic coronary heart disease. Geriatrics 40:45–47, 50–54.
3. Fleg JL. 1991. Angina pectoris in the elderly. Cardiol Clin 9:177–187.
4. Grüntzig A. 1978. Transluminal dilatation of coronary artery stenosis (letter to the editor). Lancet 1:263.
5. Faro RS, Golden MD, Javid H, et al. 1983. Coronary revascularization in septuagenarians. J Thorac Cardiovasc Surg 86:616–620.
6. Hochberg MS, Levine FH, Daggett WM, et al. 1982. Isolated coronary artery bypass grafting in patients seventy years of age and older: early and late results. J Thorac Cardiovasc Surg 84:219–223.

7. Horneffer PJ, Gardner TJ, Manolio TA, et al. 1987. The effects of age on outcome after coronary bypass surgery. Circulation 76 (Suppl V):V6–V12.
8. Horvath KA, DiSesa VJ, Peigh PS, et al. 1990. Favorable results of coronary artery bypass grafting in patients older than 75 years. J Thorac Cardiovasc Surg 99:92–96.
9. Grondin CM, Thornton JC, Engle JC, et al. 1989. Cardiac surgery in septuagenarians: Is there a difference in mortality and morbidity? J Thorac Cardiovasc Surg 98:908–914.
10. Dorros G, Lewin RF, Daley P, et al. 1987. Coronary artery bypass surgery in patients over age 70 years: report from the Milwaukee Cardiovascular Data Registry. Clin Cardiol 10:377–382.
11. Tsai T-P, Chaux A, Kass RM, et al. 1989. Aortocoronary bypass surgery in septuagenarians and octogenarians. J Cardiovasc Surg 30:364–368.
12. Holt GW, Sugrue DD, Bresnahan JF, et al. 1988. Results of percutaneous transluminal coronary angioplasty for unstable angina pectoris in patients 70 years of age and older. Am J Cardiol 61:994–997.
13. Simpfendorfer C, Raymond R, Schraider J, et al. 1988. Early and long-term results of percutaneous transluminal coronary angioplasty in patients 70 years of age and older with angina pectoris. Am J Cardiol 62:959–961.
14. Dorros G, Lewin RF and Mathiak LM. 1989. Percutaneous transluminal coronary angioplasty in patients over the age of 70 years. Cardiology Clin 7:805–812.
15. Jeroudi MO, Kleiman NS, Minor ST, et al. 1990. Percutaneous transluminal coronary angioplasty in octogenarians. Ann Intern Med 113:423–428.
16. Bentivoglio LG, Van Raden MJ, Kelsey SF, et al. 1984. Percutaneous transluminal coronary angioplasty (PTCA) in patients with relative contraindications: results of the National Heart, Lung, and Blood Institute PTCA Registry. Am J Cardiol 53 (Suppl): 82C–88C.
17. Kelsey SF, Miller DP, Holubkov R, et al. 1990. Results of percutaneous transluminal coronary angioplasty in patients ≥65 years of age (from the 1985 to 1986 National Heart, Lung, and Blood Institute's Coronary Angioplasty Registry). Am J Cardiol 66:1033–1038.
18. Holmes DR Jr, Holubkov R, Vlietstra RE, et al. 1988. Comparison of complications during percutaneous transluminal coronary angioplasty from 1977 to 1981 and from 1985 to 1986: the National Heart, Lung, and Blood Institute Percutaneous Transluminal Coronary Angioplasty Registry. J Am Coll Cardiol 12:1149–1155.
19. Holland KJ, O'Neill WW, Bates ER, et al. 1989. Emergency percutaneous transluminal coronary angioplasty during acute myocardial infarction for patients more than 70 years of age. Am J Cardiol 63:399–403.
20. Cannon AD and Dean LS. 1991. PTCA or CABG in the elderly? 1991. Cardiology 124–137.
21. Mock MB, Holmes DR Jr, Vlietstra RE, et al. 1984. Percutaneous transluminal coronary angioplasty (PTCA) in the elderly patient: experience in the National Heart, Lung, and Blood Institute PTCA Registry. Am J Cardiol 53 (Suppl):89C–91C.
22. Cook C and Hubner PJB. 1989. Percutaneous transluminal coronary angioplasty in elderly patients: a comparison with younger patients. Age Ageing 18:219–222.
23. Mills TJ, Smith HC and Vlietstra RE. 1989. PTCA in the elderly: results and expectations. Geriatrics 44:71–72, 77–79.
24. Bedotto JB, Rutherford BD, McConahay DR, et al. 1991. Results of multivessel percutaneous transluminal coronary angioplasty in persons aged 65 and older. Am J Cardiol 67:1051–1055.
25. McCallister BD, Hartzler GO, Reed WA, et al. 1983. Percutaneous transluminal coronary angioplasty in elderly patients: a comparison with coronary artery bypass surgery (abstract). J Am Coll Cardiol 1 (Suppl 2):656.
26. Mukherjee S, Faxon DP, Garber GR, et al. 1989. Early risks of revascularization in the elderly: PTCA versus CABG. Circulation 80 (Suppl II):II-261.
27. Tofler GH, Muller JE, Stone PH, et al. 1988. Factors leading to shorter survival after acute myocardial infarction in pateints ages 65 to 75 years compared with younger patients. Am J Cardiol 62:860–867.
28. Bayer AJ, Chadha JS, Farag RR and Pathy MS. 1986. Changing presentation of myocardial infarction with increasing old age. J Am Geriatr Soc 34:263–266.
29. Wittry MD, Thornton TA and Chaitman BR. 1989. Safe use of thrombolysis in the elderly. Geriatrics 44:28–30, 33–36.

30. Gruppo Italiano per lo Studio della Streptochinasi nell'Infarto Miocardico (GISSI). 1986. Effectiveness of intravenous thrombolytic treatment in acute myocardial infarction. Lancet 1:397–402.
31. The ISAM Study Group. 1986. A prospective trial of intravenous streptokinase in acute myocardial infarction (ISAM). N Engl J Med 314:1465–1471.
32. AIMS Trial Study Group. 1988. Effect of intravenous APSAC on mortality after acute myocardial infarction: preliminary report of a placebo-controlled clinical trial. Lancet 1:545–549.
33. ISIS-2 (Second International Study of Infarct Survival) Collaborative Group. 1988. Randomised trial of intravenous streptokinase, oral aspirin, both, or neither among 17, 187 cases of suspected acute myocardial infarction: ISIS-2. Lancet 2:349–360.
34. Wilcox RG, von der Lippe G, Olsson CG, et al. 1988. Trial of tissue plasminogen activator for mortality reduction in acute myocardial infarction: Anglo-Scandinavian Study of Early Thrombolysis (ASSET). Lancet 2:525–530.
35. Rich MW. 1991. Thrombolytic therapy in the elderly. Cardiovasc Rev Rep: 11–13.
36. O'Keefe JH Jr, Rutherford BD, McConahay DR, et al. 1989. Early and late results of coronary angioplasty without antecedent thrombolytic therapy for acute myocardial infarction. Am J Cardiol 64:1221–1230.
37. Lee TC, Laramee LA, Rutherford BD, et al. 1990. Emergency percutaneous transluminal coronary angioplasty for acute myocardial infarction in patients 70 years of age and older. Am J Cardiol 66:663–667.
38. Lee L, Bates ER, Pitt B, et al. 1988. Percutaneous transluminal coronary angioplasty improves survival in acute myocardial infarction complicated by cardiogenic shock. Circulation 78:1345–1351.
39. Vogel RA, Tommaso CL and Gundry SR. 1988. Initial experience with coronary angioplasty and aortic valvuloplasty using elective semipercutaneous cardiopulmonary support. Am J Cardiol 62:811–813.
40. Kahn JK, Rutherford BD, McConahay DR, et al. 1990. Supported "high risk" coronary angioplasty using intraaortic balloon pump counterpulsation. J Am Coll Cardiol 15: 1151–1155.
41. Sketch MH Jr, O'Neill WW, Tcheng JE, et al. 1990. Early and late outcome following coronary transluminal extraction-endarterectomy: a multicenter experience (abstract). Circulation 82 (Suppl III):III–310.
42. Safian RD, Gelbfish JS, Erny RE, et al. 1990. Coronary atherectomy: clinical, angiographic and histological findings and observations regarding potential mechanisms. Circulation 82:69–79.
43. Robertson GC, Simpson JB, Selmon MR, et al. 1991. Experience of directional coronary atherectomy over four years (abstract). J Am Coll Cardiol 17:384A.
44. U.S. Directional Coronary Atherectomy Investigator Group. 1990. Directional coronary atherectomy: multicenter experience (abstract). Circulation 82 (Suppl III):III–71.
45. U.S. Directional Coronary Atherectomy Investigators Group. 1990. Restenosis following directional coronary atherectomy in a multicenter experience (abstract). Circulation 82 (Suppl III):III–679.
46. Selmon M, Rowe M, Simpson J, et al. 1990. Directional coronary atherectomy for angiographically unfavorable lesions (abstract). J Am Coll Cardiol 15:58A.
47. Whitlow PL, Robertson GC, Rowe MH, et al. 1990. Directional coronary atherectomy for failed percutaneous transluminal coronary angioplasty (abstract). Circulation 82 (Suppl III):III–1.
48. Vetter JW, Simpson JB, Robertson GC, et al. 1991. Rescue directional coronary atherectomy for failed balloon angioplasty (abstract). J Am Coll Cardiol 17:384A.
49. Leon, MB. Directional coronary atherectomy. In CJ White and SR Ramee (eds), Interventional Cardiology. Clinical Application of New Technology. New York: Raven Press. 1991, pp 149–172.
50. Buchbinder M, O'Neill W, Worth D, et al. 1990. Percutaneous coronary rotational ablation using the rotablator: results of a multicenter study (abstract). Circulation 82 (Suppl III):III–309.
51. Kalman PG and Johnston KW. 1985. Outcome of failed percutaneous transluminal dilation. Surg Gynecol Obstet 161:43–46.
52. Dorros G, Cowley MJ, Simpson J, et al. 1983. Percutaneous transluminal coronary

angioplasty: report of complications from the National Heart, Lung, and Blood Institute PTCA registry. Circulation 67:723–730.

53. Bredlau CE, Roubin GS, Leimgruber PP, et al. 1985. In-hospital morbidity and mortality in patients undergoing elective coronary angioplasty. Circulation 72:1044–1052.

54. Cowley MJ, Dorros G, Kelsey SF, et al. 1984. Emergency coronary bypass surgery after coronary angioplasty: the National Heart, Lung, and Blood Institute's percutaneous transluminal coronary angioplasty registry experience. Am J Cardiol 53:22C–26C.

55. Sigwart U, Urban P, Golf S, et al. 1988. Emergency coronary artery stenting for acute post-PTCA occlusion: an alternative to surgery? (Abstract.) Circulation 78 (Suppl II): II-406.

56. Roubin GS, Douglas JS Jr, Lembo NJ, et al. 1988. Intracoronary stenting for acute closure following percutaneous transluminal coronary angioplasty (PTCA) (abstract). Circulation 78 (Suppl II):II-407.

57. Fajadet JC, Marco J, Cassagneau BG, et al. 1991. Emergency coronary stenting for acute dissection during PTCA (abstract). J Am Coll Cardiol 17:53A.

58. Leimgruber PP, Roubin GS, Hollman J, et al. 1986. Restenosis after successful coronary angioplasty in patients with single-vessel disease. Circulation 73:710–717.

59. Holmes DR, Vlietstra RE, Smith HC, et al. 1984. Restenosis after percutaneous transluminal coronary angioplasty (PTCA): a report from the PTCA Registry of the National Heart, Lung, and Blood Institute. Am J Cardiol 53:77C–81C.

60. Sigwart U, Puel J, Mirkovitch V, et al. 1987. Intravascular stents to prevent occlusion and restenosis after transluminal angioplasty. N Engl J Med 316:701–706.

61. Serruys PW, Strauss BH, Beatt KJ, et al. 1991. Angiographic follow-up after placement of a self-expanding coronary-artery stent. N Engl J Med 324:13–17.

62. Fajadet JC, Marco J, Cassagneau BG, et al. 1991. Restenosis following successful Palmaz–Schatz intracoronary stent implantation (abstract). J Am Coll Cardiol 17:346A.

63. Buchwald A, Unterberg C and Werner G. 1991. Initial clinical results with the Wiktor Stent: a new balloon expandable coronary stent. Clin Cardiol 14:374–379.

64. Litvack F, Grundfest WS, Goldenberg T, et al. 1989. Percutaneous excimer laser angioplasty of aortocoronary saphenous vein grafts. J Am Coll Cardiol 14:803–808.

65. Margolis JR, Litvack F, Grundfest W, et al. 1989. Excimer laser coronary angioplasty: results of a multicenter study (abstract). Circulation 80 (Suppl II):II-477.

66. Litvack F, Eigler NL, Margolis JR, et al. 1990. Percutaneous excimer laser coronary angioplasty. Am J Cardiol 66:1027–1032.

67. Sanborn TA, Hershman RA, Torre SR, et al. 1989. Percutaneous excimer laser coronary angioplasty. Lancet 2:616.

68. Karsch KR, Haase KK, Mauser M, et al. 1989. Initial angiographic results in ablation of atherosclerotic plaque by percutaneous coronary excimer laser angioplasty without subsequent balloon dilatation. Am J Cardiol 64:1253–1257.

69. Karsch KR, Mauser M, Voelker W, et al. 1989. Percutaneous coronary excimer laser angioplasty: initial clinical results. Lancet 2:647–650.

70. Karsch KR, Haase KK, Voelker W, et al. 1990. Percutaneous coronary excimer laser angioplasty in patients with stable and unstable angina pectoris: acute results and incidence of restenosis during 6-month follow-up. Circulation 81:1849–1859.

71. Spears JR, Reyes VP, Wynne J, et al. 1990. Percutaneous coronary laser balloon angioplasty: initial results of a multicenter experience. J Am Coll Cardiol 16:293–303.

72. O'Keefe JH, Vlietstra RE, Bailey KR, et al. 1987. Natural history of candidates for balloon aortic valvuloplasty. Mayo Clin Proc 62:986–991.

73. Cormier B, Luxereau P, Bloch C, et al. 1988. Prognosis and long-term results of surgically treated aortic stenosis. Eur Heart J 9 (Suppl E):113–120.

74. Levinson JR, Akins CW, Buckley MJ, et al. 1989. Octogenarians with aortic stenosis: outcome after aortic valve replacement. Circulation 80 (Suppl I):I-49–I-56.

75. Cheitlin MD. 1989. Severe aortic stenosis in the sick octagenarian: a clear indicator for balloon valvuloplasty as the initial procedure. Circulation 80:1906–1908.

76. Schneider JF, Wilson M and Gallant TE. 1987. Percutaneous balloon aortic valvuloplasty for aortic stenosis in elderly patients at high risk for surgery. Ann Intern Med 106:696–699.

77. Carbello BA. 1991. Timing of surgery in mitral and aortic stenosis. Med Clin North Am 9:229–238.

78. Desnoyers MR, Salem DN, Rosenfield K, et al. 1988. Treatment of cardiogenic shock by emergency aortic balloon valvuloplasty. Ann Intern Med 108:833–835.
79. Fields CD and Isner JM. 1988. Balloon valvuloplasty in adults. Cardiol Clin 6:383–419.
80. Isner JM, Samuels DA, Slovenkai GA, et al. 1988. Mechanism of aortic balloon valvuloplasty: fracture of valvular calcific deposits. Ann Intern Med 108:377–380.
81. Reynolds DJM, Stone DL, Wells FC, et al. 1987. How does aortic balloon valvuloplasty work? Br Heart J 57:70.
82. Block PC and Palacios IF. 1987. Comparison of hemodynamic results of anterograde versus retrograde percutaneous balloon aortic valvuloplasty. Am J Cardiol 60:659–662.
83. Isner JM, Salem DN, Desnoyers MR, et al. 1988. Dual balloon technique for valvuloplasty of aortic stenosis in adults. Am J Cardiol 61:583–589.
84. Lewin RF, Dorros G, King JF, et al. 1989. Percutaneous transluminal aortic valvuloplasty: acute outcome and follow-up of 125 patients. J Am Coll Cardiol 14:1210–1217.
85. Cribier A, Berber LI and Letac B. 1990. Percutaneous balloon aortic valvuloplasty: the French experience. In EJ Topol (ed), Textbook of Interventional Cardiology. Philadelphia: W.B. Saunders, pp 849–867.
86. Dorros G, Lewin RF, Stertzer SH, et al. 1990. Percutaneous transluminal aortic valvuloplasty:—The acute outcome and follow-up of 149 patients who underwent the double balloon technique. Eur Heart J 11:429–440.
87. Safian RD, Berman AD, Diver DJ, et al. 1988. Balloon aortic valvuloplasty in 170 consecutive patients. N Engl J Med 319:125–130.
88. Block PC and Palacios IF. 1988. Clinical and hemodynamic follow-up after percutaneous aortic valvuloplasty in the elderly. Am J Cardiol 62:760–763.
89. Safian RD, Kuntz RE and Berman AD. 1991. Aortic valvuloplasty. Cardiol Clin 9: 289–299.
90. Banks AK and Laird JR. Balloon aortic valvuloplasty. In CJ White and SR Ramee (ed), Interventional Cardiology: Clinical Application of New Technologies. New York: Raven Press. 1991, pp 199–221.
91. Inoue K, Owaki T, Nakamura T, et al. 1984. Clinical application of transvenous mitral commissurotomy by a new balloon catheter. J Thorac Cardiovasc Surg 87:394–402.
92. Kaplan JD, Isner JM, Karas RH, et al. 1987. In vitro analysis of mechanisms of balloon valvuloplasty of stenotic mitral valves. Am J Cardiol 59:318–323.
93. McKay RG, Lock JE, Safian RD, et al. 1987. Balloon dilation of mitral stenosis in adult patients: postmortem and percutaneous mitral valvuloplasty studies. J Am Coll Cardiol 9:723–731.
94. McKay RG, Lock JE, Keane JF, et al. 1986. Percutaneous mitral valvuloplasty in an adult patient with calcific rheumatic mitral stenosis. J Am Coll Cardiol 7:1410–1415.
95. Abascal VM, Wilkins GT, Choong CY, et al. 1988. Mitral regurgitation after percutaneous balloon mitral valvuloplasty in adults: evaluation by pulsed doppler echocardiography. J Am Coll Cardiol 11:257–263.
96. Berman AD, Weinstein JS, Safian RD, et al. 1988. Combined aortic and mitral balloon valvuloplasty in patients with critical aortic and mitral valve stenosis: results in six cases. J Am Coll Cardiol 11:1213–1218.
97. Roth RB, Block PC and Palacios IF. 1988. Mitral regurgitation after percutaneous mitral valvuloplasty: predictors and follow-up (abstract). Circulation 78 (Suppl II):II-488.
98. Palacios IF and Block PC. 1988. Percutaneous mitral balloon valvotomy (PMV): update of immediate results and follow-up (abstract). Circulation 78 (Suppl II):II-489.
99. Vahanian A, Michel P-L, Vitoux B, et al. 1988. Follow up of patients with mitral stenosis after successful percutaneous commissurotomy (abstract). Circulation 78 (Suppl II):II-489.
100. Block P. 1988. Early results of mitral balloon valvuloplasty (MBV) for mitral stenosis: report from the NHLBI Registry (abstract). Circulation 78 (Suppl II):II-489.
101. Inoue K, Nobuyoshi M, Chen C, et al. 1988. Advantage of Inoue-balloon (self-positioning balloon) in percutaneous transvenous mitral commissurotomy (abstract). Circulation 78 (Suppl II):II-490.
102. Cequier A, Bonan R, Dyrda I, et al. 1988. Percutaneous mitral valvuloplasty: long-term clinical and hemodynamic follow-up (abstract). Circulation 78 (Suppl II):II-529.
103. Vahanian A, Michel P, Cormier B, et al. 1990. Percutaneous balloon aortic valvuloplasty:

the French experience. In EJ Topol (ed), Textbook of Interventional Cardiology. Philadelphia: W.B. Saunders, pp 868–886.

104. Inoue K and Hung J. 1990. Percutaneous tranvenous mitral commissurotomy (PTMC): the Far East experience. In EJ Topol (ed), Textbook of Interventional Cardiology. Philadelphia: W.B. Saunders, pp 887–899.

105. Hung JS, Chern MS, Wu JJ, et al. 1991. Short- and long-term results of catheter balloon percutaneous transvenous mitral commissurotomy. Am J Cardiol 67:854–862.

106. Block PC, Tuczu EM and Palacios IF. 1991. Percutaneous mitral balloon valvotomy. Cardiology Clin 9:271–287.

107. John S, Bashi VV, Jairaj PS, et al. 1983. Closed mitral valvotomy: early results and long-term follow-up of 3724 consecutive patients. Circulation 68:891–896.

108. Ellis LB, Singh JB, Morales DD, et al. 1973. Fifteen- to twenty-year study of one thousand patients undergoing closed mitral valvuloplasty. Circulation 48:357–364.

109. Ellis LB, Harken DE and Black HB. 1959. A clinical study of 1000 consecutive cases of mitral stenosis two to nine years after mitral valvuloplasty. Circulation 19:803–820.

110. John S, Perianayagam WJ, Abraham KA, et al. 1978. Restenosis of the mitral valve: surgical considerations and results of operation. Ann Thorac Surg 4:316–321.

111. Housman LB, Bonchek L, Lambert L, et al. 1977. Prognosis of patients after open mitral commissurotomy. Actuarial analysis of late results in 100 patients. J Thorac Cardiovasc Surg 73:742–745.

112. Cohn LH, Allred EN, Cohn LA, et al. 1985. Long-term results of open mitral valve reconstruction for mitral stenosis. Am J Cardiol 55:731–734.

24. SURGERY IN THE AGED

JAMES R. DOUGLAS, JR.
JOHN L. OCHSNER

Elderly is defined in Webster's New Collegiate Dictionary as being "rather old, past middle age" [1]. This definition appears vague. Since there are really no means of measuring physiologic age, it is difficult to state what age signifies elderly. To add to the difficulty and confusion, particularly in regard to surgery, the definition of *elderly* varies from 45 years to more than 80 years in different reports. However, most authorities today believe that people older than age 65 are elderly, since following this age there is a fairly rapid and constant decline in general health.

Because of the increasing life span and decreasing birth rate, the elderly segment is becoming one of the most rapidly growing of our population. Operations on patients in this age group have become a major concern. The aging process is such that all organs are affected. The ability of a patient to resist the stress of an operation is related to *organ reserve* and the faculty to restore homeostasis after alteration created by stress. Measurement of organ reserve in relation to age shows an almost linear decline beginning at about age 30 [2]. Hence, the proficiency of organs to rebound from the stress of surgery declines with age. The limited reserve of organs and the propensity of the elderly to have multiple chronic diseases account for the increased risk of death and postoperative complications with major surgery. Persons age 70

Franz H. Messerli (ed.), CARDIOVASCULAR DISEASE IN THE ELDERLY (Third Edition). Copyright © 1993 Kluwer Academic Publishers. ISBN 0-7923-1859-5. All rights reserved.

or older have the highest incidence of coronary artery disease, the highest death rate from various cardiovascular diseases, and the highest mortality rate with acute myocardial infarction.

One often hears physicians state that chronologic and physiologic age differ. We agree with this hypothesis to a certain extent but also realize that *physiologic* age is a vague term. One must take into consideration many factors in determining the physiologic status of an elderly person, such as the activity of the patient before operation, the presence of associated diseases, the patient's mental orientation to the environment, and the motivation and desire of the patient to return to active life. Therefore, additional contraindications to surgery might be limited life expectancy due to senility or the lack of will to live.

Very few problems in medicine tax the wisdom of decision making and technical acuity of the surgeon and anesthesiologist more than operating on the elderly. Yet surgery of the aged is relatively common today. There are a number of reasons for this: 1) the percentage of elderly people has increased; 2) many of the elderly are in generally good health; 3) the operations are safer because of precise methods for measuring and monitoring body functions during surgery; and 4) advancements in anesthesia have been developed. Because there is an increased risk associated with surgery in elderly people [3,4], it behooves those of us charged with their care to determine precisely the risk involved, and the need for and types of operations involved. Having made these decisions, we must then execute the proper performance in operative and postoperative care. Although one should not be lax in the preparation for and performance of any operation, even greater care should be taken when dealing with the elderly. Minor derangements following the stress of anesthesia and operation might transform a functioning but borderline organ to a nonfunctioning one. This is particularly true in patients undergoing extracorporeal circulation, which is never as effective as the normal pulsatile flow. Furthermore, organs that are functionally impaired by occlusive vascular disease may be irreversibly damaged during extracorporeal circulation.

PREOPERATIVE EVALUATION

Since anesthetic and surgical risks increase with age, they must be weighed against the relative benefits to the patient. Preoperative evaluation and perioperative management play a major role in reducing risk to its minimal level. The anesthetic preoperative evaluation of the elderly is similar to that of younger patients. The rigor required, though, is increased because there is an increased likelihood that physiologic and pathologic abnormalities will be present and that medications will be used to control them among the elderly. The preoperative evaluation must include a thorough history, with particular emphasis on current medical problems and drugs being taken. Also of great importance is information indicating tolerance to exertion in daily life—that is, walking up stairs or around the block. Not infrequently, a single medical condition restricts physical activity to such a degree that more life-threatening disease remains occult (e.g., claudication on walking preventing manifestation of exertional angina).

Physical findings

The physical examination must particularly document the current cardiovascular and pulmonary status. Arteriosclerosis is a process of aging and is a generalized disease. Time should be spent not only in recording the history of symptoms, but also in a physical examination thorough enough to detail cardiovascular abnormalities. Of particular importance is the status of cerebral blood flow. The most common postoperative complication we have encountered in operating on the elderly is cerebral vascular insufficiency, which may vary from limited mental confusion to a hemispheric stroke. A good evaluation of the patient's preoperative mental status serves as a solid background against which to evaluate postoperative mental status changes. It is essential to listen for carotid bruits, and should one be present, a cerebral vascular evaluation is in order to determine its significance. Carotid bruits must be differentiated from the murmur transmitted from aortic stenosis. Calcific aortic stenosis is another condition seen with increasing frequency with advancing age. Special attention is required to elicit its murmur. Any history of significant musculoskeletal problems, as might relate to difficulties in intubating or positioning the patient, should be identified. Multiple documentation of the patient's "normal" blood pressure is important to prevent and treat dangerous hypertension in the perioperative setting. It is equally important to note the patient's normal and physiologic blood pressures. Attention to this will frequently prevent intraoperative and postoperative ischemic insults to the kidney and the brain due to inadequate perfusion pressures. We have found that determining the normal blood pressure in patients undergoing outpatient surgery or surgery on the same day as admission to the hospital is becoming increasingly difficult. The shortened preoperative time reduces the number of opportunities available to obtain measurements of preoperative pressures, which are required to establish a true baseline pressure.

Laboratory evaluation

Multiple studies in the general population now support more limited use of preoperative "screening" laboratory evaluations than in the past. The use of such screening evaluations in asymptomatic or low-risk patients is seldom cost-beneficial. In the elderly, chronic medical diseases that the patient manifests and those for which the patient is at high risk, as well as chronic drug therapy and the specific risks of the surgery planned, usually dictate the appropriate laboratory evaluation. In general, the laboratory evaluation should be designed to detect abnormalities in serum electrolytes, glucose, blood urea nitrogen, and creatinine. Renal function decreases with aging, as indicated by a progressive decline in the glomerular filtration rate. There is also a decreased ability to conserve sodium or water during a deficit and to excrete sodium or water during excess intake. Physical and laboratory evidence of inadequate hydration is of particular importance in preventing perioperative renal dysfunction. Because many elderly patients take diuretics for one reason or another, their sodium, potassium, and chloride levels may be abnormal. Patients undergoing extracorporeal circulation need special attention paid to their coagulation profile. Platelet count, prothrombin time, partial thromboplastin time, and bleeding time are necessary to detect any clotting problems. If these tests are all normal, it is unlikely that any bleeding problems will occur. Patients who are taking antiplatelet aggregation drugs (including aspirin) should discontinue the drug three weeks before surgery. If this is not practical, fresh platelets may be made available at the time of operation. If the family history suggests von Willebrand's disease, the factor VIII level should be measured.

Pulmonary function

In patients with a history of pulmonary risk factors or patients undergoing surgery of the thoracic or abdominal cavities, a chest x-ray and pulmonary function screening test are indicated to document the patient's current status, identify any significant compromise to ventilatory function, and plan postoperative management. Since chronic obstructive lung disease is often a problem in the aged, one must be sure the patient has adequate pulmonary function. If it is depressed enough to produce hypoxia or hypercarbia, the operation should be delayed until treatment with bronchodilatation and respiratory training can improve function to a safer level. Wheezing, hypercarbia, hypoxia, or serious depression of pulmonary mechanics all herald significant postoperative lung problems and warrant medical evaluation. Aging itself poses significant changes on the neuromuscular and skeletal aspects of breathing. Unfortunately, these changes interact synergistically with postoperative change brought on by the surgical incision and the presence of pain. Aggressive and innovative postoperative pain management, using epidural local anesthetics or morphine and patient-controlled intravenous analgesia, is having a major impact in reducing postoperative respiratory morbidity.

Electrocardiogram

The electrocardiogram (ECG) must be closely examined for unknown cardiac problems and recent evolution of old problems. Evidence of ischemia or rhythm and conduction problems must be examined closely and treated if possible. History and onset of a myocardial infarction have a significant role in predicting operative risk and hence are important in the decision whether and when to operate. A recent ECG in an asymptomatic elderly patient would seem a reasonable screening test despite its relative insensitivity in younger patients.

RISK ASSESSMENT

Age

In 1970, Cole [5] estimated that operative mortality increases from fourfold to eightfold in patients over age 70, compared to the mortality of their younger counterparts having the same surgery [6]. In patients over 80 years of age, Djokovic and Hedley-Whyte [6] reported an overall mortality of 6.2% within one month of surgery. A mortality rate of 7.5% has been reported by Michel et al. [7] in a group of 225 nonagenarians [7]. Goldman et al. [8] were able to define age >70 as an independent risk factor. Much of the risk associated with aging, though, clearly rests with associated disease processes [9,10].

ASA class

The American Society of Anesthesiology (ASA) classifies patients on the following scale:

I. Healthy patient (i.e., hernia repair in an otherwise healthy patient)
II. Mild systemic disease
III. Severe systemic disease that limits patient's activity
IV. Severe systemic disease that is constantly life-threatening and incapacitating
V. Moribund patient not expected to live

To any of these classes can be added the designation "E" to indicate an emergency operation, which would signify an added risk. Numerous studies have correlated an increase in operative mortality with an increasing ASA physical status scale. In the study of Djokovic and Hedley-Whyte [6], only 1 of 187 patients classified as ASA class II died, whereas 25% of the ASA class IV patients died within one month of surgery.

Surgical site

Peak morbidity rates of 20% or higher are associated with thoracic, abdominal, and major vascular surgical sites. Operations that do not invade the celomic cavity have a lesser risk. The most important factor is the ability to maintain homeostasis during operation. Operations of greater magnitude, particularly those in which larger volumes of blood may be lost, are to be feared. Because of the decrease in organ reserve in the elderly, the so-called "domino effect" can be produced when one target organ is insulted to a degree that causes failure. In efforts to repair damage and recover from this organ failure, other organs may deteriorate and eventually fail.

Urgency of operation

Anderson and Ostberg [11] reported that an elective herniorrhaphy had a 0.6% mortality compared to a 13.8% mortality for emergency repair in the elderly. Hence, when decisions are made whether or not to perform elective surgery, one must always bear in mind the consequences of emergency surgery. Although the patient is at risk because of increased age, the risk will increase greatly should the operation become necessary as an emergency. Therefore, the probability of the condition requiring emergent therapy must be weighed in the decision not to operate.

Occult coronary artery disease

In asymptomatic elderly patients without severe physical limitations, it is unlikely that extensive screening for occult coronary artery disease will prove beneficial, particularly for low-risk procedures. Unfortunately, physical and medical limitations frequently exist, and the elderly increasingly undergo major surgical procedures. In one group of patients, such screening clearly would seem justified. Patients undergoing major vascular surgery but without symptomatic coronary artery disease may benefit from preoperative cardiac evaluation using thallium–dipyridamole scans. Such scans have been shown to improve the identification of patients at risk for postoperative myocardial infarction [12].

Previous myocardial infarction

Tarhan et al. [13] reviewed 32,887 medical records of patients undergoing some type of operative procedure. In a group of 422 patients who had a previous remote myocardial infarction, almost 7% had another infarction during the first week after surgery. When the operation was performed within three months of the infarction, the reinfarction rate was 37%; at 3 to 6 months, it was 16.7%; and it remained at 5% when the infarction had occurred more than six months earlier. Such reinfarction is associated with a very high mortality rate (approximately 50%) [13–15]. In a patient with an acute myocardial infarction, six months might well be considered a minimal waiting period for noncardiac surgery.

In patients for whom delay of surgery itself carries unacceptable risks, aggressive perioperative hemodynamic monitoring and pharmacologic intervention may reduce the risks from reinfarction [16]. Similarly, aggressive coronary anatomic evaluation preoperatively and angioplastic or surgical treatment may improve outcome.

In contrast to the rule of delaying noncardiac surgery for six months following a myocardial infarction, the patient in need of myocardial revascularization may best be treated immediately at the time of infarction if the pathoanatomy of the coronary arteries and ventricular function are known and amenable to percutaneous coronary angioplasty (PTCA) or corrective surgery. If this information is unavailable, the operation should be delayed depending on the clinical course. Patients with evolving myocardial infarction (symptomatic or within six hours after the onset in asymptomatic patients) undergo emergency thrombolytic therapy, angiography, and percutaneous transluminal angioplasty. Referral for operations involves 1) failure to restore patency with thrombolysis; 2) unsuccessful angioplasty; 3) left main coronary artery disease; and 4) multivessel disease with complex lesions not amenable to PTCA.

In patients convalescing from an acute myocardial infarction, all patients with a non-Q-wave infarction or those with a positive low-level treadmill test undergo early coronary angiography before discharge from the hospital. They have an increased risk of myocardial infarction at a later date and a high morbidity. As in patients with an evolving myocardial infarction, in these patients coronary bypass grafting is performed when the results of PTCA are inadequate or the indications for PTCA are inappropriate. The very old and infirm—that is, those older than age 75 with concomitant disease—are exempt from this logic. They are followed and subject to further study only if the postinfarction signs and symptoms signify impending diaster.

Stable angina

If angina is truly stable, it does not in and of itself seem to be a major risk factor for morbidity or mortality. Patients with angina should be evaluated preoperatively with a treadmill stress test to clearly define the workload and reserve available before surgery. Measurement of ventricular function by radioactively labeled red blood cells and ventricular reaction to stress can determine the extent of myocardial impairment. Risk is clearly increased if the ejection fraction is markedly decreased with exercise. In such cases, delineation of the coronary pathoanatomy is warranted to establish the degree of the myocardium at risk for ischemic injury. Thallium imaging of the heart (with exercise or with dipyridamole) can indicate regions of the myocardium at risk for ischemic injury.

Unstable angina

Unstable angina represents a significant risk factor. Obviously, elective noncoronary surgery is not performed on patients with unstable angina [17]. When surgery is necessary, the status of the coronary artery must be determined. The character of the lesion, its location, and the amount of myocardium in jeopardy will dictate the appropriateness of angioplastic or surgical revascularization. On occasion it may be necessary to perform coronary surgery and noncardiac surgery at the same time.

Prior myocardial revascularization

Patients who have undergone previous aortocoronary artery bypass surgery (or angioplasty) are reported to do well when operated upon for other reasons. Their risk is considerably less than that of patients with similar intrinsic coronary artery disease but without the benefit of bypass surgery (0% myocardial infarction in the aortocoronary bypass group versus 5% perioperative myocardial infarction in the group without bypass) [18]. Experience at the Ochsner Clinic has shown improved operative risk after myocardial revascularization. In a study from 1970 to 1979, 96 patients who had previously had myocardial revascularization at the Ochsner Clinic later had a total of 136 noncardiac operations [19]. There were no postoperative myocardial infarctions and only one noncardiac death. Transitory postoperative arrhythmias occurred in 3.6% of patients. This study suggests that myocardial revascularization protects the cardiac patient from myocardial infarction and cardiac-related deaths during and after noncardiac operations. Since coronary surgery itself is associated with mortality and morbidity, some of the decreased morbidity in the postbypass patients subjected to further noncardiac surgery may reflect prior selection.

Conduction abnormalities
Patients with single bundle branch blocks or bifasicular blocks (right bundle and either left anterior or left posterior hemiblock) do not need pacemaker implantation prior to surgery. However, in the presence of a prolonged P-R interval, a patient with a complete right bundle branch block and either a posterior or anterior left hemiblock should probably have a pacemaker implanted preoperatively. Similarly, patients with complete or third-degree heart block require a pacemaker preoperatively. It is wise to treat patients with recent onset of bundle branch block as if they had recently had a myocardial infarction and to delay surgery for at least six months, since this conduction change may represent an ischemic event. Placement of a pulmonary artery catheter for intraoperative monitoring is associated with a high incidence of right bundle branch block. Patients with a left bundle branch block who require pulmonary artery catheterization should have readily available a means of temporary pacing. Pulmonary artery catheters with pacing capabilities are available and effective.

Arrhythmias
Arrhythmias are frequent in the elderly and should be evaluated preoperatively. Underlying causes should be sought and treated before operation. An understanding of the patient's stable preoperative rhythm (frequent unifocal premature ventricular contractions not requiring treatment) is of importance to prevent unwarranted postoperative medical therapy. Ventricular dysrhythmias of a dangerous type (multifocal, R or T, runs of two or more, or six or more a minute) should be controlled medically if reversible causes, such as myocardial ischemia or congestive heart failure, are not found. The ventricular response in atrial fibrillation should be controlled at an acceptable rate (60 to 90 per minute).

Hypertension

Preoperative hypertension has been shown by several authors to be a major morbidity risk factor. This has recently been questioned. Goldman and associates [8,20] failed to isolate hypertension as an independent risk factor. Their patients, however, were subjected to aggressive intraoperative and postoperative medical management of hypertension. Thus, smooth blood pressure control seems to be desirable before surgery.

Congestive heart failure

Decreasing cardiovascular reserve is manifested by an inability to maintain cardiac output and/or blood pressure. Likewise, there is a diminished capacity to augment cardiac output when required. This may be the result of decreased sensitivity to catecholamine at receptor sites or a decreased number of receptor sites. A delayed response of the sympathetic nervous system to the required reflex action may also play a role. Patients with clinical heart failure have little or no reserve for anesthesia and surgery. Goldman and coworkers [8] found that an S_3 gallop or jugular venous distension was associated with a 39% cardiac morbidity or mortality (14% nonfatal cardiac complication and 25% fatal). In order to assess the degree of failure and the response to therapy, noninvasive diagnostic tests may be of use preoperatively. Two-dimensional echocardiography and cardiac nuclear scanning are of particular assistance. Both can generate an estimate of heart size, regional wall motion, and ejection fraction.

Valvular heart disease

Clinically significant valvular heart disease occurs in approximately 15% of elderly people. In patients being operated on for noncardiac conditions, aortic stenosis is the valvular lesion that causes the majority of deaths. This is because of the high incidence of calcific aortic stenosis in the elderly and the frequently silent nature of the condition. On the other hand, valvular lesions such as aortic insufficiency, mitral stenosis, and mitral insufficiency usually cause detectable signs and symptoms before they reach a stage where they produce myocardial decompensation. In the elderly, aortic stenosis presenting after age 65 is most commonly due to a calcified bicuspid valve; however, we are encountering more elderly patients with significant aortic stenosis with trileaflets, in whom the stenosis results from calcific immobility of the valve leaflets. Idiopathic hypertropic subaortic stenosis is another form of aortic outflow obstruction that can first be noted in the aged. Two-dimensional echocardiography is rapidly proving to be an excellent noninvasive tool to demonstrate the presence of a valvular lesion. Transthoracic imaging is a well-established tool. Transesophageal imaging has markedly improved the resolution of cardiac valvular lesions. The advances in color flow Doppler and pulsed-wave Doppler techniques that apply to both imaging modes have further enhanced noninvasive estimation of the hemodynamic significance of valvular lesions. However, cardiac catheterization may be required to define the magnitude of a valvular lesion.

Pulmonary status

For surgical procedures involving the thorax or abdomen, a marked reduction in vital capacity (of more than 50%) can be expected postoperatively. Patients with a marginal preoperative vital capacity may require ventilator support postoperatively for varying lengths of time. Patients with a preoperative vital capacity less than 25 ml/kg should be considered at increased risk for respiratory complications. Preoperative elevations of pCO_2 indicate significantly diminished ventilatory drive and capacity. Potentially reversible risk factors should be addressed preoperatively (i.e., cessation of smoking, preoperative pulmonary toilet, and bronchodilator therapy).

One of the most significant recent advances in overall patient care and comfort has been the introduction of epidurally administered narcotics for pain during the postoperative period. Numerous studies now confirm its general benefit in patient comfort and, more importantly, improved ventilatory status. Its use should be considered for all patients with increased risk of pulmonary complications.

General poor health

Goldman et al. [8] found that this index correlated well with postoperative cardiac risk, defined by various indicators of noncardiovascular systems dysfunction (i.e., PO_2 less than 60, liver failure, renal failure, etc.).

PREOPERATIVE MANAGEMENT

Medications

With rare exceptions, if a patient's homeostasis is maintained by drug therapy (for example, beta-blockers for the control of angina), this therapy should be continued until the time of operation. Monoamine oxidase inhibitors should be withheld for two weeks prior to surgery if possible due to interaction with anesthetic agents. Preoperative medication of elderly patients with heart disease must be tempered and doses reduced because these patients may have increased central nervous system and cardiovascular sensitivity. Cautious intravenous administration of a narcotic intraoperatively is preferred over inadvertent premedicant overdose and resultant hypotension or respiratory depression. With this caveat in mind, the selection of the premedication is best made on the basis of familiarity with the agents. When extracorporeal circulation is to be employed during operation, it is imperative that drugs used to alter clotting be discontinued. This includes not only anticoagulants but also drugs that alter platelet function, such as aspirin and dypridamole. However, one should not use antagonist drugs to reverse anticoagulation but instead allow for gradual reduction in medication. The urgency of the need for operation will dictate this decision. It is particularly important not to acutely reverse anticoagulation in patients with prosthetic heart valves for fear of valve thrombosis.

Monitoring

Pulse oximetry and capnography

Pulse oximetry is routinely used to monitor all patients undergoing general anesthesia, regional anesthesia, or conscious sedation. Capnography is utilized for all patients requiring assisted or controlled ventilation.

Electrocardiogram

ECG monitoring should be standard in all aged patients. The standard lead II (right arm to left leg) is most frequently used, since it detects change in atrial activity and allows for the most accurate determination of rhythm. Monitoring ischemic changes, which occur most often in the precordial area of V5, requires either conventional monitoring of this lead or a modification of the limb lead position to approximate a poor man's V5. This modification involves placement of the left arm lead on the precordium at the V5 position and monitoring of limb lead I. Changes in S-T segment are best determined from hard copy calibrated at 1 mv/mm. Increasingly, operative monitors include S-T-segment trend analysis, which may significantly improve the detection of ischemia.

Body temperature

Temperature regulation in the elderly is extremely important. The patient's temperature must be monitored and maintained through the routine use of warming blankets. Hypothermia places an increased demand on the limited myocardial reserves of elderly patients and can induce ischemia.

Central venous pressure

In view of the critical role that volume status plays in the response of the aged to any anesthetic technique, the use of central venous pressure (CVP) lines is to be encouraged where possible. Cardiotonic drugs, which are frequently administered to the elderly, are more safely and accurately administered via a CVP line. Obviously, risks due to insertion must be weighed against benefits. Sites with low risks include the antecubital vein of the arm when a long catheter or the external jugular veins are used. Although CVP lines in these sites are placed with fewer complications, they are frequently unsuccessful. The internal jugular and subclavian veins continue to be the mainstays of central venous access. From any position, to be considered central, the venous line must aspirate blood freely and the fluid column fluctuate with respiration. Chest x-ray confirmation of position should be obtained as soon as possible.

Arterial pressure

Intra-arterial pressure monitoring is frequently necessary. The combination of peripheral vascular disease and blood pressure lability often makes accurate determination of the blood pressure difficult with use of a standard cuff. Also, intraoperative and postoperative arterial blood gas, hematocrit, and serum electrolyte values further support the use of arterial lines for major surgery in the elderly. Our choice of site for line placement is the radial artery, and then the dorsal or posterior tibial arteries. The use of other sites, such as the femoral and brachial arteries, requires considerable caution because of the potential for serious complications. If possible, care should be taken to assess the presence of adequate collateral circulation. Complications of intra-arterial monitoring, primarily thrombosis and distal embolization, are reduced by the use of small-caliber catheters made of minimally thrombogenic material. A 1.5-inch, 20-gauge, Teflon-coated, nontapered catheter inserted percutaneously has proven to be very acceptable. The more atraumatic the insertion and the shorter the duration of the cannulation, the lower the probability of complications. Improved transducer and catheter technology has resulted in the increasing use of 22-gauge catheters, which probably further reduce risk.

Pulmonary arterial pressure

In cases of severe myocardial depression or minimal cardiopulmonary reserve, pulmonary artery catheterization is indicated. Monitoring of left ventricular filling pressure via pulmonary artery wedge pressure allows for careful adjustments in volume replacement. Thermodilution cardiac outputs measured with the pulmonary artery catheter provide for early diagnosis and aggressive therapeutic intervention. Preoperative augmentation of low or borderline cardiac output has proven effective in decreasing the operative risks of these high-risk patients. Recent advances in pulmonary artery catheters, including mixed venous O_2 saturation monitoring, allow for further improved monitoring of high-risk patients, particularly those at risk for pulmonary problems postoperatively.

Other monitoring techniques

Intraoperative transesophageal echocardiographic (TEE) monitoring is an increasingly accepted modality of patient monitoring both in cardiac surgical procedures and in high-risk vascular procedures. TEE monitoring allows for rapid assessment of 1) ventricular filling and vascular volume; 2) global ventricular function and contractility; 3) segmented wall motion as an indicator of coronary ischemia; and 4) intracardiac air. At Ochsner we have found the instrument a valuable adjunct in the performance of thoracoabdominal aneurysm repairs, liver transplants, and various cardiac procedures. New color flow Doppler technology has particularly improved our assessment of valvular lesions before and after repair.

Intraoperative electroencephalogram (EEG) monitoring has evolved over the last several decades, and several major institutions find it beneficial in reducing cerebral vascular injury. In general, though, this technology has not found wide application, partly because of conflicting methodology for analysis and display of the information. Most vascular injury is focal in nature, and the technology has not evolved with sufficient resolution to easily monitor such focal reduction in cerebral blood flow.

SELECTION OF ANESTHETIC TECHNIQUE

Local anesthesia

Appropriate infiltration of a local anesthetic, regional nerve block (ulnar, etc.), or spinal or epidural anesthesia requires a fair amount of patient cooperation. Local infiltration with intravenous supplementation is desirable when satisfactory surgical results can be expected and patient comfort is acceptable. However, cardiac stress from inadequate analgesia or sedation may precipitate a cardiac or hypertensive crisis. Likewise, overzealous intravenous supplementation may lead to an unanticipated respiratory or cardiac emergency. At Ochsner Foundation Hospital, local anesthesia performed by the surgeon in elderly patients with cardiac risk is usually attended by anesthesia personnel who administer intravenous supplementation and are prepared to manage cardiovascular and respiratory consequences. Whenever sedation is used in the elderly, one should be aware that elderly patients have increased sensitivity to most sedatives and, because they have a lower cardiac output than young patients, the onset of drug action is delayed when administerd by most methods (orally, intramuscularly, and intravenously). Such a set of circumstances promotes overdosage, particularly for parenteral drugs. When administered correctly, nerve blocks are very useful and have proven especially efficacious in ophthalmic and orthopedic surgery. They should be used with the same cautions mentioned above.

Spinal and epidural anesthesia

Spinal and epidural anesthesia are particularly useful for urologic, orthopedic, and lower abdominal surgery in the elderly. The current literature [21,22] suggests that these techniques may be of particular benefit in hip procedures and prostate procedures, resulting in a reduced incidence of thromboembolic phenomena postoperatively. Increasing postoperative pain-management needs are also encouraging the use of epidural analgesia intraoperatively. It is also being increasingly used in conjunction with general anesthesia for high-risk patients intraoperatively. The early indications are that such techniques may reduce overall patient morbidity and the cost of care.

Occasionally, skeletal deformities make these techniques unsatisfactory. Again, patient cooperation is needed, and cautious intravenous supplementation must be used. In general, an absolute contraindication to spinal/epidural anesthesia is a clotting abnormality or hypovolemia. Relative contraindications may include a recent cerebrovascular accident or a coexisting medical condition highly associated with neurologic dysfunction. The primary physiologic stress placed on the patient by spinal/epidural anesthesia is arterial and venous dilation. If the arterial dilation is not extreme, it may improve the cardiac output of a marginally failing heart. However, this is a fine line because venous dilation results in peripheral venous pooling of blood and a decreased cardiac filling. Especially in the volume-depleted patient (i.e., chronic hypertensive or diuretic therapy), venous pooling can result in a catastrophic fall in cardiac output and blood pressure. Therefore, the patient's volume status must be known and expanded if it is inadequate. Central venous pressure monitoring is particularly useful in this situation. If adequate volume administration cannot be given, judicious use of such vasotonic agents as ephedrine and phenylephrine is indicated to improve peripheral vascular tone. For appropriate surgical procedures, spinal/epidural anesthesia can be of great utility in the cardiovascular cripple from whatever cause. In general, though, studies do not indicate much, if any, advantage in high-risk cardiac patients of using spinal/epidural techniques instead of well-administered general anesthesia. The cardiovascular effects of epidural analgesia are similar to those of spinal analgesia except that they are slower in onset because of the site of application. Because epidural anesthesia is routinely administered by continuous catheter techniques, incremental dosing and thus finer control are possible. Recently introduced microcatheters for continuous spinal analgesia may result in a resurgence of spinal analgesia.

General anesthesia

By far the greatest number of anesthetics given to the aged for major surgery are general anesthetics. In administering general anesthetics to the elderly with heart disease, the selection of the type of general anesthetic is frequently predicated on the physiology of the cardiovascular abnormality. In a patient with severe hypertension, the peripheral vasodilator action of halogenated inhalation agents (halothane, ethrane, or forane) may prove extremely beneficial in allowing for smooth intraoperative control of arterial pressure. Similarly, patients with ischemic heart disease who are not in congestive heart failure may benefit from the myocardial depressant action of these agents, which will serve to diminish O_2 requirements of the heart (analogous to the use of a beta-blocker for the treatment of angina). Even patients with a history of congestive heart failure, if compensated, may tolerate low doses of these agents.

Frequently, though, these patients, as well as those with severe congestive failure from any cause, cannot tolerate further myocardial depression. In these patients an intravenous narcotic technique is used. This technique, frequently referred to as a *balanced anesthetic technique*, utilizes an intravenous narcotic (fentanyl, sufentanyl) in conjunction with an intravenous tranquilizer (midazolam, droperidol), a muscle relaxant (pancuronium, vecuronium, atracurium, curare), and inhaled nitrous oxide (50% to 70% with O_2). In severe cases of cardiac failure, the technique may be reduced to a very-high-dose narcotic and 100% O_2. The techniques allow for remarkable cardiovascular stability with little alteration in preinduction status. Depending on the amount of narcotic and tranquilizer used, these techniques may require prolonged postoperative ventilatory support. Within the above guidelines, the choice between an inhalation anesthetic and a balanced technique is frequently made based on other considerations, such as the personal experience of the anesthetist or potential contraindications to the halogenated agent (concern over the use of halothane in liver disease, for example).

Modern anesthetic practice no longer sees a clear-cut separation of the extremes, since narcotics and tranquilizers may supplement halogenated agents. The key point is close monitoring of the cardiovascular response to the technique with adjustment as needed. The depressed cardiac output of the elderly slows down the onset of action of any intravenous agent. Diminished plasma binding of many intravenous agents as a result of lower serum albumin levels results in an increased amount of the free drug available. This and the relative increase in central nervous system sensitivity to drug-induced depression may make response to a drug more intense once it is established. Similarly, abnormal ventilation perfusion patterns in the aged lung result in slower uptake of inhalation agents.

Patients with significant valvular heart disease usually require maintenance of a stable rhythm and adequate cardiac chamber filling pressures. The major anesthetic risk is related to the state of the left ventricle. In patients undergoing operation to correct valvular dysfunction, the greatest risk frequently occurs during induction of anesthesia, and this is particularly true in patients with severe mitral insufficiency and frank congestive failure. In contrast, in patients undergoing extravalvular surgery, aortic stenosis is the most feared valvular abnormality during induction of anesthesia. In essence, management of any valvular disease must be firmly based on a thorough understanding of the hemodynamic derangement.

If atrial fibrillation is present, the ventricular rate should be controlled. This anesthetic technique must minimize dysrhythmias of all types. Because of this requirement for intraoperative cardiovascular stability, patients with severe valvular disease are most frequently anesthetized with a narcotic technique. In these patients, particular attention should be paid to antibiotic prophylaxis for endocarditis.

Patients with pacemakers

The anesthetic management of patients with pacemakers has been greatly simplified by better shielding of pacemakers and electrocautery equipment. Care should be taken not to place the bovey plate near the pacemaker battery. If possible, demand pacemakers should probably be converted to fixed mode if external programming is possible (with the magnet placed over the battery).

OPERATIVE TECHNIQUE

The general principles of operative technique should be adhered to more stringently in elderly patients than in the young. The tissues of the aged are more fragile, the blood vessels are damaged more easily, and since there is degeneration and loss of elastic and collagen tissue, the tissue strength is decreased. Consequently, in performing operative maneuvers, extra care must be taken in surgical manipulation to avoid tissue injury. Blood loss that might be of no consequence in a younger person could prove catastrophic in the aged because of their limited reserve to withstand physiologic alterations. Likewise, surgical maneuvers that may compress vital organs or impair circulation to them must be avoided. Such maneuvers are tolerated by younger patients because their organs are supple and have greater functional reserve, and their arteries are not sclerotic. The ability of these organs to return to normal following insult is very limited in the aged, and consequently irreversible damage may be provoked.

VASCULAR OPERATIONS

Occlusive vascular disease

The problems of operating for occlusive vascular disease in peripheral vessels are rarely different in the aged than in the young, except that elderly patients have more extensive disease and increased calcification in the vessel walls [23–25]. However, surgery in the chest and abdomen is usually of much greater magnitude and consequently carries an increased risk of complications. For this reason, various vascular operations have been devised in an attempt to avoid the coelomic cavities. For instance, obstructive lesions of the origin of the great vessels of the aortic arch may be corrected by using a bypass within the neck, thereby avoiding thoracotomy or mediastinotomy. In a patient with stenosis of the origin of the left carotid, one could restore flow with a left subclavian-carotid bypass. Similarly, a single iliac artery occlusion could be corrected by a femorofemoral bypass instead of an aortofemoral bypass, which involves opening of the abdomen with its inherent pain and risk. When the distal aorta and both iliac arteries are occluded, a subclavian femorofemoral bypass can circumvent an aortobifemoral bypass operation. It is essential to use surgical ingenuity to alter, modify, or devise new operations in order to lessen the risk in elderly patients.

Vascular aneurysms

The strength of the aortic wall is in the elastic tissue of the media, and destruction of this layer by arteriosclerosis diminishes the strength of the vessel wall. Incessant pulsatile intraluminal pressure on the weakened vessel produces progressive dilatation. As dilatation occurs, hydrodynamic principles contribute to progressive expansion of the aneurysm. Progressive distention and thinning of the vessel wall also lead to attenuation of vasavasorum with resultant ischemia of the vessel wall. The combination of vessel wall destruction, increased intraluminal lateral pressure, increased tension in the dilated wall, and reduced blood supply to the wall accounts for continued enlargement of the aneurysm. The natural course is progressive enlargement until rupture or until a nearby vital organ is compressed and its function impaired. The ultimate fate in either instance is death.

In estimating the probability of rupture, the anticipated longevity of the patient becomes an important factor. An elderly person has a surprisingly long life expectancy. On the average, a 65-year-old person will live an additional 15 years, a 75-year-old person will live 10 years, and an 80-year-old patient will live seven years [26]. However, most patients surviving aneurysmectomy do not have survival rates comparable to the general population, presumably because of generalized arteriosclerosis, of which the aneurysm is a harbinger. The decision to resect an aneurysm must take into account the estimated life span, the predictable illnesses of the elderly, the size of the aneurysm, the symptoms of the patient, and the other usual risk factors associated with a major operation.

Arteriosclerotic aneurysms can occur in any artery but are more common in the aorta, particularly in the abdominal aorta below the renal arteries. Repair of an aneurysm is one of the most common major operations per-formed in the elderly, particularly in men [27,28]. The techniques for repair of aneurysms of the aorta vary depending on the site. At present, for aneurysms of the ascending thoracic aorta, extracorporeal circulation is required. For those involving the arch of the aorta, extracorporeal circulation plus deep hypothermia and circulatory arrest yield the best results. In the descending thoracic aorta, many techniques are available to decompress the upper half of the body and perfuse the lower half during clamp isolation of the aneurysm for resection. Where feasible, a temporary shunt around the aneurysm best serves the purpose. Other methods are femoral vein–artery extracorporeal bypass and simple clamping of the aorta without means to perfuse the distal half of the body. Thoracoabdominal aneurysms are best treated by endoaneurysmorrhaphy with reimplantation of the visceral vessels into the prosthetic graft after it has been first sutured end-to-end to the proximal aorta; finally, distal flow is reconstituted with an end-to-end anastomosis to the distal aorta.

In the past 25 years, the mortality for abdominal aortic aneurysmectomy has decreased from 15% to 1%. There are many reasons for this decline. Foremost have been improvements in technique and in anesthesia, precise physiologic monitoring of the patient during the operation, and the use of anticoagulation during cross-clamp of the aorta. In the early days, renal failure following aneurysmectomy was frequent. However, avoidance of hypotension, renal artery trauma, and thrombosis have made this a rare complication.

Unfortunately, the operative mortality for ruptured aneurysms has decreased very little through the years [29, 30]. The mortality is directly related to the condition of the patient at the time of operation. In patients in hypovolemic shock, the mortality rate is greater than 50%. In patients who are in a stable condition at surgery, the mortality approaches that of elective aneurysmectomy. Ruptures appear to occur more often in the aged; consequently, because of limited organ reserve irreversible damage to these organs, in particular to the kidneys, usually results in postoperative death.

Patients undergoing aneurysmectomy are subject to the general complications of any major abdominal operation. Since arteriosclerosis is the cause of aneurysms, naturally the various complications associated with arteriosclerotic vascular disease are potential hazards during aneurysmectomy. The greatest danger is coronary insufficiency. It is therefore important that operations be performed in such a manner as to prevent further myocardial injury. Prophylactic digitalization is a preoperative requirement for patients with a history of congestive heart failure. Hypotensive episodes during induction of anesthesia and during surgery are particularly to be avoided. Undoubtedly, the use of systemic anticoagulation lessens the incidence of myocardial infarction during aortic surgery.

CARDIAC OPERATIONS

Myocardial revascularization

Myocardial revascularization has become one of the most common operations employed in this country. It is estimated that 250,000 coronary bypass operations are performed each year. In Ochsner Foundation Hospital, as in many other major institutions, coronary bypass surgery is performed more frequently than herniorrhaphies, tonsillectomies, and hemorrhoidectomies combined. Because the most common malady of the aged is arteriosclerosis, it is only natural that a significant segment of those undergoing coronary artery surgery are elderly. In a review of our first 3000 operations, 25% of patients operated on were older than 65 years of age. In the last 1000 operations, 40% of the patients were older than age 65. We would like to think that the elderly had results as good as those of younger patients, but this is not so.

In an unpublished review of Ochsner Foundation Hospital data, the mortality for patients younger than age 65 was 1.2% and the mortality for those over age 65 was 6.2%. However, the quality of life following operation was approximately equal, in that a similar percentage of younger and older patients were free of angina following operation. As one might expect, risk factors other than age were more pronounced in the older patients. Among patients older than age 65, 23.3% were diabetic, whereas only 14.6% of those younger than 65 were diabetic. Even more prognostic was ventricular function, which was worse in elderly than in nonelderly patients. Also, a higher percentage of older patients than younger patients required concomitant correction of a heart valve at the time of operation. Thus, the preoperative prognosis was worse for those over 65 years of age. However, most poor prognoses can be attributed to the fact that the extent and severity of coronary artery disease and concomitant diseases are worse in the aged.

Operative mortality for coronary artery disease in the aged, as reported in the literature [31–34], varies from 6% to 22%. The reason for the excessively high mortality is the advanced degree of disease in these people, because they are usually referred late in the course of their disease and only after intensive medical trial. The association of valvular disease with coronary artery disease in the aged adds to the mortality. However, improvement in operative technique and a better understanding of coronary artery disease have recently led to lower operative mortality rates.

The technique of performing myocardial revascularization in the elderly is no different from the same operation on the young. However, a few technical points of difference need emphasis. In placing the elderly patient on extracorporeal circulation, one must be careful not to tear the friable right atrial appendage when cannulating for venous return. The ascending aorta is the usual site for arterial return, and one must be cognizant of calcific plaques and soft atheromatous disease involving the intima that frequently are associated with the aged. Aortic dissection, dislodgement of atheromatous emboli, or both are likely to occur with traumatic cannulation.

Displacement of the heart is necessary in order to explore certain areas. The epicardium can easily be avulsed in the elderly patient if undue tension is employed with displacement. Because of the high incidence of diffuse calcification of the coronary arteries, the surgeon should select the least involved area for the site of anastomosis.

In creating the anastomosis, the surgeon must also prevent dissection of the atheromatous-involved intima and media from the adventitia. Likewise, for aortic anastomosis, care should be taken to avoid knocking off atheromatous debris into the lumen of the aorta.

Valve replacement

In the past, elderly patients with valvular heart disease were not offered valvular surgery because of the impression that the risk of dying was too great and the potential benefits did not warrant the risks. As recently as 1979 [35], editorials still emphasized the infeasibility of surgical treatment for valve disease in the elderly and recommended continuation of medical treatment only in the elderly. Because of such philosophy and direction, many older patients were denied cardiac surgery, or surgery was delayed until the cardiac condition deteriorated precipitously. Heart surgery has now improved to the point that individuals who have outlived the life expectancy of the general population can be offered a reasonable chance of survival and a good chance for functional improvement by valvular replacement. Experience at our institution and others has shown that elderly patients who undergo concomitant coronary bypass grafting with valvular replacement do better than those who have valve replacement alone. The status of the left ventricle is the determining factor in the outcome of valvular surgery, regardless of age.

Although the mortality is relatively low for aortic valve replacement and coronary artery surgery, the mortality is high for elderly patients who undergo concomitant coronary artery bypass and mitral valve replacement [36–38]. The reasons for increased mortality after mitral valve replacement are unclear. Stephenson et al. [39] reported that the 30-day hospital mortality related to mitral valve replacement in patients younger than age 60 years was 5.5%. For patients aged 60 to 69, the mortality was 15%; for patients over 70 years of age, the mortality was 54%.

Operative mortality in cardiac valve replacement is reported to vary from 0% to 75%. Variations in mortality are referable to the year reported and the relatively small number of patients in certain series, which can give a statistical mortality rate that is abnormally low or high.

Because hemodynamic and symptomatic improvements in elderly patients following isolated mitral valve replacement so closely paralleled those of younger patients, it is justifiable that the same operative criteria for isolated mitral valve disease be applied in all patients [40]. In essence, if left ventricular function in an older patient is the same as that in a younger patient, isolated mitral valve replacement carries the same low risk and brings about similar improvements.

One of the major problems in performing valvular replacement in the elderly is difficulty in weaning the patient from extracorporeal circulation [41]. Even in patients with normal valvular function, aging results in decreased left ventricular compliance and a decreased ability to respond to stress with an increased cardiac output. This inability is worse in those with valvular dysfunction. It has been demonstrated that means to reduce afterload are beneficial in removing the patients from extracorporeal circulation following valvular replacement or repair. If care is taken to protect the heart during surgery and medical reduction of the afterload is aggressive, we have infrequently had to resort to the use of intra-aortic balloon support to wean the patient from extracorporeal circulation.

In elderly patients, it is our present policy to use a porcine heterograft valve whenever possible. The reasons for this are twofold. Primarily, the patient does not need anticoagulation therapy postoperatively. The hazards of anticoagulation are known and are particularly severe in the elderly. Second, since the long-term longevity of an elderly person is normally less than 15 years, the possible disintegration of the valve after 15 years need not be a factor of concern.

Pacemaker therapy has been widely used for elderly patients, with excellent therapeutic results. We believe that transvenous placement of the electrodes is most applicable in elderly patients and requires only local anesthesia. The number of pacemaker operations has greatly increased in this country—96,000 were implanted in 1975 and 105,000 in 1985. At present, our policy is to implant these pacemakers under local anesthesia but in an operating room under fluoroscopic control. In the past, transvenous insertions were performed by percutaneous stick in the subclavian vein, thereby avoiding cutdown of the cephalic or other peripheral veins. The most convenient and least disturbing site for pocket implantation of the pulse generator can be selected by the patient and the physician.

REFERENCES

1. Webster's New Collegiate Dictionary, 150th ed. 1981. Springfield, MA: G&C Merriam Co., p 362.
2. Goldman R. 1979. Decline in organ functioning with aging. In I Rossman (ed), Clinical Geriatrics, 2d ed. Philadelphia: J.B. Lippincott, pp 23–59.
3. DeBakey ME and McCollum CH. 1982. Vascular grafts in the elderly. Med Instrum 16:89–90.
4. Harbrecht PJ, Garrison RN and Fry DE. 1981. Surgery in elderly patients. South Med J 74:594–598.
5. Cole WH. 1970. Medical differences between the young and the aged. J Am Geriatr Soc 18:589–614.
6. Djokovic JL and Hedley-Whyte J. 1979. Prediction of outcome of surgery and anesthesia in patients over 80. JAMA 242:2301–2306.
7. Michel SL, Stevens L, Amodeo P, et al. 1984. Surgical procedures in nonagenarians. West J Med 141:61–63.
8. Goldman L, Caldera DL, Nussbaum SR, et al. 1977. Multifactorial index of cardiac risk in noncardiac surgical procedures. N Engl J Med 297:845–850.
9. Greenburg AG, Salk RP and Pridhan D. 1985. Influence of age on mortality of colon surgery. Am J Surg 150:65–70.
10. Colapinto ND. 1985. Is age alone a contraindication to major cancer surgery? Can J Surg 28:323–326.
11. Anderson B and Østberg J. 1972. Long-term prognosis in geriatric surgery: 2–17 year follow-up of 7922 patients. J Am Geriatr Soc 20:255–258.
12. Boucher CA, Brewster DC, Darling RC, et al. 1985. Determination of cardiac risk by dipyridamole-thallium imaging before peripheral vascular surgery. N Engl J Med 312:389–394.
13. Tarhan S, Moffitt EA, Taylor WF, et al. 1972. Myocardial infarction after general anesthesia. JAMA 220:1451–1454.
14. Steen PA, Tinker JH and Tarhan S. 1978. Myocardial reinfarction after anesthesia and surgery. JAMA 239:2566–2570.
15. Tinker JH, Noback CR, Vlietstra RE, et al. 1981. Management of patients with heart disease for noncardiac surgery. JAMA 246:1348–1350.
16. Roa TLK, Jacobs KH, El-Etr AA. 1983. Reinfarction following anesthesia in patients with myocardial infarction. Anesthesiology 59:499–505.
17. Raabe DS Jr. 1982. Management of unstable angina pectoris. Geriatrics 37:40–46.
18. Mahar LJ, Steen PA, Tinker JH, et al. 1978. Perioperative myocardial infarction in patients with coronary artery disease with and without aorta-coronary artery bypass grafts. J Thorac Cardiovasc Surg 76:533–537.
19. Fudge TL, McKinnon WM, Schoettle GP, et al. 1981. Improved operative risk after myocardial revascularization. South Med J 74:799–801.
20. Goldman L and Caldera DL. 1979. Risks of general anesthesia and elective operation in the hypertensive patient. Anesthesiology 50:285–292.

21. Hendolin H, Mattila MAK and Poikolainen E. 1981. The effect of lumbar epidural analgesia on the development of deep vein thrombosis of the legs after open prostatectomy. Acta Chir Scand 147:425–429.
22. Modig J, Borg T, Karlström G, et al. 1983. Thromboembolism after total hip replacement: role of epidural and general anesthesia. Anesth Analg 62:174–180.
23. Benhamou AC, Kieffer E, Tricot JF, et al. 1981. Carotid artery surgery in patients over 70 years of age. Int Surg 66:199–202.
24. Sheelhy TW. 1979. Preoperative examination in the elderly. Resident and Staff Physician, September, pp 63–67.
25. Reichle FA, Rankin KP, Tyson RR, et al. 1979. The elderly patient with severe arterial insufficiency of the lower extremity: limb salvage by femoro-popliteal reconstruction. Circulation 60 (2, Part 2):124–126.
26. Sourcebook on Aging. 1977. Chicago: Marquis Academic Media, Who's Who.
27. Salerno TA, Hermandez P and Lynn RB. 1981. Abdominal aortic aneurysm in the elderly. Can J Surg 24:71–72.
28. Petracek MR, Lawson JD, Rhea WG Jr, et al. 1980. Resection of abdominal aortic aneurysms in the over-80 age group. South Med J 73:579–581.
29. Bosman CH and Stubbe LT. 1981. Twenty years' experience of surgical treatment of the ruptured atherosclerotic aneurysm of the abdominal aorta. Neth J Surg 33:160–164.
30. Lawrie GM, Morris GC Jr, Crawford ES, et al. 1979. Improved results of operation for ruptured abdominal aortic aneurysms. Surgery 85:483–488.
31. Hakki AHI, Iskandrian AS, Segal BL, et al. 1982. What are the indications for a coronary bypass? Geriatrics 37:37–39.
32. Hochberg MS, Levine FH, Daggett WM, et al. 1982. Isolated coronary artery bypass grafting in patients seventy years of age and older: early and late results. J Thorac Cardiovasc Surg 84:219–223.
33. Knapp WS, Douglas JS Jr, Carver JM, et al. 1981. Efficacy of coronary artery bypass grafting in elderly patients with coronary artery disease. Am J Cardiol 47:923–930.
34. Tucker BL, Lindesmith GG, Stiles QR, et al. 1977. Myocardial revascularization in patients 70 years of age and older. West J Med 126:179–183.
35. Jones TW, Thomas GI, Stavney LS, et al. 1979. Aortic valve replacement and the senior citizen. Am Surg 45:684–699.
36. Murphy ES, Lawson RM, Starr A, et al. 1981. Severe aortic stenosis in patients 60 years of age or older: left ventricular function and 10-year survival after valve replacement. Circulation 64 (2, Part 2):184–188.
37. Jamieson WR, Dooner J and Munro AL. 1981. Cardiac valve replacement in the elderly: a review of 320 consecutive cases. Circulation 64 (2, Part 2):177–183.
38. Teply JF, Grunkemeier GL and Starr A. 1981. Cardiac valve replacement in patients over 75 years of age. Thorac Cardiovasc Surg 29:47–50.
39. Stephenson LW, MacVaugh H III and Edmunds LH Jr. 1978. Surgery using cardiopulmonary bypass in the elderly. Circulation 58:250–254.
40. Hochberg MS, Derkac WM, Conkel DM, et al. 1979. Mitral valve replacement in elderly patients: encouraging postoperative clinical and hemodynamic results. J Thorac Cardiovasc Surg 77:422–426.
41. Berman ND, David TE, Lipton IH, et al. 1980. Surgical procedures involving cardiopulmonary bypass in patients age 70 or older. J Am Geriatr Soc 28:29–32.

SUGGESTED READING

Bergdahl L, Björk VO and Jonasson R. 1981. Aortic valve replacement in patients over 70 years. Scand J Thorac Cardiovas Surg 15:123–128.
Brown DL (ed). 1988. Risk and Outcome in Anesthesia. Philadelphia: J.B. Lippincott.
Craig DB, McLeskey CH, Mitenko PA, et al. 1987. Panel summary: geriatric anaesthesia. Can J Anaesth 34:156–167.
Dalby AJ, Firth BG and Forman R. 1981. Preoperative factors affecting the outcome of isolated mitral valve replacement: a 10 year review. Am J Cardiol 47:826–834.
Delin K, Aurell M, Granerus G, et al. 1982. Surgical treatment of renovascular hypertension in the elderly patient. Acta Med Scand 211:169–174.

Detsky AS, Abrams HB, Forbath N, et al. 1986. Cardiac assessment for patients undergoing noncardiac surgery. A multifactorial clinical risk index. Arch Intern Med 146:2131–2134.

Glasser SP, Spoto E Jr, Solomon DA, et al. 1979. When cardiac patient becomes surgical patient. Hosp Prac 14:165–173.

Koch J-P, Maron BJ, Epstein SE, et al. 1980. Results of operation for obstructive hypertrophic cardiomyopathy in the elderly. Septal myotomy and myectomy in 20 patients 65 years of age or older. Am J Cardiol 46:963–966.

Ochsner JL and Mills NL. 1978. Coronary Artery Surgery. Philadelphia: Lea & Febiger.

Stephen CR and Assaf RA. 1986. Geriatric Anesthesia, Principles and Practice. Boston: Butterworth.

Storstein O and Efskind L. 1979. Aortic valve replacement in elderly patients. Acta Med Scand 206:161–164.

25. CARDIAC TRANSPLANTATION IN OLDER PATIENTS: CHANGING PERSPECTIVES

HECTOR O. VENTURA
HERMAN L. PRICE
FRANK W. SMART
DWIGHT D. STAPLETON
CLIFFORD H. VAN METER

Since the first human orthotopic heart transplant performed by Christiaan Barnard in 1967 [1], further advances in different disciplines of the medical sciences have resulted in cardiac transplantation being an accepted therapy for patients with end-stage heart disease.

Strict criteria in recipient selection in the early years of cardiac transplantation were considered essential to achieve an excellent outcome. Among these criteria, age greater than 55 years was an absolute contraindication to cardiac transplantation. This contraindication was based on reports that patients over age 50 who underwent heart transplantation demonstrated an increased incidence of infections and postoperative mortality, resulting in only a 40% survival [2-4].

Although the selection criteria have been expanded in recent years, one of the major changes has been an increased age limit for cardiac transplantation. Therefore, several cardiac transplant programs, including the one at the Ochsner Medical Institutions, have extended the age limit, thereby not only making this procedure available to patients who, in the past, were considered "high risk," but also providing excellent results.

This chapter will address the changes in selection criteria that allowed the inclusion of older patients as transplant candidates, the outcome of cardiac transplantation in older patients, and the factors responsible for it.

Franz H. Messerli (ed.), CARDIOVASCULAR DISEASE IN THE ELDERLY (Third Edition). Copyright © 1993 Kluwer Academic Publishers. ISBN 0-7923-1859-5. All rights reserved.

AGE AS AN ABSOLUTE CONTRAINDICATION TO CARDIAC TRANSPLANTATION

In the early experience of cardiac transplantation, the establishment of rigid selection criteria was enforced to achieve the best results possible, since the procedure was associated with a high early mortality [2–4]. The factors responsible for this early mortality were considered to be related to an increased incidence of infection and high operative mortality. In addition, patients older than 50 to 55 years were found to have a survival rate of 40% due to infection and a decreased ability to withstand the surgery. Therefore, advanced age became an absolute contraindication to cardiac transplantation [2–4]. Subsequently, the introduction of cyclosporine, a major advance in the area of cardiac transplantation, has allowed the reduction of corticosteriod doses and has decreased the incidence of allograft rejection and infection [5]. In addition, refinement in the surgical techniques of both organ transplantation and harvest, improvements in cardiovascular anesthesia, and standardization of immunosuppression regimens have resulted in a one-year survival rate for cardiac transplantation exceeding 80% [6,7]. Consequently, these advances have led to broadening of the selection criteria, especially the age limit, making the procedure available to a greater number of patients. Several studies have confirmed that extension of the age limit is associated with excellent outcome after cardiac transplantation.

In 1986, Carrier et al. [8] reported their experience in 13 patients over 50 years of age compared to 49 patients under 50 years who underwent cardiac transplantation. They found no difference in early mortality (16% in the group over age 50 versus 18% in the group under age 50), actuarial survival at one year (72 ± 14% in the group over age 50 versus 66 ± 7% in the group under age 50), allograft rejection, or infection. The basic immunosuppressant was cyclosporine in 5 of the 13 patients older than 50 years, and ischemic cardiomyopathy was present more frequently in the older group (69% versus 15%). The authors concluded that since the results were not significantly different in patients over age 50, a rigid age limit for cardiac transplant recipients was unacceptable. They also stated that each recipient, regardless of age, should be evaluated individually in terms of risk and benefits from cardiac transplantation.

In 1988, Frazier et al. [9] reported the experience of the Texas Heart Institute with patients over 60 years of age. Twenty-eight of 200 patients over age 60 (14%) underwent cardiac transplantation from 1982 to 1987. The etiology of heart disease was predominantly ischemic in this group (64% versus 32%), and the actuarial survival at one year was 83%. The incidence of rejection was 1.21 (±1.10) episodes per patient compared to 1.70 (±1.33) episodes per patient in the younger group, and there was no difference in the incidence of infection. The survival was the same or even better, despite the fact that the older patients had other risk factors (previous cardiac surgery (55%), renal dysfunction, hyperglycemia), demonstrating the feasibility of cardiac transplantation in elderly persons. The investigators concluded that advanced age should not be considered a contraindication to cardiac transplantation. The authors also recognized the importance of expanding the donor selection criteria in order to increase the number of donor hearts, in view of the fact that increasing the age limit for heart transplantation also increases the number of potential recipients. Thus, older donor hearts that otherwise would be considered undesirable for young recipients should be considered in patients with advanced age. In 1989, three corroborating reports indicated that age should not be considered a contraindication to heart transplantation. Miller et al. [10] reported the results of eight patients older than age 55 (group 1) following orthotopic heart transplantation and compared them with 22 patients younger than age 55 (group 2). The immunosuppressive regimen was similar in both groups and consisted of cyclosporine, prednisone, and azathioprine. There was no difference in morbidity and mortality between the two groups and, interestingly, neurologic complications were very low in the older group despite their higher incidence of ischemic heart disease and vascular disease. The incidence of allograft rejection in the older group was lower (0.04 versus 0.11 per patient month); however, the incidence of infection was similar in both groups (0.04 versus 0.05 per patient month). All of the older patients studied were New York Heart Association functional class I, and all were able to return to work three months after heart transplantation. The authors concluded that this report offered encouraging data supporting cardiac transplantation to carefully selected older recipients.

Olivari et al. [11] reported the experience at the University of Minnesota of 23 patients older than age 55 compared to 34 patients younger than age 55 after orthotopic heart transplantation. They found no difference in neurologic events after heart transplantation, although the incidence of diabetes and osteoporosis was higher in the older group. Moreover, despite the similarity of rates of survival and freedom from rejection, life-threatening infections (*Cryptococcus meningitidis*, disseminated herpes simplex) were observed more frequently in older patients. This group concluded that cardiac transplantation is a valid therapeutic approach in older patients with end-stage heart disease, can be performed without increased operative risk, and is associated with excellent long-term survival. However, they also concluded that older patients are at higher risk for more serious infections and the development of steroid-related complications.

The experience from Harefield Hospital in England [12] has shown results similar to those from other centers. These investigators emphasized the benefits of extending the age range for potential cardiac donors, allowing the use of older donors to alleviate the scarce supply of donor organs caused by the increase in the age limit of the recipients.

In 1990, Defraigne et al. [13] reported their experience in 20 patients older than age 55 who underwent cardiac transplantation. They concluded that age was not a contraindication. In addition, they emphasized that a change in the recipient selection policy should lead to parallel changes in donor selection criteria.

In summary, the results of these studies demonstrate that age is not a contraindication to heart transplantation; therefore, many programs around the world have extended the age limit to 65 years of age and beyond.

FACTORS RESPONSIBLE FOR AN EXCELLENT OUTCOME IN OLDER PATIENTS

Several factors may be responsible for the excellent outcome in older patients following cardiac transplantation: 1) the introduction of cyclosporine and the development of more specific immunosuppressant agents; 2) the reduced overall incidence of infection; 3) the decreased number of rejections in older patients; and 4) the availability of newer antibiotics for treating infections in immunocompromised hosts [6]. It is also important to point out that older patients should undergo a detailed evaluation to exclude cerebrovascular, pulmonary, and gastrointestinal diseases before they are accepted as cardiac transplant candidates [6].

The influence of age on the incidence of allograft rejection was studied by Renlund et al. [14] in 57 recipients of orthotopic cardiac transplantation. Twenty-one patients were 54 years of age or older (range, 54 to 63 years) and 36 patients were 52 years of age or younger (range, 16 to 52 years). The results of this study demonstrated that following cardiac transplantation, the older patients had 100% actuarial survival and fewer rejection episodes during the first four months (0.24 ± 0.05 episodes per month versus 0.72 ± 0.09 episodes per month; $p < 0.001$) and during the total duration of follow-up (0.20 ± 0.03 episode per month versus 0.40 ± 0.07 episodes per month; $p < 0.045$) with the same level of immunosuppression. In addition, the older group experienced the first rejection later than the younger group (50.4 ± 4.0 days versus 27.7 ± 8.5 days; $p = 0.008$). In a multivariate analysis, younger age was found to add significantly as a predictor of rejection. This decrease in incidence of allograft rejection was not associated with a concomitant increase in the infection rate (67% in both groups). The investigators concluded that the decrease in allograft rejection was likely to be a manifestation of an age-associated decline in immune function and might represent an advantage in transplantation of carefully selected patients.

OCHSNER MEDICAL INSTITUTIONS' CARDIAC TRANSPLANT PROGRAM: EXPERIENCE IN OLDER PATIENTS

Between October 1985 and August 1991, 32 patients 55 years of age or older and with end stage heart disease underwent orthotopic cardiac transplantation at the Ochsner Medical Institutions (table 25-1). Eighteen patients (56%) were between 55 and 59 years of age (group 1) and 14 patients (44%) were 60 years of age or older (group 2). There were 14 males and 4 females in group

Table 25-1. Ochsner Medical Institutions' cardiac transplant program

Year	Total number of patients	Patients > 55 years of age	
		Number > 55	Percent > 55
1985	1	0	0
1986	11	1	9
1987	15	5	34
1988	13	5	38
1989	18	4	22
1990	28	13	46
1991	16	4	25
Totals	102	32	31

Table 25-2. Ochsner Medical Institutions' cardiac transplant program: Clinical characteristics

Data	Group 1 (55–59 years)	Group 2 (≥60 years)
Number of patients	18	14
Survival	16/18 (89%)	12/14 (86%)
Age (years)	57 ± 3	62 ± 3
Sex (male/female)	14/4	10/4
Etiology		
Ischemic	15/18 (83%)	11/14 (79%)
Nonischemic	3/18 (17%)	3/14 (21%)

1 and 10 males and 4 females in group 2. Eighty-three percent of patients in group 1 and 79% in group 2 underwent cardiac transplantation due to ischemic cardiomyopathy (table 25-2). All patients were treated with triple immunosuppressive therapy. The actuarial survival for the total population was 88% at one year.

Complications

Mortality: Early

Two patients in group 1 expired within 30 days of surgery. One experienced sudden cardiac death and the other had disseminated cytomegalovirus infection. One patient group 2 expired due to sepsis and renal and hepatic failure five days after surgery.

Mortality: Late

One patient in group 2 had sudden death six months after cardiac transplantation and was found to have accelerated atherosclerosis in the postmortem examination.

Table 25-3. Ochsner Medical Institutions' cardiac transplant program: Allograft rejection

Number of rejections	Group 1	Group 2
0	14	12
1	3	1
≥2	1	1
Risk of rejection/patient month	0.01	0.01

Table 25-4. Ochsner Medical Institutions' cardiac transplant program: Infections

Number of infections	Group 1	Group 2
Total infections	7	5
Herpes viruses	4	3
Cytomegalovirus	3	2
Varicella zoster	1	0
Pneumocystis carinii	0	1
Toxoplasmosis	1	2
Staphylococcus epidermis	1	0
Kliebsiella pneumoniae	1	0
Risk of infection/patient month	0.007	0.01

Allograft rejection

Fourteen of 18 patients group 1 were free of allograft rejection during the follow-up period, whereas three patients had one rejection episode and one patient had two episodes. Twelve patients in group 2 were free of allograft rejection during the follow-up period. One patient had one episode of rejection and one patient had two episodes of rejection. Both group 1 and group 2 had the same average risk of rejection—0.01 patient per month follow-up (table 25-3).

Infection

Seven infections were treated in group 1. The organisms in four cases were herpes viruses: cytomegalovirus (three patients) and varicella zoster (one patient). The other three cases involved toxoplasmosis, *Staphylococcus epidermidis* sepsis, and a pulmonary infection by *Klebsiella pneumoniae*, respectively. One patient in group 1 died secondary to disseminated cytomegalovirus infection. There were five treated infections in group 2. Toxoplasmosis was present in two patients, cytomegalovirus present in two, and *Pneumocystis carinii* in one. The risk of infection per patient month of follow-up was similar in both groups (table 25-4).

Quality of life

The effects of cardiac transplantation were assessed in all patients utilizing a validated questionnaire. Preliminary results demonstrated an improvement in the parameters of functional status in both groups [15].

Hypertension

Hypertension is a common complication in cardiac transplantations that usually occurs after several months of therapy with cyclosporine. The exact mechanisms of cyclosporine-induced hypertension are not known. In our experience, calcium channel blockers of the dihydropyridine type are particularly useful in the management of post-transplant hypertension. Among them, isradipine and nifedipine have the advantage of having no interaction with cyclosporine.

CONCLUSION

Clearly, age remains a selection criterion for patients who are candidates for cardiac transplatation. However, this chapter demonstrates that cardiac transplantation is a valid option for the treatment of end-stage heart disease in some older patients, since the outcome of these patients is similar to, or even better than, that of younger recipients. In order to offset the resultant donor shortage, it will be necessary to expand donor age criteria. Older patients should be carefully evaluated during the selection process to exclude cerebrovascular, gastrointestinal, and pulmonary diseases before these persons are accepted as candidates for cardiac transplantation. We believe that attention should be paid to physiologic rather than chronologic age and that the upper limits of age criteria will continue to expand.

ACKNOWLEDGMENT

The authors wish to express their sincere appreciation to Leda L. Lupo for editing and preparing the manuscript.

REFERENCES

1. Barnard CN. 1967. The operation. A human cardiac transplant: an interim report of a successful operation performed at Groote Schuur Hospital, Cape Town. S Afr Med J 41: 1271–1274.
2. Cabrol C, Gandjbackhck I, Pavie A, et al. 1983. Les transplantations cardiaques. Etat actuel. L'expérience de la Pitié. Ann Cardiol Angeiol (Paris) 32:429–433.
3. Griepp RB, Stinson EB, Dong E Jr, et al. 1971. Determinants of operative risk in human heart transplantation. Am J Surg 122:192–197.
4. Cooper DKC. 1984. Selection and management of the recipient. In DKC Cooper and RP Hanger (eds), Heart Transplantation. Lancaster: MTP Press, pp 15–22.
5. Copeland JG, Emery RW, Levinson MM, et al. 1986. Cyclosporine: an immunosuppressive panacea? J Thorac Cardiovasc Surg 91:26–39.
6. Ventura HO, Lavie CJ, Stapleton DD and Price HL. 1991. Cardiac transplantation. How recipients are selected. Postgrad Med 90:131–132, 135–138.
7. Kriett JM and Kaye MP. 1990. The registry of the International Society for Heart Transplantation: seventh official report—1990. J Heart Transplant 9:323–330.

8. Carrier M, Emery RW, Riley JE, et al. 1986. Cardiac transplantation in patients over 50 years of age. J Am Coll Cardiol 8:285–288.
9. Frazier OH, Macris MP, Duncan JM, et al. 1988. Cardiac transplantation in patients over 60 years of age. Ann Thorac Surg 45:129–132.
10. Miller LW, Vitale-Noedel N, Pennington DG, et al. 1988. Heart transplantation in patients over age fifty-five years. J Heart Transplant 7:254–257.
11. Olivari MT, Antolick A, Kaye MP, et al. 1988. Heart transplantation in elderly patients. J Heart Transplant 7:258–264.
12. Aravot DJ, Banner NR, Khaghani A, et al. 1989. Cardiac transplantation in the seventh decade of life. Am J Cardiol 63:90–93.
13. Defraigne JO, Demoulin JC, Beaujean MA, et al. 1990. Cardiac transplantation beyond 55 years of age. Transplant Int 3:59–61.
14. Renlund DG, Gilbert EM, O'Connell JB, et al. 1987. Age-associated decline in cardiac allograft rejection. Am J Med 83:391–398.
15. Milani RV, Ventura HO, Price HL, et al. 1991. Quality of life in cardiac transplantation: lack of improvement in measures of well-being (abstract). Chest 100:345.

treatment of, 240–241
Mitral stenosis, 239, 243–245, 247, 488,
    499, 521–523, 524, 525, 539
  aortic insufficiency distinguished
      from, 237
  cerebrovascular disease and, 349
  heart failure and, 99, 101–102, 105,
      110
  management of, 244–245
Mitral valve disease, 487, 488, *see also*
    specific diseases
Mitral valve prolapse, 86, 241–242,
    318, 488
Mitral valve replacement, 198, 242,
    245, 302, 488, 521, 550
M-mode echocardiography, 39, 40, 43,
    85, 233, 244, 245, 246
Moduretic, 482
Monapril, 142
Monoamine oxidase inhibitors, 218,
    222, *see also* specific types
Moricizine, 164, 188
Morphine, 152, 280, 485–486
MUGA scans, 279, 286–287
Multifocal atrial tachycardia (MAT),
    180, 385–386
Multiple microatheroemboli, 364–365
Multiple Risk Factor Intervention Trial
    (MRFIT), 19–20, 426
Myeloma, 306
Myocardial disease, 293–310, *see also*
    specific diseases
Myocardial infarction (MI), 80, 110,
    137, 139, 140, 142, 145, 149, 260,
    263, 264, 275–289, 500, 501, 520,
    532, 536–537, 548
  abdominal aortic aneurysms and,
      335, 336
  aortic dissection and, 339
  arrhythmias and, 166
  atherectomy and, 513
  CAD and, 253, 256, 258, 259, 266,
      389
  complications of, 284–286
  convalescent period in, 288–289
  diagnosis of, 277
  exercise and, 289, 457–460, 461,
      464–465, 486
  giant-cell arteritis and, 357
  heart failure and, 98–99, 276, 277,
      278, 285
  hypertension and, 17, 123, 144, 146,

    147, 154–155, 282, 288, 428, 468
  hypothyroidism and, 393
  intracoronary stents and, 514
  orthostatic hypotension and, 265
  pathogenesis of, 276
  prognosis and, 278–279
  psychological adaptation to, 401,
      402, 403, 404, 405, 407, 408–409
  PTCA and, 502, 505, 507–509,
      536–537
  sexual function and, 289, 408
  supported angioplasty and, 509
  treatment of, 279–284, 485–487
  tricuspid valve disease and, 246
  ventricular arrhythmias and, 189
Myocardial ischemia, 11, 49, 77, 82, 83,
    84, 140, 141, 150, 166, 181, 187,
    190, 198, 201, 266, 490
  CAD and, 260
  cardiomyopathy confused with, 491
  cerebrovascular disease and, 350
  diagnostic testing of, 80
  heart failure and, 95, 99, 100, 119
  hypertension and, 146, 152, 154–155
  hypothyroidism and, 394
  mitral regurgitation and, 238, 239
Myocardial perfusion imaging, 79–82,
    83, 112
Myocarditis, viral, 102
Myxedema, 110, 198, 393, 394, 474,
    492
Myxomas, 102, 243, 244, 247

Nadolol, 479
National Health and Nutrition
    Examination Survey (NHANES),
    14
National Health Epidemiologic
    Follow-Up Study (NHEFS), 14
Nephrectomy, 135
Nephrosclerosis, 126, 130, 134, 144, *see*
    also Renal artery stenosis
Netilmicin, 323
Nicardipine, 140
Nicotinic acid, 267
Nifedipine
  angina and, 485
  CAD and, 262–264
  cor pulmonale and, 382
  hypertension and, 140, 149–150, 156,
      481
  hypothyroidism and, 394